PRACTICAL GUIDE TO HIGH-RISK PREGNANCY AND DELIVERY

Fernando Arias, M.D., Ph.D.

Clinical Professor,
Obstetrics and Gynecology,
St. Louis University Medical School;
Director,
Division of Maternal-Fetal Medicine,
St. John's Mercy Medical Center,
St. Louis, Missouri

Second Edition

with 61 illustrations

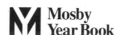 Mosby
Year Book

St. Louis Baltimore Boston Chicago London Philadelphia Sydney Toronto

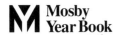

Mosby
Year Book

Dedicated to Publishing Excellence

Editorial Assistant: Colleen Boyd
Project Manager: Karen Edwards
Senior Production Editor: Gail Brower
Book Design: Jeanne Wolfgeher

SECOND EDITION

Printed in the United States of America

Mosby–Year Book, Inc.
11830 Westline Industrial Drive, St. Louis, Missouri 63146

Library of Congress Cataloging in Publication Data

Arias, Fernando, 1934-
    Practical guide to high-risk pregnancy and delivery / Fernando
Arias.—2nd ed.
        p.   cm.
    Rev. ed. of: High-risk pregnancy and delivery. 1984.
    Includes bibliographical references and index.
    ISBN 0-8016-0057-X
    1. Pregnancy—Complications.   2. Labor (Obstetrics)-
-Complications.   I. Arias, Fernando, 1934- High-risk pregnancy
and delivery.   II. Title.
    [DNLM: 1. Delivery. 2. Labor Complications. 3. Pregnancy
Complications.   WQ 240 A696h]
RG571.A75   1992
618.3—dc20
DNLM/DLC   92-12914
for Library of Congress   CIP

96 97 CL/MY 9 8 7 6

To *Judy*

PREFACE

The title of the first edition of this book, *High-Risk Pregnancy and Delivery,* has been changed to *Practical Guide to High-Risk Pregnancy and Delivery* to emphasize the practical nature of the book. Several other changes have been made to keep up with multiple new developments and to facilitate the finding of information. However, the purpose of the book remains unchanged: to provide residents in Obstetrics and Gynecology, fellows in Maternal-Fetal Medicine, obstetricians, family practice physicians, and interested nurses and medical students with a source of practical information about complications of pregnancy.

The book is now organized in different sections corresponding to well-defined areas in the subject matter. New chapters have been added on early pregnancy loss, chronic hypertension and pregnancy, fetal dysmorphology, congenital infections, and postpartum complications. With the exception of Chapter 17, which was written in collaboration with Dr. Andres Sarmiento, a former Maternal-Fetal Medicine fellow, all the chapters were written by myself, and I am responsible for all the errors, omissions, and misjudgments. The objective of single authorship was to give the reader a more cohesive view of the subjects, based on the knowledge accumulated in the literature and colored with my personal experience in the management of patients with complicated pregnancies. The problem with this approach was not only the large amount of work added to my already busy schedule, but also the significant possibility that personal biases could alter the objectivity of the recommendations formulated in some controversial areas. A conscientious effort was made to avoid this problem, but if it has happened and somebody's sensitivity was hurt, I apologize in advance.

A book is never the work of a single person. I am particularly indebted and grateful to Dr. Peter Ahlering for his help with this book. Peter is a third-year resident in Obstetrics and Gynecology at St. John's Mercy Medical Center who took time out of an extremely demanding program to read all the chapters, make valuable suggestions about their content, and try to correct my numerous grammatical and spelling errors. My deepest gratitude also to Robyn Meyer, my wonderful secretary, who word-processed the manuscript with speed and precision using many of her own evenings and weekends. I also recognize the help of Jane Dunford-Shor in the initial style editing of the book. Thanks also to Gail Brower, Senior Production Editor at Mosby–Year Book, who was a great help during the publishing process. Last, but not least, thanks to Judy. She provided constant inspiration and support and tolerated many days of solitude with a smile on her face.

Fernando Arias

CONTENTS

PART ONE

Antepartum Care

1

IDENTIFICATION AND ANTEPARTUM SURVEILLANCE OF THE HIGH-RISK PATIENT

There are two main circumstances under which the obstetrician becomes responsible for the care of a high-risk patient. In a minority of cases, the high-risk pregnant patient comes to the obstetrician with a poor obstetrical history or with a well-recognized medical complication. The most important challenge that such a patient presents is that of determining whether the severity of her problem is such that she needs to be referred to a specialist in maternal-fetal medicine rather than be managed by the general obstetrician. The majority of high-risk pregnant patients seen in daily practice, however, are women who, in the course of otherwise normal pregnancies, develop unexpected severe complications. These patients with unexpected complications frequently require difficult management decisions, and when a poor fetal or maternal outcome occurs, the obstetrician is faced with the possibility of medico-legal problems. This chapter is dedicated to analyzing systems for the identification of high-risk patients and to reviewing the methods used for the fetal surveillance of those patients who are identified as high-risk early in pregnancy. In later chapters of the book,

pertinent aspects of the prenatal care in patients who develop unexpected complications are analyzed.

◪ IDENTIFICATION OF THE HIGH-RISK PATIENT

Several high-risk identification systems have been proposed by different authors.[1-3] Each scheme consists of a list of conditions known to be poor prognostic indicators in pregnancy. All of these systems include among the high-risk factors medical complications affecting the mother and a poor obstetrical history. Most of these systems give different numerical values to the high-risk factors, depending on the severity of their effects on the pregnancy, and produce a numerical score that is supposed to reflect the seriousness of the potential problem. Some of the commercially available prenatal records have incorporated high-risk scoring systems to allow the classification of patients into high- and low-risk categories.

Identification of a high-risk pregnancy may also be achieved, without the use of scoring systems, with the careful elaboration of a medical and obstetrical history. However, an advantage of having a high-risk scoring system incorporated into the prenatal chart is that it documents the effort made to identify and analyze those high-risk factors—documentation that may be of value in the case of medico-legal problems.

The use of high-risk scoring systems should help the obstetrician not only to identify the pregnant patient at high risk, but also to elaborate a prognosis for the outcome of the pregnancy. This second objective, to elaborate a prognosis for the outcome of the pregnancy, is not accomplished frequently. This is because of the low sensitivity of the high-risk indicators and also because the outcome of the pregnancy is drastically influenced by medical intervention after the high-risk situation is identified. One ex-

ample of this limitation is care of the patient with an incompetent cervix. This condition almost certainly will lead to pregnancy loss in the absence of intervention. In this case the high-risk factor (incompetent cervix) has a high sensitivity. However, if the problem is recognized and adequately treated with a cervical cerclage, a favorable outcome almost certainly will occur. In this situation an important high-risk factor is modified by medical intervention, and a poor prognosis based on the initial risk assessment would have been incorrect. Thus a high-risk scoring system has limited use for predicting outcome.

A useful system is a modification of the high-risk scoring system proposed by Coopland et al.[4] in Manitoba, Canada (Box 1-1). This scoring sys-

---

BOX 1-1

High Risk Evaluation Form

Name _____ Age _____ Gravida _____ Para _____ Aborta _____

LMP _____ EDC _____ EDC by ultrasound _____

Reproductive history		Medical or surgical associated conditions		Present pregnancy	
Age:	<16 = 1	Previous gyneco-	= 1 __	Bleeding	
	16-35 = 0	logic surgery		<20 weeks	= 1 __
	>35 = 2 __	Chronic renal	= 1 __	>20 weeks	= 3 __
Parity:	0 = 1	disease		Anemia (<10 g %)	= 1 __
	1-4 = 0	Gestational	= 1 __	Postmaturity	= 1 __
	>5 = 2 __	diabetes (A)		Hypertension	= 2 __
Two or more	= 1 __	Class B or	= 3 __	Premature	= 2 __
abortions or history		greater diabetes		rupture of	
of infertility		Cardiac disease	= 3 __	membranes	
Postpartum	= 1 __	Other signifi-	= __	Polyhydramni-	= 2 __
bleeding or manual		cant medical		os	
removal		disorders		IUGR	= 3 __
Child >9 lb	= 1 __	(score 1 to 3		Multiple	= 3 __
Child <5 lb 8oz	= 1 __	according to		pregnancy	
Toxemia or	= 2 __	severity)		Breech or	= 3 __
hypertension				malpresentation	
Previous	= 2 __			Rh isoimmuni-	= 3 __
cesarean section				zation	
Abnormal or	= 2 __				
difficult labor					
COLUMN TOTALS	__		__		__

Total Score   _____
   (sum of the three columns)

Low risk   0-2
High risk   3-6
Severe risk   7 or more

tem takes into consideration several different factors, which are each given a numerical value from one to five, depending on their potential impact on the outcome of the pregnancy. A score of seven or more indicates, in the majority of cases, the need for referral to a maternal-fetal medicine specialist. The use of this scoring system adds little to a thorough history record and physical examination in regard to the identification of the high-risk patient. However, this system may be useful to a general obstetrician or family practice physician in determining the need for referral to the maternal-fetal medicine specialist.

There are no adequate studies providing a scientific basis for deciding whether to refer a patient with high-risk factors to a maternal-fetal medicine specialist. This decision is usually made by obstetricians and family practice physicians, who take into consideration the severity and multiplicity of the high-risk factors present in a given patient.

It seems clear that the following patients should be referred to a specialist in maternal-fetal medicine:

1. Those with conditions that may require invasive procedures for fetal diagnosis or therapy, such as:
   Rh isoimmunization
   Nonimmunologic fetal hydrops
   Fetal urinary tract obstruction
   Fetal congenital heart block
   Fetal hydrocephaly
2. Those with severe medical complications affecting the mother, such as:
   Brittle diabetes
   Cardiac disease grades III and IV
   Artificial heart valves
   Systemic lupus erythematosus
   Sickle cell disease
3. Those with recurrent poor obstetrical outcomes, such as:
   Habitual abortion
   Failed cerclages
   Recurrent stillborns
   Recurrent early rupture of membranes
   Recurrent preterm labor
4. Those with obstetrical complications that require specialized care for adequate management, such as:
   Severe preeclampsia or eclampsia with renal failure, pulmonary edema, hypertension unresponsive to treatment, in-

   tracranial bleeding or severe HELLP syndrome
   Severe fetal growth retardation
   Multiple high-risk factors

In communities where a maternal-fetal medicine specialist is not available, it will be necessary to obtain consultation from an internist to provide adequate care for some of these patients. There is no valid reason to refer patients with medical complications of pregnancy to an internist when a maternal-fetal medicine specialist is available.

Once a high-risk patient is identified, the physician must explain to the patient and her husband the potential effects of her high-risk factor(s) on the outcome of pregnancy and the effects that pregnancy may have on the maternal medical condition. In all cases the information provided to the patient should be given in simple terms.

■ PRECONCEPTION COUNSELING

Ideally, the patient with multiple or severe high-risk factors should be counseled before pregnancy occurs.[5] When preconception counseling is possible, the obstetrician should have a relaxed interview with the patient and her husband to discuss the following points:

1. The importance of high-risk factors identified in the history and physical examination of the patient
2. The potential effects that each risk factor may have on the pregnancy
3. The effect that the pregnancy may have on each of the identified risk factors
4. Potential maternal disability during pregnancy and the length of that disability
5. The special tests that will be required for monitoring maternal and fetal well-being during pregnancy
6. The prognosis for a successful fetal and maternal outcome
7. The cost of the pregnancy including additional testing and consultation required as well as the cost of neonatal intensive care if preterm delivery is a significant possibility

Although preconception counseling can be applied to all potential high-risk pregnancies, it has special importance in the care of patients with diabetes mellitus, Rh isoimmunization, history of recurrent preterm labor, and history of multiple prior pregnancy losses and in patients who have the potential to transfer genetic disorders to their offspring. It is important to advise patients who have had poor perinatal outcomes not to become pregnant again until they have reviewed the information concerning their pregnancy losses with their obstetrician and the maternal-fetal medicine specialist.

The most important requirement of preconceptional counseling is that it should be non-judgmental. The obstetrician should make an effort to avoid giving the patient an opinion about the advisability of getting pregnant. The decision to become pregnant despite significant risks is a very personal one for the patient and is based on a multiplicity of variables in addition to the medical information. The role of the obstetrician is to provide factual medical information and to support the patient's decision even if that decision does not agree with his or her personal opinion.

Another aspect of the preconception counseling is consideration of the financial burden, in terms of health-care costs as well as working disability, that parents will assume with a high-risk pregnancy. Many parents are not aware of the high cost of the complex medical technology necessary for their care, and many do not realize the limitations and intricacies of their health insurance policies.

◪ METHODS OF FETAL SURVEILLANCE FOR HIGH-RISK PATIENTS

The objectives of antepartum surveillance in the high-risk patient are:

1. To determine gestational age.
2. To discover fetal congenital abnormalities.
3. To detect abnormalities in fetal growth.
4. To detect and determine the severity of acute and chronic fetal asphyxia.

How to achieve the second of these objectives (to discover fetal congenital abnormalities) is the subject matter of Chapter 2, Antenatal Diagnosis of Congenital Diseases. At this point it is sufficient to say that all obstetrical patients should have genetic screening at the beginning of their prenatal care. A questionnaire (see Box 2-1, Chapter 2) recommended by the American College of Obstetricians and Gynecologists is useful for this purpose. A positive answer to any of the questions should be carefully investigated and may indicate the need for genetic counseling.

The method used to achieve the third objective, the detection of abnormalities in fetal growth, is fetal biometry with ultrasound. An exhaustive analysis of this method is beyond the scope of this book. In this chapter the discussion is limited to a general assessment of the value of this technique and especially to the potential pitfalls and errors that may result from its indiscriminate use. More information concerning disorders of fetal growth can be found in Chapter 17, which is dedicated to the subject of fetal growth retardation. The problems associated with excessive fetal growth are analyzed in Chapter 16, Diabetes, and Chapter 8, Prolonged Pregnancy.

Determination of gestational age

An accurate establishment of the expected date of delivery (EDD) is fundamental to the management of high-risk pregnancies. Proper assignment of the EDD is necessary to obtain and appropriately interpret laboratory tests, to plan and execute therapeutic maneuvers, and to determine the optimal management in certain difficult situations.

Clinical dating. The elements involved in the clinical estimation of gestational age are the characteristics and time of occurrence of the last menstrual period (LMP), the findings on the initial pelvic examination, the date on which fetal heart tones are first heard, and the date of the first positive pregnancy test.

The patient's menstrual history is considered adequate for the purpose of establishing the EDD only if the last menstrual period was normal in duration and amount of flow, if the prior menstrual periods came at regular intervals, and if the patient did not use oral contraceptives within 3 months of her last period. Unfortunately, approximately 30% of patients do not fulfill these criteria, making estimation of the EDD based on their LMPs unreliable. In a study of more than 11,000 pregnancies at McGill University, it was shown that LMP estimates were particularly inaccurate in patients with preterm and postterm pregnancies.[6]

Evaluation of uterine size has limited value for accurate clinical dating. Among the many variables that make assessment of the uterine size unreliable are maternal obesity, observer experience, position of the uterus, amount of amniotic fluid, multiple gestation, uterine myomatosis, and fetal growth disorders. Studies have demonstrated that physician measurements tend to underestimate the gestational age and have a preference for even numbers.[7] In patients with unreliable menstrual histories, estimation of the EDDs by measuring uterine size is useful only if it concurs with the estimation by ultrasound examination.

The date on which fetal heart tones are first audible with Doppler ultrasound devices (10 weeks) or with standard obstetrical stethoscopes (20 weeks) has also been used to determine gestational age. Similar to other clinical parameters for evaluating gestational age, the time at which fetal heart sounds are first heard is an ineffective way to assess gestational age. It has value only

when it agrees with other clinical indicators and with the ultrasound measurements.

In some patients the time at which the first positive pregnancy test was obtained may be useful for establishing the EDD. The sensitivity of the available over-the-counter pregnancy tests allows the diagnosis of pregnancy at 4 to 5 postmenstrual weeks. Thus, if a patient has a positive pregnancy test after 4 to 5 weeks of amenorrhea, the patient's dates become firmly established.

Clinical dating is not 100% accurate. Even a patient with reliable clinical criteria pointing to a given EDD should have a real-time ultrasound

TABLE 1-1 ◪ Three tolerance intervals for BPD measurements directly from the measurements

Gestational week	Tolerance intervals (mm)						
	2.5%	5%	25%	50%	75%	95%	97.5%
12	12	13	16	20	23	26	27
13	16	17	19	22	26	28	29
14	19	20	22	26	29	31	32
15	25	26	28	32	35	37	38
16	28	29	32	35	38	40	41
17	31	32	35	38	41	44	44
18	34	34	37	40	43	46	47
19	36	37	39	43	46	49	49
20	40	41	43	46	50	52	53
21	42	43	46	49	52	55	55
22	46	47	50	53	56	59	59
23	48	49	51	55	58	60	61
24	52	53	56	59	63	65	66
25	56	57	60	63	66	69	69
26	58	58	61	64	67	70	71
27	60	60	63	66	70	72	73
28	65	66	68	72	75	77	78
29	66	67	69	73	76	78	79
30	67	68	70	74	77	80	81
31	71	72	75	78	81	83	84
32	74	75	78	81	85	87	88
33	75	76	79	82	85	87	88
34	77	78	81	84	87	90	91
35	80	80	83	86	90	92	93
36	81	82	85	88	91	94	94
37	83	83	86	89	92	95	96
38	84	85	88	91	94	97	97
39	85	85	88	91	95	97	98
40	86	87	90	93	96	99	99
41	87	88	90	93	97	99	100
42	89	90	93	96	100	103	104
43	90	91	94	97	101	104	105

From Wexler S, Fuchs C, Golan A, et al: Tolerance intervals for standards in ultrasound measurements: Determination of BPD standards. *J Clin Ultrasound* 1986;14:243-250.

examination for confirmation. We have found that even patients who conceive in the course of infertility protocols may have significant errors in the estimation of their EDDs.

Dating by ultrasound. One of the most important uses of ultrasound in obstetrics is that of determining gestational age. The method most commonly used involves measurement of the biparietal diameter (BPD), the head circumference (HC), the femur length (FL), and the abdominal circumference (AC). The age in weeks corresponding to each measurement is averaged, and the mean is the estimated gestational age of the fetus. This method has replaced older techniques that used the BPD alone to determine gestational age, such as the growth-adjusted sonographic age (GASA) and the mean projected gestational age (MPGA). The results obtained by averaging several measurements (BPD, HC, FL, AC) have a better correlation with the gestational age as determined by neonatal evaluation of the newborn than any of the methods used in the past.[8] However, it should always be remembered that a single ultrasound examination for determining gestational age is unreliable after 30 weeks and that the best time to determine the age of a fetus using a single set of ultrasound measurements is between 18 and 24 weeks of gestation.

There are many tables available that provide an estimation of the number of weeks of gestation based on measurements for each of the fetal anatomical landmarks (BPD, FL, HC, and AC). It is best to use tables generated in populations studied at sea level and containing the low (5th) and high (95th) percentile values for each variable at a given gestational age. For the BPD, we prefer the table from Wexler et al.[9] shown in Table 1-1, p. 7; for the femur length, the table from Jeanty et al.[10] shown in Table 1-2; and for the head and abdominal circumferences, the tables from Hadlock et al.[11] shown in Table 1-3.

In the majority of cases, the gestational age of the fetus and the EDD will be clearly established with a single ultrasound examination if it is obtained between 18 and 24 weeks and the results agree with the clinical information. If there is more than a 1-week discrepancy between the clinical dating and the results of the ultrasound examination, the ultrasound should be repeated 4 weeks later. If the second set of ultrasound measurements agrees with the first examination, the gestational age and the EDD become clearly

TABLE 1-2 ◪ Femur length (mm)

Menstrual age (weeks)	Femur Percentile		
	5th	50th	95th
12	4	8	13
13	6	11	16
14	9	14	18
15	12	17	21
16	15	20	24
17	18	23	27
18	21	25	30
19	24	28	33
20	26	31	36
21	29	34	38
22	32	36	41
23	35	39	44
24	37	42	46
25	40	44	49
26	42	47	51
27	45	49	54
28	47	52	56
29	50	54	59
30	52	56	61
31	54	59	63
32	56	61	65
33	58	63	67
34	60	65	69
35	62	67	71
36	64	68	73
37	65	70	74
38	67	71	76
39	68	73	77
40	70	74	79

From Jeanty P, Cousaert E, Cantraine F, et al: A longitudinal study of fetal limb growth. *Am J Perinatol* 1984;1:136-144.

established. If the second set of measurements deviates more than 1 week from the first, the obstetrician should suspect an abnormality in fetal growth and use the EDD determined by the first ultrasound examination. Sonographic surveillance of the fetus should continue in order to either confirm or rule out the impression of abnormal fetal growth.

The importance of an accurate determination of the gestational age and the EDD in the high-risk patient cannot be overemphazised. The reliability of the EDD may be rated as excellent, good, or poor by using a set of criteria (Box 1-2) placed in the upper part of the first page of the prenatal record. This facilitates collecting, analyzing, and recording this important information.

TABLE 1-3 ◪ Fetal head and abdominal circumferences

Menstrual age (weeks)	Head circumference (HC)			Abdominal circumference (AC)		
	−2SD (cm)	Mean (cm)	+2SD (cm)	−2SD (cm)	Mean (cm)	+2SD (cm)
12	5.1	7.0	8.9	3.1	5.6	8.1
13	6.5	8.9	10.3	4.4	6.9	9.4
14	7.9	9.8	11.7	5.6	8.1	10.6
15	9.2	11.1	13.0	6.8	9.3	11.8
16	10.5	12.4	14.3	8.0	10.5	13.0
17	11.8	13.7	15.6	9.2	11.7	14.2
18	13.1	15.0	16.9	10.4	12.9	15.4
19	14.4	16.3	18.2	11.6	14.1	16.6
20	15.6	17.5	19.4	12.7	15.2	17.7
21	16.8	18.7	20.6	13.9	16.4	18.9
22	18.0	19.9	21.8	15.0	17.5	20.0
23	19.1	21.0	22.9	16.1	18.6	21.1
24	20.2	22.1	24.0	17.2	19.7	22.0
25	21.3	23.2	25.1	18.3	20.8	23.3
26	22.3	24.2	26.1	19.4	21.9	24.4
27	23.3	25.2	27.1	20.4	22.9	25.4
28	24.3	26.2	28.1	21.5	24.0	26.5
29	25.2	27.1	29.0	22.5	25.0	27.5
30	26.1	28.0	29.9	23.5	26.0	28.5
31	27.0	28.9	30.8	24.5	27.0	29.5
32	27.8	29.7	31.6	25.5	28.0	30.5
33	28.5	30.4	32.3	26.5	29.0	31.5
34	29.3	31.2	33.1	27.5	30.0	32.5
35	29.9	31.8	33.7	28.4	30.9	33.4
36	30.6	32.5	34.4	29.3	31.8	34.3
37	31.1	33.0	34.9	30.2	32.7	35.2
38	31.9	33.6	35.5	31.1	33.6	36.1
39	32.2	34.1	36.0	32.0	34.5	37.0
40	32.6	34.5	36.4	32.9	35.4	37.9

From Hadlock FP, Deter RL, Harrist RB: Sonographic detection of abnormal fetal growth patterns. *Clin Obstet Gynecol* 1984; 27:342-351.

BOX 1-2

Reliability of the EDD

Excellent dates

1. Patients with adequate clinical information (known, normal LMP; 28- to 30-day cycles; no recent use of oral contraceptives; uterine size in agreement with dates) PLUS ultrasound examination between 16 and 24 weeks indicating that the fetal measurements are in agreement with the clinical estimation of gestational age
2. Patients with inadequate or incomplete clinical information but with two ultrasound examinations between 16 to 24 weeks showing linear fetal growth and similar EDD

Good dates

1. Patients with adequate clinical information (as defined above) and one confirming ultrasound examination obtained after 24 weeks of gestation
2. Patients with inadequate or incomplete clinical information and two or more ultrasound examinations showing adequate growth and similar EDD

Poor dates

Any clinical situation different from those listed above

Fetal biometry with real-time ultrasound

The ability to measure different fetal anatomic landmarks and to follow their evolution during gestation is one of the most important tools that have become available to the obstetrician for the evaluation of the fetus. Fetal biometry has made it possible to determine accurately, for a large number of patients, the gestational age of the fetus and the adequacy of the fetal growth.

The fetal measurements most frequently used to follow fetal growth are the same ones used for the estimation of gestational age (BPD, FL, HC, and AC). Analysis of thousands of measurements has allowed the elaboration of curves corresponding to the development of each of these measurements throughout gestation. Most of these fetal growth curves contain the mean and the 10th and 90th percentile values. Thus the measurements obtained in a given patient can be compared with the norms, and deviations from normality can be recognized.

Fetal biometry has been fundamental for the discovery and follow-up of the fetus at high risk. However, the incorrect use of this technology has generated problems both for patients individually and for perinatal centers that have to deal with the consequences of the inadequate interpretation of fetal biometry data. The problems most frequently seen are:

1. Inadequate interpretation of fetal measurements that are thought to reveal an error in the patient's gestational age when in fact they are indicative of fetal growth retardation
2. False-positive diagnosis of fetal growth retardation
3. False-positive diagnosis of fetal anatomical abnormalities

The first of these errors has serious implications for those patients who have intrauterine growth retardation (IUGR) diagnosed in late stages, when fetal hypoxia and acidosis may already have occurred. The other two common errors have an impact on perinatal centers because these facilities may be occupied by a large number of patients unnecessarily referred for fetal surveillance or for complex diagnostic procedures.

Despite the above-mentioned problems, fetal biometry remains the most important test for following the high-risk pregnancy patient. Although there are variations in the specific nature of each high-risk pregnancy situation, all patients classified as high-risk should have serial ultrasound examinations every 4 to 6 weeks to follow fetal growth. The first of these examinations should be carried out at approximately 16 weeks of gestation.

The methods used to achieve the fourth objective in the antepartum care of the high-risk patient—that is, to detect and evaluate the severity of acute or chronic fetal hypoxia—are all biophysical in nature. They have completely replaced biochemical tests (estriol, human placental lactogen), which are now obsolete and known to be unreliable. The tests used at the present time are:

1. Nonstress test (NST)
2. Contraction stress test (CST)
3. Fetal biophysical profile (BPP)
4. Vibroacoustic stimulation test (VAST)
5. Modified biophysical profile (MBPP)
6. Umbilical and uterine Doppler ultrasound
7. Fetal movement count (FM)
8. Percutaneous umbilical blood sampling (PUBS)

Nonstress test

The nonstress test (NST) is the test most commonly used for antepartum evaluation of fetal well-being. The rationale underlying this test is that the presence of spontaneous fetal heart rate accelerations associated with fetal movements (fetal reactivity) is an indicator of fetal well-being (Figure 1-1, *A*). Likewise, the absence of fetal reactivity suggests the possibility of fetal distress and warrants further investigation (Figure 1-1, *B*). The NST is performed as described in Box 1-3.

The NST is noninvasive, easily performed and interpreted, and readily accepted by patients. The false-negative rate of the test (reactive NST in a fetus who is actually in distress) is 3.2 per 1000, indicating that the likelihood of fetal death or serious fetal morbidity following a negative reactive test is extremely low. The false-positive rate (nonreactive results in normal patients) is very high: 50% for morbidity and 80% for mortality, indicating that the probability of serious fetal problems when the test is positive (nonreactive) is low.[12] The main problems with the nonstress test are:

1. The high frequency of false-positive results.
2. The possibility that a truly abnormal result reflects an advanced rather than an early stage of fetal distress.

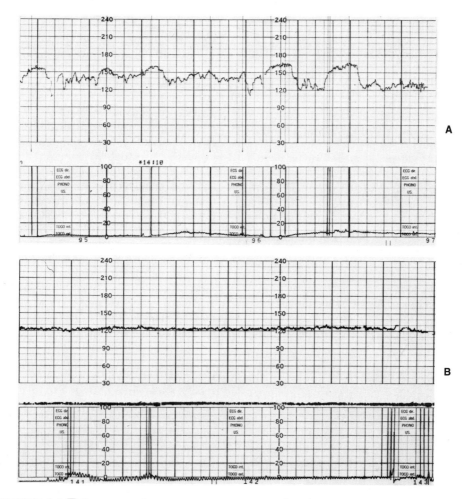

FIGURE 1-1 ◪ Reactive and nonreactive nonstress test (NST). **A,** Reactive NST. There are several accelerations of the fetal heart of 15 or more beats per minute, lasting 15 or more seconds, associated with fetal movements. **B,** Nonreactive NST. Long-term variability is absent and short-term variability is decreased; no accelerations are present in association with fetal movements.

One factor in the high frequency of false-positive results obtained with the NST is the number of accelerations of the fetal heart rate that are required to call a test "reactive." This number varies from one to five depending on the criteria adopted by each institution. Obviously, when more accelerations are required to designate the response as "reactive," the number of tests that will be designated as "nonreactive" will increase, and more false-positive results will be obtained.

Another flaw in the NST is that its interpretation relies on only one variable (i.e., the presence of accelerations of the fetal heart rate [FHR] associated with fetal movement), and it ignores other important information such as FHR variability and the presence or absence of decelerations. These observations are of value in determining the true significance of a "nonreactive" result. A "nonreactive" result in the presence of poor FHR variability or decelerations strongly suggests fetal distress. On the other hand, a "nonreactive" result when the FHR variability is normal and decelerations are absent most probably corresponds to a false-positive result.

BOX 1-3

How to Do an NST

1. Place patient in the semi-Fowler's position. Use pillows under one of her hips to displace the weight of the uterus away from the inferior vena cava. Take the patient's blood pressure every 10 minutes during the procedure.
2. Apply the tococardiographic equipment to the maternal abdomen, and observe the uterine activity and FHR for 10 minutes. Instruct the patient to push the calibration button of the uterine contraction tracing every time she feels FM.
3. A reactive test is present when two or more FHR accelerations are clearly recorded during a 20-minute period, each acceleration of 15 or more beats per minute and lasting 15 or more seconds, usually occurring simultaneously with episodes of fetal activity.
4. If no spontaneous FM occurs during the initial 20 minutes of observation, the test is continued for another 20 minutes, and during this period FM is provoked by external manipulation. If there is no acceleration with spontaneous or repeated external stimuli during a 40-minute period, the test is considered nonreactive.
5. The test is unsatisfactory if the quality of the monitor trace is inadequate for interpretation.

The NST should be analyzed taking into consideration all of the factors that provide information about the fetal well-being. An interpretation based solely on "reactivity" is incomplete and increases the incidence of false results. The variables that must be evaluated are:

1. Baseline fetal heart rate
2. Variability of the fetal heart rate
3. Presence or absence of accelerations
4. Presence or absence of decelerations

Each of these variables should be analyzed separately, and the tendency to try to produce a cumulative numerical score should be avoided.

A normal baseline heart rate is between 120 and 160 beats per minute (bpm). The abnormal alterations of this variable are tachycardia (frequency greater than 160 bpm) and bradycardia (frequency less than 120 bpm). Alterations of the baseline frequency are most often the result of maternal medications and maternal temperature,

but tachycardia and bradycardia may also occur with fetal hypoxia.

Variability is of the utmost importance in the evaluation of fetal heart monitor tracings. In the past it was believed that only direct fetal heart tracings obtained with scalp electrodes could provide adequate assessment of variability. However, modern fetal heart monitoring equipment allows, under most circumstances, adequate evaluation of variability using indirect recording of the FHR obtained with Doppler ultrasound. FHR variability depends on the interaction of the fetal sympathetic and parasympathetic systems and is influenced by gestational age, maternal medications, fetal congenital anomalies, fetal acidosis, and fetal tachycardia.

The presence of accelerations in the FHR associated with fetal movements or in response to fetal stimulation is a reliable sign of fetal health. For many years this has been used for evaluating an NST. The presence of accelerations is related to gestational age; these occur more frequently as a pregnancy approaches term. The absence of accelerations may be a sign of fetal compromise, but most commonly corresponds to periods of fetal sleep.

A problem with the definition of accelerations in the NST has been recently clarified. The study of Willis et al.[13] demonstrated that the "short criterion" (15 seconds from beginning of acceleration to return to baseline) and the "long criterion" (acceleration maintained at 15 bpm above baseline for 15 seconds) for the duration of FHR accelerations have the same sensitivity, specificity, and positive and negative predictive values. In view of these results the use of the "short criterion" is more practical.

The absence of decelerations is reassuring. The presence of moderate or severe variable decelerations or late decelerations following spontaneous contractions is worrisome and requires further evaluation.

The concern remains at the present time that the NST is not an ideal test for primary fetal surveillance because of its inability to recognize early stages of fetal distress. There is evidence, from animal experimentation and from clinical studies, that indicates that loss of FHR reactivity and loss of variability occur late in the course of chronic fetal hypoxia, whereas the presence of late decelerations is an earlier indicator. These considerations, however, have had no impact on the increasing use of the NST as the primary tool for fetal surveillance in the United States. In fact, the advantages of the NST (e.g., noninvasiveness, short duration, patient acceptance) have overridden concerns about its lack of sensitivity.

Another problem with the generalized use of the NST for primary fetal surveillance is the tendency to use the test for all patients with high-risk pregnancies without understanding that, in some situations, other tests may be more useful. One example of this situation is the use of the NST alone to follow patients with postterm pregnancies without simultaneous evaluation of the amniotic fluid volume by ultrasound.

Contraction stress test

The contraction stress test (CST) is one of the best available tests for the primary fetal surveillance of high-risk pregnancies. The test is based on experimental evidence showing that the uteroplacental blood flow decreases markedly or ceases during uterine contractions. Therefore uterine contractions cause a hypoxic stress that a normal, healthy fetus can tolerate without difficulty (Figure 1-2, A). In contrast, a fetus with chronic or acute problems will not be able to tolerate such a decrease in oxygen supply and will demonstrate this by decelerations of the FHR following the contractions (Figure 1-2, B). The protocol for performing a CST is described in Box 1-4.

The false-negative rate of the CST is 0.4 per 1000, significantly better than that of the NST.[14] However, the false-positive rate with respect to fetal morbidity is 50%, similar to that of the NST.

The end point of the CST is the presence or absence of late decelerations of the FHR following uterine contractions induced by intravenous

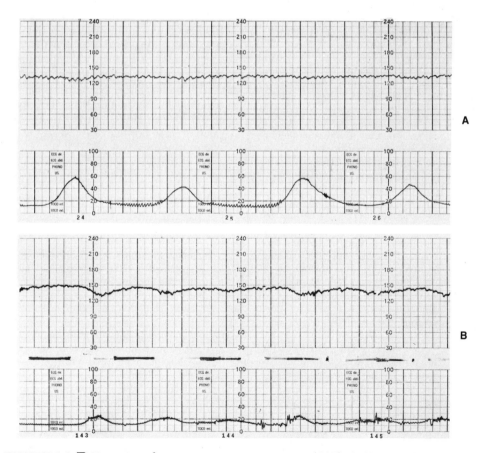

FIGURE 1-2 ◪ Negative and positive contraction stress test (CST). **A,** Negative CST. Long-term variability is absent, short-term variability is decreased, but there are no decelerations associated with the uterine contractions. **B,** Positive CST. Long- and short-term variability are decreased, and every uterine contraction is followed by a deceleration of the fetal heart rate.

oxytocin (OCT) or by nipple stimulation. As mentioned previously, late decelerations are one of the earliest indicators of fetal distress; they appear before loss of variability, decreased movement, or lack of tone. Despite being an early indicator of hypoxia, the CST is used infrequently for primary fetal surveillance. This is because of the long duration of the test, the requirement of continuous supervision by trained personnel, and the existence of risks and con-

---

BOX 1-4

How to Do a CST or an OCT

1. Place patient in semi-Fowler's position. Use pillows under the patient's hip or side to displace the weight of the uterus away from the inferior vena cava. Take the patient's blood pressure every 10 minutes throughout the test.
2. Apply the tococardiographic equipment to the maternal abdomen, and observe the uterine activity and the FHR for approximately 15 to 20 minutes. Many patients who are receiving the test because of a nonreactive NST show adequate fetal reactivity during this observation period and do not require oxytocin stimulation. Other patients show spontaneous uterine activity of sufficient frequency and duration and do not require oxytocin administration.
3. Start intravenous oxytocin administration using a Harvard pump at 0.5 mU/minute. Double the rate every 15 to 20 minutes until three contractions lasting 40 to 60 seconds occur within a 10-minute period. If late decelerations appear before this duration and frequency of contractions have been achieved, the administration of oxytocin must be interrupted. Massage of the nipples with a warm towel by the patient may be all that is necessary to provoke uterine contractions and avoid the use of oxytocin.
4. Usually the test requires between 1½ and 2 hours. The amount of oxytocin required to obtain adequate uterine contractility is generally below 16 mU/minute.
5. After completing the test, monitoring of FHR and uterine contractions should continue until they return to baseline. If uterine activity persists, the subcutaneous administration of 250 mg of terbutaline is usually sufficient to paralyze the uterus.

---

traindications associated with its performance. Presently, the CST is used mostly as the test to follow a "nonreactive" NST.

Fetal biophysical profile

The biophysical profile (BPP) is an excellent test for the evaluation of fetal well-being. It entails the observation by ultrasound of fetal breathing movements, fetal body movements, fetal tone, amniotic fluid volume, and FHR reactivity. These factors are dependent on the integrity of the fetal central nervous system and are affected in situations of fetal compromise (Box 1-5). The test is easy to perform, requires no immediate supervision by a physician, can be quickly done in the physician's office, has no contraindications, and involves no risk for the mother or the fetus. Thus it is not surprising that the BPP has gained popularity and is used with increasing frequency in the United States.

The false-negative rate of the BPP is 0.7 per 1000, a value significantly better than that of the NST and similar to that of the CST. The false-positive rate of the BPP is approximately 30%, significantly better than that of the NST or the CST.[15] The negative predictive value of the BPP is similar to that of the NST (98% for the NST, 98.5% for the BPP), but the positive predictive value of an abnormal BPP (50.8%) is better than that of a nonreactive NST.[16]

BOX 1-5

Fetal Biophysical Profile

1. *Fetal breathing movement*—30 seconds of sustained breathing movement during a 30-minute observation period
2. *Fetal movement*—Three or more gross body movements in a 30-minute observation period
3. *Fetal tone*—One or more episodes of limb motion from a position of flexion to extension and a rapid return to flexion
4. *Fetal reactivity*—Two or more FHR accelerations associated with fetal movement of at least 15 bpm and lasting at least 15 seconds in 10 minutes (reactive NST)
5. *Fluid volume*—Presence of a pocket of amniotic fluid that measures at least 1 cm in two perpendicular planes

The main problem with the BPP is the structure of the test, in which each of the five criteria (fetal breathing movements, fetal body movements, fetal tone, amniotic fluid volume, and FHR reactivity) is assigned a score of either zero or two points, despite the possibility that each of those variables may have different importance in assessing the fetal situation. The BPP variables are dependent on the activity of certain areas of the fetal central nervous system that become functional at different gestational ages. Fetal tone and movement appear between 7 and 9 weeks and require activity of the brain cortex. Fetal breathing movements begin at 20 to 21 weeks and depend on centers in the ventral surface of the fourth ventricle. FHR reactivity appears between 28 and 30 weeks and probably stems from function of the posterior hypothalamus and nucleus in the upper medulla.[14] The sensitivity of each of these centers to hypoxia is different, and those that become functional earlier in fetal development are more resistant to acute changes in fetal oxygenation. Therefore one can assume that each fetal function evaluated in the BPP has a different predictive value in indicating fetal hypoxia, an assumption that was investigated by Manning et al.[17] These investigators found that for BPP scores of 4 and 6, an abnormal NST and decreased fluid volume have higher positive predictive values than do fetal movement and fetal tone, with fetal breathing having an intermediate value. They conclude that not all abnormal biophysical profile scores are equal.

Serious consequences may ensue from improper management decisions based on the total BPP score rather than on careful evaluation of the individual test components.[18] This problem will be lessened by a recent change made by the investigators who originally developed this test: a "normal" BPP corresponds to a score of 8 or greater, but this value must include a normal amniotic fluid volume.[19] The new definition of a normal BPP will prevent the potential error associated with a score of eight when the two points are taken off in cases of markedly decreased amniotic fluid volume. Obviously, this score would be misleading because such a decrease in amniotic fluid volume is an important index of potential fetal problems, especially in postterm pregnancies. The converse may also occur. A fetus with a BPP of four consisting of two points for a reactive nonstress test and two points because of normal amniotic fluid volume is most likely perfectly normal,[20] and unnecessary intervention because of the low total score may lead to a poor perinatal outcome. To avoid errors such as those exemplified above, one must always remember that the interpretation of the biophysical profile results should be made by separate analysis of each of the individual components of the test.

Another problem with the BPP is that alterations in some of the test criteria occur relatively late in the process of fetal asphyxia. Decreased body movement and decreased fetal tone are found only when the fetal compromise is severe, and by the time of discovery, the value of intervention may be suboptimal. Other problems with the BPP are the difficulties in evaluating fetal tone, the restrictive definition of decreased amniotic fluid volume, the lack of data on the use of vibroacoustic stimulation to shorten the duration of the test, and whether prolonging the test time to increase the possibility of an adequate fetal response is permissible.

Vibroacoustic stimulation test

Vibroacoustic stimulation was originally designed to decrease the time spent in the performance of NSTs because of prolonged episodes of fetal sleep periods during the test. The results obtained with vibroacoustic stimulation have been excellent. The NST with the vibroacoustic stimulation test (VAST) is substituting the classical NST as the test most commonly used for antepartum fetal surveillance.[21] The test uses stimulation with an artificial larynx (sold in the United States by A T & T) over the fetal head for 1 to 3 seconds. This instrument produces a vibratory acoustic stimulus of approximately 80 Hz and 82 dB. A healthy fetus will respond with sudden movement (startle response) followed by acceleration of the fetal heart rate. According to Crade and Lovett,[22] fetuses of less than 24 weeks do not respond to vibroacoustic stimulation. Between 24 and 27 weeks of gestation, 30% of all fetuses will respond to the vibroacoustic stimulus. Between 27 and 30 weeks, 86% will respond, and after 31 weeks, 96% will respond to the artificial larynx. In the majority of cases, the acceleration of the fetal heart rate that follows vibroacoustic stimulation lasts for several minutes (Figure 1-3). Another normal fetal response is a series of two to five accelerations lasting 20 to 60 seconds each. Maternal perception of fetal

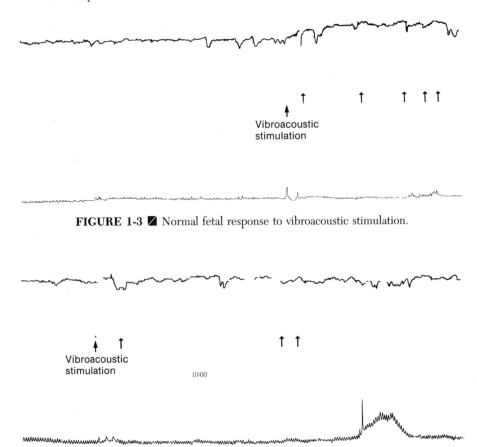

FIGURE 1-3 ◪ Normal fetal response to vibroacoustic stimulation.

FIGURE 1-4 ◪ Abnormal fetal response to vibroacoustic stimulation.

movement following vibroacoustic stimulation is another indicator of fetal well-being. If the mother does not feel the baby moving following stimulation, the fetal testing should be repeated under the conditions used for a NST.[23] An abnormal response to VAST, found in fetuses with chronic asphyxia, consists of no acceleration of the fetal heart rate or a deceleration (Figure 1-4). VAST is safe, and no evidence of hearing impairment or other abnormality has been reported in neonates exposed to VAST in utero.

There are several factors that may influence the result of VAST. Examples of these are the thickness of the maternal abdominal wall, the amount of amniotic fluid, the pressure exerted by the examiner in holding the artificial larynx against the abdomen, and the intensity of the stimulation. The influence of these factors is small, since only 2% of NSTs are nonreactive following VAST.[20] Of those NSTs that are nonreac-

tive to vibroacoustic stimulation, 17% are followed by positive contraction stress tests or by biophysical profiles equal to or less than 4.

The use of the artificial larynx in the doctor's office for fetal stimulation may become another simple measure for the antepartum surveillance of the low-risk pregnant patient. Conceivably, the use of this simple test during routine antepartum visits after 28 weeks of gestation will allow the physician to discover unsuspected cases of chronic fetal distress.

Another area of potential application of VAST is in the diagnosis of intrapartum fetal acidosis. This subject is treated extensively in Chapter 20, Birth Asphyxia.

Modified biophysical profile

Vintzileos et al.[24] were the first to propose a modification of the biophysical profile for evaluation of fetal well-being. They monitored 6543

BOX 1-6

How to Do a Modified Biophysical Profile

Start NST in the standard manner. If a spontaneous acceleration is not seen within 5 minutes, a single 1- to 2-second sound stimulation is applied in the lower abdomen with the artificial larynx. This stimulus may be repeated up to three times if necessary. Since this procedure requires two accelerations within 10 minutes for a definition of reactivity, a second stimulus is applied if 9 minutes have elapsed since the first acceleration. Accelerations are defined in the standard manner of 15 bpm amplitude from an established baseline lasting 15 seconds.

Then, a four-quadrant amniotic fluid volume is assessed by placing a linear ultrasound transducer perpendicular to the wall of the uterus and parallel to the mother's spine in four abdominal quadrants and measuring the largest vertical amniotic fluid pocket. Pockets consisting primarily of umbilical cord are disregarded. A four-quadrant sum of 5 cm or greater is considered normal.

---

high-risk fetuses with NST using VAST and estimation of amniotic fluid volume and reported no deaths of structurally normal fetuses within 1 week of their biophysical assessment. Subsequent work by Clark et al[25] has shown further the advantages of this method (Box 1-6).

The modified biophysical profile (MBPP) is the best available test for primary fetal surveillance. It combines the observation of an index of acute fetal hypoxia, the NST with VAST, and a second index indicative of chronic fetal problems, the amniotic fluid volume. The test has excellent negative and positive predictive values, is easy to interpret, has clearly defined end points, and can be performed in an average of 20 minutes.

The following guidelines are used in regard to using the MBPP as the primary test for fetal surveillance:

1. If both tests are normal, weekly fetal surveillance with MBPP is continued.
2. If both tests are abnormal (nonreactive NST, decreased amniotic fluid volume) and the pregnancy is 36 weeks or more, the patient

should be delivered. If the pregnancy is less than 36 weeks, the management is individualized. Amniocentesis, daily testing, performance of CST, or delivery may be used depending on the circumstances.
3. If the amniotic fluid volume is decreased but the NST is reactive, a search for chronic fetal conditions, particularly congenital abnormalities, is undertaken, and the frequency of testing with MBPP is increased to twice weekly.
4. If the amniotic fluid volume is normal and the NST is nonreactive, further testing with CST or full BPP is indicated.

Doppler waveform analysis of the fetoplacental and uteroplacental circulations

A recent development in maternal-fetal medicine is the ability to assess the fetoplacental and uteroplacental circulations using Doppler ultrasound. The potential application of this method for the evaluation and management of certain pregnancy complications such as fetal growth retardation and hypertensive diseases is the subject of intense investigation at the present time.

In the course of Doppler testing, fetal and maternal vessels are examined with ultrasound waves. These waves are reflected by the red cells moving inside the blood vessel. The frequency of the reflected waves is different from that of the waves emitted by the ultrasound probe. The difference in frequency between emitted and reflected waves is called the "Doppler shift." The Doppler shift is submitted to spectrographic analysis and represented graphically as a waveform. These waveforms represent changes in the velocity of the blood flowing through the vessels. Thus velocity will be greater in systole and less in diastole. Analysis of the waveforms provides a qualitative measurement of the resistance to flow in the vessels that are being examined. However, one should avoid drawing conclusions concerning the velocity or quality of the blood flowing through the vessel being examined.

There are several methods of analyzing the waveforms that provide the clinician with a numeric index of the vascular resistance. The most commonly used and simplest method is the measurement of the ratio between the peak systolic and the diastolic frequencies of the waveform (S/D ratio). Some investigators use other measurements such as the pulsatility index and the resistance index. The objective of all these methods is to obtain numerical information from the waveform analysis reflecting the resistance to blood flow in the vessel that is being examined.

It has been suggested that the presence of an elevated umbilical artery S/D ratio should alert the obstetrician to possible fetal problems.[26] An extreme situation is the presence of umbilical waveforms without diastolic flow (Figure 1-5, *B*) or with reverse flow during diastole (Figure 1-6). There is general agreement that fetuses exhibiting this abnormality are at a very high risk for death, congenital abnormalities, or significant neonatal morbidity. Conversely, a normal umbilical S/D ratio (Figure 1-5, *A*) in a pregnancy complicated by fetal growth retardation or hypertension establishes an optimistic prognosis for the outcome.[27]

The measurement of the S/D ratio in the uterine arteries may demonstrate changes indicating high vascular resistance in patients with hypertension or IUGR (Figure 1-7). Abnormal S/D ratios in the uterine arteries do not carry the same guarded prognosis about the fetal situation as do abnormal ratios in the umbilical artery. According to Fleischer et al.,[28] the presence of normal S/D ratios in both the uterine and the umbilical arteries has an excellent negative predictive value, and hypertensive patients with normal ratios have fetal outcomes that are similar to those of normotensive patients.

Umbilical and uterine Doppler waveform analysis may not produce information capable of modifying the management of high-risk obstetrical patients. Proof of the clinical utility of this technique requires randomized clinical trials.

Percutaneous umbilical blood sampling

The introduction of percutaneous umbilical blood sampling (PUBS) by F. Daffos in 1983, and the confirmation by the same investigator in 1985 of the safety of the procedure, has opened new avenues to the field of fetal diagnosis.[29] The availability of this technique has changed the management of patients with Rh isoimmunization, idiopathic thrombocytopenic purpura (ITP), toxoplasmosis, and hereditary blood disorders.

PUBS can be performed easily after 24 weeks of gestation. Attempts are being made in many centers to perform the procedure as early as 16 weeks, but in most cases it can consistently be done only after 18 weeks. PUBS can be performed at any point in the cord, but the placental insertion site is preferred. The procedure requires the use of high-resolution ultrasound equipment. Most investigators use sector scanning, free-hand technique, and a 22-gauge needle. However, many other perinatologists have similar success with linear scanning, ultrasonic needle guidance, and a 20-gauge needle.[30]

The safety of PUBS has not been completely

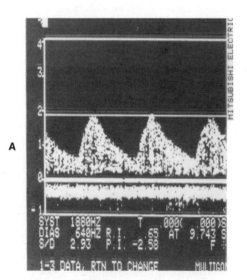
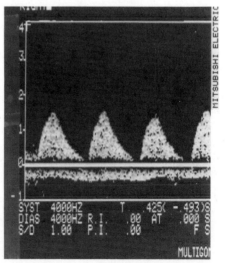

FIGURE 1-5 ■ Normal and abnormal umbilical waveforms. **A,** Normal umbilical waveforms; there is normal diastolic flow. **B,** Abnormal umbilical waveforms; there is no diastolic flow.

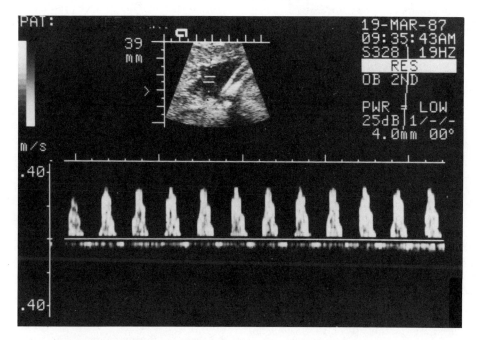

FIGURE 1-6 ▨ Reversed diastolic flow in a seriously compromised fetus.

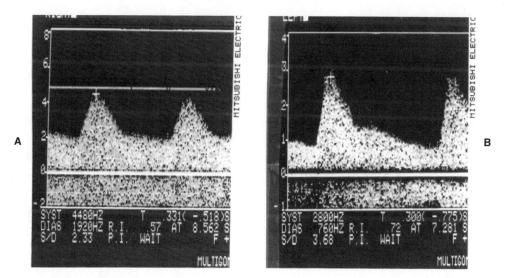

FIGURE 1-7 ▨ Normal and abnormal uterine artery waveforms. **A,** Normal uterine artery waveform with significant diastolic flow. **B,** Abnormal uterine artery waveforms with decreased diastolic flow and early diastolic notch.

BOX 1-7

Indications for Percutaneous Umbilical Blood Sampling (PUBS)

1. Rapid karyotype in fetuses with structural abnormalities discovered during ultrasound examination
2. Fetal hemolytic disease
3. Suspected fetal viral infection
4. Nonimmunologic hydrops fetalis
5. Suspected fetal thrombocytopenia
6. Diagnosis of twin-to-twin transfusion
7. Suspected fetal hemoglobinopathy

established. Preliminary reports on a few thousand samplings have indicated that the procedure has a risk of one fetal death per 300 PUBS, the same as ultrasound-guided genetic amniocentesis. Some recent information,[31] however, suggests that the mortality may be as high as 5%.

The indications for the use of PUBS will expand with further experience with the procedure. Currently, the procedure is indicated in the situations shown in Box 1-7.

Fetal movement count

The decrease or cessation of fetal movements has an ominous implication and may be associated with fetal distress or death. Thus it is not surprising that fetal movement counting has been proposed as a method for evaluating fetal health. The objective is to recognize a decrease in movement and to follow that recognition with further testing to confirm or rule out the existence of fetal distress.

The method most commonly used is the Cardiff "count of 10" or one of its modifications. Patients are instructed to begin counting the fetal movements early in the morning and continue until they count 10 movements. If 10 movements are counted in 10 hours or less, the fetus most likely is in good health. If the mother notices fewer than 10 movements in 10 hours, she should call her obstetrician and have further evaluation. Similarly, the patient should call and have additional evaluation if she notices it takes double the usual number of hours for the fetus to complete the 10 movements.

Unfortunately, trials investigating the clinical usefulness of fetal movement counting in preventing late fetal death have produced contradictory results. A study in the United States concluded that screening with the count-to-10 system is a simple and effective way to reduce fetal mortality.[32] Another study of more than 68,000 women found that formal fetal movement count did not decrease the antepartum fetal death rate when compared with informal noting of movements.[33] The main reasons for the test failure were maternal noncompliance in counting the movements and untimely late reporting of decreased fetal activity.

◢ **IMPORTANT POINTS** ◣

1. Preconception counseling of high-risk patients is important. Patients with diabetes, Rh isoimmunization, history of recurrent preterm labor, or history of recurrent pregnancy losses and patients who potentially can transfer genetic disorders to their offspring will benefit most from preconception counseling.

2. Taking a thorough history and performing a physical examination of every obstetric patient are the best ways to identify the high-risk patient.

3. The best time to determine the gestational age of the fetus by ultrasound measurements is between 18 and 24 weeks of gestation.

4. The objectives of antepartum fetal surveillance are (a) to discover congenital abnormalities; (b) to detect abnormalities in the fetal growth; and (c) to detect and evaluate the severity of acute or chronic fetal asphyxia.

5. The variables to be evaluated in the nonstress test (NST) are (a) baseline fetal heart frequency; (b) variability of the fetal heart rate; (c) presence or absence of accelerations; and (d) presence or absence of decelerations.

6. The modified biophysical profile (NST with vibroacoustic stimulation plus evaluation of amniotic fluid volume) is an excellent test for evaluation of the fetal well-being.

7. Absent or reversed end diastolic flow in the umbilical artery waveforms obtained by Doppler ultrasound is important evidence of fetal compromise and demand frequent and intensive fetal surveillance.

8. The most important indications for percutaneous umbilical blood sampling (PUBS) are the need for a rapid fetal karyotype and fetal evaluation in patients with hemolytic disease, fetal thrombocytopenia, or suspected fetal infection.

REFERENCES

1. Goodwin JW, Dunne JT, Thomas BW: Antepartum identification of the fetus at risk. *Can Med Assoc J* 1969;101:458-465.
2. Aubry RH, Pennington JC: Identification and evaluation of high-risk pregnancy: The perinatal concept. *Clin Obstet Gynecol* 1973;16:3-27.
3. Hobel CJ, Hyvarinen MA, Okada DM, et al: Prenatal and intrapartum high-risk screening: I. Prediction of the high-risk neonate. *Am J Obstet Gynecol* 1973;117:1-9.
4. Coopland AT, Peddle LJ, Baskett TF, et al: A simplified antepartum high-risk pregnancy screening form: Statistical analysis of 5459 cases. *Can Med Assoc J* 1977;116:999-1001.
5. Taysi K: Preconceptional counseling. *Obstet Gynecol Clin NA* 1988;15:167-178.
6. Kramer MS, McLean FH, Boyd ME, et al: The validity of gestational age estimation by menstrual dating in term, preterm and postterm gestations. *JAMA* 1988;260:3306-3308.
7. Alexander GR, Petersen DJ, Powell-Griner E, et al: A comparison of gestational age reporting methods based on physician estimate and date of last normal menses from fetal death reports. *Am J Pub Health* 1989;79:600-602.
8. Hadlock FP, Harrist RB, Shah YP, et al: Estimating fetal age using multiple parameters: A prospective evaluation in a racially mixed population. *Am J Obstet Gynecol* 1987;156:955-957.
9. Wexler S, Fuchs C, Golan A, et al: Tolerance intervals for standards in ultrasound measurements: Determination of BPD standards. *J Clin Ultrasound* 1986;14:243-250.
10. Jeanty P, Cousaert E, Cantraine F, et al: A longitudinal study of fetal limb growth. *Am J Perinatol* 1984;1:136-144.
11. Hadlock FP, Deter RL, Harrist RB: Sonographic detection of abnormal fetal growth patterns. *Clin Obstet Gynecol* 1984;27:342-351.
12. DeVoe LD, Castillo RA, Sherline DM: The nonstress test as a diagnostic test: A critical reappraisal. *Am J Obstet Gynecol* 1985;152:1047-1053.
13. Willis DC, Blanco JD, Hamblen KA, et al: The nonstress test: Criteria for the duration of fetal heart rate acceleration. *J Reprod Med* 1990;35:901-903.
14. Thacker SB, Berkelman RL: Assessing the diagnostic accuracy and efficacy of selected antepartum fetal surveillance techniques. *Obstet Gynecol Surv* 1986;41:121-141.
15. Vintzileos AM, Campbell WA, Ingardia CJ, et al: The fetal biophysical profile and its predictive value. *Obstet Gynecol* 1983;62:271-278.
16. Manning FA, Lange IR, Morrison I, et al: Fetal biophysical profile score and the nonstress test: A comparative trial. *Obstet Gynecol* 1984;64:326-331.
17. Manning FA, Morrison I, Harman CR, et al: The abnormal fetal biophysical profile score: V. Predictive accuracy according to score composition. *Am J Obstet Gynecol* 1990;162:918-924.
18. Vintzileos AM, Campbell WA, Nochimson DJ, et al: The use and misuse of the fetal biophysical profile. *Am J Obstet Gynecol* 1987;156:527-533.
19. Manning FA, Harman CR, Morrison I, et al: Fetal assessment based on fetal biophysical profile scoring: IV. An analysis of perinatal morbidity and mortality. *Am J Obstet Gynecol* 1990;162:703-709.
20. Sze-ya Y, Wilkerson C: Is biophysical profile (BPP) score of 4, Reactive non-stress test (NST) and adequate amniotic fluid volume (AVF) a reliable indicator of fetal well-being? *Am J Obstet Gynecol* 1991;164:363.
21. Smith CV, Phelan JP, Platt LD, et al: Fetal acoustic stimulation testing: II. A randomized clinical comparison with the nonstress test. *Am J Obstet Gynecol* 1986;155:131-134.
22. Crade M, Lovett S: Fetal response to sound stimulation: Preliminary report exploring use of sound stimulation in routine obstetrical ultrasound examinations. *J Ultrasound Med* 1988;7:499-503.
23. Arulkumaran S, Anandakumar C, Wong YC, et al: Evaluation of maternal perception of sound-provoked fetal movement as a test of antenatal fetal health. *Obstet Gynecol* 1989;73:182-186.
24. Vintzileos AM, Gaffney SE, Salinger LM, et al: The relationships among the fetal biophysical profile, umbilical cord pH and Apgar scores. *Am J Obstet Gynecol* 1987;157:627-631.
25. Clark SL, Sabey P, Jolley K: Nonstress testing with acoustic stimulation and amniotic fluid volume assessment: 5973 tests without unexpected fetal death. *Am J Obstet Gynecol* 1989;160:694-697.
26. Schulman H, Fleischer A, Stern W, et al: Umbilical velocity wave ratios in human pregnancy. *Am J Obstet Gynecol* 1984;148:985-989.
27. Rochelson B, Schulman H, Farmakides D, et al: The significance of absent end-diastolic velocity in umbilical artery velocity waveforms. *Am J Obstet Gynecol* 1987;156:1213-1218.
28. Fleischer A, Schulman H, Farmakides G, et al: Uterine artery Doppler velocimetry in pregnant women with hypertension. *Am J Obstet Gynecol* 1986;154:806-812.
29. Daffos F, Capella-Pavlovsky M, Forestier F: Fetal blood sampling during pregnancy with use of a needle guided by ultrasound: A study of 606 consecutive cases. *Am J Obstet Gynecol* 1985;153:665-670.
30. Weiner CP: Cordocentesis. *Obstet Gynecol Clin NA* 1988;15:283-301.
31. Pielet BW, Socol ML, MacGregor SN, et al: Cordocentesis: An appraisal of risks. *Am J Obstet Gynecol* 1988;159:1497-1500.
32. Grant A, Elbourne D, Valentin L, et al: Routine formal fetal movement counting and risk of antepartum late death in normally formed singletons. *Lancet* 1989;2:345-349.
33. Moore TR, Piacquadio K: A prospective evaluation of fetal movement screening to reduce the incidence of antepartum fetal death. *Am J Obstet Gynecol* 1989;160:1075-1080.

2

ANTENATAL DIAGNOSIS OF CONGENITAL DISEASES

According to the Consensus Development Conference on Antenatal Diagnosis, 100,000 to 150,000 infants are born each year in the United States with significant malformations, chromosomal abnormalities, or clearly defined genetic disorders. Fortunately, the number of these conditions that can be detected antenatally is growing at a rapid pace. This is because of the development of new techniques to obtain fetal tissue, and especially because of rapid advances in recombinant-DNA technology. The role of the obstetrician in the antenatal diagnosis of congenital diseases is of great importance and consists mainly, but not exclusively, of the following functions:

1. Identification of patients at high risk for genetic disease in their offspring
2. Discussing with such patients the implications of the problem, the technology available for diagnosis, and the alternatives available if a genetic disease is found
3. Referral of such patients to adequate facilities for expert counseling and further testing

The first part of this chapter reviews the identification of patients at risk for genetic disease. Following this is a description of three techniques most commonly used to obtain fetal tissue for genetic diagnosis—genetic amniocente-

sis, chorionic villus biopsy, and percutaneous umbilical blood sampling. These procedures are a matter of concern for most patients referred for genetic counseling, and the obstetrician should be ready to answer questions about them accurately. The third part of this chapter is a brief discussion of some of the recent advances in genetic diagnosis based on DNA technology. Last, this chapter reviews some aspects of teratology of interest to all obstetricians.

◢ IDENTIFICATION OF PATIENTS AT RISK FOR CONGENITAL DISEASE IN THEIR OFFSPRING

Patients with significant genetic risk are identified through clues provided in their histories or physical examinations, with the use of maternal serum alpha-fetoprotein (MSAFP) screening, and by abnormal ultrasound findings.

Patients with historical high-risk factors for genetic disease

In many cases the patient herself raises concern about the possibility of genetic disease in an antenatal visit. This usually happens when she has had a pregnancy with a poor outcome, when she has relatives with a congenital disease, or when she has ingested medications or has been exposed to substances that she believes may be harmful for the pregnancy. In other instances the patient is unaware of the existence of genetic high-risk factors, and they are discovered only after a thorough medical and obstetrical history is obtained.

To facilitate the identification of patients at risk, it is useful to incorporate into the antenatal record a genetic screening questionnaire suggested by the American College of Obstetricians and Gynecologists (Box 2-1, p. 24).

The following historic factors identify patients who may be candidates for further genetic testing:

1. Maternal age of 35 years or more at the expected date of delivery
2. History of a previous pregnancy with a chromosomal abnormality
3. Existence of a chromosomal abnormality in either parent
4. History of Down syndrome or other chromosomal abnormality in a family member
5. History of two or more spontaneous abortions with marked alteration in fetal development, either in the present or past marriage of either spouse
6. Previous birth of a child with multiple major malformations
7. Family history of Duchenne muscular dystrophy, hemophilia, or other genetic disease
8. Pregnancies in couples at risk for inborn errors of metabolism
9. Pregnancies at increased risk for neural tube defects
10. Pregnancies at increased risk for sickle cell disease in the offspring

Once the patient with genetic risks is identified, the obstetrician should inform her and her husband about the nature of the risks, the need for further investigation, and the availability of referral centers capable of carrying out those investigations. Because amniocentesis, chorionic villus biopsy, and fetal blood sampling may be indicated in the workup of the patient, the obstetrician should be ready to answer questions about the accuracy and safety of these procedures. The obstetrician should also be ready to discuss management alternatives if further testing demonstrates the presence of fetal genetic abnormalities. The obstetrician should not assume the role of genetic counselor because this is a field of knowledge that requires training in human genetics. The obstetrician should be ready, however, to provide adequate answers to

concerned parents at the time that genetic risks are identified and before consultation with the geneticist.

The importance of the initial discussion between the obstetrician and the patient at risk for genetic problems cannot be overemphasized. An informal and informative conversation with the physician may dissipate many of the patient's unfounded fears and generate a positive attitude toward further diagnostic tests. If the obstetrician cannot provide basic information, shows insecurity in discussing risks and benefits, or defers to later consultation with the geneticist, additional fears may result.

Pregnant women of advanced age. As shown in Table 2-1, the risk of having a child with a chromosomal abnormality increases with maternal age. This risk is 1 of 526 at age 20 and 1 of 18 at age 45.[1] The predominant chromosome defect seen is Down syndrome (trisomy 21), although trisomy 18 and trisomy 13 also occur frequently.

In view of the strong association between advanced maternal age and chromosomal defects,

TABLE 2-1 ◪ Risk of having a child with chromosomal abnormalities at different maternal ages

Maternal age	Down syndrome	Other chromosome abnormalities except 47,XXX
20	1:1923	1:526
22	1:1538	1:500
24	1:1299	1:476
26	1:1124	1:478
28	1:990	1:435
30	1:885	1:384
32	1:725	1:332
34	1:465	1:243
35	1:365	1:178
36	1:287	1:149
38	1:177	1:105
39	1:139	1:80
40	1:109	1:63
41	1:85	1:48
42	1:67	1:39
43	1:53	1:31
44	1:41	1:24
45	1:32	1:18

From Simpson JL, Golbus MS, Martin AO, et al: *Genetics in Obstetrics and Gynecology.* New York, Grune & Stratton Inc, 1982, p 58.

BOX 2-1

Genetic Screening Questionnaire

Name _____ Patient # _____ Date _____

1. Will you be 35 years or older when the baby is due? Yes ___ No ___
2. Have you, the baby's father, or anyone in either of your families ever had any of the following disorders?
   - Down syndrome (mongolism) Yes ___ No ___
   - Other chromosomal abnormality Yes ___ No ___
   - Neural tube defect, i.e., spina bifida (meningomyelocele or open spine), anencephaly Yes ___ No ___
   - Hemophilia Yes ___ No ___
   - Muscular dystrophy Yes ___ No ___
   - Cystic fibrosis Yes ___ No ___

   If yes, indicate the relationship of the affected person to you or to the baby's father: _____
3. Do you or the baby's father have a birth defect? Yes ___ No ___
   If yes, who has the defect and what is it? _____
4. In any previous marriages, have you or the baby's father had a child, born dead or alive, with a birth defect not listed in question 2 above? Yes ___ No ___
   If yes, what was the defect and who had it? _____
5. Do you or the baby's father have any close relatives with mental retardation? Yes ___ No ___
   If yes, indicate the relationship of the affected person to you or to the baby's father:

   _____

   Indicate the cause, if known:

   _____
6. Do you, the baby's father, or a close relative in either of your families have a birth defect, any familial disorder, or a chromosomal abnormality not listed above? Yes ___ No ___
   If yes, indicate the condition and the relationship of the affected person to you or to the baby's father: _____
7. In any previous marriages, have you or the baby's father had a stillborn child or three or more first-trimester spontaneous pregnancy losses? Yes ___ No ___
   Have either of you had a chromosomal study? Yes ___ No ___
   If yes, indicate who and the results: _____
8. If you or the baby's father are of Jewish ancestry, have either of you been screened for Tay-Sachs disease? Yes ___ No ___
   If yes, indicate who and the results:

   _____
9. If you or the baby's father are black, have either of you been screened for sickle cell disease? Yes ___ No ___
   If yes, indicate who and the results:

   _____
10. If you or the baby's father are of Italian, Greek, or Mediterranean background, have either of you been tested for beta-thalassemia? Yes ___ No ___
    If yes, indicate who and the results:

    _____
11. If you or the baby's father are of Philippine or Southeast Asian ancestry, have either of you been tested for beta-thalassemia? Yes ___ No ___
    If yes, indicate who and the results:

    _____
12. Excluding iron and vitamins, have you taken any medications or recreational drugs since being pregnant or since your last menstrual period? (include nonprescription drugs.) Yes ___ No ___

    If yes, give name of medication and time taken during pregnancy:

    _____

From *ACOG Technical Bulletin 108*. September, 1987.

genetic diagnostic procedures (chorionic villi sampling [CVS] or genetic amniocentesis) are routinely offered to women who are going to be 35 years old or older at the time of their delivery. The selection of 35 years of age as a cut-off point was based on risk/benefit analysis: at this maternal age the risk of chromosomal abnormalities is greater than the risk of fetal loss related to the genetic diagnosis procedures.

Unfortunately, even with generalized use of genetic diagnosis in pregnant women 35 years or older, only a maximum of 25% of all fetuses with chromosome abnormalities will be identified before birth. This low rate of detection results because the majority of pregnancies occur in a young population that is not being screened. This situation has been a powerful stimulant for researchers to design and conduct trials of biochemical markers to identify patients at risk for chromosome abnormalities. These methods of identification are described later in this chapter.

It is likely that in the near future maternal age will not be the only criterion used to determine the fetal risk for chromosomal abnormalities. Biochemical assays combined with maternal age will determine that risk and the need for additional diagnostic procedures. However, until the accuracy of the new screening methods is fully investigated, the policy of offering genetic diagnosis procedures to every pregnant woman 35 years old or more should continue. It is also important to refer for genetic counseling any pregnant woman under age 35 who requests fetal diagnosis, and if she desires, have a genetic diagnosis procedure performed afterwards.

Patients who have had a child with Down syndrome. Craniofacial features of Down syndrome include palpebral fissures, small and low-set ears, a protruding tongue, and a broad nasal bridge. Associated anomalies are common, particularly cardiac lesions and duodenal atresia. Approximately 20% to 30% of these infants die during their first year of life, and 50% are dead by the age of 5, mainly because of respiratory infections. Those who survive infancy universally have mental retardation.

In about 85% of the cases, Down syndrome results from the presence of an entire additional chromosome 21 (nondisjunctional trisomy). In 3% to 5% of the cases, Down syndrome results from translocation of a band from another chromosome (most commonly chromosome 14), and mosaic composition is the cause of only a few cases. Nondisjunctional Down syndrome is usually sporadic and shows a well-defined relationship to maternal age, whereas those cases involving translocations may be familial and unrelated to maternal age. When a pregnant woman has a history of a previous child with Down syndrome, it becomes important to know the type of chromosomal defect found in that particular child because the risk of occurrence in a future pregnancy will be different depending on the type of defect.

There is evidence suggesting that the risk of having a child with Down syndrome increases twofold when the father's age surpasses 55 years.[2] This has been refuted by recent studies[3] that found no increase in the rate of trisomic conceptions with advanced paternal age.

Information obtained with cytogenetic techniques indicated that in approximately 20% of the cases the extra chromosome 21 in infants with Down syndrome was received from the father. This information has been contradicted by recent studies using DNA technology. It has been found that the extra chromosome 21 is of paternal origin in only 5% of the patients.[4]

The recurrence risk in the case of a prior baby with trisomy 21 will also depend on the age of the mother at the time of birth of the affected child and on her age at the time of the present pregnancy.[5] If the woman was less than 30 years old at the time of the birth of the child with Down syndrome and she still is under age 30, the recurrence risk is between 2% and 3%; if she is now older than 30 years, the risk will be that corresponding to her present age (see Table 2-1) plus 1%.[1] If the mother was 30 years of age or older at the time of the birth of the child with Down syndrome, her risk in a subsequent pregnancy is no higher than that of any other woman of similar age.

The recurrence risk when the Down syndrome was caused by an unbalanced translocation will vary depending on the chromosomal composition of the parents. If both parents have a normal karyotype, the translocation in the affected child occurred de novo, and the risk of another affected child is less than 1%. If the mother's karyotype is normal but the father has a balanced 13/21, 14/21, 15/21, or 21/22 translocation, the risk of another affected child will be 2% to 3%. If the father's karyotype is normal and the mother is the carrier of a balanced 13/21, 14/21, 15/21, or 21/22 translocation, the probability

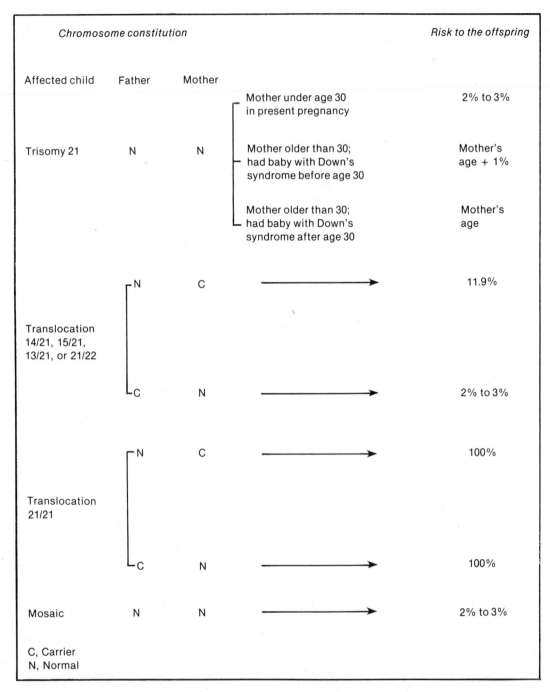

FIGURE 2-1 ◪ Recurrence risk of Down syndrome.

of having another affected child is 11.9%, which is much less than the theoretical risk of 33%. If either parent has a balanced 21/21 translocation, the risk of having an affected child in a future pregnancy will be 100%. The risk of recurrence when a previous child has been born with Down syndrome resulting from mosaicism is unknown, but is probably small (2% to 3%). Figure 2-1 summarizes the risk of recurrence for Down syndrome. In all these cases the risk of recurrence is greater than the risk of genetic diagnosis, and these patients should be advised to seek genetic counseling and to have genetic diagnosis.

Patients who have had a child with a neural tube defect. Neural tube defect (NTD) is a generic name designating malformations that result from the failure of the neural tube to close in the first 4 weeks after conception. NTDs are among the most common major malformations of the central nervous system, and their incidence changes with race and geographic location. The incidence of NTD in the United States is 1.2 to 1.7 per 1000 births overall, and it is 0.9 per 1000 for the black population.[6] In Wales and Ireland, with mostly white populations, the overall incidence of NTD is higher, with almost 1% of the pregnant population being affected.[7]

The recurrence risk for NTD, a multifactorial defect, is lower than for most chromosome abnormalities (Box 2-2). The most frequently quoted recurrence risk figures come from studies performed in England, where the prevalence of the disease is elevated. In the United States, where the frequency of NTD is lower, the recurrence risk is 1.5% to 3% when one prior child has been affected and 4% to 6% when two prior children have been affected.[8]

The prenatal assessment of patients with a history of NTD in a prior pregnancy requires the use of ultrasound, MSAFP, and amniocentesis. With endovaginal and transabdominal ultrasound, it is possible to rule out the possibility of fetal anencephaly as early as 12 weeks. To rule out spina bifida, a level II ultrasound examination by an experienced sonographer should be performed at 16 weeks. A level II examination will detect 80% to 90% of fetuses with open spine defects. Therefore a normal level II ultrasound will significantly reduce the recurrence risk of 4% (Box 2-2), especially if the MSAFP is normal. For example, a woman with a prior baby with NTD who has a normal level II examination and a MSAFP result of less than 2.0 multiples of

the median (MOM) will have a risk less than 1 in 310. Therefore, following a normal level II ultrasound, the patient should be informed of her decreased risk and offered the options of having or not having genetic amniocentesis. A MSAFP result of 2.0 MOMs or greater in a patient with a prior baby with NTD indicates the need for amniocentesis, even if the level II ultrasound is normal.[9]

The purpose of amniocentesis in patients at risk for having a fetus with NTD is to measure the concentration of alpha- fetoprotein (AFP) in the amniotic fluid. Amniotic fluid AFP concentration decreases with gestational age (Figure 2-2) and will be higher than 2.5 MOMs in 90% of patients carrying a fetus with NTD. The other

BOX 2-2 Recurrence Risk of Neural Tube Defects	
Family members affected	Anencephaly or spina bifida (%)
No siblings	
Neither parent	0.3
One parent	4.5
Both parents	30.0
One sibling	
Neither parent	4.0
One parent	12.0
Both parents	38.0
Two siblings	
Neither parent	10.0
One parent	20.0
Both parents	43.0
One sibling and one second-degree relative	
Neither parent	7.0
One parent	18.0
Both parents	42.0
One sibling and one third-degree relative	
Neither parent	5.5
One parent	16.0
Both parents	42.0

From ACOG: Maternal serum alpha-fetoprotein. *Interactions* 1989; 2(4), Hamilton, Ontario, Decker Electronic Publishing.

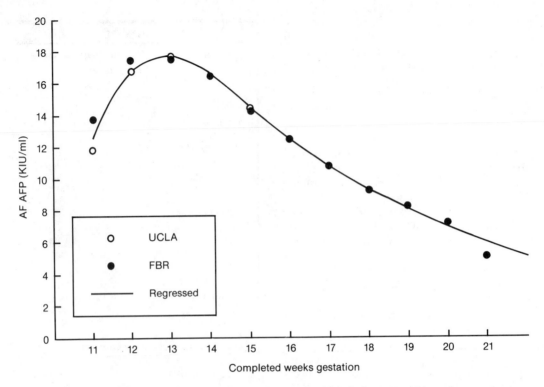

FIGURE 2-2 ◤ Median amniotic fluid alpha-fetoprotein levels from 11 to 31 weeks gestation. (Redrawn from Haddow JE [ed], Palomaki G, Knight GJ, et al: Prenatal screening for major fetal disorders in *The Foundation for Blood Research Handbook*, vol 1, Fetal disorders associated with elevated MSAFP values, 1990.)

10% of affected infants will have closed defects, and the AFP concentration will be normal. The false-positive rate for amniotic fluid AFP is 0.1% and in most cases is caused by contamination of the amniotic fluid sample with fetal serum, which has a high AFP concentration.

When the amniotic fluid AFP concentration is 2.5 MOMs or greater, it is necessary to measure the concentration of acetylcholinesterase in the fluid. A negative acetylcholinesterase assay makes highly improbable the presence of a fetal NTD. If the acetylcholinesterase assay is positive, the high-resolution ultrasound by an expert sonographer should be repeated, and if no NTD can be seen during the ultrasound examination, a second amniocentesis should be carried out to confirm the elevation of AFP and acetylcholinesterase. If the second determination is normal, the first value most probably was false-positive. False-positive acetylcholinesterase results occur infrequently in amniocentesis specimens ob-

tained before 15 weeks.[10] If the second amniocentesis shows an elevated amniotic fluid AFP level and a positive acetylcholinesterase assay, it is possible that a small open defect is present in the sacral spine that cannot be seen clearly with high resolution ultrasound. The situation should be discussed extensively with the parents, and the pregnancy should not be terminated unless the parents fully understand that it is possible that the fetus may be normal.

Ninety percent of all cases of NTD occur in families with no previously affected members and under circumstances in which genetic studies are not indicated. As discussed later, maternal serum AFP screening will be useful in discovering the majority of these affected fetuses.

In the case of patients who have had a baby with encephalocele, it is necessary to know if there were associated abnormalities such as polycystic kidneys, polydactyly, cleft palate, or congenital heart defects present. This information is important because the recurrence risk is different when the defect is isolated than when there are associated findings. When one or more associated abnormalities are present, the correct diagnosis may be Meckel-Gruber syndrome, which is an autosomal recessive condition with a 25% chance of recurrence.

There is a controversy about the value of multivitamin/folic acid supplementation in early pregnancy for the prevention of NTDs. Milunski et al.[11] looked retrospectively to the pregnancy outcome of 22,776 pregnancies and found a prevalence of NTD of 3.5 per 1000 among women who did not use multivitamins after conception. The prevalence of NTD was 0.9 per 1000 for women who used folic acid containing vitamins during the first 6 postconceptional weeks. Another group of investigators[12] in a retrospective cohort study concluded that the rate of multivitamin use among mothers of infants with neural tube defects, women who had had a stillbirth or a conceptus with another malformation, and women who had had a normal conceptus was not significantly different and that the periconception use of multivitamins or folate-containing supplements did not decrease the risk of having an infant with NTD. However, a recent prospective, randomized, double-blind trial has conclusively demonstrated that supplementation with 4 mg daily of folic acid in the periconception period protects against the development of neural tube defects.[12a]

Patients who have had a child with hydrocephaly. Adequate counseling of parents who have had a child with hydrocephaly depends on a precise diagnosis of the abnormality because the recurrence risk is different depending on the etiology. For example, the recurrence risk for X-linked aqueductal stenosis is 12% if the fetus is a male. The recurrence risk for aqueductal stenosis resulting from cytomegalic virus or toxoplasmosis infection is very low. A Dandy-Walker syndrome of multifactorial origin will have approximately a 5% chance of recurrence, whereas the risk associated with Dandy-Walker syndrome associated with a chromosome disorder may be as high as 25%.

The most important test in patients at risk for recurrent fetal hydrocephaly is serial ultrasound assessment of the fetal intracranial anatomy. Modern high-resolution ultrasound equipment allows precise measurements of the ventricular width from the beginning of the second trimes-

ter of pregnancy and detection of ventricular enlargement before the cranium becomes enlarged. It seems that the best method to evaluate the fetal ventricular size is measuring the width of the lateral ventricle atria.[13] This measurement remains fairly constant below 1 cm from 16 weeks until the end of the pregnancy. There is more information about fetal hydrocephaly in Chapter 17, Fetal Dysmorphology.

Patients who have had a child with congenital heart disease. Congenital heart disease occurs in 1 or 2 of every 1000 newborns. The most common types of congenital heart problems are ventricular septal defects, atrial septal defects, tetralogy of Fallot, patent ductus arteriosus, and pulmonary stenosis. Table 2-2 shows the risk of recurrence for several congenital heart problems.[14] The literature indicates that the risk of recurrence if one sibling is affected is from 2% to 4%, depending on the type of defect. When two prior children are affected, the risk of recurrence is from 6% to 12%. The recurrence risk may be higher than generally accepted.

Mothers who have had a child with congenital heart disease should have an ultrasound examination of the fetal heart (fetal echocardiogram, or fetal ECHO). This technique has developed to a point at which most structural heart anomalies can be accurately diagnosed between 18 and 28 weeks of gestation. Antepartum diagnosis of

TABLE 2-2 ◪ Recurrence risk of some congenital heart diseases

Anomaly	Risk (%)	
	One sib	Two sibs
Ventricular septal defect	3.0	10
Atrial septal defect	2.5	8
Tetralogy of Fallot	2.5	8
Patent ductus arteriosus	3.0	10
Pulmonic stenosis	2.0	6
Aortic stenosis	2.0	6
Aortic coarctation	2.0	6
Hypoplastic left heart	2.0	6
Transposition	1.5	5
Endocardial cushion	3.0	10
Fibroelastosis	4.0	12
Pulmonary atresia	1.0	3

From Nora JJ: *Am J Med Gen* 1988;29:137.

the anomaly makes it possible to plan the medical and surgical management that will be instituted immediately after birth. It also provides time for the adequate coordination of the different specialists that will be involved in the care of the newborn.

A fetal ECHO should be obtained also for other patients at risk of congenital heart disease in their offspring, such as insulin-dependent pregnant patients with diabetes, and for patients who have ingested drugs with cardiac teratogenic potential (lithium, Valium, Librium, Dilantin) during early organogenesis. Fetal ECHO use is also important in conditions associated with increased risk of fetal cardiac abnormalities such as fetal cardiac arrhythmias, hydrops fetalis, chromosomal abnormalities, and polyhydramnios.

A final important indication for fetal ECHO is the finding of certain extracardiac malformations that are frequently associated with congenital heart defects. The malformations most commonly associated with cardiac anomalies are esophageal atresia, tracheoesophageal fistula, diaphragmatic hernia, omphalocele, horseshoe kidney, bilateral renal agenesis, and Meckel-Gruber syndrome.[15]

Patients who have had a child with cystic fibrosis. Cystic fibrosis (CF) is characterized by pancreatic insufficiency, pulmonary abnormalities, and elevated sweat electrolyte levels. The fundamental biochemical defect seems to be an alteration in the regulation of chloride transport. CF is a relatively common disorder among whites, affecting approximately 1 of every 2000 newborns. An estimated 1 of every 20 white persons is a carrier for the abnormal gene. The disease is transmitted as an autosomal recessive trait. The risk of having a child with CF is shown in Table 2-3.[3] The disease is rare in Orientals and blacks.

Although the morbidity of patients with CF has improved significantly, more than 50% of these patients die before they reach 20 years of age. Individuals who have been exposed to the emotional trauma of seeing a family member suffering and dying of this disease frequently look for genetic counseling and antepartum screening.

The application of molecular genetic technology to the diagnosis of CF has been extremely productive. Researchers found that the CF gene is located in the middle part of the long arm of

chromosome 7 and extends over approximately 250 DNA kilobases. The membrane protein coded by the CF gene contains 1480 amino acids. Approximately 20 mutations capable of producing CF have been identified. The most common mutation found in the United States, affecting 70% to 75% of white carriers, has been named delta F508. This mutation corresponds to the loss of a trinucleotide codon and results in the loss of a phenylalanine amino acid originally situated in position 508 in the CF protein. The mutation causing CF varies with the population being studied. For example, delta F508 is present in only 30% of Ashkenazi Jews with CF.

DNA analysis is necessary to determine whether the fetus of a mother who had a prior child with CF is affected by the condition. Fetal DNA can be obtained by CVS or by amniocentesis and amplified using the polymerase chain reaction. In the majority of cases the parents will be carriers of the delta F508 mutation, and the fetal DNA analysis will consist of a search for this mutation using a specific DNA probe. If the affected child or the parents are not carriers of the delta F508 mutation, fetal DNA analysis will require the use of different DNA probes and eventually the use of restriction fragment length polymorphisms (RFLP) linked to the CF gene.

RFLPs are mutations without phenotypic expression that are transmitted from parent to child as is any other phenotypically observable marker. If an RFLP is closely linked to an abnormal gene, the RFLP will be coinherited with the abnormal gene, and the abnormal gene may be indirectly recognized in a given person by find-

TABLE 2-3 ■ Risk of having a child with cystic fibrosis (CF)

One parent	Other parent	Risk of CF in each pregnancy
No CF history	No CF history	1:1600
No CF history	First-degree relative with CF	1:240
No CF history	Sib with CF	1:120
No CF history	Has CF	1:40
Sib with CF	Sib with CF	1:9

Modified from Bowman BH, Mangos JA: *N Engl J Med* 1976; 274:937.

ing the RFLP with which it is linked. To use RFLPs for prenatal diagnosis, it is necessary to have access not only to fetal DNA but to DNA from both parents and from one affected child.

Determination of microvillar enzyme activity in the amniotic fluid is an indirect method for the prenatal diagnosis of CF that may be useful in situations in which DNA analysis is not possible. The enzymes most commonly used for this assay are gamma-glutamyl transpeptidase, aminopeptidase-M, and alkaline phosphatase. In fetuses affected by CF, the activity of these enzymes is decreased. This method is approximately 90% reliable[16] with a false-positive rate of 1% to 4% and a false-negative rate of 6% to 8%.

Cystic fibrosis is the most common inherited disease in the United States. Therefore the need for a screening test for CF that could be used in the overall obstetrical population is apparent. Unfortunately, the most common mutation responsible for CF is present in only 70% of the carriers, and the use of this mutation for screening purposes will bring about a significant number of false-negative results. Mainly because of this reason, the American Society of Human Genetics and a panel from the National Institutes of Health do not recommend screening of individuals with a negative family history of CF. However, other investigators believe that it is not necessary nor is it desirable to deny access to the general public to a test that is capable of detecting approximately 76% of the carriers and more than 50% of the couples in which both members are carriers.

Patients at risk for having a baby with sickle cell disease. Ten percent of the black population in the United States is heterozygous for the hemoglobin S gene. If two heterozygous persons conceive, the chance of that child having sickle cell disease is 25%. Today precise antenatal diagnosis of fetal sickle cell disease can be made by applying molecular genetic technology to fetal DNA obtained through chorionic villus biopsy or amniocentesis.[17]

The difference between normal B-globin and sickle cell globin is the substitution of glutamine for valine in the sixth amino acid position of the protein. This, in turn, is the result of a single nucleotide change in the DNA coding for the protein; the nucleotide sequence GAG, which codes for glutamine, has suffered a mutation to GTG, which is the code for valine. It is fortunate that there are restriction endonucleases that split a

DNA chain in all places with the sequence GT-NAG, where N = any base. A normal globin gene will be split into two fragments by the restriction endonuclease. The sickle cell gene coding for the globin change will not be split into two fragments because of the mutation it has suffered and will produce only one DNA fragment after incubation with the enzyme. This difference in the number of DNA splitting products can be recognized by means of DNA hybridization techniques.

Patients at risk of having a child with metabolic disease. Inborn errors of metabolism are infrequent. However, there is a constantly increasing number of these hereditary metabolic defects that can be diagnosed antenatally by amniocentesis, CVS, fetal biopsy, or fetal blood sampling (Table 2-3). Prenatal diagnosis is useful because in some cases the fetal condition may be altered by changes in the maternal diet and also because it makes it possible to initiate adequate treatment of the newborn shortly after birth.

As shown in Box 2-3, different types of fetal tissues should be obtained depending on the specific condition that the physician is attempting to diagnose. Patients with a history of a prior child affected by a metabolic disorder should be referred to a perinatal center for adequate evaluation of the type of genetic analysis required.

Patients at risk for having a child with Tay-Sachs disease. Tay-Sachs disease is an inborn error of metabolism characterized by the accumulation, primarily in the neurons, of a glycolipid identified as GM_2 ganglioside. This substance accumulates because of a deficiency in the synthesis of the alpha subunit of the isoenzyme hexosaminidase A. The disease causes a progressive deterioration of neurologic function until the child dies, usually between 3 and 4 years of age.

Tay-Sachs disease occurs predominantly in Jews of Ashkenazi ancestry (central and eastern Europe). One of every 30 Ashkenazi Jews is a carrier for the abnormal gene, and well over 90% of all American Jews are of Ashkenazi origin. Fortunately, the heterozygous state can be recognized by a blood test, and this makes it possible to screen the population at risk. Also, the homozygous state can be recognized antenatally by amniocentesis, culture of fetal fibroblasts, and analysis of their production of hexosaminidase A. Also, fetal DNA analysis can identify any of the three specific mutations caus-

---

BOX 2-3

Inborn Errors of Metabolism That Can Be Diagnosed Antenatally

CVS, culture, and enzyme assay

3-Hydroxy-3-methylglutaric aciduria
Maple syrup urine disease
Cytochrome *c* oxidase deficiency
Galactosemia
Alpha-1, 4-glucosidase deficiency
Menkes disease
Mucolipidosis, type II

Amniocyte culture and enzyme assay

Glutaric aciduria, type I
Isovaleric acidemia
Beta-ketothiolase deficiency
3-Hydroxy-3-methylglutaric aciduria
Medium chain acyl-CoA dehydrogenase
Long chain acyl-CoA dehydrogenase deficiency
Maple syrup urine disease
Phenylketonuria
Tyrosinemia
Ornithine-transcarbamoylase deficiency
Citrullinemia
Argininosuccinicaciduria
Cytochrome *c* oxidase deficiency
Pyruvate carboxylase deficiency
Pyruvate dehydrogenase deficiency
Galactosemia
Glycogen storage disease, type III
Holocarboxylase synthetase deficiency
Menkes disease
Mucolipidosis, type II

Amniotic fluid analysis

Methylmalonic acidemia
Propionic acidemia
3-Hydroxy-3-methylglutaric aciduria
Medium chain acyl-CoA dehydrogenase
Long chain acyl-CoA dehydrogenase deficiency
Maple syrup urine disease
Citrullinemia
Argininosuccinicaciduria
Cerebrohepatorenal syndrome (Zellweger syndrome)
Holocarboxylase synthetase deficiency
Mucolipidosis, type II

Fetal liver biopsy and enzyme assay

Ornithine-transcarbamoylase deficiency
Glucose-6-phosphatase deficiency

Maternal urine

3-Hydroxy-3-methylglutaric aciduria

RFLP mapping

Phenylketonuria
Ornithine-transcarbamoylase deficiency

Immunoblot analysis

Glycogen storage disease, type III

From Iafolla AK, McConkie-Rosell A: Prenatal diagnosis of metabolic disease. *Clin Perinatol* 1990;17:761-777.

---

ing Tay-Sachs disease: exon 11 4bp insertion mutation, intron 12 splice-junction mutation, and exon 7 mutation.[18]

Ideally, all Jews of Ashkenazi ancestry should be screened before marriage and pregnancy. If this has not been done and the wife is already pregnant, the husband should be screened. If the husband has normal serum hexosaminidase activity, there is no risk to the fetus. If the husband is a carrier, it is necessary to determine the mother's status by measuring the enzyme activity in her leukocytes, since serum screening is unreliable during pregnancy. If the mother is negative, there is no risk to the fetus. If she is positive, amniocentesis should be carried out to measure hexosaminidase A activity, or fetal DNA

should be obtained and analyzed for the presence of specific mutations.

Patients at risk for having a child with mental retardation. On rare occasions, the obstetrician is faced with the need to answer questions that patients have about the risk of recurrence of mental retardation. In the majority of cases, complete answers to these questions require careful analysis and counseling by the geneticist. However, the obstetrician may alleviate some of the couple's anxiety by providing them some general information about this subject before their visit to the geneticist.

There are several etiologic categories of patients with mental retardation. About 20% of these patients are mentally retarded as a conse-

TABLE 2-4 ◪ Recurrence risk for mild, idiopathic mental retardation

Number of retarded subjects		Recurrence risk %
Parents	Children	
0	1	6
1	1	20
2	1	42

quence of a chromosomal abnormality, predominantly Down syndrome; about 20% are retarded males who have X-linked mental retardation (fragile X); 10% to 15% are mentally retarded because of a point mutation, a category that includes patients with inborn errors of metabolism; and 5% to 15% are patients with multifactorial conditions such as intrauterine or neonatal infections and birth trauma. Finally, in 5% to 15% of the cases, particularly in individuals with mild to moderate mental retardation, no clearly defined etiologic agent may be found. Obviously, the chances of recurrence of mental retardation in a given family will depend on the etiologic diagnosis. In the idiopathic group, which may represent individuals who belong to the lower end of the normal intelligence distribution curve, there is a strong family tendency for mild mental retardation (IQ of 50 to 75), as shown in Table 2-4.

Patients who have had a child with cleft lip or cleft palate. Cleft lip and cleft palate occur with relatively high frequency (1 of every 1000 newborns), so most obstetricians should expect to be questioned a few times during their professional life about the recurrence risk of these facial abnormalities.

The genetics and etiology of cleft lip, with or without cleft palate, are different from those of isolated cleft palate. The recurrence risk for the former is 4% with one prior affected child, 10% with two prior affected children, and 10% if one parent and one prior child are both affected. The risk is higher in males, and if the cleft involves both the lip and the palate or is bilateral, the risk is greater than if it is unilateral or involves only the lip.[19] For cleft palate alone, the recurrence risk is 2.3% if either one or two prior children are affected. If the parent and one child are affected, the risk of having a second child

with cleft palate is 15%. Cleft palate is not predominant among males.[16]

Cleft lip and cleft palate can be detected by examination with high-resolution ultrasound as early as 16 weeks of gestation. However, the usefulness of antenatal diagnosis of these defects is in question: there are no ways to correct the problem before birth, and the decision to terminate a pregnancy because of the presence of these defects is, to say the least, very difficult.

Patients with abnormal MSAFP screening

The second largest group of patients at risk for genetic disease have been discovered as a result of the incorporation of MSAFP testing into the prenatal care of American women. This testing started in May of 1985 when the American College of Obstetricians and Gynecologists recommended that all pregnant women should be offered MSAFP testing. Obstetricians have followed this recommendation, and as a result, MSAFP screening is today a component of routine prenatal care.

The original purpose of MSAFP screening was the prenatal detection of patients at risk for fetal neural tube defects.[20] That the test was even more valuable was demonstrated in 1984 by Merkatz et al.[21] These investigators demonstrated an association between low MSAFP levels (less than 0.4 MOM) and the presence of autosomal trisomies in the fetus. Therefore MSAFP screening will identify two groups of patients at risk for genetic disease: those with values of 2.5 MOM or greater that are at high risk for neural tube defects and those with values of 0.4 MOM or lower that are at high risk for autosomal trisomies. The problem is that MSAFP testing has a high rate of false-positives; only a small fraction of those patients with abnormally high or low MSAFP values will actually have babies with genetic disease. Therefore it is necessary to follow a series of steps in the analysis of patients with low or high MSAFP levels to avoid incorrect diagnosis.

Maternal serum alpha-fetoprotein (MSAFP) screening is usually carried out between 15 and 20 weeks of gestation, a time when the concentration of alpha-fetoprotein in the maternal serum is increasing with advances in gestational age (Figure 2-3). Most large laboratories and referral centers correct the values obtained for maternal weight (obese mothers have lower MSAFP levels than do patients of normal

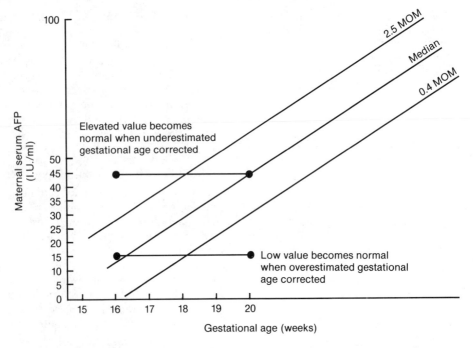

FIGURE 2-3 ◪ Maternal serum alpha-fetoprotein. Effects of correcting gestational age on interpretation of results. (Redrawn from Gabbe SG, Niebyl JR, Simpson JL [eds]: *Obstetrics: Normal and Problem Pregnancies.* New York, Churchill Livingston, 1986.)

weight), diabetes (diabetic mothers have lower MSAFP levels than nondiabetic mothers) and race (black women have higher MSAFP levels than do white women). After correction, the value obtained is compared with those values previously defined by the laboratory for each week of gestation between 15 and 20 weeks in a normal population.

Patients with elevated MSAFP levels. MSAFP values above 2.5 MOM are considered abnormal. When a patient has an elevated MSAFP level, an ultrasound examination should be performed. This need not be a level II and can be carried out in the obstetrician's office. The reason for this examination is that it can detect several of the most common nongenetic reasons causing high MSAFP values. An elevated MSAFP value may result from an error in the dating of the pregnancy. MSAFP concentration increases with gestational age, and a high value may become normal when an underestimated gestational age is corrected (Figure 2-3). Recognition of a dating error and reassignment to a more advanced gestational age will make further

testing unnecessary in about 20% to 25% of all patients with elevated MSAFP levels.

Ultrasound will also be useful in ruling out a multiple gestation. In fact, approximately 15% of patients with elevated MSAFP levels have multiple pregnancies, and once this is discovered, they will not need further testing.

A third cause of an elevated MSAFP level that can be discovered with ultrasound evaluation is undiagnosed fetal demise that may be present in as many as 5% of the patients with elevated MSAFP levels. Severe oligohydramnios, which is also easily observable with ultrasound, may also cause elevated MSAFP.

Finally, a level I ultrasound scanning is all that will be necessary to explain the elevated MSAFP levels in another 2% to 3% of patients, whose fetuses have obvious anatomical defects such as anencephaly, large spina bifida, and large omphaloceles. Occasionally, the level I ultrasound examination will demonstrate fetal hydrops caused by B19 parvovirus infection, another rare cause of elevated MSAFP.

After ruling out error in dating, multiple preg-

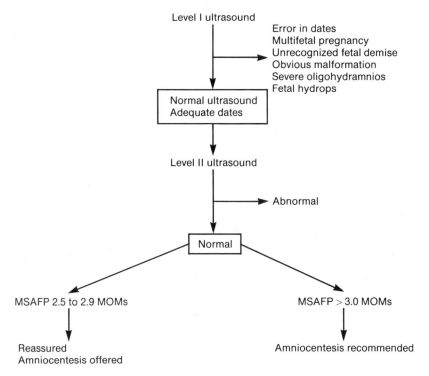

Level I ultrasound

Error in dates
Multifetal pregnancy
Unrecognized fetal demise
Obvious malformation
Severe oligohydramnios
Fetal hydrops

Normal ultrasound
Adequate dates

Level II ultrasound

Abnormal

Normal

MSAFP 2.5 to 2.9 MOMs

MSAFP > 3.0 MOMs

Reassured
Amniocentesis offered

Amniocentesis recommended

FIGURE 2-4 ◪ Management of patients with elevated MSAFP.

nancy, fetal demise, oligohydramnios, and gross congenital abnormality of the fetus, one should send the patient to a perinatal center to have a level II ultrasound examination performed by an experienced sonographer. Some investigators advise repeating the MSAFP test before performing the level II ultrasound examination, but most likely this is unnecessary.[22]

Patients with MSAFP values between 2.5 and 2.9 MOM and a normal level I ultrasound examination have approximately a 1 in 100 chance of carrying a fetus with an open spina bifida. This risk decreases to approximately 1 in 666 if a level II ultrasound examination shows no abnormalities. Under these circumstances amniocentesis is offered, but not strongly recommended.[23-25] For MSAFP values of 3.0 MOM or greater, the corrected risk is higher than the procedural risk, and amniocentesis is recommended.

The objective of genetic amniocentesis in patients with elevated MSAFP is to determine the concentration of alpha-fetoprotein (AFP) in the amniotic fluid. Amniotic fluid AFP determination is a diagnostic test, in contrast to maternal

serum alpha-fetoprotein determination, which is a screening test. If the amniotic fluid AFP concentration is normal for the gestational age of the fetus (see Figure 2-2), an open neural tube defect is highly unlikely, and there is no need for further testing. The patient must be informed, however, that unexplained elevations in MSAFP levels are associated with an increased risk of spontaneous abortion, stillbirth, prematurity, fetal growth retardation, and neonatal death.[26] The risk of obstetrical complications is directly related to the magnitude of the MSAFP elevation.[27] These patients should also know that other central nervous system malformations such as hydrocephalus occur more frequently in patients with unexplained elevated MSAFP levels. Since these patients are at high risk for poor fetal outcomes, they should be monitored closely to detect the onset of complications as early possible. The sequence of steps necessary to follow patients with elevated MSAFP is shown in Figure 2-4.

Patients with elevated amniotic fluid AFP should have a measurement of acetylcholinesterase and pseudocholinesterase activity in the amniotic fluid. If acetylcholinesterase is present in the amniotic fluid, the likelihood of an open neural tube defect is very high.[28] In patients with NTD, the ratio of acetylcholinesterase to butyrylcholinesterase levels is 0.14 or more. In cases of abdominal wall defects this ratio is less than 0.14.[29]

A patient with an elevated amniotic fluid AFP level and positive acetylcholinesterase should have a second level II ultrasound examination to identify the site of the lesion. Unfortunately, even in the best hands, not all open spine defects are recognized. If no defects are identified after high resolution scanning of the spine, a second amniocentesis should be carried out 1 week after the first one to assess the possibility of fetal blood contamination causing the elevated amniotic fluid AFP. If contamination with fetal blood is the reason for the elevated amniotic fluid AFP

level, the concentration of AFP in the fluid will decrease significantly in the second amniocentesis.

If the amniotic fluid AFP and acetylcholinesterase are abnormal in the repeated amniocentesis, patients are placed in the difficult position of making a decision involving the continuation or termination of their pregnancy in the absence of echographic confirmation of a fetal open spine defect. In this situation, the role of the obstetrician is of the utmost importance. The patient needs friendly, unbiased, and continuing support from all the members of the health team, regardless of her decision. A summary of the steps recommended to care for a patient with an elevated amniotic fluid AFP level is shown in Figure 2-5.

In most centers, chromosome analyses are performed on all amniotic fluids obtained because of elevated maternal serum MSAFP levels. When

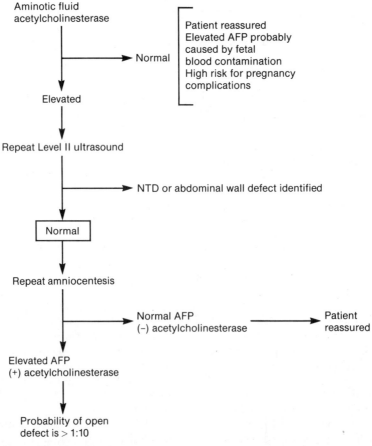

FIGURE 2-5 ▨ Management of patients with elevated amniotic fluid AFP.

the amniotic fluid AFP level is elevated, chromosome analysis is of value, since a significant proportion of fetuses with neural tube defects also have chromosomal abnormalities. Also, knowledge of the karyotype may be important for parents considering termination of pregnancy.

Patients with low MSAFP levels. The discovery of an association between low MSAFP and autosomal trisomies has made it possible to extend the screening for these chromosome defects to the overall obstetrical population. Before MSAFP screening, the only known association of autosomal trisomies was with maternal age. On this basis, all women who would be 35 years of age or older at the time of delivery were advised

to undergo genetic amniocentesis. With the availability of MSAFP screening, the search for autosomal trisomies has been extended to the obstetrical population younger than 35 years of age. With the extensive application of MSAFP and other biochemical markers such as beta protein, human gonadotropin (hCG), and estriol for the screening of the younger obstetrical population, it is expected that approximately 80% of all autosomal trisomies will be discovered.

Most tertiary centers in the United States combine maternal age and MSAFP screening for the evaluation of the risk for autosomal trisomies (Table 2-5). If the combined evaluation indicates that a woman has a risk equal to or greater than

TABLE 2-5 ◼ Risk of Down syndrome at birth for given maternal age and maternal serum alpha-fetoprotein°

Maternal age	MSAFP level (MOM)							
	Any	≤1.0	≤0.9	≤0.8	≤0.7	≤0.6	≤0.5	≤0.4
20	1923	1125	1004	882	762	613	498	415
21	1695	991	885	777	671	541	439	366
22	1538	900	803	705	609	491	398	332†
23	1408	824	736	646	558	449	365	304
24	1299	760	679	596	515	415	336†	281
25	1205	705	630	553	478	385	312	260
26	1124	658	587	516	445	359†	291	243
27	1053	616	550	483	417	336	273	228
28	990	579	517	454	392	316	257	214
29	935	547	489	429	371	299	242	202
30	885	518	463	406	351†	283	229	191
31	826	483	432	379	328	264	214	179
32	725	424	379	333†	288	232	188	157
33	592	347†	310†	272	235	189	154	128
34	465	272	243	214	185	149	121	101
35	365	214	191	168	145	117	95	79
36	237†	168	150	132	114	92	75	63
37	225	132	118	104	90	72	59	49
38	177	104	93	82	71	57	46	39
39	139	82	73	64	56	45	37	31
40	109	64	57	50	44	35	29	24
41	85	50	45	39	34	28	23	19
42	67	40	35	31	27	22	18	15
43	53	31	28	25	22	18	14	12
44	41	24	22	19	17	14	11	10
45	32	19	17	15	13	11	9	8
46	25	15	14	12	10	9	7	6
47	20	12	11	10	9	7	6	5
48	16	10	9	8	7	6	5	4
49	12	7	7	6	5	5	4	3

°Each number in the table is the denominator of the risk with a standard numerator of one.

†Numbers below the lines indicate risks greater than the maternal age 35 risk (one in 365).

1:365 of having a baby with Down syndrome, amniocentesis for determination of the fetal karyotype is recommended. The rationale behind this approach is that 1:365 is the risk of having a fetus with chromosome abnormality for a woman that is 35 years old and for many years it has been accepted that this risk is large enough to justify the performance of genetic amniocentesis. Obviously, if a young woman has a risk of 1:365 of carrying a baby with Down syndrome, as determined by a combined evaluation of her age and her MSAFP level, genetic amniocentesis is equally justified.

It has been found that maternal serum levels of unconjugated estriol are lower in pregnancies affected by Down syndrome than in normal pregnancies.[30] However, whether this information increases our ability to detect more fetuses with Down syndrome is questionable.[31] More effective in Down syndrome screening is the determination of maternal serum hCG, its beta subunit, or the free beta subunit (beta protein). The combined use of maternal age and these biochemical markers is of significant value in defining more precisely the risk of having a baby with Down syndrome and in reducing the number of genetic amniocenteses that are being performed. The detection rate can be increased to more than 60% with the use of MSAFP, hCG, and maternal age[32] or by using a combination of serum unconjugated estriol, MSAFP, hCG, and maternal age.[33,34] Recently, it has been shown that the detection rate for Down syndrome may be as high as 80% using a combination of MSAFP, maternal age, and free beta-protein concentration.[35]

When a low MSAFP level is detected, a repeated blood sample SHOULD NOT be obtained. This is because when a test is repeated, the second value will have a tendency to move toward the mean value for the population being tested. In the case of a low MSAFP level, the means of the normal and the abnormal populations are relatively close. The result of a repeated test will move toward higher values in both affected and nonaffected pregnancies. A low MSAFP value from an affected pregnancy will probably be higher if a second serum sample is obtained, giving a false sense of security and precluding further investigation of the problem.

When a low MSAFP value is reported after correction for maternal weight, maternal diabetes, and race, the first step the obstetrician

should take is to perform an ultrasound examination to confirm the patient's gestational age. As shown in Figure 2-3, MSAFP levels increase with gestational age, and a low value may become normal if ultrasound examination demonstrates that the gestational age of the patient was underestimated. Many abnormally low MSAFP values become normal after correction for gestational age. Also, if the ultrasonic dating shows that the gestational age is less than 15 weeks, the abnormally low value should be rejected, and MSAFP determination should be repeated between 16 and 18 weeks because there are no adequate norms to evaluate low MSAFP values before 15 weeks. The ultrasound examination also will be useful in recognizing missed abortions and blighted ova that may be associated with low MSAFP levels.

Genetic amniocentesis is recommended for those patients with low MSAFP levels who have an ultrasound examination confirming their dating. Patients with MSAFP below 0.25 MOM and normal karyotype have an increased incidence of spontaneous abortion, fetal death, hydatidiform mole, and choriocarcinoma. Therefore, if the fetal karyotype is normal and the MSAFP level is less than 0.25 MOM, the patient should be informed that there is a significant probability (approximately 30%) of an abnormal outcome for the pregnancy.[21,36]

It will be desirable if MSAFP screening for Down syndrome can be performed at less than 16 weeks. It seems that there is a strong correlation between low maternal levels of MSAFP in samples obtained between 8 and 12 weeks and the presence of autosomal trisomies.[37] These initial results are encouraging, and if the detection efficiency of MSAFP at 8 to 12 weeks is proven to be adequate, first-trimester MSAFP screening may replace the present system of screening at 16 to 20 weeks.

There has been great interest in the use of ultrasound for the screening of women under 35 years of age with the purpose of identifying Down syndrome fetuses. The sonographic findings proposed for the identification of Down syndrome fetuses are the presence of a short femur[38] and short humerus[39] and increased nuchal skinfold thickness.[40] There is considerable debate about the accuracy of these indicators, and up to the time of this writing, biochemical screening with MSAFP and free beta protein are the methods commonly used for Down syndrome screening. However, the finding of a short femur, short humerus, or thickened nuchal fold during a second-trimester ultrasound examination increases significantly the risk for having a Down syndrome fetus, and the mother should have adequate counseling when this occurs.

Patients with abnormal fetal ultrasound findings

The development of obstetrical ultrasound technology has generated a new objective in prenatal care, that of detection of structural abnormalities of the fetus. To achieve this, a majority of obstetricians in the United States have acquired office equipment for the performance of prenatal ultrasound, and observation of the fetus has become a part of routine prenatal care. As a consequence, more fetuses with anatomic abnormalities and in need of special diagnostic and therapeutic procedures are being discovered every day.

There is a wide variation in the nature of fetal defects detected in routine ultrasound examinations as well as in the accuracy of the findings and in the gestational ages at which the defects are found. Although not all fetal defects are detected before birth, undiagnosed malformations are being seen less frequently.

Patients with fetal anomalies discovered in the course of routine ultrasound examinations should be referred to a tertiary center for confirmation of the diagnosis, counseling, and establishment of a plan of management for the present as well as for future pregnancies. A large number of patients with fetal malformations will need karyotyping through amniocentesis or umbilical blood sampling. The reason for this is the high frequency (30%) of chromosomal disorders associated with some of the most frequently discovered anomalies.

Chapter 17 of this book is dedicated to the fetal abnormalities most frequently found during routine ultrasound in the obstetrician office.

◪ GENETIC AMNIOCENTESIS

Genetic amniocentesis is an outpatient procedure usually performed at 16 weeks of gestation but that is increasingly being done between 12 and 14 weeks of gestation (early genetic amniocentesis). Genetic amniocentesis is usually preceded by adequate counseling by a geneticist, a perinatologist, or by the obstetrician. This counseling includes, in addition to a discussion about the indications for the amniocentesis, a description of the procedure, its risks, and its complications.

Traditional genetic amniocentesis at 16 weeks

This procedure should be preceded by determination of the maternal blood group and Rh factor. This is important in determining the patient's eligibility for Rh immune globulin administration after the amniocentesis. The genetic amniocentesis also should be preceded by a level II ultrasound examination to:

1. Determine the number of fetuses
2. Measure the biparietal diameter, femur length, and abdominal and head circumferences
3. Visualize extremities, bladder, kidneys, and spine; the four chambers of the heart; and the intracranial anatomy
4. Locate the placenta

Measurements of the fetus are important for confirmation of the gestational age. The ultrasound examination before amniocentesis is also important for ruling out the presence of major congenital malformations such as anencephaly, meningomyelocele, large open spina bifida, limb reduction defects, omphalocele, polycystic kidneys, cystic hygromas, duodenal atresia, and hydrocephaly. Identification of the placental location is also an important step because if the placenta is anterior, a search must be made for a place where the needle can be inserted without puncturing the placenta. If there is no area free of placenta, a thin area, away from the center of the organ and its large vessels, should be selected and a 22-gauge needle used to withdraw the amniotic fluid. Before an amniocentesis is performed, the area selected for inserting the needle should be examined with color Doppler to be certain that a large placental vessel is not present.

Once the level II ultrasound examination is finished and an adequate puncture site has been selected, a sterile preparation of the maternal lower abdomen is performed. Local anesthesia is unnecessary although it helps relieve some of the patient's anxiety. A 22- or 23-gauge needle should always be used; larger needles offer no advantages and are more painful and traumatic. Under continuous ultrasound visualization using sector or linear transducers placed inside a sterile plastic bag, the needle is inserted in two rapid, successive steps. The first step will carry the tip of the needle into the subcutaneous tissue. The second step will place the needle inside the amniotic cavity. The two steps are necessary because many patients involuntarily contract the muscles of the anterior abdominal wall when they feel the needle in contact with their skin, and this may cause the needle to deviate from its intended route. Thus it is better to introduce the needle through the skin and the subcutaneous tissue first and then after the patient relaxes the anterior abdominal wall, to insert the needle into the uterus. When a linear transducer is used for amniocentesis, only the tip of the needle is visualized. However, with the sector transducer one can see the whole length of the needle. When the needle is inside the amniotic cavity, the stylet is removed, and fluid should come out freely from the needle. Then a plastic connecting tube is placed between the hub of the needle and the 10-ml syringe used to aspirate the fluid. The connecting tube will avoid movements of the needle caused by the physician when the syringe is directly connected to the needle. The plastic connecting tube also allows the needle to move passively within the amniotic cavity, making it extremely unlikely that the fetus will sustain a significant injury if the needle is hit by the fetus during episodes of fetal movements.[41]

The fluid is aspirated with a sterile syringe, and the first milliliter is discarded because of possible contamination with maternal cells. Two 10-ml aliquots of fluid are withdrawn, placed into two separate sterile plastic tubes, and transported to the laboratory for cytogenetic analysis and amniotic fluid AFP determination. After the fluid is removed, the needle is withdrawn, and fetal heart motion is observed with real-time ultrasound.

The amniocentesis involves separate puncture and analysis of the amniotic fluid of each sac when multiple sacs are present. After drawing fluid from the first sac, 0.5 to 1.0 ml of indigo carmine and 0.1 ml of air are mixed into 5 ml of amniotic fluid and injected into the first sac. The bubbles contained in the fluid will delineate the first sac and will allow a better selection of the second needle insertion site. Withdrawl of fluid free of dye will confirm insertion into the second sac. In some cases it is possible to draw fluid from a first sac, advance the needle through the membrane separating the sacs, and draw amniotic fluid from the second sac without the need for a second needle insertion.

Genetic amniocentesis is a safe procedure. However, it entails certain maternal and fetal risks as well as some potential technical problems. The main maternal risks associated with genetic amniocentesis are Rh isoimmunization in the Rh negative mother and infection. To prevent Rh isoimmunization, the maternal Rh factor should always be known before the procedure, and if the patient is Rh negative, 150 mg of Rh immune globulin should be administered intramuscularly following the amniocentesis. The risk of maternal infection is low, probably less than 1:1000.

The fetal risks associated with genetic amniocentesis have been assessed in several studies involving thousands of patients, both in the United States and in other countries. The results of these studies show that the danger to the fetus is extremely low, although the procedure is not entirely risk-free. Regarding the risk of abortion following genetic amniocentesis, the National Institute of Child Health and Human Development collaborative study[42] and the Canadian collaborative study[43] show no increase in spontaneous abortion following the procedure. The British collaborative study[44] shows a 1.5% increase in the abortion rate over that of control subjects. In the study of Golbus et al.,[45] the rate of spontaneous abortion was 1.5%. However, the rate of spontaneous abortion was 1.2% in the week before the procedure in patients who had made appointments for counseling and amniocentesis but did not have the procedure performed. In conclusion, the risk of fetal loss resulting from genetic amniocentesis seems to be between 0.3% and 0.5%. Most of this risk is for patients who have the placenta located in the anterior aspect of the uterus and who require transplacental amniocentesis.

The risk of fetal loss is increased in those patients who have brown and/or green amniotic fluid at the time of amniocentesis. This problem occurs in 1.6% to 6.7% of midtrimester amniocentesis. The discoloration of the fluid is due to the presence of blood breakdown products caused by an episode of intraamniotic bleeding. The majority of these patients had episodes of bleeding or spotting before the amniocentesis, which was the result of chorioamniotic separation. The fetal loss following amniocentesis in these patients varies from 5.0%[46] to 9.0%.[47]

Other complications associated with genetic amniocentesis are: (1) amniotic fluid leakage, reported by less than 1% of patients and usually disappears with bed rest; (2) unexplained fetal death following the procedure (0.7 of 1000 cases); (3) skin puncture of the fetus (1 of 929 cases); and (4) fetal trauma from the needle, reported in only a few cases.

The technical problems associated with genetic amniocentesis have to do with the occasional inaccuracy of the test and with the rare failure of the amniotic fluid cells to grow adequately in vitro. The test is extremely accurate, with an overall error rate of 0.4%. More than half of the errors are caused by contamination of the cultures with maternal cells. The culture failure rate is about 3.2%. In these cases, a second genetic amniocentesis should be performed.

It is important to inform patients that the findings of a normal fetal karyotype and a normal amniotic fluid AFP level do not guarantee the birth of a normal newborn, since there are causes of birth defects and mental retardation that cannot be detected through amniocentesis. The possibilities of this occurrence are, however, very low—most probably under 1%.

Box 2-4 shows the consent form for genetic amniocentesis used in the Genetics Unit, Department of Obstetrics and Gynecology, St. John's Mercy Medical Center, St. Louis, Missouri. The form contains comprehensive infor-

---

BOX 2-4

Consent for Amniocentesis for Diagnosis of Fetal Disorder

Amniocentesis is a test which can detect some birth defects and hereditary disorders. The test is done by withdrawing a sample of fluid from the bag of water surrounding the fetus (baby). This fluid is obtained by introducing a needle through the abdomen and uterus (womb). Some slight discomfort is experienced when the needle is introduced.

I, _____, have been informed of the following risks and limitations of amniocentesis for the diagnosis of fetal disorders, and have had the opportunity to question and discuss these with my physician and his or her assistants.

1. When the test is being performed in a stage of pregnancy when spontaneous miscarriage sometimes occurs, amniocentesis has not been shown to increase the chance of miscarriage.
2. The possibility of injuring the fetus or umbilical cord with the needle exists; however, the chance of this happening is considered to be very small.
3. As in all surgical procedures, there is a possibility of infection. If serious enough, this could cause loss of pregnancy. This risk is very low and every precaution is taken to maintain a sterile technique.
4. Ultrasound is performed to localize the placenta (afterbirth), to determine whether twins are present, and to visually guide the needle into the bag of water. It is also used to visualize fluid pockets and to evaluate fetal heart motion before and after the test.
5. In two thirds of patients, the placenta is located on the front of the uterus. In these cases it may be necessary to pass the needle through the placenta in order to obtain amniotic fluid. This could result in fetal bleeding. Although fetal bleeding is rare, it has been known to occur.
6. It is rare that the test cannot be successfully completed because of an inability to get an adequate sample of fluid.
7. An occasional complication is leakage of either clear or blood-tinged fluid from the vagina shortly after the tap. This leakage is not considered to be a serious complication and it should cease within 24 hours. If leakage persists beyond 24 hours, it is recommended that you notify your physician.
8. In some cases, the fetal cells do not grow in culture after an amniocentesis and the procedure may have to be repeated. This occurs in not more than one in fifty patients.
9. Since the test screens only for selected birth defects, the results do not guarantee the birth of a normal child. It is understood that there is a slight possibility that the laboratory tests could incorrectly assess the baby's health.
10. I believe the benefits of my having amniocentesis outweigh these potential risks associated with the procedure. I have had the opportunity to discuss any and all questions about the procedure and give my consent to have the procedure performed.

mation about risks, accuracy of the procedure, and possible technical problems. Ideally, the form should be given to the patient several days before the amniocentesis is performed and should be discussed with the patient before the procedure.

Early genetic amniocentesis at 12 to 14 weeks

Traditionally, genetic amniocentesis is performed at 16 weeks of gestation, and the results of the test become available in the eighteenth week. By this time, fetal movements may have already been noticed, making the option of termination of pregnancy, in the case of an abnormal result, particularly distressing for most patients. Also, if the patient decides to terminate the pregnancy, it is difficult to find a place where she can have a safe dilation and evacuation of the uterus, and in most cases termination will be performed with prostaglandins, which have significant side effects. These facts have generated a need for fetal genetic diagnostic procedures that could be performed at an earlier gestational age. The procedures now available for early genetic diagnosis are early amniocentesis and chorionic villi biopsy. These procedures may be used in almost all patients who are candidates for traditional amniocentesis at 16 weeks.

Early amniocentesis is becoming increasingly popular. First, most studies have demonstrated that the fetal and maternal risks are similar to those of traditional amniocentesis.[48] Second, with the development of better laboratory techniques, the fear that the amniocytes collected early in pregnancy would be difficult to culture has disappeared. Third, early genetic amniocentesis allows the physician to give results to the patient at a gestational age at which termination of the pregnancy can be performed at minimum risk and without the deep emotional conflict attached to this procedure once fetal movements have been perceived by the mother.

The objections to early amniocentesis—fundus not palpable, not enough fluid, inadequate cell growth in tissue culture—are unfounded.[49] In the hands of an experienced operator, early genetic amniocentesis can be performed in a large number of patients with no more risk than traditional amniocentesis at 16 weeks.[39,50,51] The procedure can be performed as early as 10 weeks and is easily done after 12 weeks.

The technique of early amniocentesis is slightly different from that used for traditional amniocentesis at 16 weeks in that the volume of aspiration should not exceed 1.0 to 1.5 ml for each week of gestation. Culture time is approximately the same as that of the traditional genetic amniocentesis at 16 weeks.

A patient having early genetic amniocentesis should be scheduled for a level II ultrasound when she reaches the sixteenth to eighteenth week of her pregnancy, because at 10 to 13 weeks of gestation, visualization of fetal anatomy is imprecise and it is difficult to rule out the presence of some congenital malformations. Not all centers have developed adequate standard curves for AFP in amniotic fluid samples obtained before 16 weeks, and in this situation patients having early amniocentesis should also have MSAFP determination at 16 to 20 weeks.

◢ CHORIONIC VILLI SAMPLING

Chorionic villi sampling (CVS) is a procedure for prenatal genetic diagnosis that is performed between 9 and 12 weeks. Therefore CVS avoids some of the problems associated with traditional amniocentesis at 16 weeks such as advanced gestational age when results are given to the patient and the medical and emotional problems associated with late pregnancy termination. For these reasons, from its beginnings in the early 1980s, CVS has been performed more frequently, and it is used to diagnose more genetic conditions.

Chorionic villi for antenatal diagnosis can be obtained by transcervical catheter aspiration (transcervical CVS), transabdominal needle aspiration (transabdominal CVS), and by transvaginal aspiration (transvaginal CVS).

Transcervical CVS

Similar to amniocentesis, CVS starts with a real-time ultrasound examination. The position of the uterus, the number of gestational sacs, the gestational age of the fetus, the presence of fetal heart activity, and the localization of the chorion frondosum are determined.

To perform CVS, two people are required. One person does the sonography while the other performs the sampling. While the sonographer keeps the uterus visualized at all times, the operator inserts a sterile speculum in the patient's vagina and cleans the vagina and the cervix with an antiseptic solution. A sterile polyethylene catheter with a malleable metal obturator is inserted into the endocervical canal and advanced toward the chorion frondosum. The position of the uterus and the angle between the cervix and the uterus can be modified by manipulating the speculum. Occasionally a single-tooth tenaculum should be applied to the anterior lip of the cervix to help in the manipulation of the uterus. The catheter should be inserted parallel to the chorion frondosum, and the tip of the catheter should be near its end before the sample is obtained. Once the tip of the catheter is in the desired position, the obturator is removed, a syringe with a small amount of cell culture medium is connected to the catheter, and negative pressure is applied while the catheter is slowly removed. The sample of tissue obtained is analyzed immediately with the use of an inverted microscope. An adequate sample consists of 20 mg or more of placental tissue. Most patients report no discomfort during the procedure. Vaginal spotting occurs frequently after CVS but usually disappears in 2 to 3 days.

The main risk associated with CVS is pregnancy loss after the procedure. A collaborative study in the United States[52] and a randomized study in Canada[53] have compared chorionic villi biopsy and amniocentesis at 16 weeks. They found a rate of fetal loss following transcervical CVS 0.8% greater than the rate after amniocentesis. Another significant risk is that of severe limb reduction defects when transcervical aspiration is performed between 8 and 9.5 weeks.[53a] It was also found that cramping, spotting, and bleeding after the procedure were more common after CVS. The conclusion is that CVS entails a slightly higher risk of fetal loss than does amniocentesis.

Another initial concern about transcervical CVS was the possibility of introducing bacteria into the uterus and causing chorioamnionitis. However, the incidence of infection has been lower than expected. Chorioamnionitis occurs in only 0.2% to 0.3% of patients undergoing CVS. Only two cases of life-threatening maternal infections after CVS have been reported.

Other potential risks of transcervical CVS are rupture of the membranes that occurs in approximately 0.3% of patients and severe vaginal bleeding, which occurs rarely. Rh negative women may become immunized after CVS and should receive prophylactic Rh immune globulin. Also, it is possible that a large increase in Rh antibodies after CVS may have an unfavorable effect in patients who are sensitized to the Rh factor, and CVS is not recommended in these patients. Immediately after CVS, 8.0% of the patients will experience light vaginal bleeding, and

---

BOX 2-5

Contraindications to Transcervical Chorionic Villi Sampling

Positive *Neisseria gonorrhoeae* culture of the cervix
Active genital herpes
Active bleeding
Maternal coagulopathy
Cervical stenosis
Severe cervicitis
Uterine myomata
IUD inside the pregnant uterus

---

by the end of the week after the procedure, as many as 39% will have some spotting or bleeding. However, this is usually unconsequential.

In summary, the advantages of transcervical CVS are:

1. Genetic diagnosis is achieved at an early gestational age minimizing the anxiety of the parents and facilitating termination of pregnancy for patients who choose this option.
2. It is comfortable for the patient since no pain or discomfort are involved.
3. It is technically simple.

The disadvantages of transcervical CVS are:

1. It has a slightly higher risk of fetal loss (0.8%) than traditional amniocentesis.
2. The chromosome composition of the chorionic villus is occasionally (1.3% of the cases) different from the chromosome composition of the fetal cells.
3. The enzyme composition of the chorionic villus cells may be different from the fetal cells.
4. It is difficult if the placenta is fundal.
5. There are some contraindications to transcervical CVS (Box 2-5).

Transabdominal CVS

Transabdominal CVS grew out of the need to obtain chorionic villi from patients who had contraindications to the performance of transcervical CVS and the need to reduce the potential risk of infection associated with the vaginal procedure. The transabdominal approach requires the use of real-time ultrasound for guidance, and either a one- or a two-needle technique can be used. In the latter technique, an 18-gauge needle is inserted into the chorion frondosum. The stylet of the needle is then removed, and a 20-gauge needle, 1.5 cm longer than the first one, is inserted through the first needle. The stylet of the second needle is removed, and the needle is connected to a 20-ml syringe containing 2 to 5 ml of culture medium. The syringe is attached to an aspiration device to facilitate suction. The second needle is moved slowly back and forth several times in the chorion frondosum while suction is applied with the syringe and then removed. The tissue obtained is placed in a Petri dish and examined with an inversion microscope. If the amount of tissue obtained is inadequate, the procedure can be easily repeated because the first needle remains in place. In most cases, one or two insertions yield an adequate amount of tissue. The tissue usually has little contamination with maternal decidua, blood, or mucus.

The single-needle technique requires the use of a 17- or 18-gauge needle, which is inserted using a "free-hand" technique or a needle guiding device that attaches to the ultrasound transducer. The technique is similar to that used with two needles, except that if the amount of tissue is inadequate, a new needle should be reinserted.

The risk of fetal loss after transabdominal CVS is similar to the risk of amniocentesis. The literature suggests that this risk may be minimized if transabdominal CVS is performed only after 12 weeks.[54]

The advantages of transabdominal CVS are:
1. Minimal risk of infection
2. Does not cause vaginal bleeding
3. Can be performed or in the second and third trimesters

The disadvantages of transabdominal CVS are:
1. The amount of tissue obtained is less than with transcervical CVS.
2. Patient discomfort is greater than with transcervical CVS or amniocentesis.
3. It is difficult to perform if the placenta is posterior.
4. It is technically more difficult than transcervical CVS.

Transvaginal CVS

There are some patients in whom transabdominal and transcervical CVS are difficult to perform because of extreme uterine retroversion, presence of myomas, or placental localization. In some of these patients, chorionic villi may be obtained using transvaginal aspiration under guidance with an endovaginal probe.[55]

Laboratory aspects of CVS

After chorionic villi are identified, they are picked out of the Petri dish and transferred to a second dish where they are washed, cleaned, and separated from any decidual tissue. The villi are now ready for direct cytogenetic analysis or for long-term tissue culture.

The direct cytogenic analysis of the chorionic villi is made possible by the presence of viable and actively dividing trophoblastic cells. The process of cell division is arrested by Colcemid, and the cells in metaphase are analyzed after adequate staining. The original technique for direct analysis required approximately 4 hours between the time the tissue sample was obtained and the time of the result. This has been modified, and most of the current techniques require 12 to 48 hours of incubation before the harvest of chromosomes.

The morphology of the chromosomes obtained for direct analysis is slightly different from that of those obtained after prolonged tissue culture. However, chromosomes obtained from direct analysis are useful for detecting numeric abnormalities and major rearrangements.

A problem associated with CVS is the observation of chromosomal mosaicisms complicating the interpretation of the test. Mosaicism is the presence of two or more different cell lines with different karyotypes. Mosaicism occurs in approximately 1.5% of CVS specimens. There are several mechanisms that may lead to mosaicism. One of these is contamination with maternal cells, which occurs more frequently in the cultured than in the direct preparations. Mosaicism also may result from in vitro influences on the growing cells, and in this case the problem will be apparent in the cell cultures and not in the direct preparations. Last, nondisjunction during embryogenesis with formation of aneuploid cells in the extraembryonic tissues but not in the fetus may cause mosaicism.

The majority of the mosaics in CVS occur in the direct preparations and rarely are confirmed in the fetus. This suggests that the majority of CVS mosaics are limited to the extraembryonic tissues. Therefore, when a mosaic is present in the direct preparation, it is necessary to wait for the culture results. If the mesenchymal cell culture is normal, the parents should be reassured that the fetal chromosomes are also normal. If the cell culture also shows mosaicism, it is necessary to perform fetal blood sampling to confirm the diagnosis.[56] Fetal blood is necessary because even if the mosaicism is found in amniotic cells, it may not be confirmed in the fetus or in the neonate. There is evidence suggesting that the perinatal outcome of patients with placental mosaicism is guarded.[57]

◼ PERCUTANEOUS UMBILICAL BLOOD SAMPLING

Percutaneous umbilical blood sampling (PUBS) is the latest procedure available to obtain fetal tissue for genetic analysis. The procedure was described in 1983 by Fernand Daffos and his collaborators.[58] Their initial report was followed 2 years later by a comprehensive description[59] of the complications and risks associated with the procedure, based on their experience with more than 600 cases. PUBS was originally designed to study the fetal transmission of toxoplasmosis, but it became evident that it could be used to investigate a wide range of fetal disorders (see Box 1-7). The most frequent indication for PUBS in the United States is for the investigation of fetuses with anatomical deformities or other conditions frequently associated with chromosomal abnormalities.

The main advantage of using fetal blood instead of amniotic fluid for the diagnosis of chromosome abnormalities is that it is possible to obtain a high-quality karyotype in 48 to 72 hours (rapid karyotype) rather than in the 10 to 14 days that are needed for amniotic cell culture. PUBS is useful for obtaining karyotype in patients who have fetal abnormalities detected by ultrasound (cases of fetal growth retardation or polyhydramnios) and also for the diagnosis of other genetic defects such as hereditary deficiencies of the hemostatic system, hemoglobinopathies, and metabolic disorders.

PUBS is a procedure similar to amniocentesis. It is performed as an outpatient procedure and does not require local or regional anesthesia. It can be done easily after 24 weeks of gestation and, in the hands of highly skilled operators, done as early as 18 weeks of gestation. The procedure begins with an ultrasound examination to find the placental insertion of the umbilical cord, the best place to obtain the blood sample. Color Doppler is invaluable for the correct localization of the cord origin. Once the cord placental insertion is found, a 23- to 20-gauge spinal needle of adequate length is inserted and advanced to the umbilical vein. Free-hand technique or a needle guide attached to the sector transducer may be used. The vessel is penetrated, and the necessary

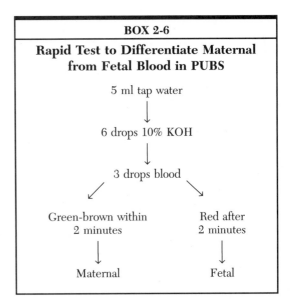

BOX 2-6

Rapid Test to Differentiate Maternal from Fetal Blood in PUBS

5 ml tap water
↓
6 drops 10% KOH
↓
3 drops blood
↙   ↘
Green-brown within 2 minutes   Red after 2 minutes
↓   ↓
Maternal   Fetal

volume of blood needed for a rapid karotype, usually 1 ml, is removed. Another small sample is sent to the laboratory for Kleihauer-Betke stain and for determination of the mean corpuscular volume (MCV) of the erythrocytes, which is always higher in fetal than in maternal blood. We also use a rapid test with potassium hydroxide (Box 2-6) to confirm the fetal origin of the blood sample.

The studies reported so far in the literature, involving more than 1400 cases, indicate that PUBS has a procedure-related fetal mortality rate of approximately 1%, but other investigators report up to 5% frequency of procedure-related deaths.[60] The complications most frequently observed with PUBS are bleeding from the puncture site, which occurs in approximately 30% of patients, and fetal bradycardia, which occurs in about 5%. Both are usually transient, but occasionally they may be severe and require emergency cesarean delivery.

◼ THE IMPACT OF THE "NEW GENETICS" ON ANTENATAL DIAGNOSIS

In the last few years, a series of techniques used primarily in molecular biology research have been succesfully applied to the solution of clinical problems in medical genetics. The knowledge generated with the use of molecular genetic technology has been called the "new genetics." The impact of these techniques on prenatal diagnosis has been spectacular, and there is a realistic promise of further advances that may lead to the treatment and correction of genetic diseases.

The technologic advances that have had the largest contribution to the new genetic knowledge are:

1. *The discovery of restriction endonucleases.* Restriction endonucleases are bacterial enzymes that recognize specific "restriction sites" in the double-stranded DNA chain of the gene and cleave the DNA molecule at that particular site. The "restriction sites" are made of short nucleotide sequences. More than 100 different restriction endonucleases, each one recognizing specific base-pair sequences, have been discovered. The importance of these enzymes is that they permit the splitting of chromosomal DNA into similar fragments each time the DNA is incubated with the same restriction enzyme and that these fragments have a size that permits further manipulation and analysis.
2. *The ability to isolate and identify specific DNA fragments using gel electrophoresis followed by hybridization with radioactively labeled complementary DNA.* This technique, called Southern blotting, has allowed direct and indirect detection of several genetic disorders in human chromosomes.
3. *The use of restriction fragment length polymorphisms (RFLP).* RFLPs are DNA variations or neutral mutations that do not have phenotypic expression and are transmitted from parent to child as is any other genetic marker. If an RFLP is closely linked to an abnormal gene, both the RFLP and the abnormal gene will be coinherited, and the abnormal locus can be identified indirectly by recognizing the closely linked RFLP. RFLPs may be used to distinguish between affected individuals, carriers, and normal patients. This technology has been successfully used for the diagnosis of cystic fibrosis, adult polycystic kidney disease, and Duchenne muscular dystrophy, among many others.

   The use of RFLPs for the diagnosis of genetic diseases depends on the recognition of particular patterns in a given family. Therefore the use of RFLPs requires the availability of DNA from an affected individual in the family under study. Once the polymorphic fragment containing the affected locus is

characterized, other members of the family can be studied for carrier status, and prenatal diagnosis becomes feasible for any pregnant member of the family. As more and more polymorphisms are recognized and more restriction enzymes are discovered, the possibility of diagnosing all monogenic disorders becomes more and more of a reality.

4. *The ability to synthesize complementary DNA chains that are exact copies of parts of the genome and to insert them into bacteria to obtain clones of these DNA fragments.* This technology allows one to multiply the amount of a given DNA fragment thousands of times, and this amplification makes it possible to carry out structural studies that could not be performed using smaller amounts of material.
5. *The DNA polymerase chain reaction is a biochemical process that permits the reproduction of a DNA segment several thousand times.* This selective amplification has been automatized, and today it is theoretically possible to obtain the necessary amounts of DNA for complex biochemical studies starting from the DNA of a single cell.[61]

◪ SOME ANSWERS TO TERATOLOGIC QUESTIONS

Society in general and patients individually are concerned about teratogenic influences. The wide publicity given to the diethylstilbestrol (DES) problem and the thalidomide tragedy are responsible to a large extent for this widespread concern about fetal safety from medications and environmental influences. Thus patients frequently ask the obstetrician about possible embryotoxic or fetotoxic effects of drugs, nutrients, or other influences. The most frequently asked questions deal with (1) the teratogenicity of diagnostic x-ray procedures; (2) the teratogenicity of certain medications prescribed during pregnancy; and (3) the teratogenicity of some other factors such as coffee, alcohol, and vaginal spermicides.

Diagnostic radiation and pregnancy

Fewer than 5 of each 1000 pregnant women are exposed to radiation during pregnancy. This happens because of the increased awareness of both patients and physicians with respect to the potential fetal effects of radiation and because of the replacement of many obstetric radiologic procedures with ultrasound. However, occasion-

TABLE 2-6 ◼ Fetal dose° during some x-ray examinations

Type of examination	Dose (rads per exam)	
	Mean	Range
Flat plate of the abdomen	0.144	0.024-1.416
X-ray of the pelvis	0.158	0.008-1.587
Intravenous pyelogram	0.448	0.024-3.069
Barium enema	0.574	0.005-9218
Upper gastrointestinal series	0.091	0.001-1.228
Lumbar spine	0.068	0.002-2.901

From Hoffman D, Felton R, Cyr W: *Effects of ionizing radiation on the developing embryo and fetus: A review,* HHS publication FDA 81-8170. Rockville, Md, US Dept of Health and Human Sciences, Public Health Service, Food and Drug Administration, Bureau of Radiological Health, 1981.

°Assuming that fetal dose is similar to ovarian dose.

ally the obstetrician must counsel a patient who has had radiologic procedures during gestation and wants to know the fetal risks associated with those procedures.

The effects of x-ray on the fetus are highly variable and depend on multiple factors, the most important being gestational age at the time of exposure and amount of radiation received by the fetus. Gestational age is important because the chances of affecting the fetus are greater in early than in late pregnancy. Particularly important seems to be the period of organogenesis, 2 to 7 weeks postconception, or 4 to 9 weeks from the last menstrual period, because ionizing radiation may interfere with organ development and cause malformations. The amount of radiation received by the fetus is also an important variable that depends on the type of x-ray examination, the number of pictures taken, the type of equipment used, and the area of the body toward which the x-ray beam was directed. As shown in Table 2-6, the amount of radiation received by the fetus in the course of most routine diagnostic examinations rarely exceeds 5 rads and is often less than 2 rads. Obviously, the possibility of adverse effects on the fetus at these radiation doses is minimal.

In counseling patients who have received radiation during pregnancy, one must reassure them that the risk of malformation is not greater than the population risk unless the patient has re-

ceived a dose larger than 10 rads. Naturally, it is impossible to guarantee that the fetus will not have a congenital malformation.

Potential teratogenicity of medications used during pregnancy

In 1978 the Food and Drug Administration established five categories of medications with respect to potential effects on the fetus or to the outcome of the pregnancy:

1. Controlled studies show no risk
2. No evidence of risk in humans
3. Risk cannot be ruled out
4. Positive evidence of risk
5. Contraindicated during pregnancy

Few drugs have been classified in one of these categories. This happens because although associations between certain drugs and fetal malformations have been found, few definite cause-and-effect relationships have been demonstrated. Also, multiple confounding variables make it difficult to analyze the effects of medications during pregnancy, and ethical constraints preclude the design and performance of randomized or cohort studies of potential teratogenic agents.

Box 2-7 shows some proven teratogenic drugs. Box 2-8 shows some nonteratogenic drugs that frequently are the subject of patient's questions and concerns. Some of the compounds shown in both tables are discussed in more detail.

BOX 2-7

Proven Human Teratogens

Compound	Major effect
Thalidomide	Phocomelia
DES	Genital tract abnormalities
Warfarin	Nasal hypoplasia, bone stippling
Androgens	Masculinization of female fetus
Folic acid antagonists	Craniofacial defects, growth retardation
Anticonvulsants	Craniofacial defects, NTD, developmental delay
Retinoic acid	Craniofacial, cardiac, thymic defects
Alcohol	Craniofacial defects, developmental delay

BOX 2-8

Nonteratogenic Agents

Progesterone	Cephalosporins
Aspirin	Penicillin
Spermicides	Ampicillin
Tylenol	Erythromycin
Heparin	General and local anesthetics
Thiazides	Benzodiazepines
Diazepam	Barbiturates
Indomethacin	Propranolol
Codeine	Narcotics
Prednisone	Aspartame
Caffeine	Video terminals

Anticonvulsant agents. Anticonvulsant therapy is frequently required during pregnancy in patients affected by seizure disorders. Unfortunately, several of the most popular anticonvulsants (phenytoin, valproic acid, carbamazepine, and trimethadione) are associated with the development of craniofacial anomalies, growth retardation, and developmental delay. The most commonly used anticonvulsant, phenytoin, causes a twofold to fivefold increase in the frequency of congenital malformations. The most common malformations constitute the "fetal hydantoin syndrome" that affects approximately 10% of those pregnant patients who use the medication. It is characterized by growth retardation, mental retardation, upward slant of the eyebrows, hypoplasia of the fingers and toenails, hernias, and a depressed nasal bridge. Other anticonvulsants, valproic acid, carbamazepine, and trimethadione are strongly associated with neural tube defects, craniofacial and digit abnormalities, and delay in psychomotor development.

In view of the strong evidence indicating embryotoxicity of anticonvulsant drugs, the present recommendation is not to use anticonvulsants during pregnancy. If these medications are required, the first choice should be phenobarbital, which is not associated with fetal malformations. If phenytoin is necessary, it should be used in the smallest dose that provides adequate clinical response.

The obstetrician should be careful in the interpretation of the above guidelines. To indiscriminately discontinue anticonvulsants may represent a health hazard for many patients. Discontinuing the medications if the patient has not

had seizures for the prior 2 years and her electroencephalogram is normal usually presents no problems. Patients with difficult or inadequate seizure control before pregnancy will likely have increased seizure activity if their medications are discontinued. They should be informed about the potential fetal effects of the anticonvulsants and also about the possibility of increased seizure activity if they stop the medications. The patient should participate actively in the decision to continue or to withhold the medications.

It is possible that in the near future it will be possible to make a decision about discontinuation of hydantoin on a more scientific basis. In fact, recent studies indicate that the risk of hydantoin fetopathy depends on the fetal capacity to eliminate the oxidative metabolites of the anticonvulsant drug by means of the enzyme epoxide hydroxylase. This enzyme seems to be regulated by a single gene with two alleles. Fetuses who are homozygous for the recessive allele will have low epoxide hydroxylase activity and will be at risk if exposed to hydantoin. Epoxide hydroxylase can be measured in fetal cells obtained by amniocentesis.[62]

Ethanol. The fetal alcohol syndrome was described in 1973 in 11 children with similar dysmorphic features whose mothers drank heavily during pregnancy.[63] The abnormalities noted in these children include fetal growth retardation, microcephaly, mental retardation, decreased length of the palpebral fissures, epicanthal folds, and flattened maxilla. Follow-up studies, 10 years later, showed continuation of the growth deficiency and dysmorphic features.[64]

No cases of fetal alcohol syndrome have been reported in women who had occasional consumption of small amounts of alcohol during pregnancy. Although it is advisable to avoid alcoholic drinks during pregnancy, the obstetrician should reassure patients who feel guilty after occasional ingestion of a small amount of alcohol and tell them that the possibility of doing harm to the fetus is minimal.[65]

Corticosteroids. Although glucocorticoids are potent palatal teratogens in experimental animals, there is no evidence that they cause congenital malformations in humans. This fact should help to relieve the anxiety of some mothers in whom glucocorticoid treatment is being considered to improve fetal lung maturation. Also, when glucocorticoids are given to accelerate the production of pulmonary surfactant, they are administered late in gestation, several weeks after organ and limb development have taken place.

Diazepam. It has been theorized that diazepam ingestion during pregnancy increases the risk of cleft lip, with or without cleft palate, in the offspring. However, case control studies indicate that exposure to diazepam during the first trimester of pregnancy does not increase the fetal risk of oral defects.[66]

Aspirin. Aspirin is one of the medications most commonly used during pregnancy. Women taking high doses of aspirin during pregnancy have prolonged pregnancies, longer duration of labor, and more bleeding during parturition than control patients.[67] Occasional consumption of aspirin has no harmful fetal or maternal effects. The use of low-dose aspirin (80 mg daily) during pregnancy is probably useful in the prevention of preeclampsia. There is no evidence that aspirin causes fetal malformations, specifically cardiac anomalies.[68] The theoretical concern about aspirin causing closure of the ductus has not been confirmed.

Progesterone. Progesterone is commonly administered to pregnant women during the first trimester for the prevention of early pregnancy loss caused by insufficient progesterone production by the corpus luteum. The medication is administered by vaginal suppositories, orally (micronized progesterone), or by injection (17-alpha hydroxyprogesterone caproate). The scientific evidence accumulated during the last few years indicates that no developmental toxicity of progesterone exists. Specifically, there is no risk of cardiac anomalies or limb reduction defects.[69,70]

Metronidazole. Metronidazole (Flagyl) is used during pregnancy for the treatment of symptomatic *Trichomonas vaginalis* infections. There is no evidence that this drug has teratogenic effects on the human fetus.

Other alleged teratogenic factors

Vaginal spermicides. A prospective study[71] found an excess of limb reduction deformities and chromosome abnormalities among the infants of women who used vaginal spermicides in the 10 months before conception when compared with control patients. However, the accumulated evidence of the last few years has failed to substantiate such an association.[72]

Coffee. In 1980, the United States Food and Drug Administration, concerned about the possi-

bility of caffeine causing limb reduction defects, advised pregnant women to avoid caffeine-containing food and drugs. Two subsequent studies[73,74] have presented convincing evidence suggesting that coffee consumption has no effect on the outcome of the pregnancy.

Visual display terminals. The possibility that the electromagnetic fields produced by video display terminals may cause adverse pregnancy outcome has been a matter of discussion for the last decade. However, a recent controlled study has failed to demonstrate that association.[75]

Aspartame. Aspartame is an artificial sweetener widely used in a variety of soft drinks and food products. It is a dipeptide made by combining aspartic acid and phenylalanine. A concern has been raised about the potential effects of elevated maternal serum phenylalanine levels following the ingestion of food or soft drinks containing aspartame. The following facts demonstrate that there should be no concern: (1) phenylalanine serum levels of less than 60 μmol/dl have not been associated with mental retardation; (2) the acceptable daily intake of aspartame is 50 mg/kg and this corresponds to approximately 62 cans of soda sweetened with aspartame; (3) the ingestion of twice the acceptable daily dose (100 mg/kg) by volunteer heterozygotes for phenylketonuria raised their phenylalanine blood level to 42 μmol/dl, well below the 60 μmol/dl associated with fetal toxicity.[76]

◪ IMPORTANT POINTS ◩

1. Most patients at risk for congenital disease in their offspring are identified by clues found in the histories and physical examinations, as a result of MSAFP screening, or because abnormalities are found in routine ultrasound examinations.

2. One reason to make MSAFP screening widely available is that only 25% of fetuses with chromosome abnormalities will be found if prenatal diagnosis is limited to women 35 years or older at the time of delivery.

3. An MSAFP of 2.2 MOM or higher requires amniocentesis in a patient with a history of a child with NTD, even if her level II ultrasound examination was negative.

4. Universal screening for cystic fibrosis is not recommended at this time. However, parents of an affected child should be offered prenatal diagnosis.

5. Patients with MSAFP between 2.5 and 3.5 MOM and no family history of NTD should have a level II ultrasound examination. If the ultrasound examination is normal, the risk for NTD should be reevaluated, and the option of not having amniocentesis should be offered.

6. Patients with abnormally high or low MSAFP and normal genetic studies are at higher risk for a poor pregnancy outcome and require careful prenatal follow-up.

7. In the next decade a tendency toward first-trimester genetic diagnosis probably will surface. Early amniocentesis and CVS will replace traditional amniocentesis at 16 weeks for most of the current indications for genetic diagnosis.

8. CVS is performed between 9 and 12 weeks. The chorionic villi can be obtained under ultrasound guidance after transabdominal, transcervical, and transvaginal approaches. The method used will depend on the placental location, the position of the uterus, and the presence of complicating factors.

9. Mosaicism occurs in approximately 1.5% of CVS specimens. The majority of mosaics are present in the direct preparation and are not confirmed in mesenchymal and fetal cell cultures.

10. The most common indication for PUBS is rapid karyotype in fetuses with abnormalities found in ultrasound examination.

11. Serious fetal accidents occur in about 1% of PUBS procedures.

12. The use of RFLP for prenatal genetic diagnosis ideally requires DNA from the parents, the fetus, and an affected sibling.

13. The risk of causing fetal malformations with the radiation involved in making a chest x-ray film or a flat plate of the abdomen is negligible.

14. Most studies have shown no developmental toxicity for progesterone given in the first trimester of pregnancy.

15. There is no evidence that caffeine, aspirin, corticosteroids, diazepam, aspartame, occasional ingestion of an alcoholic beverage, vaginal spermicides, and visual display terminals cause developmental toxicity.

REFERENCES

1. Simpson JL, Golbus MS, Martin AO, et al (eds): *Genetics in Obstetrics and Gynecology.* New York, Grune & Stratton Inc, 1982, p 58.
2. Matsunaga E, Tonamura A, Oishi H, et al: Reexamination of paternal age effect in Down's syndrome. *Hum Genet* 1978;40:259.
3. Martin RH, Rademaker AW: The effect of age on the frequency of sperm chromosomal abnormalities in normal men. *Am J Hum Genet* 1987;41:484-492.
4. Antonarakis SE, et al: Parental origin of the extra chromosome in trisomy 21 as indicated by analysis of DNA polymorphisms. *N Engl J Med* 1991;324:872-876.
5. Mikkelson M, Stene J: Genetic counseling in Down's syndrome. *Hum Hered* 1970;20:457.
6. *Congenital malformations surveillance report, July 1976-June 1977.* Atlanta, Center for Disease Control, Dec, 1977, p 25.
7. Carter CO, Lawrence KM, David PA: The genetics of the major central nervous system malformations, based on the South Wales socio-genetic information. *Dev Med Child Neurol* 1967;13(suppl):30.
8. Simpson JL, Golbus MS, Martin AO, et al (eds): *Genetics in Obstetrics and Gynecology.* New York, Grune & Stratton Inc, 1982, p 80.
9. Thornton JG, Lilford RJ, Newcombe RG : Tables for estimation of individual risks of fetal neural tube and ventral wall defects, incorporating prior probability, maternal serum alpha-fetoprotein levels, and ultrasonographic examination results. *Am J Obstet Gynecol* 1991;164:154-160.
10. Burton KB, Nelson LH, Pettenati MJ: False-positive acetylcholinesterase with early amniocentesis. *Obstet Gynecol* 1989;74:607-610.
11. Milunski A, Jick H, Jick SS, et al: Multivitamin/folic acid supplementation in early pregnancy reduces the prevalence of neural tube defects. *JAMA* 1989;262:2847-2852.
12. Mills JL, Rhoads GG, Simpson JL, et al: The absence of a relation between the periconceptional use of vitamins and neural-tube defects. *N Engl J Med* 1989;321:430-435.
12a. MRC Vitamin Study Research Group: Prevention of neural tube defects: Results of the Medical Research Council Vitamin Study. *Lancet* 1991;338:131-137.
13. Siedler DE, Filly RA: Relative growth of the higher fetal brain structures. *J Ultrasound Med* 1987;6:573.
14. Nora JJ, Nora AH: Update on counseling the family with a first-degree relative with a congenital heart defect. *Am J Med Gen* 1988;29:137.
15. Copel JA, Pilu G, Kleinman C: Congenital heart disease and extracardiac anomalies: Associations and indications for fetal echocardiography. *Am J Obstet Gynecol* 1986;154:1121-1132.
16. Szabo M, Munnich A, Teichmann F, et al: Discriminant analysis for assessing the value of amniotic fluid microvillar enzymes in the prenatal diagnosis of cystic fibrosis. *Prenatal Diagnosis* 1990;10:761-769.

17. Embury SH, Scharf SJ, Saiki RK, et al: Rapid prenatal diagnosis of sickle cell anemia by a new method of DNA analysis. *N Engl J Med* 1987;316:656-661.

18. Triggs-Raine BL, Feigenbaum AJ, Natowicz M, et al: Screening for carriers of Tay-Sachs disease among Ashkenazi Jews. *N Engl J Med* 1990;323:6-12.

19. Habib Z: Genetic counseling and genetics of cleft lip and cleft palate. *Obstet Gynecol Surv* 1978;33:441.

20. Macri JN, Hadow JE, Weiss RR: Screening for neural tube defects in the United States: A summary of the Scarborough Conference. *Am J Obstet Gynecol* 1979;133:119.

21. Merkatz IR, Nitowsky HM, Macri JN, et al: An association between low maternal serum alpha-fetoprotein and fetal chromosome abnormalities. *Am J Obstet Gynecol* 1984;148:886.

22. Fourth report of the United Kingdom Collaborative Study on alpha-fetoprotein in relation to neural tube defects: Estimating an individual's risk of having a fetus with open spina bifida and the value of repeated alpha-fetoprotein testing. *J Epidemiol* 1982;36:87-95.

23. Schell DL, Drugan A, Brindley BA, et al: Combined ultrasonography and amniocentesis for pregnant women with elevated serum alpha-fetoprotein. *J Reprod Med* 1990;35:543-546.

24. Richards DS, Seed JW, Katz VL, et al: Elevated maternal serum alpha-fetoprotein with normal ultrasound: Is amniocentesis always appropriate? A review of 26,069 screened patients. *Obstet Gynecol* 1988;71:203.

25. Nadel AS, Green JK, Holmes LB, et al: Absence of need for amniocentesis in patients with elevated levels of maternal serum alpha-fetoprotein and normal ultrasonographic examinations. *N Engl J Med* 1990;323:557-561.

26. Milunski A, Jick SS, Bruell CL, et al: Predictive values, relative risks, and overall benefits of high and low maternal serum alpha-fetoprotein screening in singleton pregnancies: New epidemiological data. *Am J Obstet Gynecol* 1989;162:291-297.

27. Nelson LH, Bensen J, Burton BK: Outcomes in patients with unusually high maternal serum alpha-fetoprotein levels. *Am J Obstet Gynecol* 1987;157:572-576.

28. Milunski A, Sapirstein VS: Prenatal diagnosis of open neural tube defects using amniotic fluid acetylcholinesterase assay. *Obstet Gynecol* 1982;59:1.

29. Loft AGR, Mortensen V, Hangaard J, et al: Ratio of immunochemically determined amniotic fluid acetylcholinesterase to butyrylcholinesterase in the differential diagnosis of fetal abnormalities. *Br J Obstet Gynaecol* 1991;98:52-56.

30. Wald NJ, Cuckle HS, Densen JW, et al: Maternal serum unconjugated estriol as an antenatal screening test for Down's syndrome. *Br J Obstet Gynaecol* 1987;95:3.

31. Macri JN, Kasturi RV, Krantz DA, et al: Maternal serum Down syndrome screening: Unconjugated estriol is not useful. *Am J Obstet Gynecol* 1990;162:672-673.

32. Petrocik E, Wassman RE, Kelly JA: Prenatal screening for Down syndrome with maternal serum human chorionic gonadotropin levels. *Am J Obstet Gynecol* 1989;161:1168-1173.

33. Wald NJ, Cuckle HS, Densen JW, et al: Maternal serum screening for Down's syndrome in early pregnancy. *Br Med J* 1988;297:883-887.

34. MacDonald ML, Wagner RM, Slotnick RN: Sensitivity and specificity of screening for Down syndrome with alpha-fetoprotein, hCG, unconjugated estriol and maternal age. *Obstet Gynecol* 1991;77:63-68.

35. Macri JN, Kasturi RV, Krantz DA, et al: Maternal serum Down syndrome screening: Free beta-protein is a more effective marker than human chorionic gonadotropin. *Am J Obstet Gynecol* 1990;163:1248-1253.

36. Simpson JL, Baum LD, Depp R, et al: Low maternal serum alpha-fetoprotein and perinatal outcome. *Am J Obstet Gynecol* 1987;156:852-862.

37. Milunski A, Wands J, Brambatti B, et al: First-trimester maternal serum alpha-fetoprotein screening for chromosome defects. *Am J Obstet Gynecol* 1988;159:1209-1213.

38. Lockwood C, Benacerraf B, Krinsky A, et al: A sonographic screening method for Down syndrome. *Am J Obstet Gynecol* 1987;157:803-808.

39. Benacerraf B, Neuberg D, Frigoletto F: Humeral shortening in second-trimester fetuses with Down syndrome. *Obstet Gynecol* 1991;77:223-227.

40. Benacerraf B, Gelman R, Frigoletto R: Sonographic identification of second-trimester fetuses with Down syndrome. *N Engl J Med* 1987;317:1371-1376.

41. Veanty P, Rodesch F, Romero R, et al: How to improve your amniocentesis technique. *Am J Obstet Gynecol* 1983;146:593-596.

42. National Institute of Child Health and Human Development National Amniocentesis Group: Midtrimester amniocentesis for prenatal diagnosis—safety and accuracy. *JAMA* 1976;236:1471.

43. Simpson JL, Dallaire L, Miller JR, et al: Prenatal diagnosis of genetic disease in Canada: Report of a collaborative study. *Can Med Assoc J* 1976;115:739.

44. Medical Research Working Party on Amniocentesis: An assessment of the hazards of amniocentesis. *Br J Obstet Gynaecol* 1978;85:1.

45. Golbus MS, Loughman WD, Epstein Ed et al: Prenatal genetic diagnosis in 3000 amniocentesis. *N Engl J Med* 1979;300:157.

46. Allen R: The significance of meconium in midtrimester genetic amniocentesis. *Am J Obstet Gynecol* 1985;152:413-417.

47. Zorn EM, Hanson FW, Greve C, et al: Analysis of the significance of discolored amniotic fluid detected at midtrimester amniocentesis. *Am J Obstet Gynecol* 1986;154:1234-1240.

48. Johnson A, Godmilow L: Genetic amniocentesis at 14 weeks or less. *Clin Obstet Gynecol* 1988;31:345.

49. Elejalde RB, Elejalde MM, Acuna JM, et al: Prospective study of amniocentesis performed between weeks 9 and 16 of gestation: Its feasibility, risks, complications and use in early prenatal diagnosis. *Am J Med Genet* 1990;35:188-196.

50. Hanson FW, Happ RL, Tennant FR, et al: Ultrasonography-guided early amniocentesis in singleton pregnancies. *Am J Obstet Gynecol* 1990;162:1376-1383.

51. Penso CA, et al: Early amniocentesis: Report of 407 cases with neonatal follow-up. *Obstet Gynecol* 1990;76:1032-1036.

52. Rhoads GG, Jackson LG, Schlesselman SE, et al: The safety and efficacy of chorionic villus sampling for early prenatal diagnosis of cytogenetic abnormalities. *N Engl J Med* 1989;320:609-617.

53. Canadian Collaborative CVS-Amniocentesis Clinical Trial Group: Multicentre randomized clinical trial of chorion villus sampling and amniocentesis. *Lancet* 1989;1:6.

53a. Firth HV, Boyd PA, Chamberlain P, et al: Severe limb abnormalities after chorion villus sampling at 56-66 days' gestation. *Lancet* 1991;337:762-763.

54. Saura R, Longy M, Horovitz J, et al: Risks of transabdominal chorionic villus sampling before the 12th week of amenorrhea. *Prenatal Diagnosis* 1990;10:461-467.

55. Sidransky E, Black SH, Soenksen DM, et al: Transvaginal chorionic villus sampling. *Prenatal Diagnosis* 1990;10:583-586.

56. Gosden C, Nicolaides KH, Rodeck CH: Fetal blood sampling investigation of chromosome mosaicism in amniotic fluid cell culture. *Lancet* 1988;1:613-617.

57. Johnson A, Wapner RJ, Davis GH, et al: Mosaicism in chorionic villus sampling: An association with poor perinatal outcome. *Obstet Gynecol* 1990;75:573-577.

58. Daffos F, Capella-Pavlovsky M, Forrestier F: A new procedure for fetal blood sampling in utero: Preliminary results of 53 cases. *Am J Obstet Gynecol* 1983;146:985.

59. Daffos F, Capella-Pavlovsky M, Forrestier F: Fetal blood sampling during pregnancy with use of a needle guided by ultrasound: A study of 606 consecutive cases. *Am J Obstet Gynecol* 1985;153:665.

60. Pielet BW, Socol ML, McGregor SN, et al: Cordocentesis: an appraisal of risks. *Am J Obstet Gynecol* 1988;159:1497-1500.

61. Saiki RK, Gelfand DH, Stoffel S, et al: Primer-directed enzymatic amplification of DNA with a thermostable DNA polymerase. *Science* 1988;239:487-491.

62. Buehler BA, Delimont D, Van Waes M, et al: Prenatal prediction of the fetal hydantoin syndrome. *N Engl J Med* 1990;322:1567-1572.

63. Jones KL, Smith DW, Ulleland CN, et al: Pattern of malformation in offspring of chronic alcoholic mothers. *Lancet* 1973;1:1267-1271.

64. Streissguth AP, Clarren SK, Jones KL: Natural history of the fetal alcohol syndrome: A 10-year follow-up of 11 patients. *Lancet* 1985;2:85-91.

65. Mills JL, Graubard BI: Is moderate drinking during pregnancy associated with an increased risk for malformations? *Pediatrics* 1987;80:309-314.

66. Rosenberg L, Mitchell AA, Parsells JL, et al: Lack of relation of oral clefts to diazepam use during pregnancy. *N Engl J Med* 1983;309:1282-1285.

67. Lewis RB, Schulman JD: Influence of acetylsalicylic acid, an inhibitor of prostaglandin synthesis, on the duration of human gestation and labor. *Lancet* 1973;2:1159.

68. Werler MM, Mitchell AA, Shapiro S: The relation of aspirin use during the first trimester of pregnancy to congenital cardiac defects. *N Engl J Med* 1989;321:1639-1642.

69. Katz Z, Lancet M, Skoenik J, et al: Teratogenicity of progestogens given during the first trimester of pregnancy. *Obstet Gynecol* 1985;65:775-780.

70. Wiseman RA, Dodds-Smith IC: Cardiovascular birth defects and antenatal exposure to female sex hormones: A reevaluation of some base data. *Teratology* 1984;30:359-370.

71. Jick H, Walker AM, Rothman KJ, et al: Vaginal spermicides and congenital disorders. *JAMA* 1981;245:1329.

72. Bracken MB: Spermicidal contraceptives and poor reproductive outcomes: The epidemiological evidence against an association. *Am J Obstet Gynecol* 1985;151:552-556.

73. Linn S, Schoenbaum SC, Monson RR, et al: No association between coffee consumption and adverse outcomes of pregnancy. *N Engl J Med* 1982;306:141.

74. Rosenberg L, Mitchel AA, Shapiro S, et al: Selected birth defects in relation to caffeine-containing beverages. *JAMA* 1982;247:1429.

75. Schnorr TM, Grajewski BA, Hornung RW, et al: Video display terminals and the risk of spontaneous abortions. *N Engl J Med* 1991;324:727-733.

76. Sturtevant FM: Use of aspartame in pregnancy. *Int J Fertil* 1985;30:85-87.

PART TWO

Pregnancy Complications

3

EARLY PREGNANCY LOSS

Human reproduction is a relatively inefficient process. Some investigators have demonstrated that only 57% of all conceptions advance beyond 20 weeks. Of those lost, 75% occur before implantation, and only 25% are clinically recognizable.[1] Recent investigations have found an overall pregnancy loss of 31% with 22% occurring before implantation.[2] Although the number of pregnancies wasted before implantation is very large, most of them are not recognized clinically, and in practice the problem of early pregnancy loss is limited to those pregnancies aborted after implantation.

The risk of spontaneous abortion for a woman with no history of reproductive wastage is about 15%. The study of Poland et al.[3] indicates that the likelihood of a repeated abortion after a first spontaneous abortion for a woman with no living children is 19%. If there is a history of two consecutive spontaneous abortions, the risk increases to 35%, and if the history is of three consecutive spontaneous abortions, the likelihood of a repeated abortion is 47%. These figures show a higher risk for recurrent abortion than those commonly quoted from the work of Warburton and Fraser,[4] which was limited to women who

had at least one liveborn child. When there is at least one liveborn child, the risk of subsequent abortion is 24% to 32% irrespective of the number of prior abortions. This information is summarized in Table 3-1.

◢ DEFINITION AND CLASSIFICATION

For the purpose of this discussion, a spontaneous abortion is defined as any recognized, involuntary pregnancy loss occurring before fetal viability, 24 weeks. Approximately 80% of all spontaneous abortions occur before 12 weeks and are called early abortions. The rest occur between the thirteenth and the twenty-fourth week and are called late abortions. The classification of abortions as early and late has some clinical value because the majority of early abortions correspond to anembryonic pregnancies or blighted ova, whereas most of the abortions with a fetus present occur in the second trimester. However, many blighted ova do not give symptoms and are not discovered until after 12 weeks, and some abortions with a fetus present occur before 12 weeks.

Fortunately, the introduction of ultrasound has made it possible to differentiate embryonic

TABLE 3-1 ◪ Risk of spontaneous abortion

Number of consecutive abortions	Risk of subsequent abortion (%)
No previous liveborn child	
0	12.3
1	19.0
2	35.0
3	47.0
At least one liveborn child	
0	12.3
1	23.7
2	26.2
3	32.2

from anembryonic pregnancies before abortion occurs. This has simplified the counseling of patients with threatened abortions and of patients who had one or more spontaneous abortions. According to the clinical and echographic findings, it is possible to separate early pregnancy losses into two groups:

1. *Blighted ova*—those early pregnancy losses in which fetal development is not observed with ultrasound and fetal tissue is absent on the histologic examination of the products of conception
2. *Early fetal demise*—those early pregnancy losses in which fetal development is clearly observed by ultrasound and fetal tissue is found on the histologic examination

The differentiation between these two types of abortions is of fundamental importance. The lack of development of fetal structures defines a subset of abortions of genetic origin. In contrast, the early interruption of fetal life is a complex phenomenon with multiple etiologies. Therefore, couples with blighted ova do not require extensive workup, whereas patients who have aborted cytogenetically normal fetuses need an extensive search for nongenetic factors responsible for the pregnancy loss.

There is a strong tendency for consecutive abortions to be of the same type. If a previous spontaneous abortion was a blighted ovum, a subsequent abortion has a 70% chance of also being anembryonic. If an apparently normal fetus was seen in the products of conception, the probability that a following abortion will be similar is 85%.[5]

◪ ETIOLOGY

Usually, an explanation can be found for the large majority of spontaneous abortions. The most frequent causes are:

1. Genetic abnormalities, 50% to 60% of cases
2. Endocrine abnormalities, 10% to 15%
3. Chorioamniotic separations, 5% to 10%
4. Incompetent cervix, 8% to 15%
5. Infections, 3% to 5%
6. Abnormal placentation, 5% to 15%
7. Immunologic abnormalities, 3% to 5%
8. Uterine anatomic abnormalities, 1% to 3%
9. Unknown reasons, less than 5%

Genetic causes

Genetic anomalies are the most frequent and important causes of early pregnancy losses. The majority of genetically originated abortions occur before 8 weeks and are blighted ova. The abnormal zygote found in a blighted ovum results from an error in maternal or paternal meiosis I or II, from superfecundation of an egg by two spermatozoids, or from a chromosome division in the absence of cytoplasmic division.

To determine the parental origin of an abnormal zygote is expensive and complex. Furthermore, even if the origin of the abnormal gamete is known, the information may not be useful because it probably happened by chance.

It is not unusual to find a normal 46,XY or 46,XX karyotype in the chorionic villi analysis of blighted ova. In these cases the lack of fetal development may be the result of a lethal molecular mutation that cannot be identified with the present methods of analysis.

The chromosomal abnormalities most frequently found in abortions are[6]:

autosomal trisomy This nondisjunctional defect is found in approximately 60% of blighted ova with abnormal karyotypes. The trisomy predominantly affects chromosomes 16, 21, and 22, although it may affect any other of the autosomes. Trisomy 16 is most frequently found in abortus material, and in these cases the sac is completely empty.

triploidy This defect, which consists of a mean chromosomal count of 69, occurs in 15% to 20% of all abortions with abnormal chromosomes. In many cases the sac is empty, but if a fetus is present, it has obvious abnormalities (omphalocele, syndactyly, cleft lip and palate, etc.). In about 50% of the cases, hydropic degeneration of the placenta is present. In humans, the most common reason for triploidy is double fertilization of a single ovum. In triploidy without molar degeneration, the extra chromosomal set is probably maternal.

monosomy X   About 25% of all abortions with chromosomal abnormalities have a karyotype 45,X. About one of every 15 fetuses with 45,X karyotype will not be aborted and will be identified at birth as an individual with Turner's syndrome. Some of the abortion specimens with 45,X karyotypes are sacs containing a small umbilical cord that inserts into an amorphous mass of embryonic tissue. Monosomy X may be the result of the loss of an X chromosome at the time of fertilization, or it may be the result of nondisjunction during either male or female meiosis.

tetraploidy   This anomaly, consisting of a mean chromosomal count of 92, is found in 3% to 6% of blighted ova with abnormal chromosomes. In these cases abortions usually occur very early in pregnancy, and the embryo cannot be recognized in the specimen. This condition probably results from a failure of cytoplasmic division after a chromosome division in the germinal cells.

structural rearrangement of the chromosomes
This subset consists of unbalanced translocations and inversions and accounts for 3% to 5% of abortions with abnormal chromosomes. Couples that have abortions with structural rearrangements of the chromosomes should have karyotype analysis because 5% will be carriers of the rearranged chromosome. Couples having abortions with numerical abnormalities of the chromosomes usually have normal karyotypes.

Chromosomal abnormalities are found in approximately 80% of blighted ova and 5% to 10% of the abortions in which a fetus is present. In the later case autosomal trisomies predominate, but fetuses with triploidy and monosomy X are occasionally recognized.

There are cases of early fetal death in which extensive investigations, including karyotype, give negative results. In such cases it is unavoidable to suspect the existence of a lethal mutation undetectable with the present methods of analysis. In fact, it is possible that lethal mutations similar to those found in experimental models may be present in humans. Animal experiments using insertional mutagenesis (insertion and integration within the genome of a DNA fragment, which causes disruption of the function of one or several genes) have provided evidence indicating that inactivation of the genes containing the information for collagen synthesis causes an arrest in development and embryonic death.[7]

Fetal death may also be the result of mutations affecting genes that control the expression of other genes at the transcriptional level (homeobox genes) or mutations that cause excessive concentration of products and embryonic cell toxicity.

Endocrine abnormalities

A series of complex hormone interactions provide adequate support for the development of early pregnancy. Failure in any of the hormones involved in this process theoretically may lead to spontaneous abortion.

Progesterone deficiency. Progesterone deficiency has been an obvious candidate as an etiologic factor of early pregnancy loss because of its well-known effect in maintaining uterine quiescence. Unfortunately, progesterone deficiency is overdiagnosed, and progesterone supplementation is overused.

Most of the evidence incriminating progesterone deficiency in early pregnancy loss comes from studies demonstrating that luteal phase deficiency occurs more frequently in patients with recurrent abortions than in control patients.[8-10] A rigorous diagnosis of corpus luteum defect requires histologic confirmation of endometrium out of phase by 2 or more days during the secretory period of the menstrual cycle. Because endometrial biopsies are not obtained during pregnancy, the only possible method of documenting a corpus luteum deficiency during gestation is by measuring the serum progesterone concentration.[11] However, progesterone production by the corpus luteum is pulsatile and is characterized by marked fluctuations in serum levels.[12] As a result, many studies have shown a poor correlation between serum progesterone levels and endometrial biopsy findings.

Another problem with the use of serum progesterone levels for the diagnosis of progesterone deficiency in patients with first trimester bleeding or with a history of multiple pregnancy losses is that patients with blighted ova have a low serum progesterone concentration.[13] In these patients, low serum progesterone concentration is the result rather than the cause of the abortion. Because blighted ova are so frequent, patients with low progesterone concentrations in early pregnancy must be examined for blighted ova rather than treated for corpus luteum deficiency.

It has been suggested that measurement of

17-hydroxy progesterone, a substance almost exclusively produced by the corpus luteum, could be a better marker than progesterone. In a recent study, measurements of serum 17-hydroxy progesterone in patients conceiving after the use of ovulation-inducing agents could discriminate patients that miscarried from those that did not.[14] Unfortunately, measurement of this substance did not differentiate aborters from nonaborters in patients that did not receive ovulation induction.

There are few maternal side effects of progesterone administration, and several studies have demonstrated the lack of teratogenic effects of this hormone. For these reasons treatment with progesterone is frequently dispensed on the assumption that a deficiency is present, without attempting to demonstrate a low serum progesterone. The most common uses for progesterone supplementation are in patients with symptoms of threatened abortion, in patients conceiving after ovulation induction, in those with a serum level less than 15 ng/ml, or in those with a history of early pregnancy losses.

Thyroid deficiency. Measurements of thyroid-stimulating hormone (TSH) and free thyroxine are almost routine in patients with a history of repeated pregnancy losses. However, it is rare that a deficiency or an excess of thyroid hormone is the etiology of early pregnancy loss. Patients with thyroid dysfunction are affected instead by preterm labor, usually occurring after 24 weeks.

Diabetes. Controversy surrounds the question of whether women with insulin-dependent diabetes have a higher than normal risk of spontaneous abortion. Some investigators believe that diabetes is not a cause of early pregnancy loss.[15,16] However, a large multicenter, controlled study found that diabetics with both an elevated blood glucose and hemoglobin A_{1C} in the first trimester have a significantly increased risk of spontaneous abortion, whereas those with good metabolic control had a risk similar to that of control subjects.[17] The frequency of fetal congenital abnormalities is larger in diabetics, but most of these abnormalities do not cause early fetal losses.

Increased androgen. A rare endocrine etiology for early pregnancy losses is maternal hyperandrogenicity.[18] Apparently the excessive androgen produces corpus luteum dysfunction.

Patients are usually hirsute and have elevated serum levels of testosterone and dehydroepiandrosterone sulfate (DHEAS). The pregnancy loss is usually an early fetal demise occurring at about 14 weeks.

Polycystic ovary syndrome. Spontaneous abortions occur more frequently in patients with polycystic ovary syndrome (PCO) than in normal control subjects.[19] It seems that the elevated serum luteinizing hormone concentration that characterizes this syndrome has a deleterious effect on the corpus luteum.[20] Pituitary suppression with gonadotropin-releasing agonists followed by hCG administration has been found to be useful in the prevention of this type of miscarriage.[21]

Infection

Infection is a relatively uncommon cause of early pregnancy loss. Infections causing abortion are usually ascending and facilitated by some degree of cervical incompetence. In a minority of patients hematogenous infections with varicella, parvovirus, rubella, toxoplasmosis, herpes simplex, treponema, listeria, chlamydia, and mycoplasma are an unexpected finding on fetal autopsy or in histologic or bacteriologic examination.

Patients with ascending infection usually develop temperature elevation and uterine cramps after 14 weeks. This is followed rather quickly by the onset of uterine contractions or by rupture of the membranes. At the time of arrival at the hospital, the cervix is usually dilated 3 cm or more, and the products of conception are protruding through the cervix. Histologic examination of the placenta shows severe chorioamnionitis. The bacteria isolated from the placenta are a mixture of anaerobic and aerobic organisms with predominance of group B streptococci and *Escherichia coli*. Ascending infections frequently recur in subsequent pregnancies, suggesting the presence of a defect in the cervix facilitating uterine invasion by the vaginal flora.

Mycoplasma hominis and *Ureaplasma urealyticum* are occasionally found in cultures of aborted products of conception.[22] This is in contrast with the high frequency of positive cervical and endometrial ureaplasma cultures found in patients with a history of repeated spontaneous abortions or infertility.[23] Also, there are uncontrolled studies suggesting that diagnosis and treatment of mycoplasma infection before pregnancy prevents recurrent abortion.[24] Despite these observations, the evidence linking infection with mycoplasmas to early pregnancy loss is unconvincing. Even more tenuous is the possibility of a causal relationship between early pregnancy loss and chlamydia infection.

Anatomic abnormalities of the uterus

Anatomic abnormalities of the uterus cause approximately 10% to 15% of all abortions with adequate fetal development. Uterine anatomic abnormalities may be acquired, such as in patients with uterine synechiae, or may be the result of a developmental error, such as in patients with müllerian fusion defects or DES-induced lesions. Incompetent cervix is a uterine anatomic abnormality that may be congenital, but in the majority of cases it results from a traumatic injury to the cervix.

Uterine synechiae. The association between uterine synechiae and early pregnancy losses has been known since the original work of Asherman in 1947. Uterine synechiae are bandlike structures between the walls of the uterus causing minimal to almost complete obliteration of the uterine cavity. Histologically, these bands are made of fibrous tissue, myometrium, and endometrium. The endometrium around these adhesions is usually atrophic with distorted gland openings.

In the majority of cases, synechiae are the result of intrauterine infection combined with surgical trauma after the retention of products of conception following abortion or delivery. Schenker and Margalioth[25] found that in 66% and 22% of 1856 patients, intrauterine adhesions were associated with postabortal and postpartum curettage, respectively. In the same study, it was noticed that 14% of patients with synechiae had a history of multiple pregnancy losses.

The diagnosis of uterine synechiae is usually made by hysterosalpingogram or by direct observation with the hysteroscope. Treatment requires surgical division of the fibrous bands, placement of an intrauterine device to avoid contact between the ends of the adhesions, and treatment with estrogen to stimulate endometrial growth.

There are no randomized, controlled studies comparing the efficacy of hysteroscopic-guided division with blind ablation of the uterine bands

in preventing abortion. However, most studies using historic controls suggest that there is a substantial reduction in the number of spontaneous abortions after treatment.

Müllerian abnormalities. Septate uterus and bicornuate uterus are examples of müllerian fusion abnormalities associated with early pregnancy losses. Some other abnormalities such as double uterus and unicornuate uterus are manifested more commonly by preterm labor, characteristically occurring later with each successive pregnancy. It has been suggested that septate and bicornuate uteri are associated with early pregnancy losses because of inadequate blood supply to the conceptus when the pregnancy is implanted in the relatively avascular septum. Another mechanism of pregnancy loss in these patients is incompetent cervix, an abnormality that is frequently present in patients with abnormal uterine anatomy. That is the reason it has been suggested that a prophylactic cervical cerclage should be used in all pregnant patients with congenital uterine anomalies.[26]

DES exposure in utero. Approximately 70% of women exposed in utero to diethylstilbestrol (DES) have a small, T-shaped uterus and an abnormally high frequency of poor pregnancy outcomes.[27] Early abortion is not a frequent complication in these patients. Rather, they tend to lose their pregnancies between 20 to 28 weeks because of incompetent cervix. Patients exposed in utero to DES should have a cervical cerclage between 12 and 16 weeks to improve the chance of a normal pregnancy outcome.

Incompetent cervix. Incompetent cervix is a well-recognized cause of pregnancy loss in the late second trimester. The main clinical feature of this condition is painless cervical dilation. Typically, these patients seek care because of a sensation of vaginal pressure. Speculum examination reveals bulging membranes, as well as various degrees of cervical dilation. Most patients also notice the onset or an increase in mucous vaginal discharge in the preceeding days. Frequently the mucous discharge has a slight blood stain.

Incompetent cervix is usually the result of cervical trauma, most commonly overzealous mechanical dilation during a pregnancy termination or a diagnostic curettage. However, deep cervical lacerations during vaginal delivery and extensive conization for the treatment of cervical dysplasia are also relatively common etiologic factors. As mentioned, cervical incompetence may also be congenital, occurring in patients with müllerian fusion abnormalities and in patients exposed to DES in utero.

The diagnosis of incompetent cervix is easy when the physician has the opportunity to see the patient with bulging membranes and painless cervical dilation. However, this is not possible in the majority of patients. When the diagnosis is unclear in nonpregnant patients, the increased compliance of the cervix can be demonstrated by passing a No. 8 Hegar or a No. 15 Pratt dilator or a Foley catheter filled with 1 ml of water through the internal cervical os. During pregnancy, the diagnosis should be suspected in patients with a history of second trimester pregnancy losses and an increased amount of vaginal discharge. In these patients ultrasound examination may also demonstrate funneling of the membranes into the endocervical canal or a diameter of the internal os greater than 23 mm.[28]

When the diagnosis of incompetent cervix is known, the best approach is to place a cervical cerclage at between 12 and 16 weeks. The surgical techniques most commonly used are the Shirodkar and the McDonald procedures. In the first, the vaginal mucosa is opened in the anterior and the posterior aspects of the cervix and a 5-mm Mersilene band is tied as close as possible to the internal cervical os and buried under the vaginal mucosa. In the McDonald method, a 4-mm Mersilene or 5-mm silk suture is tied in a purse-string fashion around the cervix. The Shirodkar operation is technically more involved and takes longer to perform, but has a lower failure rate.

Surgical correction of an incompetent cervix with dilation and herniated membranes is more difficult than the prophylactic procedure and has a higher failure rate. In some of these cases amniocentesis is necessary to rule out infection and to remove amniotic fluid, facilitating the reduction of the amniotic sac. In many of these patients the cervix is significantly effaced making dissection of the vaginal mucosa for a Shirodkar cerclage difficult; therefore most obstetricians use the McDonald method in such cases. Novy et al.[29] have described some modifications to the classical Shirodkar cerclage that facilitate its application in patients with dilated cervices.

The most common complications after emergency cerclage are acute chorioamnionitis and rupture of the membranes. Once the membranes have been exposed to the vaginal flora, the patient should be considered infected and aggressive antibiotic treatment started. If signs of overt chorioamnionitis develop, the suture should be removed and the patient delivered. Rupture of the membranes may occur in as many as 45% of patients who have emergency cerclage, usually occurring 1 to 3 days after surgery. The management of patients with preterm rupture of membranes (PROM) after cerclage is complex and controversial. Some investigators believe that the cerclage should be removed, but others have reported significant prolongation of pregnancy allowing the suture to remain.

Patients that fail a Shirodkar operation or patients with little cervix left after extensive conization are candidates for transabdominal cerclage. In this procedure the internal os of the cervix is reached by laparotomy, and a Mersilene band is tied at this level.

Subchorionic hematomas and chorioamniotic separations

A relatively frequent cause of first-trimester vaginal bleeding, but an uncommon cause of pregnancy loss, is the separation of the fetal membranes. The bleeding may occur between the amnion and the chorion (chorioamniotic separation) or between the chorioamnion and the decidua (subchorionic hematoma). Patients with these abnormalities have first-trimester vaginal bleeding that may vary in severity. Usually they have minimal or no cramping. Ultrasound shows a normal, active fetus and an area of membrane separation usually opposite to the placental implantation site. Often a thin membrane can be seen floating between the uterus and the fetus in cases of chorioamniotic separation. In subchorionic hematomas the membrane is thick and has limited mobility.

In the majority of these patients, bleeding stops spontaneously a few days after its onset. However, some patients continue bleeding in small amounts for several weeks, and a few abort or become infected. Some of these patients show discoloration of the amniotic fluid with blood pigments when they have genetic amniocentesis in the second trimester.

The cause of such bleeding and membrane separation is unknown. The course of the problem is not related to the severity of the initial bleeding episode. However, estimation of the hematoma size by ultrasound seems to be of prognostic value.[30] Most patients with a severe initial episode do well, and the pregnancy continues without problems after a few days of spotting, but persistent bleeding has a guarded prognosis.

Defective placentation

During normal placentation the spiral arteries undergo adaptive changes characterized by loss of the normal musculoelastic arterial wall and replacement by fibrinoid material containing throphoblastic cells. These changes transform the narrow, thick-walled arteries into wide-open, tortuous vascular channels that provide the necessary blood flow for the developing conceptus. The lack of these changes has been named abnormal placentation and is a feature shared by patients with preeclampsia, severe growth retardation, and preterm labor and also by some patients with early fetal deaths.[31] Abnormal placentation occurs with similar frequency in patients with chromosomally normal and abnormal fetuses, but is not a finding in patients with blighted ova. Patients with recurrent abortions caused by abnormal placentation that are able to prolong a pregnancy beyond the second trimester remain at high risk for preeclampsia, preterm labor, and fetal growth retardation.

Immunologic causes of abortion

The possibility of an immunologic rejection of the conceptus is frequently used as an explanation for recurrent spontaneous abortions. However, few patients fullfill rigorous criteria, suggesting that their pregnancies are lost as a result of an immunologic process.

The best-defined patients with immunologic pregnancy losses are those with antiphospholipid antibody syndrome. A less well–defined group is that with repeated pregnancy losses and weakly positive antinuclear antibodies titers. The less clearly defined group corresponds to those patients suspected of having pregnancy losses caused by alloantibodies. These three groups are analyzed separately as follows.

Antiphospholipid antibody syndrome. In 1957 Laurell and Nilsson described a patient with five prior intrauterine deaths who had a biologically false-positive syphilis test and an anticoagulant antibody. Later it was found that the circulating anticoagulant and the molecule responsible for the false-positive serology were antiphospholipid antibodies. In the last 25 years numerous investigators have further described the association between antibodies that bind phospholipid molecules and repetitive pregnancy losses. Antiphospholipid antibodies account for 3% to 5% of patients with repetitive pregnancy losses. The frequency of fetal death and recurrent abortion in untreated patients with antiphospholipid antibodies is greater than 90%.

There are several antiphospholipid antibodies. The most relevant to the obstetrician are the lupus anticoagulant (LAC), the anticardiolipin antibody (ACA), and the antibody that causes false-positive syphilis test (BFP-ST). The obstetric significance of antibodies against phosphatidylserine, phosphatidylethanolamine, and phosphatidylinositol is not clear yet.

The name lupus anticoagulant was derived from the fact that this antibody was found first in patients with lupus and acted as an anticoagulant by prolonging the partial thromboplastin time (PTT). This name was a poor choice because soon it was found that LAC was present in many patients who did not have lupus and that in the majority of patients the antibody was responsible for episodes of thrombosis rather than anticoagulation. In the laboratory, LAC is not measured directly. It is assessed by its effects on the PTT and the kaolin clotting time.[32] Typically, patients with LAC have a prolonged PTT. When this occurs, most laboratories repeat the test after mixing the patient plasma with an equal volume of normal plasma. If the normal plasma does not correct the PTT within 4 seconds of the control value, an antiphospholipid antibody is likely present. Unfortunately, a normal PTT does not exclude the possibility of LAC, and if the clinical suspicion is strong and the PTT is normal, a Kaolin clotting time or a dilute Russell viper venom time[33] should be performed.

It has been found that some patients with LAC and recurrent abortions have elevated values of serum IgM (normal value 40 to 260 mg/dl). For this reason, it has been suggested that a determination of IgM concentration should be a part of the evaluation of patients with recurrent abortions.[34]

The anticardiolipin antibody is the antiphospholipid antibody most commonly found in patients with repetitive early pregnancy losses. ACA is found in 90% of patients with LAC, but the majority of patients with positive ACA do not have LAC. ACA is measured in the laboratory by means of an enzyme-linked immunosorbent assay (ELISA) test, and IgG, IgM, and IgA antibodies can be demonstrated. The clinical significance of the IgM and IgA antibodies is unknown. A serum IgG antibody titer greater than 20 U is significant.

The less common antiphospholipid antibody is BFP-ST. BFP-ST and ACA measure antibody against cardiolipin, but they are not the same. Some patients with BFP-ST do not have ACA, and most patients with positive ACA have nonreactive syphilis serology.

The presence of any or several of the three antiphospholipid antibodies is associated with recurrent early pregnancy losses, episodes of venous and arterial thrombosis, severe preeclampsia of early onset, severe intrauterine growth retardation (IUGR), and chorea gravidarum. Other associations are a history of ischemic stroke, transient ischemic episodes, migraine headaches, and early onset preeclampsia. Patients with antiphospholipid antibodies may develop serious postpartum complications. Pulmonary infiltrates, fever, and cardiac symptoms may appear after delivery and have life-threatening severity.[35] Rarely, pulmonary complications occur before delivery.

Typically, these patients give a history of a live fetus documented by ultrasound or by Doppler before demise or abortion occurs. The majority of the pregnancy losses occur between 14 and 18 weeks. As many as 28% of these patients have a history of thrombosis.[36]

Fetal death in these patients is caused by extensive thrombosis of the placental vessels, and the placenta is usually smaller than expected for the gestational age. On microscopic examination, the spiral arteries show absence of adaptive changes and contain thrombi, many of which are recanalized indicating a chronic process. The placenta also shows infarcts, frequently extensive, and accelerated maturity of the chorionic villi.[37] There are several hypotheses about the mechanism of systemic and placental thrombosis in these patients. A popular theory is that the antiphospholipid antibody interacts with the vascular endothelium inhibiting prostacyclin synthesis.[38] However, investigations have shown that antiphospholipid antibodies do not inhibit prostacyclin synthesis even in damaged endothelial cells.

Patients with asymptomatic antinuclear antibodies. Investigators have reported significantly greater prevalence of low-titer antinuclear antibodies (ANA) in patients with unexplained fetal losses before viability than in normal control subjects.[39] This high frequency of positive ANA titers also occurs in patients with fetal losses caused by nonimmunologic factors such as uterine anatomic malformations and luteal phase defect.[40,41] These findings are not universally accepted, and there are studies showing no difference in the prevalence of ANA and anti-DNA antibodies in habitual aborters versus normal control subjects.[42]

In these patients the ANA titer is between 1:20 and 1:160, and the fluorescent pattern is usually speckled or homogenous. Other than for the abnormal serology and the history of prior pregnancy losses, these patients have no signs or symptoms and do not fullfill established criteria for the diagnosis of lupus. However, on close interrogation, sometimes it is possible to elicit a history of nasal or oral ulcerations, skin sensitivity, or unexplained recurrent musculoskeletal pain.

A positive ANA titer in a patient with prior early pregnancy losses indicates the need for further investigation of autoimmune factors, as well as a search for LAC, ACA, and BFP-ST, and anti-DNA antibodies should be initiated. If any of these tests is positive, autoimmunity is most probably responsible for the pregnancy losses, and adequate treatment may be instituted. A more difficult management problem is the patient who has negative results of these tests, because the treatment is controversial.

Alloimmune etiology of early pregnancy losses. The possibility that some abortions result from maternal immunologic rejection of the fetal allograft is intellectually appealing. Unfortunately, it is difficult to define this mechanism of abortion in terms of its clinical and laboratory characteristics, and as a consequence, many patients are submitted to potentially dangerous, unproven, and expensive forms of therapy to modify their immune response.

One of the immunologic theories of abortion is that there are allotypic antigens in the fetal membranes. Animals injected with human trophoblasts produce identifiable antibodies to those allotypic antigens that are cytotoxic to peripheral blood leukocytes. For this reason the trophoblast antigens have been called trophoblast/lymphocyte cross-reactive (TLX) antigens. If the embryo inherits from the father TLX antigens that do not exist in the mother, the mother will recognize those antigens and will mount a protective response, and the pregnancy will not be aborted. If the TLX antigens of the father and the mother are similar, the embryo will inherit paternal TLX antigens that will not stimulate the maternal immune system to produce the protective response, and the pregnancy will be aborted. This theory further proposes that the similarity in TLX antigens between the parents can be demonstrated in some patients because they share several human leukocyte antigens (HLA). However, HLA sharing is not a condition for TLX sharing. This theory is highly controversial, and there is evidence indicating that HLA sharing is no more common in patients with increased pregnancy losses than in normal control subjects.[43] Also, there is not a clear definition of the nature of the embryonic protective factors that are produced during normal pregnancy and allegedly absent in couples sharing HLA antigens.

Another component of the same theory is that the mother produces antipaternal blocking antibodies that have complement-dependent or antibody-dependent lymphocytotoxicity. These antibodies would have a protective effect and would avoid pregnancy rejection.[44,45] Blocking antibodies can be detected by mixing lymphocytes of the mother and the father (MLC assay). Under normal circumstances the lymphocytes will recognize each other as foreign, and this will lead to cell proliferation and increase uptake of radioactive DNA precursors by the nuclei of the dividing cells. This reaction will be absent or minimal in primary aborters that have never carried a pregnancy to term. Secondary aborters, those patients that have had one or more children before they began to have spontaneous abortions, have a high concentration of antipaternal blocking antibodies. These findings have been interpreted to indicate that the primary aborter does not mount a protective immunologic reaction to the pregnancy, whereas the secondary aborter mounts an exaggerated response that is cytotoxic to the trophoblast. There are multiple problems with this theory. First, the MLC test is not reproducible, and the results have wide variation. Second, the molecular mechanism of action of these antipaternal blocking antibodies has not been elucidated. Finally, there is evidence that pregnancy and abortion may occur irrespective of the presence or absence of blocking antibodies.[46]

Despite the lack of scientific and clinical data supporting the alloimmune theory of spontaneous abortion, immunotherapy with paternal or donor pool leukocytes is being promoted as a solution for this emotionally charged disorder. Most of the immunotherapy studies are affected by imprecise definition of the patients being studied, absence of histologic and genetic data to define the nature of prior pregnancy losses, and lack of randomized double-blind trials. At this time, immunotherapy with leukocyte transfusion for repeated pregnancy losses is purely experimental and potentially dangerous. Rigorous research in this area is urgently needed to clarify some of the conflicting information.

Figure 3-1 summarizes the diverse etiology of early pregnancy losses.

◼ DIAGNOSIS AND MANAGEMENT

A fundamental aspect of the care of patients with early pregnancy losses is to be certain that a etiologic diagnosis is made. To sign out a patient's chart as "first-trimester abortion," "spontaneous abortion," or "missed abortion" is inadequate. Abortion is the common result of many different disorders, and ideally, the underlying cause of each pregnancy loss should be discovered. The importance of this is apparent when a patient experiences repeated early pregnancy loss.

The most common situations that the obstetrician encounters regarding early pregnancy losses are the patient with first-trimester vaginal bleeding, the patient with fetal death or second-trimester abortion, and the patient that has a history of multiple early pregnancy losses. Each of these situations is analyzed separately.

First-trimester vaginal bleeding

Clinical assessment. The most common symptom of a patient with impending abortion is vaginal bleeding. There are benign conditions that cause first-trimester vaginal bleeding, but the obstetrician should always assume the worst and carefully investigate all patients with this complaint. In most patients there is an interval of several days between the onset of symptoms and the actual miscarriage. However, in some the symptoms progress rapidly, and there is little time for diagnostic procedures. Because it is impossible to know in advance if there is sufficient time for testing, the obstetrician should examine patients with first-trimester bleeding within a reasonable time.

The most important information from the initial assessment is the gestational age of the preg-

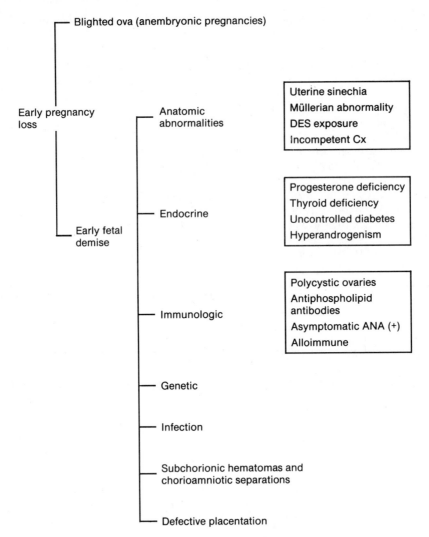

FIGURE 3-1 ◪ Etiology of early pregnancy losses.

nancy. If the pregnancy is less than 6 weeks as estimated by clinical dating and by assessment of the uterine size, it is probably better to measure the serum hCG to decide whether an ultrasound examination should be performed and how to interpret its results. Speculum examination will rule out cervical or vaginal lesions that are occasionally the reason for bleeding. Bimanual examination of the uterus will determine whether the uterine size is consistent with the clinical dating. A large uterus may indicate a hydatidiform mole, whereas a small uterus suggests a blighted ovum. The presence of a tender adnexal mass suggests an ectopic pregnancy. Also, the pelvic examination may show cervical changes if the process is advanced.

Hormonal assessment. Determination of serum hCG, progesterone, and estradiol levels are particularly useful in patients with vaginal bleeding at less than 6 weeks. One of the most important aspects of the management of these patients is determining whether the pregnancy is intrauterine. This diagnostic dilemma is easily solved if the ultrasound examination shows a gestational sac inside of the uterus. However, as shown in Table 3-2, it is possible to see a gesta-

TABLE 3-2 ◪ Time table of ultrasound and hormonal findings during normal embryologic development

Gestational age (GA) (weeks)	Postconcept GA (days)	Mean sac diameter (mm)	Yolk sac	Embryo	Approx. hCG level (μIU/ml)
4	14	5	(−)	(−)	1000
5	21	12	(+)	(−)	6000
6	28	18	(+)	(+)	17000
7	35	24	(+)	(12 to 18 mm)	47000
8	42	30	(+)	(head, trunk, limbs)	88000

Abnormal signs:
10-mm sac without yolk sac
18-mm sac without fetal pulse
24-mm sac without embryo

tional sac inside of the uterus using an endovaginal transducer only when the quantitative hCG determination is 1000 μIU/ml or more. To visualize an intrauterine gestational sac transabdominally, the serum hCG must be approximately 3000 μIU/ml.

Patients with first-trimester bleeding and serum hCG values below this critical value should have a repeated quantitative hCG evaluation 3 days after the initial one. If the second result indicates a doubling of the hCG concentration, then the pregnancy is likely to be intrauterine, and there is a high probability of a normal outcome. If the hCG value does not double and the initial progesterone and estradiol concentrations are low (progesterone less than 15 ng/ml, estradiol less than 200 ng/ml), then the pregnancy is abnormal, either a blighted ovum or an ectopic. The predictive accuracy of low values for hCG, progesterone, and estradiol is 90% to 95%, and most patients exhibiting this combination have spontaneous abortions or tubal pregnancies. The prediction of a normal outcome based on favorable hormone concentrations early in gestation is accurate in approximately 80% of the cases.

Ultrasound assessment. After the initial examination, the patient with first-trimester vaginal bleeding should have an ultrasound of the pelvis using both abdominal and endovaginal transducers. The abdominal ultrasound should visualize a sac if the gestational age is 5.5 weeks or more and the hCG concentration is greater than 3000 μIU/ml. Vaginal ultrasound will demonstrate a sac at 4.5 weeks if the hCG concentration is 1000 μIU/ml or greater.[47] The gestational sac,

fetal pole with heart motion, and the yolk sac should be seen at 6 weeks.[48] The fetal heart rate is less than 100 beats per minute at 6 weeks, increasing to 140 or more at 7 weeks. The yolk sac and the fetal pole appear almost simultaneously, at 6 to 7 weeks.[48] The presence of a yolk sac in the absence of fetal pole is almost pathognomonic of the diagnosis of blighted ovum. However, it is possible to see the yolk sac a few days before fetal heart motion is recognized. In these cases, however, the sac is small.

The predictive accuracy of normal pelvic ultrasound findings before 9 weeks of gestation is greater than 90%.[49] In some cases it is necessary to repeat the ultrasound examination to be certain of the diagnosis of an abnormal pregnancy. Repeated examinations are necessary more often when the patient complains of bleeding before 6 weeks. If no fetal heart motion is seen by 7 weeks or 2 weeks after the initial visualization of the gestational sac, the pregnancy is abnormal. As mentioned, simultaneous determinations of hCG, progesterone, and estradiol levels are useful in reaching a correct diagnosis soon.

Sonographic evidence of normal fetal cardiac activity in the patient with first-trimester vaginal bleeding indicates a low risk for abortion. In fact, Simpson et al.[50] demonstrated that the fetal loss rate after documenting the presence of fetal heart motion by ultrasound at 8 weeks is only 3.2%. This finding has been confirmed by other investigators.[51]

Management. Patients with first-trimester vaginal bleeding as well as reassuring ultrasound and hormonal findings should be told that the possibility of spontaneous abortion is small (2.5%

to 3.2%) and that most likely the outcome of the pregnancy will be normal. Bed rest is indicated as long as bleeding persists, and progesterone supplementation may be prescribed if the serum value is less than 15 ng/ml.

Patients with blighted ova should be advised to have chorionic villi biopsy for chromosome analysis. If this is impossible, a piece of placental tissue should be sent to the genetic laboratory at the time of evacuation of the uterus. The information provided by the chromosome analysis is important, and the patient should be discouraged from continuing the pregnancy and possibly miscarrying at home, thereby losing a sample for genetic analysis. If the karyotype of the blighted ovum reveals an autosomic trisomy, the patient will be at higher than normal risk for a subsequent trisomy offspring, and genetic amniocentesis should be recomended in subsequent pregnancies. Similarly, if the karyotype of the blighted ovum shows structural rearrangement of the chromosomes, the mother and the father should have chromosome analysis to rule out the possibility that one is a carrier of a translocation or inversion.

Early fetal demise

The differential diagnosis of the causes of fetal death or abortion when there is adequate fetal development is complex and requires meticulous analysis of clinical and laboratory information.

Clinical assessment. The most common reasons for early fetal demise or abortion with well-formed fetuses are chromosome abnormalities, antiphospholipid antibody syndrome, ascending infection, incompetent cervix, uterine anatomic abnormalities, subchorionic hematomas, and abnormal placentation. The history and physical examination will help focus the investigation on a few diagnostic possibilities. However, in many cases the history and the physical examination are unrevealing, and it is necessary to make extensive use of laboratory testing.

Laboratory assessment. Histologic and microbiologic examination of the placenta is a fundamental part of the evaluation of these patients. The placenta will show extensive acute inflammatory changes in patients with ascending infection and typical lesions in patients with chronic villitis caused by cytomegalic virus infection. Examination of the decidual tissue attached to the placenta will reveal physiologic changes in the spiral arteries. Thrombosis of fetal and maternal vessels will be apparent in patients with protein C deficiency or other alterations of the hemostatic system. The placenta may also show changes suggestive of the possibility of fetal chromosome abnormalities.

A careful fetal autopsy, preferably performed by someone interested in fetal pathology, may also provide valuable information about the etiology of the late abortion. Anatomic abnormalities suggestive of a genetic syndrome or histologic changes suggestive of an infectious process may be discovered. Fetal blood should be obtained by cardiac puncture and used for karyotyping the fetus as well as for bacteriologic cultures for *Mycoplasma, Ureaplasma, Chlamydia,* and *Listeria*. A radiologic examination of the fetus may reveal skeletal abnormalities resulting from genetic syndromes.

A mother having a second trimester fetal demise or abortion should have a Kleihauer-Betke test to rule out the possibility of extensive fetomaternal hemorrhage. The search for connective tissue disorders includes an ANA titer, anticardiolipin antibody, and lupus anticoagulant. If any of these tests is positive, further laboratory analysis will be necessary. A TORCH titer may reveal unexpected elevation of cytomegalovirus (CMV), herpes or toxoplasma IgG antibodies, suggesting an intrauterine infection with one of these organisms.

Unless there is an obvious cause for the problem, all mothers having a second-trimester abortion, particularly those with ascending infection and incompetent cervix, should have a hysterosalpingogram a few weeks after their miscarriage to rule out a uterine anomaly.

Management. Patients with early fetal demise should ideally have an induction with laminaria tents for cervical dilation followed by prostaglandin suppositories or high-dose oxytocin rather than uterine evacuation and curettage. The former procedure will provide an intact fetus and placenta that may be analyzed by the pathologist, the geneticist, and the microbiologist. With evacuation and curettage the products of conception are usually fragmented, and anatomic abnormalities cannot be recognized.

Patients with recurrent early pregnancy losses

Approximately 1 of every 100 to 200 women experience three consecutive first-trimester losses, thus fulfilling the classic definition of habitual abortion. However, today most women seek help after they have experienced two consecutive miscarriages. Unfortunately, the counseling and management of patients with repeated early pregnancy losses is frequently affected by inadequate documentation of the clinical events surrounding each abortion and by deficient investigation of the losses. Because of the lack of information, the physician cannot, in many cases, provide an adequate explanation to these patients, and they fall prey to individuals advocating unproven therapies.

Clinical assessment and diagnostic workup. The majority of patients with repetitive early pregnancy losses have had recurrent aneuploidic abortions or blighted ova. There are several indices that suggest recurrent blighted ova in patients with repetitive abortions:

1. The finding of molar degeneration in the histologic examination of the products of conception of a prior abortion. This is suggestive of triploidy.
2. Previous abortions showing empty sacs on ultrasound examination. This is suggestive of trisomy 16.
3. History of a malformed infant in the pedigree. This suggests balanced translocation in one of the parents.
4. Interval infertility, another finding suggestive of balanced translocation in the parents.
5. Repetitive abortions occurring before 12 weeks.

Patients with a history of repetitive aneuploidic abortions do not need extensive workups unless they are suspected of having a translocation. The nature of the genetic error leading to the production of blighted ova should be explained clearly to them. The probability of a successful pregnancy in the next attempt will be 62%[52] without any treatment, and they should be discouraged from undergoing experimental treatments unless they are conducted under a controlled, randomized protocol.

The analysis of patients having had an early fetal demise is more complex than that of patients with repetitive blighted ova. The factor to be ruled out first is anatomic abnormalities of the uterus and cervix. The anatomy of the uterus should be examined by means of a hysterosalpingogram. Cervical incompetence should not be a major problem in the differential diagnosis because of its distinctive clinical features.

The possibility of infection causing repetitive early pregnancy losses will be valid only if the patient is a carrier of the organism causing the infection and only if there is a break in the natural barriers that prevent infection from reaching the inside of the uterus. Therefore individuals with repeated ascending infections should have group B streptococci cultures from the rectum and the outer third of the vagina and should be critically evaluated for cervical incompetence. Also, cervical cultures for *Mycoplasma*, *Ureaplasma*, and *Chlamydia* may be obtained and the patient then treated if the tests are positive, although the significance of such findings in relation to repetitive early pregnancy losses is questionable.

A corpus luteum deficiency causing progesterone deficiency may result in pregnancy loss in the first trimester, especially between 8 and 12 weeks, when the production of progesterone switches from the corpus luteum to the developing placenta. Typically, these patients have uterine contractions for several days preceding the onset of bleeding and the abortion. The possibility that a given patient is affected by this condition may be investigated by endometrial biopsy or serum progesterone determinations during the secretory phase of the cycle.

As discussed earlier, polycystic ovarian syndrome and hyperandrogenism are other endocrine conditions associated with repeated early pregnancy losses. They can be easily diagnosed by determining the serum luteinizing hormone/follicle-stimulating hormone (LH/FSH) ratio and total testosterone concentration. Thyroid gland dysfunction is a cause of preterm labor rather than early pregnancy loss, but this is an endocrine abnormality that is easy to diagnose and to treat.

A fetal demise caused by abnormal placentation should be suspected in cases of growth-retarded but chromosomally normal fetuses. However, making the definite diagnosis of abnormal placentation causing repetitive early pregnancy losses is difficult. The best opportunity to do so is at the time of delivery when it is easy to obtain a biopsy of the placental implantation area with a Novak curette. The biopsy will show the lack of physiologic changes in the spiral arteries. In other cases there is some decidua attached to the maternal side of the placenta, and an interested pathologist can find the characteristic histologic features of the condition.

Patients with repetitive early fetal deaths should also be investigated for the possibility of autoimmune disorders. They should have determinations of ANA titer, lupus anticoagulant, venereal disease (VDRL), anticardiolipin, and SS-A antibodies. They should be discouraged from testing for other immunologic etiologies such as shared (HLA) or antipaternal antibodies because the results of these tests likely have no relation to the problem and are useless in establishing a prognosis.

Treatment. The treatment of patients with multiple early pregnancy losses depends on the etiology. Some patients with anatomic abnormalities of the uterus will benefit from hysteroscopic surgery. Patients with incompetent cervix will benefit from a cerclage. Patients with recurrent ascending infections will benefit from cerclage and antibiotic treatment. Patients with corpus luteum deficiency will need progesterone supplementation during pregnancy. Patients with polycystic ovarian syndrome may benefit from pituitary suppression with gonadotropin-releasing (GnR) analogues and induction of ovulation with hCG. Patients with hyperandrogenism of adrenal origin will benefit from treatment with prednisone, and those with recurrent abnormal placentation may benefit from low-dose aspirin and dipyridamole.

The treatment most frequently used for patients with antiphospholipid antibodies is low-dose aspirin and prednisone. The treatment is started as soon as the diagnosis of pregnancy is made, ideally a few days after a menstrual period is missed. Others recommend treatment before conception, but there is no information demonstrating that this approach is better. The aspirin dose is 80 mg daily; the prednisone dose varies between 40 and 60 mg daily. Another treatment protocol consists of low-dose aspirin and subcutaneous heparin. The heparin dose is usually 5000 U every 12 hours, although some investigators have used as much as 24,000 U daily.[53]

Treatment of patients with lupus anticoagulant should normalize their PTT. Treatment of patients with anticardiolipin antibody should suppress any increase in the antibody concentration and maintain a normal platelet count.

Treatment with a regimen of low-dose aspirin and prednisone or aspirin and heparin is approximately 80% successful. In those pregnancies that advance beyond the second trimester, fetal growth retardation is common, as is early onset preeclampsia.

The main complications of prednisone therapy are increased weight gain, moon facies, acne, marked striae, and abnormal glucose tolerance. The main problems with heparin include compliance, formation of painful nodules and ecchymuses at the injection sites, and occasional epistaxis and hematuria. Major complications of these medications such as osteoporosis, aseptic necrosis of the femoral head, optic nerve damage, and heparin-induced thrombocytopenia are extremely rare during pregnancy.

◪   IMPORTANT POINTS   ◪

1. Human reproduction is relatively inefficient. Only 57% of all conceptions advance beyond 20 weeks. Of those lost, 75% occur before implantation, and only 25% are clinically recognizable.

2. Approximately 80% of all spontaneous abortions occur before 12 weeks. The large majority of them are anembryonic pregnancies, or blighted ova.

3. The differentation between embryonic and anembryonic abortions is of fundamental importance. Anembryonic pregnancies (blighted ova) have a genetic origin, usually an error in maternal or paternal meiosis I or II. In contrast, embryonic abortions have multiple etiologies.

4. Patients with blighted ova usually have low-serum progesterone that is the result rather than the cause of abortion. The presence of a blighted ovum should be ruled out in every patient with threatened abortion and low-serum progesterone.

5. Ascending infections that recur in subsequent pregnancies strongly suggest the presence of a cervical defect that facilitates uterine invasion by the vaginal flora.

6. The most common complications following emergency cerclage for incompetent cervix are rupture of the membranes and acute chorioamnionitis. Once the membranes have been exposed to the vaginal flora, the patient should be considered infected and treated aggressively with antibiotics.

7. Abnormal placentation with inadequate changes in the spiral arteries is a common feature for patients with preeclampsia and severe growth retardation and is also shared by many patients with preterm labor, premature ruptured membranes, and early fetal demise.

8. The best-defined subset of patients with immunologic pregnancy losses are those with

antiphospholipid antibody syndrome. The most relevant of these antibodies to the obstetrician are the anticardiolipin antibody (ACA), the lupus anticoagulant (LAC), and the antibody that causes false-positive syphilis test (BFP-ST).

9. The presence of any or several of the three antiphospholipid antibodies is associated with recurrent early pregnancy losses and stillbirths, severe preeclampsia, severe IUGR, episodes of venous and arterial thrombosis, and severe postpartum complications.

10. The possibility that some abortions result from maternal immunologic rejection of the fetus is highly controversial and has little clinical and experimental support. Immunotherapy with leukocyte transfusion for repeated pregnancy losses is experimental and potentially dangerous.

11. Histologic and microbiologic examination of the placenta is a fundamental part of the evaluation of patients with early fetal demise. Also, a carefully performed fetal autopsy may provide invaluable information about the etiology of the abortion.

12. The obstetrician should investigate each pregnancy loss until the underlying cause is discovered. Otherwise, the diagnosis and management of patients with repetitive early pregnancy losses will be affected by inadequate information about the nature of their prior abortions.

REFERENCES

1. Miller JF, Williamson E, Glue J, et al: Fetal loss after implantation: A prospective study. *Lancet* 1980;2:554.
2. Wilcox AJ, Weinberg CR, O'Connor JF, et al: Incidence of early loss of pregnancy. *N Engl J Med* 1988;319:189-194.
3. Poland BJ, Miller JR, Jones DC, et al: Reproductive counseling in patients who have had a spontaneous abortion. *Am J Obstet Gynecol* 1977;127:685.
4. Warburton D, Fraser FC: Spontaneous abortion risks in man: Data from reproductive histories collected in a medical genetics unit. *Am J Hum Genet* 1964;16:1.
5. Warburton D, Kline J, Stein Z, et al: Does the karyotype of a spontaneous abortion predict the karyotype of a subsequent abortion? Evidence from 273 women with two karyotyped spontaneous abortions. *Am J Hum Genet* 1987;41:465-483.
6. Eiben B, Bartels I, Bahr-Porsch S, et al: Cytogenetic analysis of 750 spontaneous abortions with the direct-preparation method of chorionic villi and its implications for studying genetic causes of pregnancy wastage. *Am J Hum Genet* 1990;47:656-663.
7. Lohler J, Timpl R, Jaenisch R: Embryonic lethal mutation in mouse collagen alpha-1 (I) gene causes rupture of blood vessels and is associated with erythropoietic and mesochymal cell death. *Cell* 1984;38:597.
8. Tho PT, Byrd JR, McDonough PG: Etiology and subsequent reproductive performance of 100 couples with recurrent abortion. *Fertil Steril* 1979;32:389.
9. Botella-Llusia J: The endometrium in repeated abortion. *Int J Fertil* 1962;7:147.
10. Balasch J, Creus M, Marquez M, et al: The significance of luteal phase deficiency on fertility: A diagnostic and therapeutic approach. *Hum Reprod* 1986;1:145.
11. Hernandez Horta JL, Gordillo-Fernandez J, Soto de Leon B, et al: Direct evidence of luteal insufficiency in women with habitual abortion. *Obstet Gynecol* 1977;49:705-708.
12. Filicori M, Butler JP, Crowley WF: Neuroendocrine regulation of the corpus luteum in the human. *J Clin Invest* 1984;73:1638.
13. Yuen BH, Livinston JE, Poland BJ, et al: Human chorionic gonadotropin, estradiol, progesterone, prolactin, and B-scan ultrasound monitoring of complications of early pregnancy. *Obstet Gynecol* 1981;57:207-214.
14. Check JH, Vaze MM, Epstein R, et al: 17-Hydroxyprogesterone level as a marker for corpus luteum function in aborters vs nonaborters. *Int J Fertil* 1990;35:112-115.
15. Crane JP, Wahl N: The role of maternal diabetes in repetitive spontaneous abortion. *Fertil Steril* 1981;36:477.
16. Stray-Pedersen B, Stray-Pedersen S: Etiologic factors and subsequent reproductive performance in 195 couples with prior history of habitual abortion. *Am J Obstet Gynecol* 1984;140:2.
17. Mills JL, Simpson JL, Driscoll SG, et al: Incidence of spontaneous abortion among normal women and insulin-dependent diabetic women whose pregnancies were identified within 21 days of conception. *N Engl J Med* 1988;319:1617-1623.
18. Badarau L, Gavrilita L, Iuschevici C: A microscopic study of placenta and uteroplacental membranes in repeated abortion due to hyperandrogenism. *Rev Fr Gynecol Obstet* 1972;67:685-697.
19. Sagle M, Bishop K, Ridley N, et al: Recurrent early miscarriage and polycystic ovary. *Br Med J* 1988;297:1027-1028.
20. Regan L, Owen EJ, Jacobs HS: Hypersecretion of luteinising hormone, infertility, and miscarriage. *Lancet* 1990;336:1141.
21. Johnson P, Pearce JM: Recurrent spontaneous abortion and polycystic ovary disease: Comparison of two regimens to induce ovulation. *Br Med J* 1990;300:154-156.
22. Sompolinsky D, Solomon F, Elkinal L, et al: Infections with mycoplasma and bacteria in induced midtrimester abortion and fetal loss. *Am J Obstet Gynecol* 1975;121:610-616.
23. Stray-Pedersen B, Eng J, Reikvan TM: Uterine T-mycoplasma colonization in reproductive failure. *Am J Obstet Gynecol* 1978;130:307.
24. Qinn PA, Chewchuck AB, Suber J, et al: Efficacy of antibiotic therapy in preventing spontaneous pregnancy loss among couples colonized with genital mycoplasma. *Am J Obstet Gynecol* 1983;145:239-244.

25. Schenker JG, Margalioth EJ: Intrauterine adhesions: An updated appraisal. *Fertil Steril* 1982;37:593-610.

26. Golan A, Langer RM, Wexler B, et al: Cervical cerclage: Its role in the pregnant anomalous uterus. *Int J Fertil* 1990;35:164.

27. Kaufman RH, Noller K, Adam E, et al: Upper genital tract abnormalities and pregnancy outcome in diethylstilbestrol exposed progeny. *Am J Obstet Gynecol* 1984; 148:973.

28. Feingold M, Brook I, Zakutt H: Detection of cervical incompetence by ultrasound. *Acta Obstet Gynecol Scand* 1984;63:407.

29. Novy MJ, Haymond J, Nichols M: Shirodkar cerclage in a multifactorial approach to the patient with advanced cervical changes. *Am J Obstet Gynecol* 1990;162:1412-1420.

30. Pedersen JF, Mantoni M: Large intrauterine haematomata in threatened miscarriage: Frequency and clinical consequences. *Br J Obstet Gynaecol* 1990;97:75.

31. Khong TY, Liddell HS, Robertson WB: Defective hemochorial placentation as a cause of miscarriage: A preliminary study. *Br J Obstet Gynaecol* 1987;94:649-655.

32. Exner T, Richard KA, Kronenberg H: A sensitive test demonstrating lupus anticoagulant and its behavioural patterns. *Br J Haematol* 1978;40:143-151.

33. Thiagarajan P, Pengo V, Shapiro SS: The use of the dilute Russell viper venom time for the diagnosis of lupus anticoagulant. *Blood* 1986;68:869-874.

34. Gleicher N, Friberg J: IgM gammopathy and the lupus anticoagulant syndrome in habitual aborters. *JAMA* 1985;253:3278-3281.

35. Kochenour NK, Branch DW, Rote NS, et al: A new postpartum syndrome associated with antiphospholipid antibodies. *Obstet Gynecol* 1987;69:460-468.

36. Branch DW: Antiphospholipid antibodies and pregnancy: Maternal implications. *Semin Perinatol* 1990;14:139-146.

37. De Wolf F, Carreras LO, Moerman P, et al: Decidual vasculopathy and extensive placental infarction in a patient with repeated thromboembolic accidents, recurrent fetal loss, and lupus anticoagulant. *Am J Obstet Gynecol* 1982;142:829-833.

38. Reece EA, Gabrielli S, Cullen MT, et al: Recurrent adverse pregnancy outcome and antiphospholipid antibodies. *Am J Obstet Gynecol* 1990;163:162-169.

39. Garcia-de la Torre, Hernandez-Vasquez L, Angulo-Vasquez J, et al: Prevalence of antinuclear antibodies in patients with habitual abortion and in normal and toxemic pregnancies. *Rheumatol Int* 1984;4:87-89.

40. Xu L, Chang V, Murphy A, et al: Antinuclear antibodies in sera of patients with recurrent pregnancy wastage. *Am J Obstet Gynecol* 1990;163:1493-1497.

41. Cowchock S, Smith B, Gocial B: Antibodies to phospholipids and nuclear antigens in patients with repeated abortions. *Am J Obstet Gynecol* 1986;155:1002-1010.

42. Petri M, Golbus M, Anderson R, et al: Antinuclear antibody, lupus anticoagulant and anticardiolipin antibody in women with idiopathic habitual abortion: A controlled, prospective study of 44 women. *Arthritis Rheum* 1987;30:601-606.

43. Caudle MR, Rote NS, Scott JR, et al: Histocompatibility in couples with recurrent spontaneous abortions and normal fertility. *Fertil Steril* 1983;39:793-798.

44. Rocklin RE, Kitzmiller JL, Carpenter CB, et al: Maternal-fetal relation: Absence of an immunological blocking factor from the serum of women with chronic abortion. *N Engl J Med* 1976;295:1209-1213.

45. Oksenberg JR, Persitz E, Amar E: Mixed lymphocyte reactivity nonresponsiveness in couples with multiple spontaneous abortions. *Fertil Steril* 1983;39:525.

46. Park MI, Edwin SS, Scott JR, et al: Interpretation of blocking activity in maternal serum depends on the equation used for calculation of mixed lymphocyte culture results. *Clin Exp Immunol* 1990;82:363-368.

47. Bree RL, Edwards M, Bohm-Velez M, et al: Transvaginal sonography in the evaluation of normal early pregnancy: Correlation with HCG levels. *AJR* 1989;153:75-79.

48. Warren WB, Timor-Tritsch I, Peisner DB, et al: Dating the early pregnancy by sequential appearance of embryonic structures. *Am J Obstet Gynecol* 1989;161:747-753.

49. Goldstein I, Zimmer EA, Tamir A, et al: Evaluation of normal gestational sac growth: Appearance of embryonic heartbeat and embryo body movements using the transvaginal technique. *Obstet Gynecol* 1991;77:885.

50. Simpson JL, Mills JL, Holmes LB, et al: Low fetal loss rates after ultrasound-proved viability in early pregnancy. *JAMA* 1987;258:2555-2557.

51. Siddiqui TA, Caligaris JT, Miodovnik M, et al: Rate of spontaneous abortion after first trimester sonographic demonstration of fetal cardiac activity. *Am J Perinatol* 1988;5:1-4.

52. Howert-de Jong MH, Termijtelen A, Eskes TKAB, et al: The natural course of habitual abortion. *Eur J Obstet Gynecol* 1989;33:221-228.

53. Rosove MH, Tabsh K, Wasserstrum N, et al: Heparin therapy for pregnant women with lupus anticoagulant or anticardiolipin antibodies. *Obstet Gynecol* 1990;75:630-634.

4

PRETERM LABOR

◪ INTRODUCTION AND DEFINITIONS

Preterm labor is an important problem associated with high perinatal mortality and morbidity. It is defined as the onset of labor in patients with intact membranes before 37 weeks.

The medical literature on preterm labor may be difficult to understand because of changing definitions. In 1948 the first World Health Assembly of the League of Nations defined *prematures* as all infants with birth weights under 2500 g. This definition was useful because it identified a group of newborns at high risk for neonatal complications and death. Unfortunately, the definition is incorrect because the correlation between infant weight and functional maturity is poor. Many infants with birth weights under 2500 g show evidence of advanced maturity and should not be called premature. On the other hand, some babies may be developmentally immature in spite of having large birth weights.

In an attempt to correct the deficiencies of the 1948 definition, the World Health Organization recommended in 1972 that the term *premature* not be used and instead that newborns should be described in terms of either birth weight or gestational age. Any infant weighing less than 2500 g at birth should be called *low birth weight*, and any infant born before 37 completed weeks from the first day of the mother's last menstrual period (LMP) should be called *preterm*. Unfortunately, basing the definition of *preterm* on the mother's LMP is not adequate because a large number of obstetric patients cite unreliable dates. An assessment of gestational age based on clinical and neurologic examination of the newborn is much more precise[1] and has become standard in modern studies on preterm labor.

When the correlation between birth weight and gestational age was analyzed, it was found that any newborn, term or preterm, could be small for gestational age (SGA), adequate for gestational age (AGA), or large for gestational age (LGA).[2] This classification of the newborn on the basis of birth weight and gestational age is used in the majority of modern studies on this subject.

The definitions most frequently used in the discussion of preterm labor are:

prematurity   Term used in the past to designate infants with birth weights under 2500 g. The term implies birth before maturity and should not be used.

preterm   Infant born before 37 completed weeks of gestation. The weeks of gestation may be determined by calculating from the mother's LMP, a procedure that is frequently in error; by clinical dating plus ultrasound examination, which is the gold standard in obstetrics; or by examination of the newborn.

low birth weight   Newborn weighing less than 2500 g at birth. Low birth weight infants may be preterm or postterm, more than 42 weeks of gestation.

adequate for gestational age (AGA)   Newborn with somatic development (weight, length, head circumference) adequate for his or her gestational age as determined by neonatal examination. AGA infants may be preterm, term, or postterm.

small for gestational age (SGA)   Newborn with somatic development below the 10th percentile for his or her gestational age as determined by neonatal examination. SGA infants may be preterm, term, or postterm.

large for gestational age (LGA)   Infant with somatic development above the 90th percentile for his or her gestational age as determined by neonatal examination. LGA infants may be preterm, term, or postterm.

premature labor   Term that implies labor before maturity and should not be used.

preterm labor   Labor (regular, painful, frequent uterine contractions causing progressive effacement and dilation of the cervix) occurring before 37 completed weeks of gestation.

A predominant source of confusion, particularly in evaluating the effectiveness of labor-inhibiting drugs, is the definition of preterm labor. Most investigators require the presence of progressive effacement and dilation of the cervix to make this diagnosis, but sometimes definitions that omit cervical changes are used.

Another source of confusion is that old studies group together patients with preterm rupture of the membranes (PROM) and patients with preterm labor and intact membranes. These are two closely related but different syndromes that should be analyzed independently.

◪ MATERNAL AND FETAL CONSEQUENCES OF PRETERM LABOR

Maternal mortality and morbidity as a consequence of preterm labor is rare. The most common maternal effects are feelings of inadequacy at fulfilling a reproductive role. These feelings are most common in women who have suffered repeated pregnancy losses. A second relatively common maternal problem is the development of postpartum endometritis. However, most patients who develop endometritis respond rapidly to the administration of antibiotics.

In contrast to the good maternal prognosis after preterm labor, the effect of this condition on the fetus is devastating; neonatal mortality is high, and neonatal morbidity is frequent and severe.

Perinatal mortality

The continuous improvement in neonatal care makes it difficult to precisely evaluate the contribution of preterm labor to perinatal mortality and morbidity. In one study carried out in South Africa,[3] preterm labor was responsible for almost half of preterm deliveries and for 52% of all early neonatal deaths. In a similar study from England,[4] preterm labor caused 38% of the preterm neonatal deaths. This difference in the contribution of preterm labor to neonatal mortality most probably reflects differences in neonatal care. Unfortunately, no mention is made in these two studies about PROM; patients with this condition were probably included in the preterm labor group introducing unreliability to their figures. We found that preterm labor accounted for 24.5% of all preterm deliveries in a population made of 60% indigents and 40% medium socioeconomic class in the midwest of the United States.[5] The same analysis in a predominantly mid and high socioeconomic group revealed an incidence of 19.2% preterm delivery resulting from preterm labor. This is not surprising because there is a wide variation in the occurrence of preterm labor among different ethnic and socioeconomic groups.

Neonatal survival for preterm infants is directly related to their gestational ages and birth weights. Table 4-1 shows the neonatal survival

TABLE 4-1 ◪ Approximate neonatal survival of preterm infants born in a tertiary care center

Gestational age (weeks)	Weight range (grams)	Survivors (%)
24 to 26	500 to 750	50.0
26 to 28	750 to 1000	74.5
28 to 30	1000 to 1400	91.2
30 to 32	1400 to 1800	96.5
32 to 34	1800 to 2200	99.0
> 34	> 2200	100.0

rates that should be expected in institutions with adequate intensive neonatal care facilities. Despite all advances in neonatology, the most efficient system for decreasing perinatal mortality and morbidity is to keep the fetus inside the uterus until it reaches at least 1500 g of weight or 32 weeks of gestational age.

Perinatal morbidity

To cover adequately the large number of problems that may occur in preterm infants as a consequence of being delivered too early is beyond the scope of this book. However, it is necessary to look closely at neonatal respiratory distress syndrome (RDS) and intraventricular hemorrhage (IVH) because these two problems are the most significant causes of neonatal mortality and morbidity in the preterm infant.

Neonatal respiratory distress syndrome. Neonatal RDS is a situation characterized by grunting, intercostal retraction, nasal flaring, cyanosis in room air, and requirement of oxygen to maintain adequate arterial oxygen pressure. There are multiple causes of neonatal RDS. They include (1) transient tachypnea of the newborn (TTN), caused by wet lungs or by transient intrapartum asphyxia; (2) congenital pneumonia that results from intraamniotic infection; (3) pulmonary hypertension; and (4) congenital defects such as diaphragmatic hernia or pulmonary hypoplasia caused by Potter's syndrome. However, the most frequent cause of neonatal RDS is hyaline membrane disease (HMD). Chest x-ray examination is essential in differentiating HMD from other causes of RDS.

HMD occurs because of inadequate production of pulmonary surfactant by the type II alveolar cells of the newborn. The surfactant spreads in the lung tissue–air interface, preventing alveolar collapse during expiration and allowing the alveoli to open easily at the next inspiration. If surfactant is not present in adequate amounts, the alveoli will collapse during expiration and each inspiration will require considerable effort. This situation rapidly leads to fatigue, decreased respiratory effort, hypoxia, cyanosis, acidosis, and eventually death.

The pulmonary surfactant is a heterogeneous mixture of lipids and protein. Dipalmitoylphosphatidylcholine (DPPC) is the main component of the pulmonary surfactant. After its synthesis, DPPC accumulates in osmophilic structures called lamellar bodies that consist of multiple, closely packed phospholipid bilayers. The lamellar bodies are released from the cells into the alveolar fluid, and from there they go into the amniotic fluid. This makes it possible to assess the biochemical maturation of the fetal lungs by studying the amniotic fluid phospholipid composition. The incorporation of this fact into the day-to-day management of obstetrical patients has been one of the most significant advances in reproductive medicine in this century.

Tests for the assessment of fetal pulmonary maturity. The first reliable test to determine the biochemical maturation of the fetal lungs was the measurement of the *lecithin to sphingomyelin ratio (L/S ratio)* in the amniotic fluid.[6] This determination involves extraction of the amniotic fluid with chloroform/methanol, precipitation of surface-active phospholipids with cold acetone, and determination of the L/S ratio by thin-layer chromatography. The finding of a mature L/S ratio, 2.3 or greater, predicts with 95% accuracy the absence of HMD. The 5% of cases in which the prediction is incorrect usually are infants of diabetic mothers or infants born after significant intrapartum asphyxia. The L/S ratio is not a good predictor of pulmonary immaturity, and when the L/S ratio is less than 2.3, only 54% of the newborns will develop HMD. This high proportion of false predictions of pulmonary immaturity is a serious defect of the L/S ratio because pregnancies in which early delivery is desirable may be prolonged unnecessarily. The L/S ratio is noninformative also if the amniotic fluid is contaminated with blood or meconium or is collected from a vaginal pool.

The 5% false-positive answers obtained with the L/S ratio can be decreased by simultaneously determining the presence of *phosphatidylglycerol (PG)* in the amniotic fluid sample. According to Kulovich et al.,[7,8] if PG is present in a sample with a mature L/S ratio, the infant will not develop HMD even if the pregnancy is complicated by maternal diabetes or by intrapartum asphyxia. PG appears in the amniotic fluid usually after 36 weeks and is a marker of the final biochemical maturation of the fetal lungs. How PG works is not precisely known, although it has been suggested that it may stabilize the surfactant complex. The measurement of PG in the amniotic fluid has been facilitated by the availability of immunologic slide testing that allows a rapid, precise, and inexpensive evaluation.[9] However, the immunologic test is not as sensitive for detecting small amounts of PG as the chromatographic technique.

When the amniotic fluid specimen is contaminated with blood or meconium, a quantitative determination of DPPC may be used instead of the L/S ratio to assess fetal pulmonary maturity.[10] DPPC is not present in blood or meconium or in vaginal secretions. DPPC can be separated from other phospholipids because its unsaturated fatty acid can be selectively oxidized and this changes its chromatographic migration. A DPPC concentration greater than 500 µg/dl is predictive of fetal lung maturity. A comparison between DPPC and L/S ratio[10] showed significant advantages for the DPPC method, which had a 97% positive predictive value (90% for the L/S ratio) and an 83% negative predictive value (55.5% for the L/S ratio). When the fluid is stained with blood, meconium, or vaginal products, DPPC may be the best way to evaluate pulmonary maturity. Despite its advantages, DPPC determination is not commonly used.

Fluorescence polarization of the amniotic fluid is another available test for the assessment of fetal pulmonary maturity. This method, introduced by Shinitzky et al.,[11] measures the microviscocity of the amniotic fluid phospholipids in fluorescence polarization units. Unfortunately, the test is unreliable if the fluid is contaminated with blood or meconium and is inaccurate when used before 34 weeks of gestation.[12]

The *Abott TDx Fetal Lung Maturity (FLM) test* is another application of the fluorescence polarization test that is rapidly gaining acceptance as an index of fetal lung maturity. The test is based on the competitive binding between albumin and surfactant for a ligand named PC16. This substance exhibits high fluorescence polarization when bound to albumin that decreases when it is bound to surfactant. Since the albumin concentration in the amniotic fluid remains relatively constant during the third trimester of pregnancy, decreases in fluorescence polarization of the fluid reflects increased concentration of surfactant. This test is rapid, requires a small amount of fluid, is quantitative, and has predictive values similar or better than the L/S ratio. An FLM concentration of greater than 70 mg/g has a 95% predictive value for fetal pulmonary maturity.[13]

A simple and inexpensive method for the evaluation of fetal lung maturity is the measurement of the *amniotic fluid optical density at 650 nm.*[14] Unfortunately, this method is affected by con-

tamination of the fluid with blood or meconium, by variations in the speed of centrifugation, and by refrigeration of the sample. Under ideal conditions, a mature optical density at 650 nm will correctly predict a mature L/S ratio in 92% of the cases. An immature optical density at 650 nm will predict an immature L/S ratio in 72% of the cases.[15] It has been suggested that optical density at 650 nm may be used as a screening test and that values between 0.10 and 0.20 should prompt further evaluation with additional fetal lung maturity tests.[16]

Some other tests have been used as substitutes for the L/S ratio. One of them, the *shake test*, is easy to perform, and when it predicts maturity, its accuracy is close to 100%. Unfortunately, a negative test is not a good predictor of pulmonary immaturity, and further testing is necessary if the test is negative. The shake test estimates qualitatively the stability of the bubbles formed after shaking a mixture of amniotic fluid with ethanol.

Some of the disadvantages of the shake test have been overcome with the development of the *foam stability index (FSI)*. This is a semiquantitative measure of the surfactant present in a sample of amniotic fluid.[17] In this test the fluid is mixed with ethanol in the necessary amounts to achieve alcohol concentrations ranging from 44% to 50%. The risk of RDS is 73% when the test is negative and no bubbles are produced in the mixture at 44%. The risk of RDS is 29% if the test is positive at ethanol concentrations of 44%, 45%, and 46%. The chances of developing RDS is 0.35% if bubbles are produced when the ethanol concentration is 47%. Thus a positive FSI at an ethanol concentration of 47% is a better predictor of fetal pulmonary maturity than a mature L/S ratio, but the L/S ratio is a better predictor at intermediate ranges. Both tests have a similar predictive value when the L/S ratio is less than 1.5 and the FSI is negative.

Another rapid and inexpensive alternative test for assessing fetal pulmonary maturity is the *tap test.*[18] The test is performed by mixing 1 ml of amniotic fluid with one drop of 6N hydrochloric acid and then adding 1.5 ml of diethyl ether. The test tube is briskly tapped creating bubbles in the ether layer. If the fetus is mature, the bubbles will rise to the surface and break down. If the fetus is immature, the bubbles are stable or break down slowly. Similar to the other available tests to assess fetal lung maturity, the tap test has an excellent positive predictive value, 98% to

100%, but the negative test is not a good predictor of lung immaturity.

Acceleration of fetal pulmonary maturity with steroids. It is possible to accelerate the maturation of the fetal lungs in patients at high risk for preterm delivery. The classic study on this area was by Howie and Liggins in New Zealand.[19] They had 411 patients in a betamethasone-treated group and 410 in a control group. The incidence of RDS was 8.8% in the treated vs. 28.7% in the control group—a significant difference (p<0.001). The perinatal mortality was significantly lower in the corticosteroid-treated group. Similar studies in other parts of the world have confirmed the original observation of Howie and Liggins.

Several questions are frequently asked about glucocorticoids and fetal lung maturity. One is the minimal time required after administration of the drug before a protective effect on the fetus is obtained. According to Howie and Liggins' study, 24 hours seems to be the minimal time necessary to obtain a significant effect.

Another question is the duration of the drug effect. In the study by Howie and Liggins, when infants were delivered between 7 and 21 days after treatment, there was a higher incidence of RDS in betamethasone-treated infants (21.2%) than in the control group (7.1%). These data suggest that the glucocorticoid effect is transient and treatment should be repeated if delivery is delayed more than 7 days after the initial dose.

Another frequent question concerns the gestational age at which glucocorticoid treatment is effective. According to the data of Howie and Liggins shown in Table 4-2, the effect of therapy is best in infants between 30 and 32 weeks, but there is also a significant reduction in the incidence of RDS in babies under 30 and between 32 and 34 weeks. Thus glucocorticoids should be administered in any situation in which fetal lung maturity is desirable from viability to 34 weeks of gestation. After 34 weeks, the drug seems to have little influence on the respiratory outcome of the newborn. This may be because of lack of responsiveness to the medication. Also, since a majority of babies at 34 weeks have adequate lung maturity, to demonstrate an effect of glucocorticoid therapy in those that have immature lungs will require a number of patients much larger than that used by Howie and Liggins in their study.

The possibility of harmful effects of glucocorticoids on fetus or mother is minimal. In more

TABLE 4-2 ☑ Incidence of RDS in live born infants delivered 24 hours to 7 days after treatment with betamethasone or placebo

Gestational age at delivery (weeks)	% with RDS		
	Betamethasone	Placebo	p
Under 30	27.8	57.7	0.04
30 to 32	8.7	56.0	0.001
32 to 34	0.0	12.9	0.04
34+	5.5	5.4	NS

From Howie RN, Liggins GF: In Anderson A, et al (eds): *Preterm Labor.* London, Royal College of Obstetricians and Gynecologists, 1977, p 281.

than 14 years of extensive use of glucocorticoids to accelerate fetal lung maturity, not a single case has been reported demonstrating any significant problems associated with this therapy.

Surfactant replacement therapy. The outcome of babies with HMD has changed dramatically with the development of surfactant replacement therapy. In 1980, Fujiwara[19a] reported a spectacular improvement in gas exchange in infants with severe HMD treated with a modified bovine surfactant. This observation stimulated the development of clinical trials, and today surfactant treatment is a well-established therapeutic modality for infants with HMD.[20]

Surfactant is a complex mixture of phospholipids and proteins. The most important phospholipids are DPPC and PG. The most important proteins are surfactant-associated proteins A, B, and C.

Both natural and artificial surfactants have been used for the treatment of neonatal HMD. Natural surfactant can be obtained from human amniotic fluid and cow, calf, and pork lungs. The process of preparation of animal surfactants causes the loss of apoprotein A. The best known of the natural surfactants is *Survanta*, which is obtained from bovine lungs. The artificial surfactants contain no associated proteins. They are made of mixtures of DPPC and PG with or without emulsifiers. The best known are *Exosurf* and *ALEC*.

Surfactant can be used as soon as a preterm baby is delivered and before the development of symptoms and signs of HMD. It also can be used after symptoms have developed.[21] It is administered via endotracheal tube. It is given in one or multiple doses according to different protocols.

The response to surfactant administration is immediate and results in a decrease in the oxygen concentration necessary to ventilate the infant and in a decrease in ventilatory pressure. The effect may be transient and repeated doses are necessary. The use of surfactant has been an important factor in the present survival rate of preterm infants (see Table 4-1). Survival rates of 70% for newborns of 24 weeks are not uncommon today. However, surfactant use has not decreased the rate of intraventricular hemorrhage (IVH), necrotizing enterocolitis (NEC), and bronchopulmonary dysplasia. There is no increase in neurodevelopmental impairments in preterm survivors after surfactant treatment.[22]

Intraventricular hemorrhage. Several central nervous system lesions are associated with preterm delivery, and most of them have the common denominator of hemorrhage and necrosis. The most common site of hemorrhage is the subependymal germinal matrix.[23] There is an abundance of plasminogen activator in the germinal tissue causing locally excessive fibrinolysis, and this may be the reason why bleeding frequently continues until the blood fills the ventricular system. However, not all subependymal hemorrhages progress into the ventricular system, and 40% are confined to their place of origin.

Several studies[24,25] have tried to identify preventable obstetric events placing the fetus at high risk for IVH. It has been found that mode of delivery, breech presentation, PROM, and vaginal bleeding do not increase the likelihood of IVH. The most common associations are extreme prematurity, birth weight less than 1500 g, and neonatal complications. Also, labor, intrapartum hypoxia, and blood pressure fluctuations are important factors associated with intraventricular and subarachnoid hemorrhage in the preterm infant.[26-28] Hypoxia causes damage to the vascular endothelium of the fragile veins of the preterm infant, and this, along with the venous congestion also caused by hypoxia, may result in rupture of blood vessels. A contributory factor may be elevated plasma osmolarity produced by over-enthusiastic use of sodium bicarbonate in the course of the infant's resuscitation.

Anderson et al.[29] investigated the association between IVH in newborns with birth weights less than 1500 g and multiple intrapartum events. They found that the incidence of IVH and the progression of IVH from grade I to grade III or IV was related to the active phase of labor rather than to the route of delivery.

The severity of IVH can be estimated by examination of the infant, by ultrasound scanning of the baby's head, and by computed tomography. Mild and even moderate degrees of bleeding are usually associated with good prognosis and with recovery without neurologic sequelae. In contrast, severe bleeding is frequently fatal, and survivors frequently develop hydrocephaly.

Prevention of IVH. The obstetrician plays a role in the prevention of IVH by avoiding and aggressively treating intrapartum hypoxia. A liberal policy of cesarean section should dominate the intrapartum management of patients in premature labor. Also, avoidance of labor may be of critical importance for the prevention of IVH.

There are indications that prenatal administration of phenobarbital and vitamin K_1 are useful for the prevention of IVH. Phenobarbital is used in a single dose of 10 mg/kg body weight (minimum 500 mg; maximum 700 mg) as a constant IV infusion for 30 minutes when delivery appears imminent.[30] Vitamin K_1 is given in an initial dose of 10 mg intramuscularly (IM) followed by 20 mg orally daily until delivery.[31] The good results obtained with prenatal administration of phenobarbital are in contrast to the conflicting results obtained when the medication is given to the baby after birth.

Another drug being investigated as a preventative agent for the development of IVH is indomethacin. There is evidence from animal studies and from uncontrolled human experiences that this medication, given in the neonatal period, may be useful for the prevention of IVH. However, no studies have been published demonstrating a preventative effect of indomethacin when given before delivery.

◼ ETIOLOGY OF PRETERM LABOR
Chorioamnionitis

Evidence accumulated in the last few years indicates that chorioamnionitis is the cause of 20% to 30% of all cases of preterm labor. Armer and Duff[32] reviewed all English language papers published between 1980 and 1990 describing results when amniocentesis was performed at the time of admission of patients in preterm labor. They found than 13% had chorioamnionitis demonstrated by positive amniotic fluid cultures.

An additional 10% will have positive fluid cultures if the amniocentesis is repeated at the time of delivery.[33]

The mechanism responsible for the initiation of labor in patients with an infected uterus has not been completely clarified. The work of Romero[33,34] strongly suggests that initiation of parturition is controlled by the host that reacts to bacterial aggression with the production of intermediate substances such as interleukin-1, tumor necrosis factor, and platelet activating factor that activate prostaglandin production by the decidua and the amniotic membranes.

Intraamniotic infection causing preterm labor may exist without fever, leukocytosis, uterine tenderness, fetal tachycardia, or any of the classic signs commonly described for severe infections of the pregnant uterus. Preterm labor, usually resistant to conventional treatment with beta-mimetic agents, and advanced cervical dilation may be the only signs indicating the presence of an infectious process.

Our present understanding of intrauterine infection causing preterm labor may be summarized as follows: for reasons that are poorly understood, the barrier between the uterine cavity and the vagina breaks allowing the entrance of bacteria into the uterus. These bacteria replicate slowly in the decidua and eventually reach the necessary concentration to colonize the amniotic membranes and infect the amniotic fluid, the umbilical cord, and other fetal tissues. Patients in preterm labor with fetal tachycardia, uterine tenderness, and mild temperature elevation have reached a final stage in the progression of uterine infection. In these cases preterm labor is a mechanism of fetal and maternal protection and should not be interrupted. The opportunities to modify the course of preterm labor of infectious origin probably are in the initial stages of infection, when bacteria are still localized in the decidua and have not invaded the amniotic membranes.

No test is available to diagnose the earlier stages of infection leading to preterm labor. There are several tests for diagnosing infection once it has reached the amniotic cavity. Their value is to inform the obstetrician that the infection has reached an end point at which the only therapeutic alternative is delivery. These tests are:

Amniotic fluid Gram stain
Amniotic fluid limulus amebocyte lysate assay
Amniotic fluid gas liquid chromatography
Amniotic fluid bacterial cultures
Amniotic fluid leukocyte count
Amniotic fluid acridine orange stain

The *Gram stain* of the amniotic fluid is a simple and rapid test for the diagnosis of amniotic fluid infection.[35] It can be performed in both spun and unspun specimens. Some prefer to spin the fluid in a clinical centrifuge (approximately 3000 rpm) for 5 minutes, decant the supernatant, and use one or two drops of the fluid and sediment remaining at the bottom of the tube for Gram staining. The presence of any bacteria is indicative of infection (positive predictive value of 100%). A negative Gram stain does not rule out the possibility of an early infection localized in the decidua and not shedding bacteria into the amniotic fluid.

The *limulus amebocyte lysate assay* is the most sensitive test available for the detection of gram-negative endotoxin. The test is also useful in certain gram-positive intraamniotic infections.[36] The test is easy to perform and is relatively inexpensive. When this test is combined with the Gram stain, the sensitivity for the detection of intraamniotic infection is greater than 95%.

Gas liquid chromatography is a technique that identifies fatty acid chains elaborated by microbial metabolism.[37] Although the sensitivity of this method is high, it is time-consuming and requires relatively expensive laboratory equipment.

Bacterial cultures of aerobic and anaerobic germs provide definite evidence of the presence of amniotic fluid infection. The infection frequently is mixed. The most common offenders are:

Ureaplasma urealyticum
Gardnerella vaginalis
Group B *Streptococcus*
Escherichia coli
Bacteroides sp
Mycoplasma hominis
Fusobacterium sp
Listeria monocytogenes
Lactobacillus sp
Peptostreptococcus sp
Chlamydia trachomatis

In a recent study the isolates found most frequently in the placentas of infants delivered prematurely were *Ureaplasma urealyticum* (47% of the cases) and *Gardnerella vaginalis* (26% of the cases).[38]

The presence of leukocytes in the amniotic fluid is a relatively insensitive test for amniotic fluid infection. When the infection is still localized in the decidua and has not spread into the amniotic fluid, it may cause an increase in amniotic fluid leukocytes. Also, leukocytosis in the absence of bacteria suggests the possibility of mycoplasma infection.

The acridine orange stain allows visualization of mycoplasma in amniotic fluids with leukocytosis and without bacteria seen in the Gram stain. The test is easy to perform.

The existence of amniotic infection causing preterm labor may be recognized postpartum by *histologic examination of the placenta,* which should be routine in every case of preterm labor. Safarti et al.[39] found histologic evidence of infection in 27% of placentas and membranes obtained after preterm delivery as compared to 4.7% when the placentas and membranes were obtained from normal patients delivering at term. In the work of Hillier et al.[38] microorganisms were isolated from the area between the chorion and the amnion in 61% of women who delivered before 37 weeks and in only 21% of those delivering at term.

The most important question to be answered in the upcoming years is that of the nature of the alteration in the cervix and its mucous plug that allows the passage of microorganisms into the uterus. It is possible that aggressive treatment of vaginal and endocervical gland infections before pregnancy or during the first trimester of pregnancy may be useful for the prevention of ascending infection. It is also possible that prophylactic cerclage may be useful for patients with repetitive second-trimester pregnancy losses caused by ascending infection and preterm labor.

Infections outside of the uterus

Maternal infections outside of the uterus are a relatively frequent cause of preterm labor. Approximately 5% to 10% of patients in preterm labor have an infection outside of the uterus, most commonly in the urinary tract. Romero and Mazor[33] has presented evidence suggesting that extrauterine infections may cause preterm labor by a mechanism involving the production of interleukins and tumor necrosis factor by maternal macrophages, which in turn will trigger the production of prostaglandins by the amnion.

The strongest association of preterm labor is with urinary tract infection (UTI). In one study,

25% of patients admitted to the hospital because of preterm labor had a urinary sediment suggestive of UTI, although culture-proven infection was documented in only half of them. In another study the presence of group B streptococcus in the urine was associated with preterm labor, and treatment to prevent recolonization reduced the incidence of the problem.[40] Frequently, trichomonads are seen in the microscopic examination of the urine in patients with preterm labor. Vaginal trichomoniasis is also a common finding in patients in preterm labor.

The data from the Collaborative Perinatal Project have clearly demonstrated the existence of an association between culture-proven UTI during pregnancy and preterm delivery. The association between asymptomatic bacteriuria and preterm delivery is controversial. Kaas[41] suggested that asymptomatic patients with two or more urine cultures having more than 100,000 colonies of pathogenic bacteria per milliliter of urine have 2 to 3 times more risk of preterm labor than do controls with negative cultures. Some investigations have supported Kaas's findings, whereas others have reached different conclusions. The overall weight of the evidence, however, seems to favor the existence of a strong association between UTI and preterm labor.[42]

Placental abnormalities

Preterm labor occurs frequently in pregnancies with abnormalities in the morphology, implantation, or function of the placenta.

Anatomic abnormalities such as battledore placenta, circumvallate placenta, and marginal insertion of the umbilical cord are frequently associated with preterm labor. These are uncommon problems; for example, the incidence of battledore placenta is approximately 1 of 1000 deliveries. The mechanism of preterm labor caused by placental anatomic abnormalities is unknown.

Preterm labor is common in patients with placenta previa. It is tempting to speculate that bleeding results from uterine contractions causing some degree of placental separation. In the majority of patients with placenta previa, contractions disappear with bed rest or after treatment with tocolytic agents. In some cases contractions and bleeding persist, and delivery is then necessary.

Patients with severe abruptio placentae usually have rhythmic uterine contractions superimposed on tetanic contracture of the uterus, and most of them deliver shortly after the onset of symptoms. Other patients presenting with preterm labor have small degrees of placental separation associated with minimal external bleeding. The placentas of patients delivering prematurely frequently show small peripheral placental separation.

A significant number of patients in preterm labor deliver infants that have advanced maturation and require little support in the neonatal intensive care unit. In these cases the placenta usually is small, has extensive fibrosis and calcification, and in some cases separates with difficulty from the uterus, requiring manual removal and postpartum curettage. Histologic examination shows inadequate development of spiral arteries, spiral artery thrombosis, accelerated maturation, and placental infarcts. These patients most probably represent a subgroup in which preterm labor is the result of placental vascular insufficiency. The mechanism of labor in patients with placental insufficiency is unknown.

Intravascular volume expansion is frequently inadequate in patients who develop preterm labor.[43] Patients with conditions that decrease the uteroplacental blood flow frequently have low birth weight babies and preterm labor. Doppler studies, which reflect the fetoplacental circulation, are frequently abnormal in patients in preterm labor.[44] Finally, if fetuses from term and preterm labor are compared, the incidence of fetal growth retardation is greater in the preterm labor group.[45] All these facts emphasize the important contribution of placental vascular insufficiency to preterm labor.

The following signs suggest that preterm labor may be caused by placental insufficiency:

1. Absence of infection (negative Gram stain, negative amebocyte lysate assay, negative culture, no leukocytes in the fluid)
2. Amniotic fluid analysis showing a mature L/S ratio or positive PG at a gestational age at which fetal pulmonary maturity is not expected
3. Fetal size 1 or 2 weeks behind the patient's gestational age
4. Therapeutic response to intravascular volume expansion

Preterm labor resulting from anatomic or functional impairment of the placenta has a survival value for the fetus.

Anatomic abnormalities of the uterus

Congenital abnormalities of the uterus and cervix account for 1% to 3% of all cases of preterm labor. The most important of these conditions are the septate and the bicornate uterus. In these patients the incidence of spontaneous abortion is 27%, and the incidence of preterm labor, if the pregnancy continues beyond 20 weeks, varies between 16% and 20%. Leiomyomas are an acquired anatomic abnormality that is also associated with preterm labor. It is important that these conditions are diagnosed, because once they are identified, it is possible to adopt corrective measures to avoid preterm labor and pregnancy losses. The mechanism of preterm labor in patients with anatomic abnormalities of the uterus is unknown.

Congenital abnormalities of the uterus, cervix, and vagina result from failure in the fusion, canalization, or absorption of the müllerian ducts during embryonic development. Women born to mothers who ingested diethylstilbesterol (DES) during pregnancy have a high incidence of anatomic abnormalities of the uterus demonstrable by hysterosalpingography.[46] A large number of DES patients also have incompetent cervix. The possibility that a congenital malformation of the uterus is present should be considered in every patient with history of recurrent spontaneous abortions or recurrent preterm labor and in patients with recurrent malpresentations, such as breech and transverse lie. About 50% of the patients will benefit from surgical correction.

Fetal pathology

The possibility that the mother is carrying a fetus with major congenital abnormalities should always be considered when dealing with patients in preterm labor. Neural tube defects and inborn errors of metabolism, such as hyperalaninemia, are some of the birth defects found to be associated with preterm labor.

Anencephaly is a congenital defect traditionally associated with prolonged gestation. However, there is a wide range of gestational ages at delivery in anencephalic infants, and many of them are born after preterm labor. Potter's syndrome is another condition in which a majority of infants deliver early because of preterm labor.

Uterine overdistention

Stretching of the uterine muscle because of multifetal pregnancy or an excessive amount of amniotic fluid is another relatively common cause of preterm labor. Amniocentesis in these patients shows an elevated intrauterine pressure.

Preterm labor of unknown origin

It is not possible to establish precisely the etiology of preterm labor in approximately 20% to 30% of these patients. The search for the trigger of parturition in these patients is an area of active investigation.

◢ EPIDEMIOLOGY OF PRETERM LABOR

There are few studies on the epidemiology of preterm labor. Most of the available information is in relation to low birth weight deliveries or preterm births, but not specifically to preterm labor. In the material that follows, some of the variables associated with low birth weight or preterm deliveries are analyzed, and emphasis is placed on any existing relation between those variables and preterm labor.

Socioeconomic and ethnic factors

There is a strong association between low birth weight and low socioeconomic status. The best evidence on this association comes from England, where pregnant patients are classified according to their socioeconomic levels. Patients in classes I and II are in professional and managerial positions, those in class III are clerical workers, and those in classes IV and V are semiskilled and unskilled workers. The British Perinatal Mortality Survey[47] demonstrated that mothers in classes IV and V had a 10.9% incidence of preterm deliveries, in contrast to a 4.3% incidence in classes I and II. What is not known is how much of this increase is the consequence of preterm labor and how much is the consequence of an increased number of SGA infants. In developing countries as many as 50% of all low birth weight infants are SGA rather than preterm.

In the United States, low birth weight infants are more common in blacks (12.4%) and Puerto Ricans (9.1%) than in whites (5.8%). It is not known if the large incidence of low birth weight infants in the first two ethnic groups reflects a genetic or biologic predisposition or is a consequence of lower income, poor nutrition, less education, more physically demanding jobs, and other socioeconomic variables.

Maternal characteristics

An important maternal variable strongly associated with the birth of a baby weighing less than 2500 g is the weight of the mother before pregnancy. Women weighing less than 112 lb before pregnancy have 3 times as many low birth weight infants as mothers who weigh more than 126 lb before pregnancy.

Another significant association with low birth weight is maternal smoking during pregnancy. The incidence of births under 2500 g is twice as great for smokers as for nonsmokers. When large populations are compared, the mean decrease in infant birth weight for smokers is between 150 and 250 g, and the weight reduction is proportional to the number of cigarettes smoked per day.

A less significant association exists between birth weight and maternal age. This relation follows a reverse-J curve with a high frequency of small babies (15.8%) being born to mothers under 15 years of age. The incidence of low birth weight decreases with maternal age, reaching a minimum between 25 and 29 years of age (6.1%). Then it starts to rise, reaching a new peak (9.9%) when the maternal age is between 45 and 49 years.

The relation of occupation to low birth weight and preterm labor has been the subject of multiple studies. It seems that the specific conditions of a given work are more important than the fact of working during pregnancy. Some studies indicate that prolonged standing, longer hours of work, and physical fatigue during work are strong predictors of preterm labor.[48] It seems also that work at home is a risk factor as important as work outside of home.[49] However, another study suggests that working long hours in a stressful occupation has little effect on pregnancy outcome.[50]

Coitus during pregnancy

There is anecdotal evidence as well as some scientific data suggesting the existence of an association between coital activity during pregnancy and preterm labor. Goodlin et al.[43] found that the incidence of orgasms after 30 weeks of gestation was significantly higher in women delivering preterm than in a control group delivering at term. The same investigator asked five gravidas who claimed to be able to achieve orgasm at will to initiate orgasms with the purpose of inducing labor when they were at term. Four of these women were admitted in labor within 9 hours following orgasm, and the fifth had an episode of false labor. Naeye,[51] using data from the Collaborative Perinatal Project, has shown that the frequency of amniotic fluid infection in the presence of intact membranes was significantly larger in mothers who had coitus once or more per week during the month before delivery than in those mothers who did not have coitus. The implication of this study is that coital activity during pregnancy may be a factor facilitating the production of preterm labor. Other investigators also using the data from the Collaborative Perinatal Project have failed in demonstrating an association between coitus and adverse outcome of pregnancy.[52]

Obstetric factors

An important maternal variable associated with birth weight is weight gain during pregnancy. Mothers who gain between 25 and 30 lb during pregnancy have the best outcome, not only in terms of infant birth weight, but also in terms of neonatal morbidity and mortality. In contrast, lack of weight gain or weight loss during pregnancy is important indicator of the possibility of an SGA baby.

Another important correlation is the weight of a prior baby. If the prior baby had a birth weight under 2500 g, the possibility of having a small baby is 24.8% if the patient is white and 33% if the patient is black. This is in contrast to an incidence of 5.8% if the prior baby's weight was greater than 2500 g.

Another important factor is neonatal outcome in the prior pregnancy. If the last pregnancy ended in neonatal death, the chances of having a low birth weight baby are 21.8%. If the baby from the prior pregnancy is alive, the risk of a low birth weight baby is only 6.6%.

Other important historic factors associated with preterm birth are the number of spontaneous abortions, the number and characteristics of prior induced abortions, and the number of prior preterm deliveries. With respect to prior spontaneous abortions, the British data[53] indicate that the incidence of preterm delivery is not increased if the maternal history reveals only first-trimester abortions but increases significantly if there are as few as one mid-trimester abortion. In contrast, studies in the United States[54] have

shown that there is a 2.5 times increase in the incidence of low birth weight in women with a history of at least one spontaneous abortion.

With respect to the relation between induced abortions and preterm birth, the information in the literature is controversial. Initial reports from Hungary indicated a low birth weight incidence of 9.3% in mothers with no prior pregnancy termination. This incidence raised to 13% after one termination and to over 20% with three or more induced abortions. Studies from the United States contradict the Hungarian findings and suggest that there is no difference in pregnancy outcome between patients with and without histories of prior pregnancy terminations. It is possible that the discrepancy between these studies reflects differences in the technique used for pregnancy termination, the degree of forcible dilation of the cervix, and the existence of small but perhaps significant variations in gestational age at the time of abortion.

Everyone agrees that the highest risk for preterm birth exists in the woman with a history of one or more preterm deliveries. The risk of delivering a low birth weight infant is 36.7% for women with histories of preterm delivery plus one or more abortions and is 70% for women with histories of two or more preterm births.

◪ DIAGNOSIS OF PRETERM LABOR

The diagnosis of preterm labor has three components: (1) the identification of patients at risk for preterm labor, (2) the detection of early warning signs of preterm labor, and (3) the diagnosis of established preterm labor.

Identification of the patient at risk for preterm labor

The best predictor of preterm labor is a poor past reproductive performance. This makes it difficult to identify nulliparous patients at risk. This is disappointing because more than 40% of all preterm labor patients are nulliparous and the impact of preventative measures will not be optimal if they remain undetected.

Several factors associated with preterm labor were organized into a high-risk scoring system by Papiernik.[55] This scoring system was slightly modified by Gonik and Creasy[56] (Table 4-3). A patient with a score of 10 or more in the Papiernik scoring system is classified as being at high risk for preterm labor. It is controversial as

TABLE 4-3 ◪ Scoring system to identify patients at high risk for preterm labor

Points	Socioeconomic factors	Previous medical history	Daily habits	Aspects of current pregnancy
1	Two children at home Low socioeconomic status	Abortion × 1 Less than 1 yr since last birth	Works outside	Unusual fatigue
2	Maternal age < 20 yr or > 40 yr Single parent	Abortion × 2	Smokes more than 10 cigarettes per day More than 3 flights of stairs without elevator	Gain of < 5 kg by 32 wk
3	Very low socioeconomic status Height < 150 cm Weight < 45 kg	Abortion × 3	Heavy or stressful work that is long and tiring Long daily commuting Extensive traveling	Breech at 32 wk Weight loss Head engaged at 32 wk Febrile illness
4	Maternal age < 18 yr	Pyelonephritis		Bleeding after 12 wk Short cervix Opened internal os Uterine irritability
5		Uterine anomaly Second-trimester abortion DES exposure Cone biopsy		Placenta previa Hydramnios
10		Preterm delivery Repeated second-trimester abortion		Twins Abdominal surgical procedure

Adapted from Papiernik E: *Clin Obstet Gynecol* 1984;11:315 and Gonic B, Creasy RK: *Am J Obstet Gynecol* 1986; 154:3-8.

to whether the use of the Papiernik scoring system followed by intensive patient education and prenatal attention is effective in decreasing the incidence of preterm labor. Some investigators[57] have found this approach to the problem to be useful, whereas others[58,59] have found no benefit.

Early warning symptoms of preterm labor

The majority of patients who develop preterm labor have some of the warning symptoms shown in Box 4-1 several days or even weeks before the onset of regular contractions.[60,61] These warning symptoms are subtle, and the patient frequently ignores their importance. Every pregnant patient, and especially those identified by the Papiernik scoring system, should be taught to rec-

ognize these symptoms and to call their obstetricians when they occur. Women are 75% accurate in their ability to recognize warning symptoms of preterm labor.[62] However, the warning symptoms are unspecific and frequently are disregarded as a minor complaint or attributed to *round ligament pain* or *gastrointestinal flu.*

All obstetrical patients should be alerted early in the course of their pregnancies to:
1. The importance of excessive uterine activity and the early warning signs of preterm labor.
2. The dangers of using names to describe their contractions that give a false sense of security such as *false labor* and *Braxton-Hicks contractions.*[63]
3. Avoid attributing pelvic or abdominal discomfort to organs other than the uterus.

4. Report to the obstetrician immediately when early warning symptoms of excessive uterine activity are detected.

Cervical examination

If any of the warning symptoms or a combination of them occur, the obstetrician should proceed to a pelvic examination. This examination will help determine whether the patient's complaints are indicative of preterm labor or correspond to a minor problem. There are several studies indicating that patients destined to develop preterm labor can be identified by means of pelvic examination several weeks before the onset of major symptoms.[64,65]

During pelvic examination the obstetrician should assess the position, the length, and the consistency of the cervix and the development of the low uterine segment. When examined between 20 and 34 weeks of gestation, the large majority of nulliparous patients have cervices pointing posteriorly, closed, at least 2 cm long, and harder in consistency than any other vaginal or uterine tissues palpated during the examination. In the multiparous patient, the cervix may have varying degrees of effacement and dilation. However, multiparous patients with cervices 2 to 3 cm dilated by 28 weeks will have a 27% incidence of deliveries before 34 weeks compared with 2% in patients with cervices that are open 1 cm or less.[66]

All pregnant patients, regardless of their parity, stretch or develop their low uterine segments before parturition. When the low segment is not developed, it is possible to introduce the fingers into the vaginal fornices without problems. In contrast, when the low uterine segment is developed, the examiner will find that the upper third of the vagina is filled with the thinned low uterine segment. In many patients, development of the low segment occurs simultaneously with the engagement of the presenting part. The finding of a soft, short cervix and a developed low uterine segment indicates that contractions are affecting the cervix and tocolysis is necessary.

The importance of cervical changes as a predictor of preterm labor and delivery is such that it has been proposed that cervical examinations should be performed in all pregnant patients at every prenatal office visit during the late second and the early third trimesters. This practice is part of the routine antepartum care in several European countries, but not in the United States. Studies indicate that routine cervical examinations identify some patients before signs of preterm labor appear.[65,67,68] The sensitivity of this method in predicting preterm labor is 63% for nulliparous and 53% for multiparous patients.[69]

It is possible to obtain a more precise definition of cervical changes before preterm labor using ultrasound.[70] Transabdominal and endovaginal transducers may be used for this purpose, but the endovaginal method is better because the cervical length is not affected by the degree of bladder filling. The cervical length remains relatively constant between 12 and 36 weeks at 4.0 +/− 1.2 cm. Patients at risk for preterm labor show shortening of the cervix below 3 cm, widening of the endocervical canal, thinning of the low uterine segment, and bulging of the membranes in the endocervical canal.

Home monitoring of uterine activity

Home monitoring of uterine activity using data transmission devices has been recently introduced as a solution for the early detection of excessive uterine activity. The most important reason for the use of daily home monitoring is that many women, especially those with multifetal pregnancies, do not recognize their own uterine activity.[71] This makes it impossible for them to detect the increased number of contractions that precede preterm labor.[72] One controlled study[73] and a few uncontrolled observations have given support to the use of this system. Other controlled studies[74,75] have shown no difference in the rate of preterm labor and preterm delivery between patients monitored at home with telemetry devices and patients receiving education about preterm labor and using self-palpation for monitoring uterine activity.

For most patients, home uterine monitoring is not better than frequent nursing contact and support. However, patients who cannot recognize adequately the presence of contractions will certainly benefit from home monitoring. The inability to perceive contractions is particularly high in patients with multifetal pregnancies and with uterine overdistention caused by an excessive amount of fluid.

Home uterine monitoring is expensive. Its general application should wait for proof of its effectiveness and for cost-benefit analysis as compared with simpler and less expensive methods.

Diagnosis of established preterm labor

The diagnosis of established preterm labor is simple. It requires abnormal uterine activity and changes in cervical effacement and dilation. When this diagnosis is made, the chances for a significant prolongation of pregnancy are limited.

◼ MANAGEMENT OF PRETERM LABOR

The management of preterm labor depends on the presentation of the patient at the time the problem is identified. The majority of patients will belong to one of the following groups:

1. Patients at high risk for preterm labor (patients who have scores greater than 10 in the Papiernik scoring system)
2. Patients who develop warning symptoms of preterm labor
3. Patients in established preterm labor

Management of patients at high risk for preterm labor

Patients identified as high-risk for preterm labor by means of the scoring system of Papiernik require special attention during pregnancy. The following measures are recommended.

Education about preterm labor. The patient should be given a detailed explanation about the subtle nature of the early symptoms and signs of excessive uterine activity. The patient should be instructed to avoid self-diagnosis of *round ligament pain, false labor, Braxton-Hicks contractions,* and *intestinal flu* and to call

in the event of any pain or discomfort below the costal margin. Smoking should be prohibited.

Aggressive treatment of vaginal and cervical infections. Treating infections may be the most important preventative measure in patients at risk for preterm labor. Women with bacterial vaginosis are prone to develop intraamniotic infection.[76] Patients at risk for preterm labor should have a speculum examination, and vaginitis or chronic cervicitis should be treated immediately.

Vaginal infections with *Gardnerella vaginalis* should be treated aggressively. Characteristically, this infection does not produce any burning or pain, and the most significant symptom is the presence of a watery discharge that sometimes has a foul smell. On examination, the vaginal pH is 5.0 or more, and the wet smear shows a large number of bacteria, few leukocytes, and clue cells. The treatment of choice is metronidazole, 500 mg twice daily for 7 days. This medication is safe during pregnancy after 12 weeks of gestation. The second choice for the treatment of *Gardnerella vaginalis* is ampicillin, 500 mg 4 times daily for 7 days. For penicillin-sensitive patients, ampicillin may be substituted by erythromycin, 250 mg 4 times daily for 7 days.

It is very important to obtain clinical and bacteriologic evidence of the success of the treatment in patients treated for vaginitis or cervicitis. If the infection persists, it is necessary to reevaluate the microbiology of the infection, to use a different treatment, or to treat the husband who may be a source of reinfection.

Occasionally, the only evidence of cervical infection is the presence of thick, yellow mucus that is very adherent to the endocervical glands and bleed when removed with a piece of cotton. These findings should raise the suspicion of *Chlamydia* infection. All pregnant patients and especially those at high risk for preterm labor should have diagnostic tests for *C. trachomatis* at the initial visit and be treated with amoxicillin or erythromycin if the test is positive.[77]

Even if there is no evidence of infection of the vagina or the cervix on visual inspection, cultures should be obtained for group B streptococcus, and chlamydia. Group B streptococcus is sensitive to treatment with penicillin. Chlamydia responds well to erythromycin, 250 to 500 mg 4 times daily for 7 days. Alternative treatment is trimethoprim/sulfamethoxazole, 160 and 800 mg respectively, twice daily for 10 days.

A recent study[78] found no correlation between antepartum cultures for *Ureaplasma urealyticum* and preterm labor, preterm delivery, or preterm rupture of the membranes. Another study found no difference in outcome in patients with *U. urealyticum,* treated or not with erythromycin.[79] Therefore, cervical cultures for *Ureaplasma* and mycoplasma are not recommended at this time.

Frequent pelvic examinations. All patients at high risk for preterm labor, and especially those who *do not* complain of excessive uterine activity, should have pelvic examinations at each prenatal visit. Some patients have difficulty perceiving or identifying contractions, and the only way to find out that they are occurring is by periodic pelvic examinations or by home uterine monitoring.

Serial ultrasound examinations. The patient at high risk for preterm labor should be monitored by means of ultrasound examinations every 4 weeks starting at 16 weeks. The purpose of these examinations is to detect inadequate fetal growth, decreased amniotic fluid, or a prematurely calcified placenta. These are signs suggesting that placental insufficiency is the reason behind the patient's tendency toward preterm labor. Also, evaluation of cervical length with ultrasound seems to be a promising approach for the identification of patients at high risk.

Coital abstinence. There is evidence suggesting the existence of a relationship between coital activity during pregnancy and preterm labor. This should be explained to the woman at risk for preterm delivery and to her husband. Discontinuation of coital activity is mandatory if the patient has noticed strong contractions after coitus or at the time of orgasm.

Limitation of physical activity. Most pregnant women at risk for preterm delivery notice a relationship between increased physical activity and the occurrence of preterm contractions. They should be counseled to avoid strenuous activities, to avoid exercise, and to rest in the lateral supine position every time they have an opportunity to do so.

Change in working conditions. There are studies indicating that working conditions are related to preterm labor. Modification of working conditions is indicated in pregnant women who:

Work 8 or more hours without interruption
Work more than 5 days per week
Work standing up on their feet most of the time

BOX 4-2

Management of Patients at Risk for Preterm Labor

Education about preterm labor
Aggressive treatment of cervical and vaginal infections
Frequent pelvic examinations
Serial ultrasound examinations
Coital abstinence
Limitation of physical activity
Change in working conditions

Work with vibrating instruments
Perform monotonous, repetitive work (assembly lines, factories)

A summary of the management measures for patients at risk for preterm labor is shown in Box 4-2.

Management of patients with warning signs of preterm labor

Patients who develop warning signs of preterm labor have reached a dangerous stage because progression of the symptoms will lead to established preterm labor and decreased opportunity for effective treatment. Pharmacologic intervention at this stage is necessary.

Antibiotics. With growing evidence indicating that in a significant number of patients preterm labor is caused by decidual-amniotic infection, intervention with antibiotics in the early stages of the process is logical. Trials of antibiotic treatment in patients in preterm labor have given contradictory results. Eschenbach et al.[79] and Newton et al.[81] found no benefits, but Morales et al.[80] and McGregor et al.[80a] demonstrated significant pregnancy prolongation in women in preterm labor treated with ampicillin and clindamycin.

It is possible that antibiotics are effective only when treatment is initiated early in the infectious process. When the infection has advanced to the point of causing focal tissue necrosis or involves the amniotic membranes, the chances of success are limited.

With respect to which antibiotics to be used, a combination of erythromycin and clindamycin will adequately cover the large majority of the bacteria implicated in the production of preterm labor. Metronidazole and trimethoprim/sulfamethoxazole are good second choices.

Prophylactic tocolysis. Tocolysis is indicated in patients with warning signs of preterm labor because stopping uterine contractions may prevent further cervical effacement and the loss of the mucous plug. Administration of tocolytic agents under these circumstances has been designated as *prohylactic* and is discouraged by many authorities because of the lack of evidence proving their efficacy. Despite this lack of support from the academic community, the prophylactic use of tocolytic agents is generalized throughout the world. Patients feel that their contractions are being treated, and doctors feel that they are doing something for their patients.

All pharmacologic agents used to inhibit preterm uterine contractions act by affecting intracellular calcium concentration in the myometrium. Some of them promote the extrusion of calcium from the cell (beta-adrenergic agents and indomethacin), some displace calcium (magnesium sulfate), and some block the entrance of calcium into the myometrial cells (calcium channel blockers). Indomethacin acts also by inhibiting prostaglandin production.

Beta-adrenergic agents. In the early stages of excessive uterine contractility, a low dose of any beta-adrenergic agent may be sufficient to decrease the frequency and intensity of contractions. The medications most frequently used are terbutaline, 2.5 mg orally every 6 hours, and ritodrine, 20 mg orally every 6 hours. The dosage can be increased up to 5 mg of terbutaline or 40 mg of ritodrine every 4 hours. At the higher dosage, these medications cause side effects poorly tolerated by some patients.

Patients in oral beta-adrenergic therapy should be instructed to take their pulse before each dose of medication and to postpone the new dose until the pulse rate is under 100 beats per minute (bpm). There is a direct relationship between the blood levels of these agents and the pulse rate. Patients should know that once the pulse rate reaches 120 bpm, more than 90% of their beta-2-adrenergic receptors are saturated, the benefit obtained with an additional dose of medication would be minimal, and the possibility of serious side effects would be increased. Monitoring the pulse rate is also useful for identifying the rare patient who is resistant to the pharmacologic effect of beta-adrenergic agents. If the patient reports that her pulse rate is below 80

bpm when she is due for a dose, she should be asked to monitor her pulse rate 1 hour and 2 hours after she takes the medication. If there is only an increase of 10 bpm or less in pulse rate 1 and 2 hours after taking the medication, the dose of terbutaline or ritodrine can be increased. We have occasionally seen patients taking 7.5 mg of terbutaline every 4 hours without increasing their heart rate above 100 bpm.

Calcium channel blockers. In the last few years, the calcium channel blocker nifedipine has been added to the armamentarium for the treatment of excessive uterine activity. Nifedipine is an effective tocolytic agent that is well tolerated by the majority of pregnant patients. No significant fetal problems after treatment with nifedipine have been reported up to the time of this writing. The medication is given orally and the starting dosage is 10 mg every 6 hours. The dosage can be increased up to 20 mg every 4 hours, but at this high dosage the incidence of side effects is high. The most common side effect is lowering of the blood pressure, causing patients to feel unusually tired. Another side effect seen in a small number of patients is a sensation of facial flushing. Nifedipine does not have marked effects on carbohydrate metabolism and can be given to diabetic pregnant patients without fear of hyperglycemia or hypoglycemia. It does not cause alterations in the cardiac rhythm and can be given to pregnant patients with symptomatic mitral valve prolapse or with mild or moderate supraventricular arrhythmias. Nifedipine is an excellent drug for patients with chronic hypertension and preterm contractions because the medication is also an antihypertensive agent.

Calcium channel blockers and beta-adrenergic agents have an additive effect, and low doses of both medications administered simultaneously may produce better uterine relaxation and fewer side effects than a single agent given in large doses.

Magnesium salts. Oral magnesium salts are an alternative to beta-adrenergic agents for the prophylactic treatment of preterm contractions.[82] Magnesium gluconate is used in doses of 1 g orally every 4 to 6 hours. Magnesium oxide is given in doses of 200 mg every 3 to 4 hours. Enteric-coated magnesium chloride is given in doses of 535 mg every 4 hours.[83] At this dosage the magnesium blood level does not increase beyond 2.5 mg/dl.[84] The effectiveness of oral magnesium for ambulatory tocolysis is similar to that of terbutaline and ritodrine.[81,82,84]

Oral magnesium is most commonly used in patients unable to tolerate increases in their dosage of terbutaline or nifedipine. The addition of magnesium to their treatment may be effective in arresting uterine irritability despite the marginal increase achieved in serum magnesium levels. There are no significant side effects of oral magnesium administration. The most common complaints are increased thirst and diarrhea.

Progesterone. The use of progesterone for the prevention of preterm labor is controversial. However, two recent meta-analyses of the literature indicate that progestational agents reduce the occurrence of preterm birth.[85,86] Progesterone is widely used for the prevention of miscarriages, but both meta-analyses concluded that the hormone is not useful for this purpose. Used in combination with ritodrine in a double-blind trial, progesterone significantly reduced the mean duration of the intravenous perfusion and the mean quantity of beta-adrenergic agents administered.

The tocolytic properties of progesterone are probably the result of its antagonistic effect on prostaglandin F_2-alpha,[87] to alpha-adrenergic stimulation,[88] and its ability to block the development of gap junctions necessary for the propagation of muscular activity.[89]

Natural progesterone is completely innocuous for mother and fetus. It is available in solutions for IM injection and in rectal or vaginal suppositories, micronized capsules for oral ingestion, and sublingual tablets. The micronized form is the simplest to administer and is used in a dosage of 50 mg every 8 to 12 hours.

Bed rest. Bed rest in the lateral position usually decreases the frequency and intensity of uterine contractions. Patients with warning symptoms of preterm labor frequently report significant improvement when they stop working and rest at home. However, controlled studies on the role of bed rest on preterm labor have produced conflicting results. It is possible that some of these studies involve heterogeneous patient populations, with different etiologies for their preterm labor and at different stages in the severity of the process.

Search for placental insufficiency. Placental insufficiency is the second largest cause of preterm labor. A careful search for signs of placental insufficiency is necessary in every patient

---

BOX 4-3

Management of Patients with Warning Symptoms of Preterm Labor

Antibiotics
Prophylactic tocolysis
 Oral beta-adrenergic agents
 Calcium channel blockers
 Magnesium sulfate
 Progesterone
Bed rest
Search for placental insufficiency

---

who develops warning signs of preterm labor. Signs of placental insufficiency may be subtle and require a meticulous search. The most common finding is a fetal size 1 or 2 weeks behind what is expected for the gestational age. The tendency is to consider a small discrepancy between dates and fetal size as a result of the variability of ultrasound measurements. However, in the patient with warning signs of preterm labor small discrepancies are significant. Other signs alerting the obstetrician to the possibility of placental insufficiency are the presence of a prematurely aged placenta, the presence of intravascular volume constriction, a decrease in the normal amount of amniotic fluid, and Doppler studies indicating high resistance to flow.

A summary of the management of patients with warning symptoms of preterm labor is shown in Box 4-3.

Management of patients with established preterm labor

The possibilities of obtaining a significant prolongation of pregnancy for patients admitted to the hospital with regular uterine contractions and with demonstrable cervical changes are limited. Also, in a majority of these patients, prolongation of pregnancy offers no fetal advantages because preterm labor is a protection mechanism when the fetus is threatened by problems such as infection or placental insufficiency.

Because of the inability to obtain a significant prolongation of pregnancy and the possibility that prolongation of pregnancy may be harmful to the fetus, the management of established preterm labor is usually limited to selecting those patients who may benefit from glucocorticoid

---

BOX 4-4

Management of Patients with Established Preterm Labor

Identification of patients that need to be delivered

Maternal disease
Advanced labor
Fetal congenital abnormalities
Fetal growth retardation
Chromosomal abnormalities
Adequate fetal lung maturity

Treatment

IV tocolysis
    Beta-adrenergic agents
    Magnesium sulfate
    Diazoxide
Indomethacin
Glucocorticoids
Phenobarbital
Vitamin K_1

---

therapy and to adopting measures that may decrease newborn morbidity. To accomplish these goals, it is best to follow a sequence of decision-making steps, as indicated in Box 4-4.

Identification of patients that need to be delivered. The first step in identifying patients that need to be delivered is to determine if there are maternal or fetal conditions indicating that preterm labor should not be interrupted. These conditions are discussed below.

Maternal disease. The history and physical examination are important in identifying mothers with chronic or acute illnesses that will not benefit from tocolysis. The presence of hyperthyroidism, chronic hypertension, preeclampsia, chronic renal disease, systemic lupus or any other connective tissue disorder, sickle cell disease, cardiac disease causing moderate or severe functional impairment or the finding of any acute or chronic infectious disease process or any other significant maternal medical complication will be an indication for delivery.

Advanced labor. The initial evaluation will identify patients with cervical dilation 5 cm or greater, 100% effaced, and with membranes bulging. Many of these patients are infected, the possibilities of arresting labor are limited, and the incidence of severe side effects of tocolytic

therapy is high. Therefore, labor should be allowed to continue.

Fetal congenital abnormalities. Lethal abnormalities such as anencephaly, acrania, osteogenesis imperfecta, and bilateral renal agenesis are better treated by allowing preterm labor to continue. Other abnormalities, not necessarily lethal, such as severe nonimmunological fetal hydrops, severe skeletal dysplasias, hypoplastic left heart, severe gastroschisis with herniation of the liver or heart into the amniotic cavity, microcephaly, and large meningomyeloceles are also better treated by allowing delivery. However, in situations such as diaphragmatic hernia, omphalocele, and some cardiac lesions in which the congenital defect may be treated successfully after birth, prolongation of pregnancy may help to improve survival and decrease morbidity. In general, if the fetus of a patient in preterm labor has gross congenital anatomic deformities, the advantages of prolongation of pregnancy should be critically questioned.

Fetal growth retardation. A uterine fundal height inappropriate for the gestational age, decreased amount of amniotic fluid, fetal measurements inappropiate for the gestational age, abnormal fetal femur-to-abdomen ratio or head-to-abdomen ratio, premature calcification of the placenta, and abnormal Doppler studies are findings suggestive of the possibility of fetal growth retardation. In these cases preterm labor has a survival value for the fetus and should not be interrupted.

Chromosomal abnormalities. When fetal growth retardation is detected, it is important to consider that the defective growth may be caused by a chromosomal abnormality. The presence of a lethal autosomal trisomy (11, 18) is a contraindication to inhibition of labor and to cesarean delivery.

The presence of nonlethal but severe chromosomal abnormalities (i.e., trisomy 21) requires a search for associated anatomic defects that are common in these fetuses. Preterm labor in fetuses with trisomy 21 should be managed the same way as it is in a normal fetus.

Chorioamnionitis. Overt chorioamnionitis occurs in 10% or less of patients in established preterm labor. However, it is of prime importance to rule out the presence of this condition. Patients suspected of having chorioamnionitis are those with uterine tenderness, temperature elevation, fetal tachycardia, and resistance to tocolytic agents. The presence of chorioamnionitis may be confirmed by finding bacteria in the Gram stain of the amniotic fluid. In these cases the pregnancy should be delivered.

The diagnosis of chorioamnionitis in a patient in preterm labor is an indication for discontinuation of tocolysis, initiation of antibiotic treatment, and delivery. Trials of antibiotic treatment in this situation have given disappointing results. Once the infection has reached the magnitude necessary to cause definite symptoms and signs of preterm labor, the chances of success with antibiotic therapy are limited.

Subclinical chorioamnionitis occurs in a few patients in preterm labor who have no clinical evidence of infection. Usually, these patients continue with contractions, develop PROM, or show signs of infection shortly after admission.

The patient with chorioamnionitis should be treated with IV antibiotics, and steps should be taken for delivery as soon as the diagnosis is made. There is evidence in the literature indicating that mother and baby do better when antibiotics are initiated before rather than after delivery.[90] We prefer aztreonam, 2 g intravenous piggyback (IVPB) every 8 hours, and ampicillin/sulbactam, 3 g IVPB every 8 hours.

Adequate fetal pulmonary maturity. On some occasions physical examination and ultrasound evaluation of the patient in preterm labor reveal a fetus with a size larger than expected for the gestational age. In these cases an error in dating should be suspected, and amniocentesis should be performed to determine whether the fetus is mature.

On other occasions the amniotic fluid shows adequate fetal lung maturity at an early gestational age. This usually happens in patients with placental insufficiency. If the fetal lungs are mature or close to mature, delivery is indicated.

Treatment. Patients identified as not needing delivery are a group without overt maternal or fetal infection, without advanced cervical changes, and with fetal pulmonary immaturity demonstrated by amniocentesis. Management of these patients involves tocolysis, antibiotics, glucocorticoids, phenobarbital, and delivery.

The evaluation of the patient in preterm labor is not complete until a careful search for the presence or absence of fetal breathing movements is completed. This is important for prognosis as to the likely success of tocolytic

therapy. In fact, there are several papers in the literature[91,92] indicating that when fetal breathing movements are present, the patient is responsive to therapy. The absence of fetal breathing movements correlates with unresponsiveness to tocolysis.

Intravenous tocolysis. There is no evidence that therapeutic tocolysis achieves a substantial prolongation of pregnancy.[93] However, intravenous tocolytic agents are widely used in patients in established preterm labor. The decision to use these agents in the patient in established preterm labor should be determined by the following considerations:

1. Administration of tocolytic agents should never cause severe maternal side effects.
2. The main objective of treatment is to keep patients undelivered for the short time necessary for glucocorticoid treatment.

The first consideration is of the utmost importance. IV tocolysis is a therapeutic modality of questionable efficacy that has the potential for serious maternal side effects. The principle of *primum non nocere* should always be applied when IV tocolysis is being contemplated.

BETA-ADRENERGIC AGENTS. Intravenous beta-adrenergic agents are the usual first choice for the treatment of patients in established preterm labor. These powerful medications are contraindicated in several conditions and have bothersome and potentially dangerous side effects. One of the most common contraindications is the presence of maternal cardiac disease. The decrease in afterload and the increased inotropic effect of these agents may precipitate cardiac failure in the pregnant patient with heart disease. Signs and symptoms of cardiac failure and anginal pain may complicate therapy with beta-adrenergic agents if the mother has a hyperdynamic circulation caused by hyperthyroidism or sickle cell disease.

Pulmonary edema is a serious complication of beta-adrenergic therapy. This complication occurs in patients receiving oral or intravenous treatment, although it is more frequent in the latter group. It occurs more frequently in patients who have excessive plasma volume expansion, such as those with twins or those who have received generous amounts of intravenous fluids. It also occurs more frequently in patients who have chorioamnionitis. The clinical picture is one of respiratory distress, bilateral rales on auscultation of the lungs, pink frothy sputum, and typical x-ray picture. Patients receiving IV beta-adrenergic drugs should be monitored continuously with pulse oximetry to anticipate the production of pulmonary edema.

In the majority of cases, treatment of pulmonary edema associated with beta-adrenergic therapy is simple and produces excellent results. As soon as the diagnosis is made, the patient should be given oxygen by mask or nasal prongs and treated with intravenous furosemide (20 mg initially, to be repeated several times depending on the clinical response). With these simple measures, the majority of patients have a brisk diuresis and then a dramatic response in their respiratory status.

Patients with insulin-dependent diabetes are also at high risk for complications with beta-adrenergic therapy. These patients develop significant hyperglycemia, glycosuria, and ketonuria and require considerable increases in the amount and frequency of insulin administration. This effect of beta-adrenergic agents is the consequence of exaggerated glycogenolysis and accelerated lipolysis. Usually patients with diet-controlled gestational diabetes require subcutaneous insulin, and patients with insulin-dependent diabetes usually require continuous intravenous insulin to maintain adequate blood sugar control. Beta-adrenergic agents are contraindicated in the unstable pregnant diabetic. In stable pregnant diabetic patients, they may be used, but frequent monitoring of blood sugar and electrolyte plasma concentration, as well as aggressive insulin therapy, is necessary.

Another group of patients in whom the administration of beta-adrenergic agents is contraindicated is patients with chorioamnionitis. Also, patients receiving monoamine oxidase inhibitors for the treatment of psychiatric disorders have difficulties in metabolizing these agents. Finally, asthmatic patients already taking beta-adrenergic agents may develop tachyphylaxis when receiving an increased dosage of the medication. There is evidence that prolonged use of these agents leads to destruction of beta-adrenergic receptor sites and production of drug resistance. A summary of the relative contraindications to beta-adrenergic agents is shown in Box 4-5.

To be given IV, terbutaline is dissolved in lactated Ringer's solution and started at 5 μg per minute. The initial dosage is increased gradually until a dosage adequate to stop uterine contrac-

---

BOX 4-5

Contraindications to the Use of Intravenous Beta-adrenergic Agents for the Treatment of Patients With Established Preterm Labor

Symptomatic cardiac disease, especially ventricular outflow obstruction
Symptomatic cardiac rhythm or conduction disturbances
Hyperthyroidism
Sickle cell disease
Uncontrolled insulin-dependent diabetes
Chorioamnionitis
Eclampsia or severe preeclampsia
Multifetal gestation
Severe obstetrical bleeding
Severe anemia
Patients on monoamino oxidase inhibitors
Asthmatic patients already taking beta-adrenergic agents

---

tions is found or until side effects are intolerable (Box 4-6). Another beta-adrenergic drug commonly used in the United States is ritodrine. A protocol for the intravenous use of ritodrine is in Box 4-7.

It is desirable to obtain a serum potassium determination before the initiation of IV beta-adrenergic therapy and at approximately 6-hour intervals during the duration of therapy. Serum potassium usually drops 0.5 to 1.0 mEq/L in the first few hours of treatment and remains at this level or decreases another 1.0 mEq/L during the next 24 hours. There is no agreement as to the need to treat the drop in potassium levels. Some authorities believe that it is unnecessary to give potassium and restore its plasma concentration to normal values. It is preferable to maintain the potassium serum concentration close to normal and give 40 to 80 mEq of potassium in one of the IV fluids bottles if the concentration falls under 3.0 mEq/L.

The hematocrit/hemoglobin values of patients in preterm labor should be measured before initiation of IV beta-adrenergic therapy. If moderate-to-severe anemia exists, it should be corrected because anemia decreases blood viscosity and may be an important contributory factor to high-output cardiac failure. Also, water and electrolytes are retained, and this causes decrease in

---

BOX 4-6

Use of Terbutaline in the Treatment of Preterm Labor

Preparation of solution

Dissolve 5 ampules of terbutaline (5 mg) in 500 ml of Ringer's lactate solution. This preparation contains 10 μg of terbutaline per milliliter.

Continuous intravenous infusion

Using a Harvard pump, start IV infusion at a rate of 5 μg/min (0.5 ml/min; 30 ml/hr). Increase every 10 minutes by 5 μg/min (0.17 ml/min; 10.2 ml/hr) until a rate of 15 μg/min (1.5 mL/min; 90 ml/hr) is reached. If contractions have not disappeared with this dose, a double-strength solution (5 mg in 250 ml of Ringer's lactate solution) should be prepared to avoid excessive intravenous fluid administration. Further increases should continue until contractions disappear, toxicity appears, maternal pulse rate exceeds 120 bpm, or a dose of 30 μg/min is reached. Once an adequate dose is reached, it should be maintained for 12 hours after the contractions stop. Do not taper down before switching to oral or subcutaneous treatment.

Subcutaneous treatment

Discontinue the infusion of terbutaline IV, and 15 minutes later give 250 μg subcutaneously. Continue giving the same amount every 3 to 4 hours as necessary to keep the pulse rate between 100 and 120 bpm.

Oral treatment

Give a 5 mg tablet of terbutaline, and 30 minutes later discontinue the intravenous or subcutaneous administration. Give the same dosage every 4 hours for the first 24 hours as long as the pulse rate does not exceed 120 bpm. Then adjust the dosage to 2.5 to 5.0 mg every 3 to 6 hours depending on the patient's response to therapy.

BOX 4-7

Use of Ritodrine in the Treatment of Preterm Labor

Preparation of solution

Dissolve 3 ampules of ritodrine (150 mg) in 500 ml of D_5W Ringer's lactate solution. The preparation contains 300 μg of ritodrine per milliliter.

Continuous intravenous infusion

Using a Harvard pump, start intravenous infusion at a rate of 100 μg/min (0.33 ml/min; 20 ml/hr). Increase every 10 minutes by 50 μg/min (0.17 ml/min; 10.2 ml/hr) until the contractions stop, the pulse rate exceeds 120 bpm, toxicity appears, or a maximal rate of 350 μg/min (1.17 ml/min; 102 ml/hr) is reached. Once an adequate dose is reached, it should be maintained for 12 hours after the contractions stop. Do not taper down before switching to the oral treatment.

Oral treatment

Give one tablet of ritodrine (10 mg), and 30 minutes later discontinue the intravenous infusion. Continue the administration of one tablet every 2 hours for the first 24 hours after intravenous treatment as long as the pulse rate does not exceed 120 bpm. Then adjust the dosage, and use 10 to 20 mg every 4 to 6 hours as necessary.

hematocrit/hemoglobin levels and in blood viscosity. Drops in hematocrit/hemoglobin levels during IV beta-adrenergic therapy indicate significant increase in plasma volume, which may precede the development of pulmonary edema.

The plasma glucose concentration should be measured before and every 6 hours after initiation of IV beta-adrenergic therapy. A mild elevation to levels below 200 mg/dl is almost universal. This elevation is more marked in patients with gestational and insulin-dependent diabetes. Persistent elevations above 200 mg/dl require treatment with subcutaneous or IV insulin.

CONTINUOUS SUBCUTANEOUS ADMINISTRATION OF TERBUTALINE. Continuous subcutaneous administration of low-dose terbutaline using precision minipumps is a therapeutic modality being introduced into obstetric practice without controlled studies demonstrating its usefulness, indications, and side effects. This mode of therapy is experimental, potentially dangerous, and is being aggressively marketed at an exorbitant cost for the patient.

MAGNESIUM SULFATE. The use of magnesium sulfate for the treatment of preterm labor originated because of the observation that this medication causes decrease in the frequency and intensity of contractions in preeclamptic patients in labor. Also, the medication has a quiescent effect on isolated myometrial strips. Finally, magnesium use may be indicated because patients who develop preterm labor have significantly lower magnesium levels than control patients.[94]

Magnesium sulfate in tocolysis is used mainly for patients who have contraindications to beta-adrenergic agents, particularly pregnant diabetics. Magnesium sulfate has no inotropic effect on the heart and is the first choice for preterm labor treatment in patients with cardiac abnormalities. The medication, however, is a volume expander and should be used with caution in patients with valvular disease.

The main problems with the use of magnesium sulfate as a tocolytic agent have to do with its effectiveness and with maternal and fetal side effects. One randomized study involving 156 women treated with IV magnesium sulfate in doses resulting in a mean serum concentration of 5.5 +/− 1.4 mg/L concluded that the drug was ineffective in preventing preterm delivery.[95] Other studies have reached opposite conclusions, and a comparison of magnesium sulfate vs. terbutaline and ritodrine shows that none of these drugs is more effective than the others in arresting preterm labor. This is particularly true when preterm labor has not caused more than 2 cm of cervical dilation. If the cervix is dilated beyond 2 cm, terbutaline or ritodrine is more effective than magnesium sulfate in arresting labor.

The most frequent side effects of magnesium sulfate are pulmonary edema, hypothermia, and neuromuscular toxicity. Intravenous administration of magnesium sulfate causes a significant increase in plasma osmolarity that is compensated for by mobilization of fluid into the intravascular space. This expansion of plasma volume is significant in patients with other factors predisposing them to pulmonary edema such as infection and twins.

The neuromuscular toxicity of magnesium sulfate is well known. Because of this toxicity, blood levels of the medication should be checked periodically, and maternal reflexes and respirations should be closely monitored. The neuromuscular toxicity of magnesium can be reversed quickly by intravenous administration of calcium gluconate.

Hypothermia is a rare complication of magnesium sulfate administration. When it occurs, it causes fetal bradycardia. Maternal hypothermia reverses in a few hours after discontinuation of magnesium administration.

The dosage of magnesium sulfate used for tocolysis is similar to the dosage used for the treatment of preeclampsia (Box 4-8). The initial dose is 6 g, given slowly in no fewer than 20 minutes. Maintenance dosage is usually 2 g per hour, but many patients need as much as 3 g per hour to stop their contractions. Magnesium therapy should continue for at least 48 hours in the lowest effective dose to keep the patient from having contractions.

It is important to avoid fluid overload in patients receiving IV magnesium. Total IV fluids in 24 hours should not exceed 3000 ml. Reflexes and respiration rate should be monitored every hour. Although there is no relation between the maternal serum magnesium levels and the success of tocolysis,[96] magnesium serum levels should be measured every 6 hours, and the concentration of the medication should be maintained within therapeutic range (5.5 to 7.5 mEq/L) to avoid maternal toxicity.

Magnesium concentration in the fetus and the neonate are similar to maternal levels. This translates clinically into decreased long-term fetal heart rate variability and into central nervous

---

BOX 4-8

Magnesium Sulfate for the Treatment of Patients in Established Preterm Labor

Loading dose

Six grams (50 ml of 10% solution) added to 100 ml of normal saline, given IVPB in no less than 30 minutes

Maintenance dose

Two to 3 g per hour depending on the response to therapy and the magnesium blood levels

Monitor

- Urine output (should be at least 30 ml/hr)
- Deep tendon reflexes (should be present and 1+ to 2+)
- Respiration rate (should be 15 per minute or more)
- Temperature

Magnesium blood levels

Therapeutic	5 to 8 mEq/L
Loss of deep tendon reflexes	10 mEq/L
Respiratory failure	12 mEq/L

---

system depression and hypocalcemia in the neonate. Infants of mothers treated with IV magnesium sulfate shortly before delivery are frequently hypotonic at birth and require respiratory support until the magnesium is eliminated.

DIAZOXIDE. Diazoxide is a medication structurally related to the thiazide diuretics that is used in the treatment of hypertensive crisis. Diazoxide inhibits the contractility of arterial and venous smooth muscle. The drug also inhibits respiratory, gastrointestinal, and genitourinary smooth muscle, and the latter action is responsible for its effectiveness as a tocolytic agent.

The most common maternal side effects of diazoxide administration are hypotension, tachycardia, hyperglycemia, and decreased uteroplacental blood flow caused by maternal hypotension. The most important fetal side effects are hyperglycemia and fetal distress resulting from decreased uteroplacental perfusion.

To avoid severe maternal and fetal side effects, it is necessary to expand the maternal intravascular volume before diazoxide administration. For most patients, 500 to 1000 ml of lactated Ringer's or normal saline solution constitutes adequate hydration before diazoxide administration.

The dosage of diazoxide is 5 mg/kg (300 mg for patients with weights around 130 lb, 400 mg for patients with weights around 150 lb). The medication should be given intravenously, slowly, in 15 to 30 minutes. To achieve this, 1 ampule of diazoxide is dissolved in 250 ml of half-normal saline solution and given IVPB in 30 minutes. The medication also can be given safely in small boluses of 50 to 100 mg every 5 minutes. The patient should be in the lateral recumbent or in slight Trendelenburg position while the medication is being administered. Continuous monitoring of maternal blood pressure and heart rate, uterine activity, and fetal heart rate is necessary.

In the experience of Adamsons and Wallach at the University of Puerto Rico,[97] diazoxide will totally eliminate uterine contractions within 15 minutes after its administration. The duration of action of the medication varies from patient to patient, and in many cases one single dose stops uterine activity indefinitely. If labor recurs, a second dose may be administered. If the effect of the second dose lasts for a shorter time than the first dose, further efforts with diazoxide or with any other tocolytic agents are doomed to fail, and it is better to allow the patient to deliver without further tocolytic therapy.

INDOMETHACIN. Indomethacin is the best available tocolytic agent but is not used as a first-line medication because of concerns over hemodynamic effects on the fetus. One study found that 7 of 14 fetuses of mothers taking indomethacin had constriction of the ductus arteriosus.[98] The presence of ductal constriction was inferred from Doppler measurements indicating increased blood flow velocity. Also, there are a few case reports of babies born after indomethacin treatment that have developed pulmonary hypertension and early closure of their ductus. Finally, if used for prolonged periods, indomethacin may adversely decrease fetal urinary output and cause oligohydramnios.[99] The fetal hemodynamic alterations are rapidly reversible after the medication is discontinued. Most babies born to patients treated with indomethacin during pregnancy do not show any significant cardiovascular complications.[100,101] The sensitivity of the fetal ductus to indomethacin decreases with gestational age, and the drug is probably safe when used before 32 weeks.

The initial dose of indomethacin is a 50- or 100-mg rectal suppository. This is followed by 25 mg orally every 4 or 6 hours. Treatment is usually continued for 3 days. At the end of this period, treatment may continue if the ultrasound examination shows normal fluid volume and no tricuspid regurgitation. If any of these abnormalities are present, a different tocolytic agent should be used for maintenance treatment.

ANTIBIOTICS. The use of antibiotics to arrest the infectious process causing preterm labor is ineffective when applied to patients with established preterm labor. Once the infectious process has advanced to the point of full activation of the mechanism of labor, antibiotics are ineffective in achieving prolongation of pregnancy.

GLUCOCORTICOIDS. Once the patient with established preterm labor has been started on tocolytic treatment, it is necessary to evaluate whether she is a suitable candidate for glucocorticoid treatment for the purpose of accelerating the maturation of the fetal lungs. The most common contraindication to the use of glucocorticoids is the presence of chorioamnionitis.

Depp et al.[102] have categorized the patients who are candidates for glucocorticoid administration into three groups: (1) patients deriving no benefit, (2) patients receiving minimal benefit, and (3) patients having maximal benefit. This analysis must be performed in every patient treated for preterm labor, and glucocorticoid administration should be limited to those patients who are going to obtain maximal benefit from their use.

Patients who will not receive benefit from glucocorticoid treatment include those in whom the drug is contraindicated, those with adequate fetal pulmonary maturity, and those who will deliver their babies in less than 24 hours or more than 7 days after receiving the steroid. Patients who will have minimal benefit from glucocorticoid administration are those with more than 34 weeks of gestation and an unknown state of fetal lung maturity. Patients who will have maximal benefit from glucocorticoid administration are those under 34 weeks of gestation, with immature fetal lungs, and who will deliver their babies more than 24 hours and less than 7 days after steroid treatment.

In the study of Depp et al.,[102] 84.7% of their patients at risk for preterm delivery and between 28 and 33 weeks of gestation and 94.3% of those between 34 and 37 weeks were excluded from steroid treatment. The most common reason for

exclusion was a predicted time of delivery less than 24 hours or more than 7 days from the time of treatment. This prediction was correct in a large majority of the cases. Only 10.9% of all patients were considered to be ideal candidates for glucocorticoid therapy.

A mixture of betamethasone phosphate (6 mg) and betamethasone acetate (6 mg) must be given intramuscularly in two consecutive doses 24 hours apart to those patients who will receive maximal benefit from glucocorticoid therapy. Some obstetricians prefer to use dexamethasone 4 mg IM every 6 hours for 4 doses. Since it seems that the effect of glucocorticoids on the fetal lung is transient, it may be useful to administer a *booster* dose every week to those patients who remain undelivered 7 days after the initial glucocorticoid treatment.

The blood glucose concentration should be monitored during preterm labor treatment with beta-adrenergic agents and glucocorticoids. This therapeutic combination causes profound alterations in carbohydrate and lipid metabolism, especially in the patient with diabetes. Also, glucocorticoids and beta- adrenergic agents cause water retention that may be severe and then become an important factor in the development of pulmonary edema. Patients receiving this combination of drugs should have monitoring of their body weight and their fluid input and output. Any evidence of significant intravascular volume expansion requires limitation of fluid intake and, if necessary, administration of furosemide.

PHENOBARBITAL. A considerable amount of animal experimentation and clinical evidence exists in the literature supporting the concept that administration of phenobarbital to the mother prevents intraventricular bleeding in the newborn.[103,104] Phenobarbital is given to mothers in established preterm labor with an estimated fetal weight less than 2000 g or gestational age less than 32 weeks. The dose is 10 mg/kg, 500 mg minimum and 700 mg maximal dose, given IV in 30 minutes. This dose is high enough to achieve anticonvulsant blood levels in the newborn infant.

VITAMIN K₁. There are studies indicating that administration of vitamin K_1 to patients in preterm labor reduces the incidence and severity of intraventricular bleeding in the neonate.[31,105] The validity of these observations has been questioned in view of the limited transfer of vitamin K_1 through the placenta. However, the vitamin can cross the placenta in preterm gestations, and when it is given in an initial dose of 10 mg IM followed by 20 mg orally daily, the umbilical cord levels of treated mothers are significantly higher than in control patients.[106] The medication is innocuous and should be used in every patient at risk of delivering before 32 weeks of gestation.

Delivery of the preterm infant. Labor and delivery may be a severe insult to the preterm infant. This has led to suggestions that cesarean section should be used to deliver infants under 1500 g, irrespective of their presentation. This is a controversial subject, and there is no solid evidence that cesarean is a better way of delivering very small babies, although this is a suggestive proposition.[107] Recent work by Anderson and his group[29] indicates that the *active phase of labor* rather than *delivery* is the most important factor behind the production of intracranial bleeding in the preterm infant of less than 1500 g. If that is the case, cesarean should be performed before the active phase of labor.

Preterm infants tolerate hypoxia more poorly than infants at term.[108] This implies that electronic monitoring patterns that are not a sign for intervention in a term infant do indicate intervention in the preterm baby.[61] The preterm infant is the perinatal patient with the greatest need for adequate monitoring, and significant damage could be prevented by timely intervention at the early signs of fetal distress.

If cesarean delivery is necessary for the delivery of a preterm infant and the low uterine segment has not developed, the best incision in the uterus is a low vertical incision that may be extended upwards if necessary.[59] Delivery of a preterm baby through a low transverse incision over a thick low uterine segment is as traumatic as a vaginal delivery.

◪ IMPORTANT POINTS ◪

1. Hyaline membrane disease (HMD) is the most common cause of respiratory distress syndrome in the preterm newborn. HMD occurs because of inadequate production of pulmonary surfactant by the alveolar cells type II.

2. A positive L/S ratio is a reliable test for determining fetal pulmonary maturity. Unfortunately, a negative L/S ratio is not a good predictor of pulmonary immaturity. Also,

the L/S ratio is unreliable if the fluid is contaminated with blood or meconium or collected from a vaginal pool.

3. Phosphatidylglycerol (PG) usually appears in the amniotic fluid after 36 weeks and is a marker of the final biochemical maturity of the fetal lungs. A positive PG is an excellent index of pulmonary maturity. However, a negative PG does not mean that the baby will develop HMD.

4. The FLM test is based on the competence between albumin and surfactant for a fluorescent ligand. This test is rapid, requires only a small amount of fluid, is quantitative, and has predictive values similar to the L/S ratio. A FLM concentration equal or greater than 70 mg/g has a 95% predictive value for fetal lung maturity.

5. Glucocorticoids should be used in all patients at risk of preterm delivery up to 34 weeks of gestation.

6. The outcome of babies with HMD has changed dramatically with the development of surfactant replacement therapy. Surfactant is a complex mixture of DPPC, PG, and surfactant-associated proteins A, B, and C. Natural surfactant obtained from animal lungs does not have apoprotein A. Artificial surfactants do not contain apoproteins and may or may not contain emulsifiers.

7. There are indications that prenatal administration of phenobarbital and vitamin K_1 is useful for the prevention of intraventricular bleeding in preterm newborns.

8. The most frequent etiologic agents for preterm labor are intraamniotic infection, infections outside the uterus, placental abnormalities, anatomic abnormalities of the uterus, fetal abnormalities, and uterine overdistention.

9. The best predictor of preterm labor is a poor past reproductive performance. Unfortunately, more than 40% of all patients who develop preterm labor are nulliparous.

10. Several factors associated with preterm labor have been organized in scoring systems. Patients with an elevated score are at high risk for preterm labor.

11. The majority of patients who develop preterm labor have early warning symptoms.

Patients should be taught to recognize these symptoms and call for help when they occur.

12. Patients destined to develop preterm labor can be identified by means of pelvic examinations to assess the position, length, and consistency of the cervix. This practice is part of the routine antepartum care in several European countries, but not in the United States. It is possible to obtain a precise definition of the cervical changes using vaginal ultrasound examination.

13. For most patients at risk, home uterine monitoring is not better than frequent nursing contact and support for the prevention of preterm labor. However, patients who cannot adequately perceive the presence of contractions certainly will benefit from home uterine monitoring. The inability to adequately perceive contractions occurs frequently in patients with multifetal pregnancies.

14. Aggressive treatment of vaginal and cervical infections is one important preventative measure in patients at risk for preterm labor. These patients should have cultures for group B streptococci and chlamydia in the course of their prenatal care.

15. Trials of antibiotic treatment for the prevention of preterm labor have given contradictory results. The most likely explanation is that the number of patients that benefit is low, and large numbers are necessary to demonstrate an effect.

16. Tocolysis with intravenous beta-adrenergic agents is a therapeutic modality of questionable efficacy and has potential for serious maternal side effects.

17. The objectives of the management of patients with established preterm labor are to select those patients who need to be delivered, identify those who will benefit from glucocorticoid treatment, and prepare the fetus for a preterm birth.

18. The terbutaline pump for continuous subcutaneous administration is being aggressively marketed without controlled studies demonstrating its efficacy, indications, and side effects. The use of this device is experimental and potentially dangerous.

REFERENCES

1. Dubowitz LMS, Dubowitz V, Goldberg CG: Clinical assessment of gestational age in the newborn infant. *J Pediatr* 1970;77:1.
2. Lubchenco LO, Searls DT, Braie JV: Neonatal mortality rate: Relationship to birth weight and gestational age. *J Pediatr* 1972;81:814.
3. Rush RW, Davey DA, Segal ML: The effect of preterm delivery on perinatal mortality. *Br J Obstet Gynaecol* 1978;85:806.
4. Rush RW, Keirse MJNC, Howat P, et al: Contribution of pre-term delivery to perinatal mortality. *Br Med J* 1976;2:965.
5. Arias F, Tomich P: Etiology and outcome of low birth weight and pre-term infants. *Obstet Gynecol* 1982;60:277.
6. Gluck L, Kulovich MV, Borer RC, et al: Diagnosis of the respiratory distress syndrome by amniocentesis. *Am J Obstet Gynecol* 1971;109:440.
7. Kulovich MV, Hallman MB, Gluck L: The lung profile: I. Complicated pregnancy. *Am J Obstet Gynecol* 1979;135:57.
8. Kulovich MV, Gluck L: The lung profile: II. Complicated pregnancy. *Am J Obstet Gynecol* 1979;135:64.
9. Garite TJ, Yabusaki KK, Moberg LS, et al: A new rapid slide agglutinate test for amniotic fluid phosphatidylglycerol: Laboratory and chemical correlation. *Am J Obstet Gynecol* 1983;147:681.
10. Torday J, Carson L, Lawson EE: Saturated phosphatidylcholine in amniotic fluid and prediction of the respiratory distress syndrome. *N Engl J Med* 1979;301:1013.
11. Shinitzky M, Goldfisher A, Bruck A, et al: A new method for assessment of fetal lung maturity. *Br J Obstet Gynaecol* 1976;83:838.
12. Simon NV, Levisky JS, Elser RC, et al: Influence of gestational age on prediction of fetal lung maturity by fluorescence polarization of amniotic fluid. *Obstet Gynecol* 1985;65:346.
13. Russell JC, Cooper CM, Ketchum CH, et al: Multicenter evaluation of TDx test for assessing fetal lung maturity. *Clin Chem* 1989;35:1005-1010.
14. Sbarra AJ, Michlewitz H, Selvaray RJ, et al: Relation between optical density at 650 nm and L/S ratios. *Obstet Gynecol* 1977;50:723.
15. Khouzami VA, Beek JC, Sullivant H, et al: Amniotic fluid absorbance at 650 nm: Its relation to the lecithin/sphyngomyelin ratio and neonatal pulmonary sufficiency. *Am J Obstet Gynecol* 1983;147:552.
16. Tsai MY, Josephson MW, Knox GE: Absorbance of amniotic fluid at 650 nm as a fetal lung maturity test: A comparison with the L/S ratio and tests for disaturated phosphatidylcholine and phosphatidylglycerol. *Am J Obstet Gynecol* 1983;146:963.
17. Sher G, Startland BE, Freer BE, et al: Assessing fetal lung maturity by the Foam Stability Index test. *Obstet Gynecol* 1978;52:673.
18. Socol ML, Sing E, Depp OR: The tap test: A rapid indicator of fetal pulmonary maturity. *Am J Obstet Gynecol* 1984;1148:445.
19. Howie RN, Liggins GC: Clinical trial of betamethasone therapy for prevention of respiratory distress in preterm infants, in Anderson A, Beard R, Brudenell JM, et al (eds): *Preterm labor.* London, Royal College of Obstetricians and Gynecologists, 1977; p 281.

19a. Fujiwara T, Maeta H, Chida S, et al: Artificial surfactant therapy in hyaline membrane disease. *Lancet* 1980; 1:55-59.

20. Horbar JD, Soll RF, Sutherland JM, et al: A multicenter randomized, placebo-controlled trial of surfactant therapy for respiratory distress syndrome. *N Engl J Med* 1989;320:959-965.

21. Collaborative European Multicenter Study Group: Surfactant replacement therapy for severe neonatal respiratory distress syndrome: An international randomized clinical trial. *Pediatrics* 1988;82:683-691.

22. Morley CJ, Morley R: Follow up of premature babies treated with artificial surfactant (ALEC). *Arch Dis Child* 1990;65:667-669.

23. Fujimura M, Salisbury DM, Robinson RO, et al: Clinical events relating to intraventricular hemorrhage in the newborn. *Arch Dis Child* 1979;54:409.

24. Baden HS, Koroner SB, Anderson GD, et al: Obstetric factors and relative risk of neonatal germinal layer/intraventricular hemorrhage. *Am J Obstet Gynecol* 1984;148:798.

25. Beverley DW, Chance GW, Coates CF: Intraventricular hemorrhage—timing of occurrence and relationship to perinatal events. *Br J Obstet Gynaecol* 1984;91:1007-1013.

26. Tejani N, Rebold B, Tuck S, et al: Obstetric factors in the causation of early perinventricular-intraventricular hemorrhage. *Obstet Gynecol* 1984;64:510.

27. Volpe JS: Perinatal hypoxic-ischemic brain injury. *Pediatr Clin North Am* 1976;23:383.

28. Perlman JM, Goodman S, Kreusser KL, et al: Reduction in intraventricular hemorrhage by elimination of fluctuating cerebral blood flow velocity in preterm infants with respiratory distress syndrome. *N Engl J Med* 1985;312:1353-1357.

29. Anderson GD, Bada HS, Sibai BM, et al: The relationship between labor and route of delivery in the preterm infant. *Am J Obstet Gynecol* 1988;158:1382-1390.

30. Kaempf JW, Porreco R, Molina R, et al: Antenatal phenobarbital for the prevention of periventricular and intraventricular hemorrhage: A double-blind, randomized, placebo-controlled, multihospital trial. *J Pediatr* 1990;117:933-938.

31. Morales WJ, Angel JL, O'Brien WF, et al: The use of antenatal vitamin K_1 in the prevention of early intraventricular hemorrhage. *Am J Obstet Gynecol* 1988; 159:774-779.

32. Armer TL, Duff P: Intraamniotic infection in patients with intact membranes and preterm labor. *Obstet Gynecol Surv* 1991;46:589-593.

33. Romero R, Mazor M: Infection and preterm labor. *Clin Obstet Gynecol* 1988;31:35.

34. Romero R, Brody DT, Oyarzun E, et al: Infection and labor. III. Interleukin-1: A signal for the onset of parturition. *Am J Obstet Gynecol* 1989;160:1117-1123.

35. Romero R, Emamian M, Quintero R, et al: The value and limitations of the Gram stain examination in the diagnosis of intraamniotic infection. *Am J Obstet Gynecol* 1988;159:114.

36. Romero R, Kadar N, Hobbins JC, et al: Infection and labor: The detection of endotoxin in amniotic fluid. *Am J Obstet Gynecol* 1987;157:815.

37. Gravett MG, Eschenbach DA, Speigel-Brown CA, et al: Rapid diagnosis of amniotic fluid infection by gas liquid chromatography. *N Engl J Med* 1982;306:727.

38. Hillier SL, Martius J, Krohn M, et al: A case-controlled study of chorioamnionic infection and histologic chorioammionitis in prematurity. *N Engl J Med* 1988;319:972-978.

39. Safarti P, Pageant G, Gauthier C: Le role de l'infection dans les avortements tardifs et les accouchements prematures. *Can Med Assoc J* 1968;13:1079.

40. Thomsen AC, Morup L, Hansen KB: Antibiotic elimination of group-B streptococcus in urine in prevention of preterm labour. *Lancet* 1987;1:591-593.

41. Kaas EH: Pregnancy, pyelonephritis, and prematurity. *Clin Obstet Gynecol* 1970;13:239.

42. Romero R, Oyarzun E, Mazor M, et al: Meta-analysis of the relationship between asymptomatic bacteriuria and preterm delivery/low birth weight. *Obstet Gynecol* 1989;73:576.

43. Goodlin RL, Quaife MA, Dirksen JA: The significance, diagnosis, and treatment of maternal hypovolemia as associated with fetal/maternal illness. *Semin Perinatol* 1981;5:163.

44. Brar HS, Medearis AL, DeVore GR, et al: Maternal and fetal blood flow velocity waveforms in patients with preterm labor: Prediction of successful tocolysis. *Am J Obstet Gynecol* 1988;159:947-950.

45. Westgren MD, Beall M, Divon M, et al: Fetal femur length/abdominal circumference ratio in preterm labor patients with and without successful tocolytic therapy. *J Ultrasound Med* 1986;5:243-245.

46. Kaufman R, Binder G, Gray P, et al: Upper genital tract changes associated with *in utero* exposure to diethylstilbesterol. *Am J Obstet Gynecol* 1977;128:51.

47. Baird D: Environmental and obstetrical factors in prematurity with special reference to the experience in Aberdeen. *Bull WHO* 1962;26:291.

48. Mamelle N, Laumon B, Lazar P: Prematurity and occupational activity during pregnancy. *Am J Epidemiol* 1984;119:309.

49. Launer LJ, Villar J, Kestler E, et al: The effect of maternal work on fetal growth and duration of pregnancy: A prospective study. *Br J Obstet Gynaecol* 1990;97:62-70.

50. Klebanoff MA, Shiono PH, Rhoads GG: Outcomes of pregnancy in a national sample of resident physicians. *N Engl J Med* 1990;323:1040-1045.

51. Naeye RL: Coitus and associated amniotic-fluid infections. *N Engl J Med* 1979;301:1198.

52. Klebanoff MA, Nugent RP, Rhoads GG: Coitus during pregnancy: Is is safe? *Lancet* 1984;2:914-917.

53. Butler N, Bonham D: *Perinatal Mortality*. Edinburgh, E&S Livingston, 1963, p 288.

54. Funderburk SJ, Guthrie D, Maldrum D: Suboptimal pregnancy outcome among women with prior abortions and premature births. *Am J Obstet Gynecol* 1976; 126:55.

55. Papiernik E: Prediction of the preterm baby. *Clin Obstet Gynecol* 1984;11:315.

56. Gonik B, Creasy RK: Preterm labor: Its diagnosis and management. *Am J Obstet Gynecol* 1986;154:3-8.

57. Herron MA, Katz M, Creasy RK: Evaluation of a preterm birth prevention program: Preliminary report. *Obstet Gynecol* 1982;59:452.

58. Main DM, Richardson D, Gabbe SG, et al: Prospective evaluation of a risk scoring system for predicting preterm delivery in black inner city women. *Obstet Gynecol* 1987;69:61-66.

59. Owen J, Goldenberg RL, Davis RO, et al: Evaluation of a risk scoring system as a predictor of preterm birth in an indigent population. *Am J Obstet Gynecol* 1990;163:873-879.

60. Ianes JD, Stilson R, Johnson FJ, et al: Symptoms that precede preterm labor and preterm premature rupture of membranes. *Am J Obstet Gynecol* 1990;162:486-490.

61. Katz M, Goodyear K, Creasy RK: Early signs and symptoms of preterm labor. *Am J Obstet Gynecol* 1990;162:1150-1153.

62. Kragt H, Keirse MJNC: How accurate is a woman's diagnosis of threatened preterm delivery? *Br J Obstet Gynaecol* 1990;97:317.

63. Hill WC, Lambertz EL: Let's get rid of the term *Braxton Hicks contractions*. *Obstet Gynecol* 1990;75:709-710.

64. Weekes ARL, Flynn MJ: Engagement of the fetal head in primigravidas and its relationship to duration of gestation and time of onset of labor. *Br J Obstet Gynaecol* 1975;82:7.

65. Woods C, Bannerman RHO, Booth RT, et al: The prediction of premature labor by observation of the cervix and external tocography. *Am J Obstet Gynecol* 1965;91:396.

66. Leveno KJ, Cox K, Roaik ML: Cervical dilatation and prematurity revisited. *Obstet Gynecol* 1986;68:434.

67. Stubbs TM, Van Dorsten JP, Miller MC: The preterm cervix and preterm labor: Relative risks, predictive values, and change over time. *Am J Obstet Gynecol* 1986;155:829-834.

68. Holbrook RH, Falcon J, Herron M, et al: Evaluation of the weekly cervical examination in a preterm birth prevention program. *Am J Perinatol* 1987;4:240-244.

69. Blondel B, Le Coutour X, Kaminski M, et al: Prediction of preterm delivery: Is is substantially improved by routine vaginal examinations? *Am J Obstet Gynecol* 1990;162:1042-1048.

70. Anderson FH, Ansbacher R: Ultrasound: A new approach to the evaluation of cervical ripening. *Semin Perinatol* 1991;15:140-148.

71. Newman RB, Gill PJ, Wittreich P, et al: Maternal perception of prelabor uterine activity. *Obstet Gynecol* 1986;68:765-769.

72. Katz M, Newman RB, Gill PJ: Assessment of uterine activity in ambulatory patients at high-risk of preterm labor and delivery. *Am J Obstet Gynecol* 1986;154:44-47.

73. Iams DJ, Johnson FF, O'Shaughnessy RW, et al: A prospective random trial of home uterine monitoring in pregnancies at increased risk of preterm labor. *Am J Obstet Gynecol* 1987;157:638.

74. Morrison JC, Martin JN, Martin RW, et al: Prevention of preterm birth by ambulatory assessment of uterine activity: A randomized study. *Am J Obstet Gynecol* 1987;156:536.

75. Dyson DC, Crites YM, Ray Da, et al: Prevention of preterm birth in high-risk patients: The role of education and provider contact versus home uterine monitoring. *Am J Obstet Gynecol* 1991;164:756-762.

76. Silver HM, Sperling RS, St. Clair PJ, et al: Evidence relating bacterial vaginosis to intraamniotic infection. *Am J Obstet Gynecol* 1989;161:808-812.

77. McGregor JA, French JI: Chlamydia trachomatis infection during pregnancy. *Am J Obstet Gynecol* 1991;164:1782-1789.

78. Carey JC, Blackwelder WC, Nugent RP, et al: Antepartum cultures for *Ureaplasma urealyticum* are not useful in predicting pregnancy outcome. *Am J Obstet Gynecol* 1991;164:728-733.

79. Eschenbach DA, Nugent RP, Rao AV, et al: A randomized placebo-controlled trial of erythromycin for the treatment of *Ureaplasma urealyticum* to prevent premature delivery. *Am J Obstet Gynecol* 1991;164:734-742.

80. Morales WJ, Angel JL, O'Brien WF, et al: A randomized study of antibiotic therapy in idiopathic preterm labor. *Obstet Gynecol* 1988;72:829-833.

80a. McGregor JA, French JI, Seo K: Adjunctive clindamycin therapy for preterm labor: Result of a double-blind, placebo-controlled trial. *Am J Obstet Gynecol* 1991;165:867-875.

81. Newton ER, Dinsmoor MJ, Gibbs RS: A randomized, blinded, placebo-controlled trial of antibiotics in idiopathic preterm labor. *Obstet Gynecol* 1989;74:562-566.

82. Martin KJ, Gaddy DK, Martin JN, et al: Tocolysis with oral magnesium. *Am J Obstet Gynecol* 1987;156:433-434.

83. Ricci JM, Hariharan S, Helfgott A, et al: Oral tocolysis with magnesium chloride: A randomized, controlled, prospective clinical trial. *Am J Obstet Gynecol* 1991;165:603-610.

84. Ridgway LE, Muise K, Wright JW, et al: A prospective randomized comparison of oral terbutaline and magnesium oxide for the maintenance of tocolysis. *Am J Obstet Gynecol* 1990;163:879-882.

85. Goldstein P, Berrier J, Rosen S, et al: A meta-analysis of randomized control trials of progestational agents in pregnancy. *Br J Obstet Gynaecol* 1989;96:265-274.

86. Keirse MJNC: Progestogen administration in pregnancy may prevent preterm delivery. *Br J Obstet Gynaecol* 1990;97:149-154.

87. Csapo AI: Effects of progesterone, prostaglandin F_2-alpha and its analogue ICI 81008 on the exitability and threshold of the uterus. *Am J Obstet Gynecol* 1976;124:367-378.

88. Williams LT, Lefkowitz RJ: Regulation of rabbit myometrial alpha-adrenergic receptors by estrogen and progesterone. *J Clin Invest* 1977;60:815-818.

89. Garfield RE, Puri CP, Csapo AI: Endocrine, structural, and functional changes in the uterus during premature labor. *Am J Obstet Gynecol* 1982;142:21-27.

90. Gibbs RS, Dinsmoor MJ, Newton ER, et al: A randomized trial of intrapartum versus immediate postpartum treatment of women with intraamniotic infection. *Obstet Gynecol* 1988;72:823-828.

91. Jaschevatzky O, Ellenbogen A, Anderman S, et al: The predictive value of fetal breathing movements in the outcome of premature labor. *Br J Obstet Gynaecol* 1986;93:1256-1258.

92. Besinger RE, Compton AA, Hagashi RH: The presence or absence of fetal breathing movements as a predictor of outcome in preterm labor. *Am J Obstet Gynecol* 1987;157:753-757.

93. Leveno KJ, Little BB, Cunningham FG: The national impact of ritodrine hydrochloride for inhibition of preterm labor. *Obstet Gynecol* 1990;76:12-15.

94. Kurzel RB: Serum magnesium levels in pregnancy and preterm labor. *Am J Perinatol* 1991;8:119-127.

95. Cox SM, Sherman ML, Leveno KJ: Randomized investigation of magnesium sulfate for prevention of preterm birth. *Am J Obstet Gynecol* 1990;163:767-772.

96. Madden C, Owen J, Hauth JC: Magnesium tocolysis: Serum levels versus success. *Am J Obstet Gynecol* 1990;162:1177.

97. Adamsons K, Wallach RC: Treating preterm labor with diazoxide. *Contemp OB/GYN* 1988;33:166.

98. Moise KJ, Huhta JC, Sharif DS, et al: Indomethacin in the treatment of premature labor. *N Engl J Med* 1988;319:327-331.

99. Hickok DE, Hollenbach KA, Reilley SF, et al: The association between decreased amniotic fluid volume and treatment with nonsteroidal anti-inflammatory agents for preterm labor. *Am J Obstet Gynecol* 1989;160:1525-1551.

100. Niebyl JR, Witter RF: Neonatal outcome after indomethacin treatment for preterm labor. *Am J Obstet Gynecol* 1986;155:747-749.

101. Gerson A, Abbasi S, Johnson A, et al: Safety and efficacy of long-term tocolysis with indomethacin. *Am J Perinatol* 1990;7:71-74.

102. Depp R, Boehm JJ, Nosek JA, et al: Antenatal corticosteroids to prevent neonatal respiratory distress syndrome: Risk versus benefit considerations. *Am J Obstet Gynecol* 1980;137:338.

103. Shankaran S, Cepeda EE, Ilagan N, et al: Antenatal phenobarbital for the prevention of neonatal intracerebral hemorrhage. *Am J Obstet Gynecol* 1986;154:53-57.

104. Morales WJ, Koerten J: Prevention of intraventricular hemorrhage in very low birth weight infants by maternally administered phenobarbital. *Obstet Gynecol* 1986;68:295-299.

105. Pomerance JJ, Teal JG, Gogolok JF, et al: Maternally administered antenatal vitamin K_1: Effect on neonatal prothrombin activity, partial thromboplastin time, and intraventricular hemorrhage. *Obstet Gynecol* 1987;70:235-241.

106. Kazzi NJ, Ilagan NB, Liang KC, et al: Placental transfer of vitamin K_1 in preterm pregnancy. *Obstet Gynecol* 1990;75:334-337.

107. Philip AGS, Allan WC: Does cesarean section protect against intraventricular hemorrhage in preterm infants? *J Perinatol* 1991;11:3-9.

108. Haesslein HC, Goodlin RC: Delivery of the tiny newborn. *Am J Obstet Gynecol* 1979;134:192.

5

PREMATURE RUPTURE OF THE MEMBRANES

Under normal circumstances, the fetal membranes rupture during the active phase of labor. Premature rupture of the membranes (PROM) occurs when the membranes rupture before the initiation of labor. PROM affects 2.7% to 17% of all pregnancies and in most cases happens spontaneously and without apparent cause. The wide range in the incidence of PROM most probably reflects different definitions of the problem, as well as true differences in its prevalence.

PROM is usually followed by labor. The onset of labor after PROM is directly related to the gestational age at the time of the rupture. In a study at the University of California in Los Angeles (UCLA), it was found that labor started within 24 hours of PROM in 81% of patients carrying babies larger than 2500 g.[1] The situation is markedly different when PROM occurs early in gestation. In this latter case, only 48% of the patients develop labor within 3 days after PROM.[2]

PROM is a significant obstetric problem. It is responsible for approximately 30% of all preterm deliveries[3] and causes important maternal morbidity. Unfortunately, advances in the understanding of the etiology, pathogenesis, management, and prevention of PROM have been relatively few.

▨ ETIOLOGY AND PATHOGENESIS

PROM may occur because of a reduction in membrane strength or an increase in intrauterine pressure or both. However, the possibility that extensive intrauterine pressure is an independent cause of PROM is not supported by clinical observations. Patients can tolerate intense uterine contractions and increased intrauterine pressures caused by polyhydramnios for prolonged periods without rupturing the membranes. Therefore, for all practical purposes, the cause of PROM is a reduction in membrane strength. The membranes may lose their tensile strength because of the effect of bacterial proteases, other products of bacterial metabolism, or repeated stretching caused by uterine contractions. Membranes weakened by any of these mechanisms will fail under the effect of normal pressure.

The evidence implicating infection as a fundamental factor in membrane weakening and rupture is experimental[4,5] and clinical.[6-9] Most investigators agree that the source of infection is bacteria normally present in the vagina or the cervix.[9-12] The mechanism of ascending infection is not clear. Under normal circumstances the membranes are separated from the vaginal flora by the cervix and the endocervical mucus. It is possible that unrecognized uterine activity causes cervical changes facilitating the occurrence of ascending infections. Other factors that may facilitate ascending infection are cervical incompetence, repeated pelvic examinations,[13] and coitus.[14] More clinical and laboratory research about the conditions that facilitate ascending infections is necessary.

The evidence indicating the effect of uterine contractions on membrane strength is not as direct as the effect of infection. Toppozada et al.[15] presented data indicating that repeated stretching of the membranes such as that occurring during labor causes anatomic changes and decreased tensile strength. Lavery et al.[16] demonstrated that uterine activity causes strain hardening of the membranes with development of microscopic flaws that reduce the ability to tolerate normal increases in pressure.

◪ DIAGNOSIS
Visualization of amniotic fluid in the vagina

The diagnosis of PROM is easily made when amniotic fluid is present in the vaginal vault. If no fluid is present, slight pressure on the uterus and gentle moving of the fetus may provoke leaking. Sometimes it is useful to ask the patient to cough or strain down. Fluid for laboratory tests should be collected over the lower blade of the speculum before it comes into contact with the vaginal wall.

Nitrazine test

The vaginal pH is normally 4.5 to 5.5. Amniotic fluid usually has a pH of 7.0 to 7.5. Nitrazine paper quickly will turn deep blue if the vaginal fluid has an alkaline pH. The membranes probably are intact if the color of the paper remains yellow or changes to olive-yellow (pH 5.0 to 5.5). Antiseptic solutions, urine, blood, and vaginal infections alter the vaginal pH and cause false-positive results. The Nitrazine test produces 12.7% false-negative and 16.2% false-positive results.

Fern test

Ferning results from the drying out of salts contained in the amniotic fluid. To perform the test, a sample of fluid is placed on a glass slide and allowed to dry. In patients of less than 28 weeks of gestation, it is best to heat dry thick drops of fluid with a match.[17] The preparation is observed under the microscope, looking for a crystallization pattern that resembles a fern. The accuracy of the test is affected by blood or meconium. The test may produce false-positive results if the sample is obtained from the cervix because dry cervical mucus forms an arborization pattern that may be confused with PROM. The fern test gives 4.8% false-negative and 4.4% false-positive results.[18] The diagnosis of PROM is close to 100% reliable if the vaginal fluid gives both positive Nitrazine and positive fern tests.

Evaporation test

For the evaporation test endocervical samples are heated until the water content has evaporated. If a white residue is left, amniotic fluid is present. If the residue is brown, the membranes are intact.[19,20]

Ultrasound examination

Ultrasound should not be used as the primary means of diagnosis of PROM. False-positive findings may occur in patients with oligohydramnios resulting from causes other than PROM, and false-negative may occur in patients with discrete amniotic fluid losses. However, it should be assumed that PROM has occurred if ultrasound examination shows little or no fluid in the uterus. In contrast, the presence of a normal amount of fluid makes the diagnosis of PROM unlikely.

Several semiquantitative techniques have been used for the ultrasound assessment of amniotic fluid volume. For some investigators the absence of a pocket of fluid with a vertical diameter greater than 2 cm indicates oligohydramnios. Others use the subjective qualitative impression of the individual performing the examination. The method most commonly used is the four-quadrant technique that consists of measuring the vertical diameters of the largest pockets seen in each of the four quadrants of the uterus.[21,22] The diameters are added, and the result is the amniotic fluid index. Moore[23] has demonstrated that this is a better technique than the measurement of single pockets of fluid.

Intraamniotic fluorescein

Injection of fluorescein into the amniotic cavity is rarely indicated for the diagnosis of PROM. This procedure may be performed when PROM cannot be confirmed with noninvasive techniques. In these cases, 1 ml of a sterile solution of 5% sodium fluorescein is injected into the amniotic cavity. A tampon is placed in the vagina and examined with a long-wave ultraviolet light 1 or 2 hours later. The detection of fluorescent material is equivalent to a positive diagnosis of PROM.[24] One ml of sterile indigo carmine may be used instead of fluorescein, and the tampon is inspected for the presence of a blue discoloration.

Amnioscopy

Amnioscopy is an invasive procedure rarely indicated in the diagnosis or management of PROM. It requires a distensible cervix to introduce a metallic or plastic cone for direct visualization of the membranes and the amniotic fluid. Amnioscopy may cause PROM in patients with intact membranes and may carry a large bacterial inoculum into the amniotic cavity in patients with PROM.

Diamine oxidase test

Diamine oxidase is an enzyme produced by the decidua, which diffuses into the amniotic fluid. Measurement of diamine oxidase by paper strips placed in contact with the vagina is an accurate way to diagnose PROM.[25] The test requires relatively elaborate laboratory procedures and is not ready for general use.

Fetal fibronectin

Fetal fibronectin is a large–molecular weight glycoprotein present in large amounts in the amniotic fluid. This substance can be detected in the endocervix or the vagina of patients with PROM by means of an enzyme-linked immunosorbent assay (ELISA). The test seems to be highly accurate and is not affected by blood, but meconium may interfere.[26]

Alfa-fetoprotein test

Alpha-fetoprotein (AFP) is present in high concentration in the amniotic fluid, but does not exist in vaginal secretions or in the urine. Therefore determination of this substance in the vaginal secretions is an accurate test for the diagnosis of PROM. A study using a rapid colorimetric monoclonal antibody AFP test found a sensitivity of 98% for AFP, 77% for Nitrazine, and 62% for ferning. Specificity was 100% for the AFP test.[27] The test may be unreliable at term because amniotic fluid AFP decreases with gestational age. Also, maternal blood contamination affects the accuracy of the test.

High leaks

In some cases PROM is the result of a *high leak*. This is a term used to describe a loss of fluid caused by a tear in the membranes located above the lower uterine segment. The majority of patients with high leaks have small losses and show normal amount of fluid in ultrasound examination. High leaks may seal spontaneously and are not usually associated with fetal and maternal complications. The diagnosis of a high leak is difficult.

Occasionally, patients with PROM show an intact sac at the time of delivery. These cases result from rupture of the amnion, accumulation of fluid between the amnion and the chorion, and sealing of the amnion with formation of two sacs containing amniotic fluid.[28] When the first sac, or *chorionic cyst,* ruptures, the clinical picture is that of PROM, but the true amniotic sac is intact.

◪ MATERNAL AND FETAL PROBLEMS ASSOCIATED WITH PROM
Infection

Chorioamniotic infection occurs frequently in patients with PROM, and a significant part of the patient's surveillance is directed at the early recognition of infection. The overall incidence of chorioamnionitis ranges from 4.2%[29] to 10.5%.[30] The occurrence of chorioamniotic infection after PROM seems to be greater in hospitals caring for low socioeconomic segments of the population than in institutions taking care of the affluent. The reason for this difference is not clear, but it may be because of decreased antibacterial activity in the amniotic fluid of patients of low socioeconomic conditions.[31]

The diagnosis of chorioamnionitis is clinical. It requires the presence of fever (≥100° F or 37.8° C) and at least two of the following conditions: maternal tachycardia, fetal tachycardia, uterine tenderness, foul odor of the amniotic fluid, or maternal leukocytosis.[32] Histologic chorioamnionitis, characterized by varied degrees of polymorphonuclear leukocyte infiltration of the chorioamnion, is found more frequently than the clinical disease.

The overall risk of chorioamnionitis after PROM is approximately 20%.[33] This risk is inversely related to the gestational age at the time of rupture. In the UCLA series,[1] histologic amnionitis was present in 23.8% of all patients with PROM lasting more than 24 hours if the infant's weight was 2500 g or larger; in 31.2% if the baby's weight was between 1000 and 2499 g; and in 27.5% of the cases when the infant's weight was less than 1000 g. Beydoun and Yasin[34] found an incidence of chorioamnionitis of 58.6% in patients with PROM before 28 weeks of gestation. This is in contrast with an incidence of less than 10% when PROM occurs after 36 weeks. The data from the Collaborative Perinatal Project[35] show that definite clinical infection of the neonate follows a similar pattern: the incidence of neonatal sepsis was 2.0% for infants larger than 2500 g; 4.8% for infants between 2000 and 2500 g; and 20% for infants smaller than 2000 g.

The high incidence of chorioamnionitis and neonatal infection when PROM occurs in pregnancies remote from term may be the consequence of decreased antibacterial activity of the amniotic fluid.[36,37] The antibacterial activity of the fluid is low in early pregnancy and increases with gestational age. Another factor is the limited ability of the preterm infant to fight infection.

Some investigators have found that the incidence of chorioamniotic infection after PROM is related to the duration of the latent period between rupture of the membranes and delivery of the fetus. Burchell[38] found that 1.7% of his patients developed fever within 24 hours after PROM, 7.5% between 24 and 48 hours, and 8.6% beyond 48 hours. In the UCLA series,[1] the prevalence of chorioamnionitis was 2.7% before 12 hours, 6.3% between 12 and 24 hours, and 26.4% after 24 hours of latent period. In another study,[6] 10% of the patients had histologic evidence of infection 12 hours after rupture of the membranes, 30% in 24 hours, 45% in 48 hours, and 48% in 72 hours. Newton et al.[29] determined by logistic regression analysis that the chances of developing chorioamnionitis were 20% for patients who had 20 hours of PROM and 3 hours of internal fetal monitoring. This probability increased to 40% if the latent period was 20 hours but internal fetal monitoring lasted 12 hours. Some investigators have found no increase in the incidence of infection with prolongation of the latent period.[39,40] Others have found good fetal and maternal outcomes in spite of chorioamnionitis.[41,42]

The bacteria most frequently found in the amniotic fluid and the placenta of patients with chorioamnionitis are *Ureaplasma urealyticum*, *Mycoplasma hominis*, *Bacteroides bivius*, *Gardnerella vaginalis*, group B streptococci, peptostreptococci, *Escherichia coli*, *Fusobacterium* sp., and enterococci.[43] Most of these organisms are part of the normal vaginal flora. Some of them are more virulent than others. Group B streptococcus and *E. coli* are present in only 20% of cases of chorioamnionitis but are responsible for 67% of the cases of maternal or fetal bacteremia. Anaerobes are active locally and rarely cause bacteremia.

Particular attention has been given to group B streptococcus (GBS) in its relation to PROM. This organism is frequently found in patients with subclinical amnionitis, and it may cause overwhelming neonatal infection resulting in death or severe neurologic morbidity. Patients with GBS infection commonly have PROM at an early gestational age and a shorter duration of their latent phase.[44] Several tests have been proposed for the rapid diagnosis of GBS colonization of the genital tract. Unfortunately, they are not sensitive enough for routine clinical use.[45] Culture methods require a minimum of 18 hours to detect GBS.

The risk of postpartum infectious morbidity for the mother with amnionitis is lower than the risk of infection for her neonate. Only 5.1% of all women with chorioamnionitis who have vaginal deliveries develop sepsis, whereas 10% to 20% of their babies show clinical infection.[1] Maternal infectious morbidity increases 5 times when the patient is delivered by cesarean section. Maternal infection after PROM may be severe and has an overall mortality rate of 1 in 5400 cases.[46]

Laboratory tests are useful for verifying or predicting the development of infection. The blood test most commonly used is the *maternal leukocyte count*. Patients with PROM and chorioamnionitis usually show between 12,000/mm^3 and 15,000/mm^3 white cells and a left shift. Hoskins et al.[47] found that a white cell count equal or greater than 12,000/mm^3 had a 67% sensitivity and an 82% positive predictive value for the diagnosis of amniotic infection.

Another useful blood test is the determination of *C-reactive protein* (CRP), a substance that increases markedly in patients with infection, neoplasms, and tissue necrosis. The median CRP concentration during pregnancy ranges from 0.7 to 0.9 mg/dl with no variations resulting from gestational age.[48] There is a slight elevation in CRP values during labor. The usefulness of CRP in the diagnosis of chorioamnionitis has been the object of several studies.[49-52] Unfortunately, they have used different methods and threshold values resulting in a wide variation in results. Fisk et al.[53] found CRP to be highly specific for the diagnosis of chorioamnionitis. CRP elevation usually occurs 2 or 3 days before the development of clinical signs.

The *Gram stain* of amniotic fluid is valuable for confirming the diagnosis of amnionitis. Some use a drop of the sediment obtained after centrifugation, but others use unspun fluid. The presence of any bacteria is diagnostic of infection. Common findings in patients with symptoms of overt amnionitis are gram-positive cocci in chains (group B streptococci) or gram-negative rods (*E. coli*). The accuracy of the Gram stain in the diagnosis of chorioamnionitis has been studied by Romero et al.[54] They found that a positive Gram stain has a 93.3% positive predictive value and a negative Gram stain has an 85.4% negative predictive value. The accuracy of the test depends on the concentration of bacteria at the time of sampling, and patients at early stages of infection may have a negative Gram stain. The presence of white cells in the fluid is not an accurate index of infection. However, a marked leukocytic reaction in the absence of bacteria is suggestive of *Mycoplasma* infection. If the Gram stain is negative for both bacteria and white cells, the probability of infection is less than 5%.

Another valuable amniotic fluid test is the *leukocyte esterase assay*. A positive test has a 91% sensitivity and 95% positive predictive value for the diagnosis of chorioamnionitis.[44] Also, organic acids produced by bacterial metabolism can be recognized in the amniotic fluid by gas-liquid chromatography analysis and used to confirm the diagnosis of infection.[55] Unfortunately, this sensitive technique requires sophisticated equipment and has no practical use at this time. Low amniotic fluid glucose concentration is another sign of amniotic infection. Finally, amniotic fluid cultures are valuable for identifying the bacteria causing infection and their antibiotic sensitivity.

One problem with the use of amniotic fluid in the diagnosis of chorioamnionitis is the difficulty in obtaining fluid in patients with PROM. The rate of success varies between 45% and 95%. Placing the patient in the Trendelenburg position for 3 or 4 hours before amniocentesis may be useful when no adequate pockets of fluid are seen in the initial evaluation.

Vintzileos et al.[56] originally reported the value of the *biophysical profile* (BPP) as a predictor of chorioamnionitis in patients with PROM. The absence of fetal breathing and gross body movements during a 30-minute period of observation was associated with chorioamnionitis in almost 100% of the cases. When they were present for at least one episode lasting 30 or more seconds during a 30-minute period, the possibility of infection was less than 5%. Approximately 60% of the patients had amnionitis when the episode of movements lasted only a few seconds. They also found that the first manifestations of impending fetal infection were a nonreactive nonstress test (NST) and the absence of fetal breathing movements. No cases of fetal infections were found if breathing movements were present within 24 hours before delivery. In a subsequent study they found that the efficacy of amniotic fluid Gram stain was inferior to daily BPPs in predicting the development of amnionitis.[57] They also found a better outcome for patients with PROM managed with BPP than those managed expectantly or with amniocentesis at the time of admission.[58] The value of BPP in the early diagnosis of amnionitis has been supported by other investigations[59] and questioned by some.[60,61]

The NST is also valuable in predicting chorioamniotic infection. The sensitivity, specificity, positive predictive value, and negative predictive value of a nonreactive NST in predicting infection were 78.1%, 86.3%, 65.7%, and 92.1%, respectively.[62] Patients with persistent nonreactive NST from the time of admission and those with an initially reactive NST that becomes nonreactive have the highest infection rates.

Hyaline membrane disease

Several studies have concluded that hyaline membrane disease (HMD) is the greatest threat to the fetus when PROM occurs before term. For example, in the Yale-New Haven Hospital series,[63] 29.8% of the perinatal deaths before 36 weeks were caused by HMD, 14% by complications of HMD, and 12.3% by complications of the therapy for HMD. This corresponds to a total of 56.1% of fetal deaths directly or indirectly caused by HMD.

There is an important relationship between gestational age and development of HMD and chorioamnionitis in patients with PROM. Figure 5-1, based on the data of Mercer et al.,[64] shows that HMD affects only 2% to 3% of babies with PROM at 33 to 34 weeks, whereas chorioam-

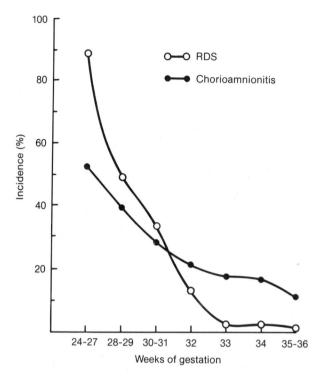

FIGURE 5-1 ◪ Graph depicting the relative risk of chorioamnionitis *(closed circles)* vs. hyaline membrane disease *(open circles)* at different gestational ages for patients with PROM. (Based on data from Mercer B, Dahmus M, Rodriguez J, et al: Perinatal outcome with preterm premature rupture of the membranes and fetal pulmonary maturity, abstract 288. San Antonio, *38th Meeting of the Society for Gynecologic Investigation*, 1991.)

nionitis complicates 18% of these pregnancies. At 32 weeks the risk of HMD is 14.8%, and the risk of infection is 22.2%. At less than 32 weeks the risk of HMD is greater than the risk of infection. It seems clear from this study that expectant management to improve fetal pulmonary maturity should dominate other considerations before 32 weeks, whereas delivery to avoid infection should be the dominant tendency after 32 weeks.

Pulmonary hypoplasia

A feared respiratory sequela of preterm PROM is pulmonary hypoplasia. This complication is frequent when PROM occurs before 26 weeks and the latent period is prolonged for more than 5 weeks. It is characterized by severe respiratory distress occurring immediately after birth and requiring maximal ventilatory support. The lungs are small and clear on x-ray examination. The course is characterized by the develop-

ment of multiple pneumothoraces and interstitial emphysema. The outcome is usually fatal, and survivors frequently suffer from chronic bronchopulmonary dysplasia.

The prenatal diagnosis of pulmonary hypoplasia is not accurate. The best method is the measurement of the thoracic-to-abdominal circumference ratio. This ratio remains constant during gestation, and when it is 0.89 or greater, the prognosis is good.[65] The absence of fetal breathing movements has been studied extensively as a predictor of pulmonary hypoplasia. Most investigations concluded that absence of fetal breathing movements is not a good predictor.

Abruptio placentae

Patients with PROM have an incidence of abruptio placentae of approximately 6%, significantly higher than the 2% found in patients with intact membranes.[66,67] Abruption usually occurs within the setting of prolonged and severe oligohydramnios. The clinical picture is that of mild-to-moderate vaginal bleeding and preterm labor. Usually the abruption is not severe enough to cause fetal demise or disseminated intravascular coagulation (DIC). The reason for the high incidence of abruption in patients with PROM is the progressive decrease in intrauterine surface area causing detachment of the placenta.

Fetal distress

Abnormal fetal heart rate monitoring patterns occur in approximately 7.9% of patients with PROM as compared with 1.5% in patients with intact membranes.[68] The most common abnormality is variable decelerations reflecting umbilical cord compression caused by oligohydramnios. As a consequence, the rate of cesarean births in patients with PROM is high.

Fetal deformities

Facial and skeletal deformities may occur as a consequence of prolonged PROM. Similar to pulmonary hypoplasia, most of these cases occur with PROM before 26 weeks and after a latent phase of 5 or more weeks.[69]

Congenital abnormalities

An important fact to consider when planning management strategies is the high incidence of major congenital malformations occurring in PROM remote from term. In the Yale-New Haven series, 4 of 20 non-RDS deaths were caused by congenital malformations.[60] Likewise, in the UCLA series, 6 of 77 perinatal deaths (8%) were caused by multiple congenital abnormalities.[1]

◪ MANAGEMENT
Identification of patients who require delivery

The first step in the management of PROM is to identify those patients who require immediate delivery. Such patients are discussed below.

Patients in labor. No effort should be made to stop labor and prolong the pregnancy if the patient is having frequent uterine contractions and the pelvic examination shows a cervix 100% effaced and dilated 4 cm or more. The use of continuous intravenous infusion of tocolytic agents in this situation is not effective and may lead to pulmonary edema.

Patients with mature fetal lungs. Patients with PROM and adequate fetal pulmonary maturity demonstrated by lecithin to sphingomyelin (L/S) ratio, phosphatidylglycerol (PG), and albumin/surfactant ratio should be delivered. Demonstration of fetal pulmonary maturity is another reason making amniocentesis desirable in the initial evaluation of patients with PROM. Up to 10% of fetuses with PROM before 32 weeks have positive PG. This increases to 25% between 32 and 35 weeks.

Patients with fetal malformations. Conservative management with its inherent risk of maternal infection is inadequate if the fetus has lethal abnormalities. Fetuses with nonlethal abnormalities should be treated as if they were normal, but parental input into the management decisions is of great importance.

Patients with fetal distress. Umbilical cord compression and cord prolapse are relatively frequent complications in PROM, especially in patients with unengaged breech presentations, transverse lies, and severe oligohydramnios. If the fetal heart rate (FHR) monitoring shows a pattern of moderate or severe variable decelerations or episodes of fetal bradycardia associated with poor beat-to-beat variability, the patient should be delivered. If the fetus is in vertex presentation, the possibility of amnioinfusion (Box 5-1), induction of labor, and vaginal delivery should be strongly considered. Cesarean section is the method of choice for the delivery of fetuses in abnormal presentations.

Patients with overt infection. The patient with chorioamnionitis should have her labor induced if there are no contraindications for vaginal delivery and if labor is not already in progress. If vaginal delivery is contraindicated (transverse lie, premature breech, etc.), a cesarean section should be performed after starting

---

BOX 5-1

Amnioinfusion Technique

1. Warm up a plastic bag containing 500 ml of normal saline solution.
2. Run the saline solution through a blood warmer keeping the solution at 37° C.
3. Connect the saline solution through the side arm of a three-way stopcock placed between the pressure transducer of the fetal monitor and the intrauterine pressure catheter.
4. Infuse the first 250 ml of saline in approximately 30 minutes. If necessary, infuse the other 250 ml in about 30 minutes.

antibiotic treatment. Several studies have demonstrated a lower rate of maternal and neonatal complications when antibiotics are given before delivery rather than postpartum.[70-72] Many use ampicillin-sulbactam, 3 g intravenously (IV) every 6 hours; aztreonam, 2 g IV every 8 hours; and clindamycin, 900 mg IV every 8 hours. With this antibiotic regimen, infection by gram-negative bacteria, gram-positive cocci, anaerobes, and enterobacteriacea is presumptively being covered.

There are different opinions about the length of time that a patient with PROM and chorioamnionitis may be in labor. Some investigators have not found a definite time after diagnosis when delivery is necessary to avoid maternal and fetal complications.[73,74] These studies, however, are not conclusive, and persistence in attempts to obtain a vaginal delivery in these patients may be potentially dangerous. Some investigators recommend to deliver by cesarean section if vaginal delivery has not occurred within 12 hours after the diagnosis of chorioamnionitis.

When chorioamnionitis is not severe and delivery is anticipated to occur in a few hours, antibiotic treatment may be postponed until the umbilical cord is clamped. In these cases, the pediatrician will obtain cultures from the baby and initiate antibiotic therapy that will be discontinued after 3 days if the cultures are negative. If the mother receives antibiotics before the cord is clamped, most pediatricians will opt for a 7-day course of antibiotics.

Patients with subclinical amnionitis. The identification of patients with subclinical chorioamnionitis is important because treatment with antibiotics and delivery may improve their outcome. Romero et al.[75] has demonstrated that approximately 40% of patients with PROM are infected at the time of admission to the hospital, but only a minority of them have signs and symptoms of overt infection.

Amniocentesis for Gram stain and culture is the accepted technique to detect subclinical chorioamnionitis. The amniotic fluid sample should be sent for Gram stain, aerobic and anaerobic cultures, and *Mycoplasma* cultures. Gas-liquid chromatography of the amniotic fluid is a promising technique for detecting subclinical infection.[52]

Patients at high risk for infection. A policy of expectancy is not adequate if the mother is at high risk for infection. The past and present medical history of the mother should be meticu-

---

> **BOX 5-2**
>
> **Patients at High Risk for Infection**
>
> Patients taking immunosuppressant drugs
> Patients with a history of rheumatic heart disease
> Patients with insulin-dependent diabetes
> Patients with sickle cell disease
> Patients with heart valve prosthesis
> Patients who have had several pelvic examinations since PROM occurred

---

lously reviewed in search of factors making her highly susceptible to infection or making it unusually dangerous for her to develop infection. Some of these factors are shown in Box 5-2. For the majority of these patients the best management is delivery.

Determination of gestational age

Once conditions indicating the need for immediate delivery have been ruled out, gestational age becomes the most important variable in the management of PROM. For a detailed discussion about assessment of gestational age, see Chapter 1. If the information collected is confusing or unreliable, the gestational age should be estimated by ultrasound examination. It is important to remember that the lack of fluid affects the accuracy of ultrasound measurements, and the gestational age is frequently underestimated.[76]

Patients with PROM after 36 weeks. Patients with PROM after 36 weeks should be delivered. There is little to be gained by conservative management when the pregnancy has advanced to a stage at which fetal pulmonary maturity is complete or almost complete. The only question remaining in regard to these patients is that of the best time for delivery, and the answer will be provided by evaluating the cervix.

Induction should start shortly after admission if the cervix is ripe. The probability that induction will fail and a cesarean section will be performed is high if the cervix is not ripe.[77] In these cases a waiting period that should not exceed 24 hours may improve the chances of vaginal delivery. Awaiting spontaneous onset of labor for 24 hours did not result in maternal and neonatal infection in the study of Conway et al.[78] It is important to determine, before this waiting period, that the vertex is engaged and that FHR monitoring shows no abnormalities. Maternal temperature should be obtained frequently, the baby should be monitored daily, and ampicillin, 500 mg every 6 hours orally, or erythromycin, 250 mg every 6 hours orally, should be given pending the results of vaginal cultures for group B streptococcus. If labor does not start spontaneously within 24 hours, labor should be induced.

Patients with PROM between 32 and 36 weeks. The most frequent complication of patients with PROM between 32 and 36 weeks is chorioamnionitis (see Figure 5-1). Therefore the dominant tendency in their management should be toward delivery. Induction with oxytocin should be initiated if the cervix is ripe. Unfortunately, in many of these patients the cervix is not ripe, and induction has a high probability of ending in cesarean delivery. A compromise between the risks of expectancy and the risks of induction may be achieved by expectant management combined with antibiotic treatment. Parsons et al.[79] reported a perinatal mortality of 0%, neonatal infection morbidity of 0%, and incidence of HMD of 2.7% in patients with PROM between 32 and 36 weeks actively delivered or expectantly managed with antibiotics. This approach is also supported by the work of Amon et al.[80] They reported a significant decrease in neonatal infection in patients with PROM managed expectantly and treated with ampicillin, 1 g intravenous piggyback (IVPB) every 6 hours, when compared with a control group. Approximately 50% of these patients had gestational ages between 31 and 37 weeks.

Patients with PROM between 26 and 32 weeks. The predominant risk for patients with PROM between 26 and 32 weeks is hyaline membrane disease (HMD). Administration of glucocorticoids and prolongation of the latent phase are beneficial for patients of this gestational age if they do not have clinical or subclinical amnionitis.

The controversy about the use of glucocorticoids in patients with PROM continues although recent evidence, including meta-analysis of the results of several trials, indicates that they are beneficial.[81]

There is evidence that prolongation of the latent period has a beneficial effect on fetal lung maturation. Yoon and Harper,[82] found a 24.6% incidence of respiratory distress syndrome (RDS) among 138 infants weighing 1001 to 2165 g delivered less than 12 hours after PROM. In contrast, RDS was present in only 12.5% of 48 infants of similar weight born more than 24 hours after PROM. Bauer et al.[83] found no cases of RDS in 10 premature infants born after more than 16 hours of latent period, whereas there were 4 cases of RDS in 7 infants born after a latent period of less than 16 hours. Richardson et al.[84] found a 64% incidence of RDS in 42 neonates with an average gestational age of 32.4 weeks delivered less than 24 hours after PROM, whereas in 22 infants with a gestational age of 30.4 weeks and with PROM lasting more than 24 hours the incidence of RDS was 32%. In another study,[60] it was found that the incidence of RDS decreased from 58% to 28% if the latent period was greater than 16 hours. However, Jones et al.[85] reviewed 16,000 births and found no association between prolongation of the latent period and decreased incidence of RDS.

Administration of tocolytic agents does not significantly prolong the latent period in patients with PROM. However, they may be useful in patients who have contractions at the time of admission and who may deliver before receiving the benefit of glucocorticoid administration.

Patients with PROM between 26 and 32 weeks should be admitted to the hospital and placed in bed rest with bathroom privileges. The fetus should be monitored daily with NST. Daily white blood cell (WBC) counts and CRP determinations will help in the assessment of infection. These patients should be treated with betamethasone (Celestone), 12 mg IM daily in two separate doses, 24 hours apart, and ampicillin, 1 g IVBP every 6 hours. Terbutaline, 2.5 to 5 mg every 6 hours orally, may be given if the mother has mild to moderate uterine activity. It is unnecessary and potentially dangerous to use intravenous tocolysis in these patients. An alternative medication if the patient does not tolerate terbutaline well is nifedipine in doses of 10 mg orally every 4 to 6 hours.

These patients should be delivered if infection develops, if labor starts, or if signs of fetal distress—mainly, variable decelerations—appear in the FHR tracing. The route of delivery will depend on the ripeness of the cervix and the FHR tracing. If the cervix is ripe, the head is deep in the pelvis, and a short labor is anticipated, the patient should deliver vaginally. If the cervix is not ripe, it is better to do a cesarean section.

When a cesarean is done at an early gestational age, the low uterine segment should be assessed as soon as the abdomen is entered, and a vertical incision performed if it is thick. To de-

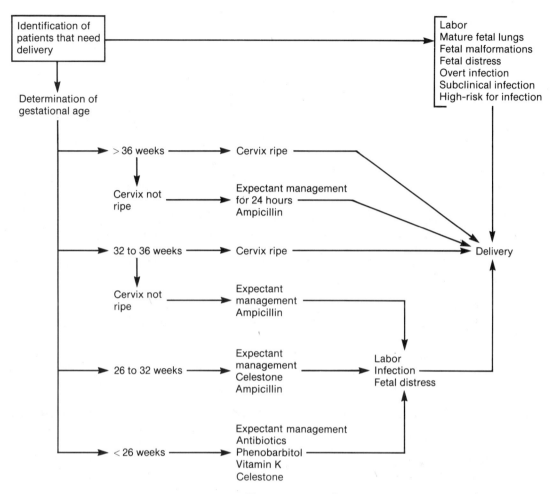

FIGURE 5-2 ◪ Management of PROM.

liver a small baby through a low transverse incision in an underdeveloped low segment may be more traumatic than a vaginal delivery.

Patients with PROM before 26 weeks. This group of patients has a poor perinatal outcome. Forty-eight percent of them will deliver within 3 days, 67% within 1 week, and 83% within 2 weeks of PROM.[86] Perinatal mortality is 60% to 90%. Approximately 50% of the mothers will have chorioamnionitis, 50% will be delivered by cesarean section, and 6.8% will have abruption. Sixteen percent of the surviving newborns will have long-term sequelae.[87] Most of the survivors are patients who extend their latent period for 2 or more weeks. Some patients have their pregnancies prolonged for several weeks after PROM without evidence of infection and with little or no fluid in the uterus. They are at high risk for fetal musculoskeletal deformities and

pulmonary hypoplasia. Deformities usually appear after 4 or more weeks of PROM.

No plan of management has been shown to improve the outcome of these pregnancies. We aggressively treat these patients with tocolytic agents, glucocorticoids, phenobarbital,[88] vitamin K, and antibiotics attempting to improve the outcome. There are methods still under investigation for the treatment of this situation, such as the PROM fence,[89] cervical caps, amnioinfusion of fluid and antibiotics, or fibrin sealing of the leak.[90]

Patients with PROM before 26 weeks should be in a tertiary center under the care of a specialist in fetal and maternal medicine.

The overall plan of management for patients with PROM is summarized in Figure 5-2. Future developments certainly will introduce modifications to this protocol.

▨   **IMPORTANT POINTS**   ◧

1. How soon labor starts after PROM is directly related to the gestational age at the time of rupture: after 36 weeks, more than 80% of the patients will be in labor within 24 hours; before 28 weeks, 48% will be in labor after 3 days of rupture.

2. The most probable cause of PROM is a reduction in membrane tensile strength caused by the effect of bacterial proteases or by repeated stretching caused by uterine contractions.

3. The method most commonly used for the ultrasound evaluation of amniotic fluid volume is the four-quadrant technique. It consists of measuring the vertical diameter of the largest pocket of fluid seen in each of the four quadrants of the uterus. The measurements are added, and the result is the amniotic fluid index. An amniotic fluid index less than 5 cm indicates oligohydramnios.

4. The diagnosis of chorioamnionitis is clinical. It requires the presence of fever (>100° F, or >37.8° C) and two of the following conditions: maternal tachycardia, fetal tachycardia, uterine tenderness, foul odor of the amniotic fluid, or maternal leukocytosis.

5. The risk of chorioamnionitis is inversely related to the gestational age at the time of PROM: it is greater than 50% when it occurs before 28 weeks, decreases to approximately 25% between 30 and 32 weeks, and remains between 12% and 20% from 32 to 36 weeks.

6. A positive Gram stain of the amniotic fluid has a 93.3% positive and an 85.4% negative predictive value for the diagnosis of chorioamniotic infection.

7. The first biophysical manifestations of impending infection in patients with PROM are a nonreactive NST and absence of fetal breathing movements. These signs are associated with chorioamnionitis in almost 100% of the cases. Patients with persistent nonreactive NST and those with an initially reactive NST that becomes nonreactive have the highest infection rates.

8. The incidence of hyaline membrane disease is inversely related to the gestational age at the time of PROM: it affects more than 80% of babies born before 28 weeks, more than 30% between 28 and 31 weeks, 14.8% at 32 weeks, 3% to 4% at 33 to 34 weeks, and very few after 34 weeks.

9. The first step in the management of PROM is to identify those patients who require delivery. They are patients in labor, patients with mature fetal lungs, with lethal fetal malformations, with fetal distress, with overt infection, or with subclinical infection, and those who are at high risk for infection.

10. Opinions vary about the length of time that a patient with PROM and overt chorioamnionitis may be in labor. Some investigators have not found a definite time after diagnosis of amnionitis when delivery is necessary to avoid maternal and fetal complications. However, persistence in attempts to obtain a vaginal delivery in these patients may be potentially dangerous. One policy is to deliver the patient no later than 12 hours after the diagnosis of chorioamnionitis has been established.

11. The predominant risk for patients with PROM between 32 and 36 weeks is chorioamnionitis. Therefore the dominant tendency in their management should be toward delivery. Unfortunately, in many of these patients, the cervix is unripe, and induction may lead to cesarean delivery.

12. The predominant risk for patients with PROM between 28 and 32 weeks is hyaline membrane disease. Administration of glucocorticoids and prolongation of the latent phase are beneficial for these patients if they do not have clinical or subclinical chorioamnionitis.

13. Administration of tocolytic agents does not significantly prolong the latent period in patients with PROM. These agents may be useful in patients with contractions at the time of admission and who may deliver before receiving the benefit of glucocorticoid treatment.

REFERENCES

1. Gunn GC, Mishell DR, Morton DG: Premature rupture of the membranes. *Am J Obstet Gynecol* 1970;106:469.
2. Moretti M, Sibai BM: Maternal and perinatal outcome of expectant management of premature rupture of membranes in the midtrimester. *Am J Obstet Gynecol* 1988; 159:390-396.
3. Arias F, Tomich P: Etiology and outcome of low birth weight and preterm infants. *Obstet Gynecol* 1982;60:277.
4. McGregor JA, French JI, Lawellin D, et al: Bacterial protease-induced reduction of chorioamniotic membrane strength and elasticity. *Obstet Gynecol* 1987;69:167-174.
5. Sbarra AJ, Thomas GB, Cetrulo CL, et al: Effect of bacterial growth on the bursting pressure of fetal membranes in vitro. *Obstet Gynecol* 1987;70:107-110.
6. Naeye RL, Peters EC: Causes and consequences of premature rupture of fetal membranes. *Lancet* 1980;2:192.
7. Miller JM, Hill GB, Welt SI, et al: Bacterial colonization of amniotic fluid in the presence of ruptured membranes. *Am J Obstet Gynecol* 1980;137:451.
8. Regan JA, Chao S, James LS: Premature rupture of the membranes, preterm delivery, and group B streptococcal colonization of mothers. *Am J Obstet Gynecol* 1981; 141:184.
9. Cederquist LL, Zervoudakis IA, Ewool LC, et al: The relationship between prematurely ruptured membranes and fetal immunoglobulin production. *Am J Obstet Gynecol* 1979;134:784.
10. Minkoff H, Grunebaum AN, Schwarz RH, et al: Risk factors for prematurity and premature rupture of membranes: A prospective study of the vaginal flora in pregnancy. *Am J Obstet Gynecol* 1984;150:965-972.
11. Gravett MG, Nelson PH, DeRouen T, et al: Independent associations of bacterial vaginosis and *Chlamydia trachomatis* infection with adverse pregnancy outcome. *JAMA* 1986;256:1899-1903.
12. Ryan GM, Abdella TN, McNeeley SG, et al: *Chlamydia trachomatis* infection in pregnancy and effect of treatment on outcome. *Am J Obstet Gynecol* 1990;162:34-39.
13. Lenihan JP: Relationship of antepartum pelvic examinations to premature rupture of the membranes. *Obstet Gynecol* 1984;63:33-37.
14. Naeye RL: Factors that predispose to premature rupture of the membranes. *Obstet Gynecol* 1982;60:93.
15. Toppozada MK, Sallam NA, Gaafar AA, et al: Role of repeated stretching in the mechanism of timely rupture of the membranes. *Am J Obstet Gynecol* 1970;108:243-249.
16. Lavery JP, Miller CE, Knight RD: The effect of labor on the rheologic response of chorioamniotic membranes. *Obstet Gynecol* 1982;60:87.
17. Borten M, Friedman EA: Amniotic fluid ferning in early gestation. *Am J Obstet Gynecol* 1986;154:628-630.
18. Tricomi V, Hall JE, Bittar A, et al: Arborization test for the detection of ruptured fetal membranes. *Obstet Gynecol* 1966;27:275.
19. Iannetta O: A new simple test for detecting rupture of the fetal membranes. *Obstet Gynecol* 1984;63:575-576.
20. Schiotz H: The evaporation test for detecting rupture of the fetal membranes. *Acta Obstet Gynecol Scand* 1987;66:245-246.
21. Phelan JP, Ahn MO, Smith CV, et al: Amniotic fluid index measurements during pregnancy. *J Reprod Med* 1987;32:601.
22. Sarno AP, Ahn MO, Phelan JP: Intrapartum amniotic fluid volume at term: Association of ruptured membranes, oligohydramnios and increased fetal risk. *J Reprod Med* 1990;35:719-723.
23. Moore TR: Superiority of the four-quadrant sum over the single-deepest-pocket technique in ultrasonographic identification of abnormal amniotic fluid volumes. *Am J Obstet Gynecol* 1990;163:762-767.
24. Smith RP: A technique for the detection of rupture of the membranes. *Obstet Gynecol* 1976;48:172.
25. Gahl WA, Kozina TS, Fuhrmann DD, et al: Diamine oxidase in the diagnosis of ruptured fetal membranes. *Obstet Gynecol* 1982;60:297.
26. Lockwood CJ, Senyei, Dische MR, et al: Fetal fibronectin in cervical and vaginal secretions as predictor of preterm delivery. *N Engl J Med* 1991;325:669-674.
27. Rochelson BL, Rodke G, White R, et al: A rapid colorimetric AFP monoclonal antibody test for the diagnosis of preterm rupture of the membranes. *Obstet Gynecol* 1987;69:163.
28. Schuman W: Double sac with secondary rupture of the bag of waters during labor: A clinical entity and its explanation from examination of the membranes. *Am J Obstet Gynecol* 1951;62:633.
29. Newton ER, Prihoda TJ, Gibbs RS, et al: Logistic regression analysis of risk factors for intraamniotic infection. *Obstet Gynecol* 1989;75:571-575.
30. Soper DE, Mayhall CG, Dalton HP: Risk factors for intraamniotic infection: A prospective epidemiologic study. *Am J Obstet Gynecol* 1989;161:562-568.
31. Tafari N, Ross SM, Naeye RL, et al: Failure of bacterial growth inhibition by amniotic fluid. *Am J Obstet Gynecol* 1977;128:187.
32. Gibbs RS, Blanco JD, St. Clair PJ, et al: Quantitative bacteriology of amniotic fluid from patients with clinical intraamniotic infection at term. *J Infect Dis* 1982;145:1-8.
33. Vintzileos AM, Bors-Koefoed R, Pelegano JF, et al: The use of fetal biophysical profile improves pregnancy outcome in premature rupture of the membranes. *Am J Obstet Gynecol* 1987;157:236-240.
34. Beydoun SN, Yasin SY: Premature rupture of the membranes before 28 weeks: Conservative management. *Am J Obstet Gynecol* 1986;155:471-479.
35. Shubeck F, Benson RC, Clark WW, et al: Fetal hazard after rupture of the membranes. *Obstet Gynecol* 1966;28:22.
36. Schlievert P, Johnson W, Galask RP: Isolation of a low molecular weight antibacterial system from human amniotic fluid. *Infect Immun* 1976;14:1156-1166.
37. Blanco JD, Gibbs RS, Krebs LF: Inhibition of group B streptoccci by amniotic fluid from patients with intraamniotic infection and from control subjects. *Am J Obstet Gynecol* 1983;147:247-250.
38. Burchell RC: Premature spontaneous rupture of the membranes. *Am J Obstet Gynecol* 1964;88:251.
39. Schreiber J, Benedetti T: Conservative management of preterm rupture of the fetal membranes in a low socioeconomic population. *Am J Obstet Gynecol* 1980;136:92.
40. Varner MW, Galask RP: Conservative management of premature rupture of the membranes. *Am J Obstet Gynecol* 1981;140:39.
41. Gibbs RS, Castillo MS, Rodgers PJ: Management of acute chorioamnionitis. *Am J Obstet Gynecol* 1980; 136:709.

42. Koh KS, Cham FH, Manfared AH, et al: The changing perinatal and maternal outcome in chorioamnionitis. *Am J Obstet Gynecol* 1979;53:730.

43. Gibbs RS, Duff P: Progress in pathogenesis and management of clinical intraamniotic infection. *Am J Obstet Gynecol* 1991;164:1317-1326.

44. Newton ER, Clark M: Group B streptococcus and preterm rupture of membranes. *Obstet Gynecol* 1988;71:198-202.

45. Skoll MA, Mercer BM, Baselski V, et al: Evaluation of two rapid group B streptococcal antigen tests in labor and delivery patients. *Obstet Gynecol* 1991;77:322-326.

46. Lebherz TB, Hellman LP, Madding R, et al: Double-blind study of premature rupture of the membranes. *Am J Obstet Gynecol* 1963;87:218.

47. Hoskins IA, Johnson TRB, Winkel CA: Leukocyte esterase activity in human amniotic fluid for the rapid detection of chorioamnionitis. *Am J Obstet Gynecol* 1987;157:730-732.

48. Watts DH, Khron MA, Wener MH, et al: C-reactive protein in normal pregnancy. *Obstet Gynecol* 1991;77:176-180.

49. Hawrylshyn P, Bernstein R, Milligan JE, et al: Premature rupture of membranes: The role of C-reactive protein in the prediction of chorioamnionitis. *Am J Obstet Gynecol* 1983;147:240-246.

50. Evans MI, Hajj SN, Devoe LD, et al: C-reactive protein as a predictor of infectious morbidity with premature rupture of membranes. *Am J Obstet Gynecol* 1980;138:648-652.

51. Farb HF, Arnesen M, Geistler P, et al: C-reactive protein with premature rupture of membranes and premature labor. *Obstet Gynecol* 1983;62:49-51.

52. Ismail MA, Zinaman MJ, Lowensohn RI, et al: The significance of C-reactive protein levels in women with premature rupture of membranes. *Am J Obstet Gynecol* 1985;151:541-544.

53. Fisk NM, Fysh J, Child AG, et al: Is C-reactive protein really useful in preterm premature rupture of membranes? *Br J Obstet Gynaecol* 1987;94:159-164.

54. Romero R, Emanian M, Quintero R, et al: The value and limitations of the Gram stain examination in the diagnosis of intraamniotic infection. *Am J Obstet Gynecol* 1988;159:114-119.

55. Gravett MG, Eschenbach DA, Speigel-Brown CA, et al: Rapid diagnosis of amniotic fluid infection by gas-liquid chromatography. *N Engl J Med* 1982;306:725-728.

56. Vintzileos AM, Campbell WA, Nochimson DJ, et al: The fetal biophysical profile in patients with premature rupture of the membranes—An early predictor of fetal infection. *Am J Obstet Gynecol* 1985;152:510-516.

57. Vintzileos AM, Campbell WA, Nochimson DJ, et al: Fetal biophysical profile versus amniocentesis in predicting infection in preterm premature rupture of membranes. *Obstet Gynecol* 1986;68:488-494.

58. Vintzileos AM, Bors-Koefoed R, Pelegano JF, et al: The use of fetal biophysical profile improves pregnancy outcome in premature rupture of membranes. *Am J Obstet Gynecol* 1987;157:236-240.

59. Goldstein I, Romero R, Merrill S, et al: The use of fetal biophysical profile as predictor of intraamniotic infection in preterm premature rupture of membranes. *Am J Obstet Gynecol* 1988;159:363-358.

60. Miller JM, Kho MS, Brown HL, et al: Clinical chorioamnionitis is not predicted by an ultrasonic biophysical profile in patients with premature rupture of membranes. *Obstet Gynecol* 1990;76:1051-1054.

61. Kivikoski AI, Amon E, Vaalamo PO, et al: Effect of third trimester premature rupture of membranes on fetal breathing movements: A prospective case-control study. *Am J Obstet Gynecol* 1988;159:1474-1477.

62. Vintzileos AM, Campbell WA, Nochimson DJ, et al: The use of nonstress test in patients with premature rupture of the membranes. *Am J Obstet Gynecol* 1986;155:149-153.

63. Berkowitz RL, Bonta BW, Warshaw JE: The relationship between premature rupture of the membranes and the respiratory distress syndrome. *Am J Obstet Gynecol* 1976;124:712.

64. Mercer B, Dahmus M, Rodriguez J, et al: Perinatal outcome with preterm premature rupture of the membranes and fetal pulmonary maturity, abstract 288. San Antonio, *38th Meeting of the Society for Gynecologic Investigation*, 1991.

65. Johnson A, Callan NHA, Bhutani VK, et al: Ultrasonic ratio of fetal thoracic to abdominal circumference: An association with fetal pulmonary hypoplasia. *Am J Obstet Gynecol* 1987;157:764-769.

66. Nelson DM, Stempel LE, Zuspan FP: Association of prolonged preterm premature rupture of membranes and abruptio placentae. *J Reprod Med* 1986;31:249.

67. Vintzileos AM, Campbell WA, Nochimson DJ, et al: Preterm rupture of the membranes: A risk factor for the development of abruptio placentae. *Am J Obstet Gynecol* 1987;156:1235-1238.

68. Oberg LJ, Garite TJ, Freeman RK: Fetal heart rate patterns and fetal distress in patients with preterm premature rupture of the membranes. *Obstet Gynecol* 1984;64:60-64.

69. Nimrod C, Varela-Gittings F, Machin G, et al: The effect of very prolonged membrane rupture on fetal development. *Am J Obstet Gynecol* 1984;148:540-543.

70. Sperling RS, Ramamurthy RS, Gibbs RS: A comparison of intrapartum versus immediate postpartum treatment of intraamniotic infection. *Obstet Gynecol* 1987;70:801-805.

71. Gibbs RS, Dinsmoor MJ, Newton ER, et al: A randomized trial of intrapartum versus immediate postpartum treatment of women with intra-amniotic infection. *Obstet Gynecol* 1988;72:823-828.

72. Gilstrap LC, Leveno KJ, Cox SM, et al: Intrapartum treatment of acute chorioamnionitis: Impact on neonatal sepsis. *Am J Obstet Gynecol* 1988;159:579-583.

73. Gibbs RS, Castillo MS, Rodgers PJ: Management of acute chorioamnionitis. *Am J Obstet Gynecol* 1980;136:709.

74. Hauth JC, Gilstrap LC, Hankins GDV, et al: Term maternal and neonatal complications of acute chorioamnionitis. *Obstet Gynecol* 1985;66:59-62.

75. Romero R, Quintero R, Oyarzun E, et al: Intraamniotic infection and the onset of labor in preterm premature rupture of the membranes. *Am J Obstet Gynecol* 1988;159:661-666.

76. O'Keefe DF, Garite TJ, Elliott JP, et al: The accuracy of estimated gestational age based on ultrasound measure-

ment of biparietal diameter in preterm premature rupture of the membranes. *Am J Obstet Gynecol* 1985;151:309-312.

77. Duff P, Huff RW, Gibbs RS: Management of PROM and unfavorable cervix in term pregnancy. *Obstet Gynecol* 1984;63:697.

78. Conway DI, Prendville WJ, Morris A, et al: Management of spontaneous rupture of the membranes in the absence of labor in primigravid women at term. *Am J Obstet Gynecol* 1984;150:947-951.

79. Parsons MT, Sobel D, Cummisky K, et al: Early delivery vs. expectant management in patients with preterm rupture of membranes at 32-36 weeks gestation, abstract 381. New Orleans, 9th Annual Meeting of the Society of Perinatal Obstetricians, 1989.

80. Amon E, Lewis SV, Sibai BM, et al: Ampicillin prophylaxis in preterm premature rupture of the membranes: A prospective randomized study. *Am J Obstet Gynecol* 1988;159:539-543.

81. Romero R, Oyarzan E, Mazor M, et al: Meta-analysis of the effect of steroids in the prevention of respiratory distress syndrome in premature rupture of membranes, abstract 360. New Orleans, 9th Meeting of the Society of Perinatal Obstetricians, February, 1989.

82. Yoon J, Harper R: Observations on the relationship between duration of rupture of the membranes and the development of idiopathic respiratory distress syndrome. *Pediatrics* 1973;52:161.

83. Bauer C, Stern L, Colle E: Prolonged rupture of membranes associated with a decreased incidence of respiratory distress syndrome. *Pediatrics* 1974;53:7.

84. Richardson C, Pomerance JJ, Cunningham MD, et al: Acceleration of fetal lung maturation following prolonged rupture of the membranes. *Am J Obstet Gynecol* 1974;118:1115.

85. Jones MD, Burd LI, Bowes WA Jr, et al: Failure of association of premature rupture of membranes with respiratory distress syndrome. *N Engl J Med* 1975;292:1253.

86. Moretti M, Sibai BM: Maternal and perinatal outcome of expectant management of premature rupture of membranes in the midtrimester. *Am J Obstet Gynecol* 1988;159:390-396.

87. Bengston JM, VanMarter LJ, Barss V, et al: Pregnancy outcome after premature rupture of the membranes at or before 26 weeks' gestation. *Obstet Gynecol* 1989;73:921-926.

88. Morales WJ, Koerten J: Prevention of the intraventricular hemorrhage in very low birth weight infants by maternally administered phenobarbital. *Obstet Gynecol* 1986;68:295-299.

89. Ogita S, Imanaka M, Matsumoto M, et al: Premature rupture of the membranes managed with a new cervical catheter. *Lancet* 1984;1:1330-1331.

90. Baumgarters K, Moser S: The technique of fibrin adhesions for premature rupture of the membranes during pregnancy. *J Perinat Med* 1986;14:43.

6

ERYTHROBLASTOSIS FETALIS

Before the discovery of the Rh system by Landsteiner in 1940, little was known about the etiology of erythroblastosis fetalis, a condition in which the fetus becomes edematous and often dies in the uterus from severe anemia and high-output cardiac failure. After this discovery, it was quickly learned that maternal rhesus blood factor (Rh) isoimmunization, with placental transfer of IgG antibodies, was the phenomenon responsible for the fetal red cell destruction. This was followed by the finding that spectrophotometric analysis of the amniotic fluid was an excellent index for measuring the severity of the fetal anemia and by the realization that early delivery and intrauterine transfusions (IUTs) could be lifesaving maneuvers for the compromised fetus. Finally, it was found that the administration of D immunoglobulin to mothers at risk is an extremely effective way of preventing the initial immune response that causes Rh isoimmunization. Therefore, the field has moved in 40 years from a stage of little knowledge about a serious disease to a situation in which preventive measures have made the occurrence of that disease a relatively rare event.

■ ETIOLOGY

Erythroblastosis fetalis is a disease in which the red blood cells of the fetus and the newborn are hemolyzed by maternal isoantibodies (anti-

bodies capable of reacting with red cells from the same species but not with red cells of the individual producing the antibodies) that have been able to cross the placenta. The resulting anemia leads to fetal heart failure, massive edema (hydrops fetalis), and intrauterine death. It also may cause varied degrees of neonatal hyperbilirubinemia (hemolytic disease of the newborn). Approximately 97% of all cases of erythroblastosis fetalis are caused by maternal immunization against the Rh(D) antigen present in the fetal red cells. The remaining cases are caused by immunization against other fetal antigenic groups such as C, c, E, e, K, k, Fy^a, M, and Jk^a. Maternal isoimmunization may be a consequence of the administration of Rh-positive blood to an Rh-negative female, but in the overwhelming majority of cases, it results from the passage of fetal Rh-positive red cells into the bloodstream of Rh-negative mothers in the course of pregnancy and especially at the time of delivery. In response to this immunologic stimulation, the mother develops IgM and IgG antibodies, the latter being able to cross the placenta and destroy the fetal red cells.

■ PATHOPHYSIOLOGY

The inheritance of blood group antigens occurs according to Mendelian laws and, with the exception of the group Xg$_a$, which is X-linked, is autosomal and codominant (both alleles are expressed in the heterozygous individual). According to the Fisher-Race paired gene theory, the Rh system is formed by six Rh genes, three carried on each chromosome. Each tri-gene complex (haplotype) is inherited from each parent with little or no crossing over. Three of the genes are dominant (C, D, E), and three are recessive (c, d, e); the most important is the D gene, which confers to the individual the characteristic of being Rh-positive. An Rh-positive person may be homozygous (DD) or heterozygous (Dd), whereas an Rh-negative individual may only be homozygous (dd). This has practical importance because a homozygous Rh-positive father (DD), if mated with an Rh-negative (dd) mother, passes to his offspring a dominant D gene, regardless of which of the two paired genes is carried over to the child. As a result, the offspring is Rh-positive in 100% of the cases. If the father is heterozygous (Dd), the chances of a child being Rh-positive are only 50%. The distinction between homozygous and heterozygous Rh-negative fathers is complicated because there is no antiserum against the d antigen, and it has to be made using genotype frequency tables based on allelic frequencies (Tables 6-1 and 6-2).

Some red cells react weakly with anti-D antibodies because they contain a gene that produces only a part of the D antigen. This variant is called D^u, and it should be absent (D^u negative) in a given individual for that person to be considered Rh-negative. A third allele of C and c has also been identified, most commonly in association with D and e, and has been called C^w. Some individuals have a rare state termed *Rh-null* in which their red cells lack Rh antigens.

The C and E Rh antigens may in rare instances initiate the reactions leading to the production of erythroblastosis fetalis. Other antigens with similar potential are the K (Kell), Fy^a (Duffy), and Jk^a (Kidd). They usually cause isoimmunization via a previous blood transfusion rather than as a consequence of a previous pregnancy. An antigen frequently found in routine antenatal testing is the Lewis group (Le^a and Le^b). The Lewis antigens do not cause erythro-

TABLE 6-1 ◪ Prevalence of Rh chromosome types in whites

Antigens	Frequency (%)
C D e	40
c d e	38
c D E	14
c D e	2.5
c d E	1.1
C d e	1.0
C D E	0.24
c d E	Very low

TABLE 6-2 ◪ Genotype frequency table

C	D	E	c	e	Type	Not excluded	%	Homo/hetero (H)(h)
+	+	−	+	+	CDe/cde	CDe/cDe	32.0	h
						cDe/Cde	2.0	H
							0.1	h
							17.0	H
+	+	−	−	+	CDe/CDe	CDe/Cde	0.8	h
							12.0	H
+	+	+	+	+	CDe/cDE	CDe/Cde	1.0	h
						cDE/Cde	0.3	h
							11.0	h
−	+	+	+	+	cDE/cde	cDE/cDe	1.0	H
						cDE/cdE	0.1	h
							2.0	H
−	+	+	+	−	cDE/cDE	cDE/cdE	0.3	h
							2.0	h
−	+	−	+	+	cDe/cde	cDe/cDe	0.1	H

blastosis fetalis and differ from all of the other red cell antigens in that they are not synthesized in the red cell membrane but are absorbed into it. There are other rare antigenic groups that may cause mild to severe erythroblastosis fetalis (Table 6-3). The interested reader may consult the paper by Weinstein.[1]

During normal pregnancy, fetal red cells cross the placenta in 5% of patients during the first trimester and by the end of the third trimester in 47% of patients.[2] In most of these cases, the number of fetal cells transferred to the mother is small and insufficient to produce a primary immune response. For this and other reasons, the incidence of antepartum primary sensitization in the course of the first Rh-incompatible pregnancy is less than 1%.[3]

In the majority of cases, maternal isoimmunization is the consequence of a fetal-maternal blood leakage happening at the time of delivery. Passage of fetal blood into the maternal circulation at the time of parturition is the rule rather than the exception, but only 10% to 15% of Rh-negative mothers who have Rh-positive husbands become sensitized at delivery. This low index of sensitization implies the existence of several factors influencing the probability of primary isoimmunization. One of these factors is the size of the inoculum; it is accepted that the greater the number of fetal cells entering the maternal circulation, the greater the possibility of maternal sensitization, although some mothers have been immunized with as little as 0.25 ml of fetal Rh-positive cells. Another factor is the coexistence of ABO incompatibility between mother and fetus; if the mother is group O and the father is A, B, or AB, the frequency of sensitization is decreased by 50% to 75% because the maternal anti-A or anti-B antibodies destroy the fetal red cells carrying the Rh antigen before they can elicit an immune response. Furthermore, 30% to 35% of Rh-negative subjects are nonresponders (cannot be immunized) to the Rh-positive antigen, a characteristic that seems to be genetically controlled but dependent to a certain extent on the amount of Rh-positive blood injected into the maternal circulation.

If an immune response is elicited during pregnancy (incidence less than 1%) or at delivery (incidence 10% to 15%) in an Rh-negative mother who carries an Rh-positive baby, the initial maternal response will be the development of anti-Rh IgM antibodies with a molecular weight too large to cross through the placenta. Unfortunately, this is followed by the synthesis of anti-Rh IgG antibodies that do cross the placenta and stick to the fetal red cells, accelerating their destruction in the infant's reticuloendothelial system. The time between the fetal-maternal bleeding and the initiation of the primary immune response is not exactly known and probably has some biologic variation, but usually is several weeks. That is the reason prophylactic administration of D immunoglobulin to the mother shortly after delivery inhibits the immune response. Even when the administration of D immunoglobulin is delayed up to 2 weeks after transfusion of Rh-positive cells, the procedure is protective in 50% of the cases.

Maternal isoimmunization is usually detected during routine antenatal screening. The antibodies are assayed in saline solution, albumin, and with Coombs' serum.[4] Antibodies capable of agglutinating red cells suspended in saline solution at 4° to 20° C are complete (IgM) antibodies.

TABLE 6-3 ◪ Irregular antibodies associated with hemolytic disease

Blood group system	Related antigen
Kell	K
	k
	K_o
	K_{pa}
	Js_a
	Js_b
Rh (non-D)	E
	e
	C
	c
Duffy	Fy^a
	Fy^b
Kidd	Jk^a
	Jk^b
	Jk3
MNSs	M
	N
	S
	s
	U
MSSs	Mi^a
	Mt^a
	Vw
	Mur
	Hil
	Hut

Modified from Weinstein L: *Clin Obstet Gynecol* 1982; 25:321.

This means that they are capable of bridging the minimal intercellular distance of 25 Å that exists between red cells in solution. As mentioned before, IgM antibodies are not capable of crossing the placenta and do not produce erythroblastosis fetalis. Incomplete (IgG) antibodies, such as the anti-Rh antibody, are not capable of bridging the intercellular distance existing between erythrocytes. This distance results from the fact that red cells repel each other because of their negative surface charge, or *zeta potential*. Therefore, to produce red cell agglutination with incomplete antibodies, it is necessary to reduce the zeta potential and decrease the intercellular distance. This is achieved in the laboratory by the addition of albumin to the suspending medium. Thus antibodies that are not capable of agglutinating red cells in saline at 4° to 20° C but are capable of agglutinating red cells at 37° C in the medium containing albumin are IgG antibodes and are important to the obstetrician because they are capable of crossing the placenta and causing fetal hemolytic disease. The Coombs' serum (containing antiglobulin antibodies) is, like albumin, capable of enhancing the agglutination of red cells coated with incomplete (IgG) antibodies or with complement.

Once Rh isoimmunity has been initiated, the individual produces large amounts of antibodies (secondary response) in response to small amounts of fetal Rh-positive blood leaking through the placenta in a subsequent pregnancy. The anti-Rh antibodies cross the placenta and attach to the infant's red cells, making them susceptible to destruction by the reticuloendothelial system. Depending on the severity of the hemolysis, the clinical picture may include congestive heart failure, hepatomegaly, splenomegaly, peripheral edema, and placental hypertrophy. The marked hepatomegaly and splenomegaly present in erythroblastotic stillborns are a consequence not only of the development of large foci of compensatory extramedullary hematopoiesis but also of the accumulation of fluid because of congestive heart failure. If untreated, about 20% to 30% of fetuses affected by erythroblastosis die in utero.

Kernicterus (bilirubin deposits in the basal nuclei of the brain) and jaundice are not components of erythroblastosis fetalis during intrauterine life, since accumulation of the pigment is prevented by its removal through the placental circulation and metabolism in the maternal liver. However, after birth the newborn liver cannot effectively handle the large amount of pigment released during the brisk hemolytic process, and this leads to rapid increases in serum bilirubin and eventual tissue deposition.

◪ MANAGEMENT

In the management of erythroblastosis fetalis the obstetrician is usually faced with one of the two following types of patients: (1) the Rh-negative nonimmunized patient or (2) the Rh-negative immunized patient. These two groups of patients are managed differently.

Management of the Rh-negative nonimmunized patient

The Rh-negative nonimmunized group is formed by primigravida and multigravida patients who are Rh negative and do not have detectable isoantibodies in the initial prenatal evaluation. It is important to remember that every Rh-negative patient who has received anti-D immunoglobulin in a previous pregnancy should have antibody screening in all subsequent pregnancies. This is because, as will be discussed later, postpartum administration of anti-D immunoglobulin does not guarantee that isoimmunization is prevented in 100% of the cases. The search for maternal isoimmunization should not be restricted to Rh-negative patients, and an antibody screening should also be obtained during the initial prenatal evaluation in Rh-positive patients who have had previous blood transfusions, unexplained fetal losses, or infants with unexplained jaundice during the previous pregnancy.

If the pregnant patient is Rh negative and the antibody screening is negative, the problems for the obstetrician are (1) to assess the chances for the patient to become isoimmunized, (2) to take measures to detect isoimmunization if it actually occurs during the present pregnancy, and (3) to use adequate prophylaxis antepartum and in the immediate postpartum period.

To assess the possibility of isoimmunization in these patients, it is necessary to know the blood group and Rh classification of the father. If the father is Rh negative, the infant will be Rh negative, and there is no need for further testing. If the father is Rh positive, the infant has a 50% (if the father is heterozygous) to a 100% (if the father is homozygous) probability of being Rh positive, and the mother may become sensitized during pregnancy. As mentioned before, the chances for sensitization to occur before delivery are about 1%, and to detect its occurrence, the

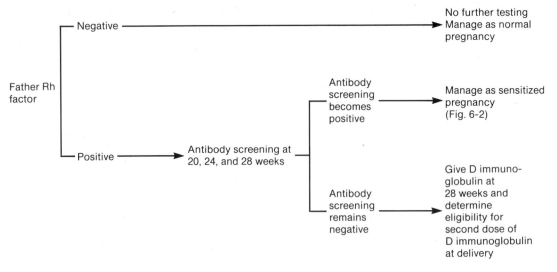

FIGURE 6-1 ◪ Management of the Rh-negative nonimmunized gravida.

antibody screening should be repeated at 20, 24, and 28 weeks of gestation. If any of these antibody screenings reveal the appearance of anti-D antibodies, the patient should be managed as an Rh-negative immunized pregnancy. If the antibody screening does not show evidence of isoimmunization, the patient should receive anti-D immunoglobulin at 28 weeks of gestation, and further antibody screenings will be unnecessary. At the time of delivery, it will be necessary to determine the mother's eligibility to receive a second dose of anti-D immunoglobulin in the immediate postpartum period.

There are three points of discussion in the previous protocol for the management of the Rh-negative nonimmunized gravida (Figure 6-1). The first point has to do with the determination of the Rh genotype in the Rh-positive husband of the Rh-negative nonimmunized pregnant woman. The reason for the omission of this test from the protocol is that the finding of heterozygosity or homozygosity in the father does not alter the plan of management. In fact, even if the father is heterozygous, the mother still has a theoretical risk of sensitization of 50% and should be screened during pregnancy and receive anti-D globulin prophylaxis at 28 weeks.

The second point of discussion in the protocol has to do with the frequency of antibody screening. Since Rh isoimmunization is so rare during the antenatal period, the question arises about

the need for antibody screening every 4 weeks until prophylactic Rh-immunoglobulin is given at 28 weeks. This frequency of testing is probably the most adequate to avoid missing the development of antibodies in the occasional patient who becomes immunized before delivery. The first immunized pregnancy rarely produces severe erythroblastosis.[5] However, a poor fetal outcome may be the result of inadequate surveillance.

The third point of discussion concerns the antepartum administration of D immunoglobulin. There is evidence that giving D immunoglobulin to Rh-negative patients at 28 weeks of gestation decreases the incidence of third-trimester immunization from 20 in 1000 to 2 in 1000 patients. After antepartum administration of D immunoglobulin, the antibody screening will detect anti-D antibodies in the patient's serum, but their amount should not be greater than 1:4 at term. The hospital blood bank should be notified at the time of antepartum administration that D immunoglobulin has been administered to facilitate the interpretation of the patient's future antibody screening. An anti-D titer of greater than 1:4 at term most probably results from isoimmunization rather than from D immunoglobulin administration.

The problem with antepartum D immunoglobulin administration is cost-effectiveness. Many women will receive one or two doses of a relatively expensive medication, and only a few will benefit from it. However, antepartum D immunoglobulin administration decreases the incidence of Rh isoimmunization and is a procedure of choice.

The Rh-negative gravida who remains unsensitized (negative antibody screenings) during pregnancy and receives D immunoglobulin antepartum should have her eligibility for postpartum administration determined immediately after parturition. D immunoglobulin should be given under the following circumstances:

1. The infant is Rh positive.
2. The direct Coombs' test on umbilical cord blood is negative. This test reveals whether the infant's red cells are covered by irregular antibodies.
3. A crossmatch between the anti-D immunoglobulin and the mother's red cells is compatible.

The usual dosage of D immunoglobulin is 300 mg. This amount of D immunoglobulin is capable of neutralizing the antigenic potential of up to 30 ml of fetal blood (about 15 ml of fetal cells) and prevents Rh isoimmunization in 90% of the cases. In the other 10% of the cases, D immunoglobulin is ineffective, probably as a consequence of a large transfusion of fetal cells into the mother and insufficient antigenic neutralization with the usual dose of medication. A large fetal-maternal hemorrhage occurs in 1 of every 300 to 500 deliveries, and it should be suspected with the birth of a pale baby, a fetal hemoglobin concentration of less than 10 g, abruptio placentae, midforceps operations, and traumatic deliveries. The clinical indicators of a large fetal-maternal hemorrhage are not completely reliable, and ideally, the transfusion volume should be quantified with the use of the Kleihauer-Betke stain. This method is based on the fact that an acid solution (citric acid phosphate buffer pH 3.5) elutes the adult but not the fetal hemoglobin from the red cells; fetal erythrocytes appear in a smear stained dark red and surrounded by colorless ghosts that are adult erythrocytes without hemoglobin. This test can detect as little as 0.2 ml of fetal blood diluted in 5 L of maternal blood.

The Kleihauer-Betke test is useful only to evaluate the volume of large fetal-maternal hemorrhages. It is not useful and should not be used to determine the need for D immunoglobulin administration. In fact, about 50% of Rh-nega-

tive mothers who become sensitized have negative postpartum Kleihauer-Betke testing.[6] The Kleihauer-Betke test is somewhat difficult to perform and may produce false-positive results as a consequence of multiple factors affecting the acid elution of hemoglobin from the red cells. Also, the presence of reticulocytes and adult red cells containing fetal hemoglobin may cause false-positive results.

In the United States, a crossmatch of the D immunoglobulin against the mother's red cells is carried out before the administration of this product. This practice had its origin in the initial trials to determine the effectiveness of D immunoglobulin treatment, at which time there was a fear of causing hemolysis in the recipient. Today it is known that the infusion of plasma containing antibodies incompatible with the recipient is innocuous and does not cause intravascular hemolysis. However, the important benefit of the D immunoglobulin crossmatching is the ability of this test to detect a large fetal-maternal hemorrhage. In fact, if more than 20 ml of fetal blood has entered the maternal circulation, the D immunoglobulin crossmatch becomes incompatible. Therefore, this crossmatch test is being used as a screening procedure to detect mothers who have had large fetal-maternal transfusions and who would not be protected by the administration of the usual 300-mg dosage of D immunoglobulin. Because of its simplicity, the D immunoglobulin crossmatch is widely used in place of the Kleihauer-Betke stain to screen mothers in need of high dosages of D immunoglobulin. However, the threshold sensitivity of the D immunoglobulin crossmatch is high, and the Kleihauer-Betke test should be the procedure of choice to assess the volume of the fetal-maternal bleeding.

D immunoglobulin should also be given to all Rh-negative women after spontaneous or induced abortions, after amniocentesis, and after ectopic pregnancies unless they are already sensitized.

D immunoglobulin can be given any time up to 4 weeks after delivery. The maximal protective effect is obtained if the antibody is administered within 72 hours after delivery. There is nothing magic, however, in this standard timing. This limit was chosen arbitrarily in the original experiments in which the value of D immunoglobulin in preventing Rh isoimmunization was proven. Other experiments have shown that administra-

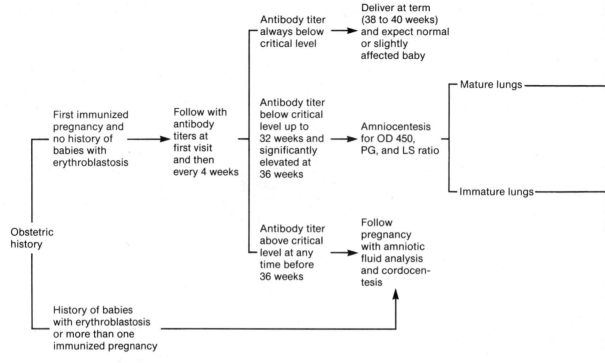

FIGURE 6-2 ◪ Management of the Rh-negative immunized gravida.

tion of D immunoglobulin several days and even weeks after delivery still has a protective effect, although the efficiency of the protection is reduced. Therefore, D immunoglobulin should be given to any eligible Rh-negative mother as soon as possible after delivery, but treatment should not be withheld if more than 72 hours have passed in the postpartum period. The administration of D immunoglobulin to eligible mothers after delivery decreases the incidence of Rh sensitization from 15% to 1% or 2%. The 1-in-10 failure rate results from undetected large fetal-maternal bleeding or from isoimmunization occurring before delivery.

Management of the Rh-negative immunized patient

The management of the immunized Rh-negative patient (Figure 6-2) is based on the adequate use of four diagnostic techniques:
1. Maternal serum antibody titers
2. Fetal assessment by ultrasound
3. Amniotic fluid bilirubin determinations
4. Fetal blood sampling

Maternal serum antibody titers. Maternal antibody titers are useful for the follow-up of patients exclusively in their first immunized pregnancy. The reason for this limitation is that the correlation between antibody titers and transfer of fetal cells into the maternal circulation that exists in most first-affected pregnancies is completely lost during subsequent gestations. Also, following the initiation of immunization, the serum antibody concentration is very low and rarely exceeds the critical level of most laboratories. The critical level means that no death resulting from erythroblastosis has occurred within 1 week of delivery when the antibody titer was at that level or lower.

The concentration of anti-D antibodies is determined by a titration procedure in which progressively double dilutions of the maternal serum are incubated with Rh-positive group 0 erythrocytes and agglutination is used as the end point. There is a wide variation in antibody titers among different Rh-immunized patients. In many of them, especially during the pregnancy immediately after the initiation of immu-

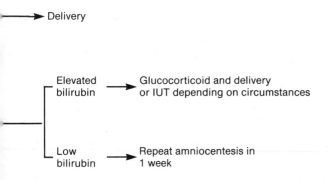

Delivery

Elevated bilirubin ⟶ Glucocorticoid and delivery or IUT depending on circumstances

Low bilirubin ⟶ Repeat amniocentesis in 1 week

nization, the concentration of antibodies is so low that they can only be detected in undiluted serum and may not appear until late in pregnancy. The explanation for those cases of late appearance of antibodies is that fetal-maternal bleeding generating a maternal antibody response is more common in the later stages of gestation.

There are variations in antibody titers among different laboratories, and the obstetrician managing an immunized pregnancy should use the same laboratory for all of the antibody titer determinations. For maximal accuracy of the test, serum samples should be stored, and the procedure should be repeated in the original sample each time that a titer is determined in a subsequent sample. Also, it is important to know the critical titer level associated with intrauterine death used by the reporting laboratory. For example, this critical level is 1:16 at the Columbia-Presbyterian Medical Center[3] and 1:32 at the University of Louisville.[7]

Patients with histories of fetal or neonatal erythroblastosis should not be monitored with antibody titers. In a study at the Boston Lying-In Hospital,[8] it was found that immunized patients with titers remaining at or below 1:64 and with negative past obstetric histories had a 4% incidence of intrauterine death before 37 weeks. In contrast, patients with similar titers but with histories of delivering erythroblastotic infants had a 32% stillbirth rate before 37 weeks. When the titer was above 1:64, the patients with negative

histories had a stillborn incidence of 17.2%, whereas those with histories of affected infants had a stillborn rate of 67.8%. Although there is a gross correlation between antibody titer and fetal outcome, in patients with similar titers the past obstetric history is the predominant indicator of the outcome. Therefore patients with histories of having given birth to infants with erythroblastosis should be managed on the basis of spectrophotometric analysis of the amniotic fluid, even if their antibody titers do not exceed the critical level.

Patients in the course of their first sensitized pregnancy should have antibody titers every 4 weeks unless the following occurs:

1. The titer is found to be at or above the critical level in the initial evaluation.
2. The titer reaches or exceeds the critical level at any time during gestation.
3. There is a significant rise (two-tube dilution) in the titer between any two consecutive samples, even if the upper dilution does not reach the critical level (e.g., an increase from 1:4 to 1:32 with a critical level of 1:64).

If any of these three conditions is fulfilled, there is no further use for antibody titers as an index for monitoring a first sensitized pregnancy. Further management will be based on examination of the amniotic fluid.

If the antibody titer remains under the critical level at all times up to 36 weeks of gestation, the patient with a first sensitized pregnancy should be delivered by elective induction of labor between 38 and 40 weeks, and the birth of a non-affected (Rh-negative) or mildly affected infant should be anticipated. The neonatologist should be notified in advance of the induction of an Rh-negative immunized mother so that evaluation and treatment of the newborn can be started in the delivery room and continued without delays.

A special group of patients are those with a first sensitized pregnancy who are being monitored with antibody titers and who have a sudden titer elevation when they are at 36 or more weeks of gestation. For such a patient, an amniocentesis should be performed, and the baby should be delivered if the indexes of lung maturity are adequate. If the fetal maturity tests indicate pulmonary immaturity and the bilirubin level is low (less than 0.05), the pregnancy should be allowed to continue as long as weekly amniocentesis tests show fetal pulmonary immaturity and low bilirubin concentration. These babies with mild hemolytic disease should be delivered as soon as their lungs have reached adequate maturation.

A different problem is posed by the patient who at 36 weeks or more of gestation has inadequate fetal lung maturity and a high bilirubin concentration in the amniotic fluid (OD 450 greater than 0.05). One approach is to give the mother glucocorticoids and to deliver the baby in 24 to 48 hours. Another approach is to proceed to fetal blood sampling and intrauterine transfusion (IUT) if the fetus is anemic. Which of these two approaches is the best to follow in a given case will depend on multiple factors such as the feasibility of performing fetal blood sampling and IUTs, the nursery facilities available, parental desires, etc.

Patients with their first sensitized pregnancy, with histories of babies with erythroblastosis or whose titers are elevated above the critical level before 36 weeks, should be monitored with serial amniocentesis and, perhaps, cordocentesis, as discussed on p. 125.

Fetal assessment by ultrasound. High-resolution ultrasound is a valuable tool in the management of sensitized Rh-negative patients. Modern equipment allows a clear visualization of the fetal structures and early diagnosis of the presence of fetal ascites, pericardial effusion, liver enlargement, and placental swelling. For these reasons, some investigators believe that the accuracy of ultrasound in detecting signs of fetal hemolytic disease is better than that of amniotic fluid bilirubin measurements.[8,9]

There are two important objections to the use of ultrasound as the main indicator of fetal hemolytic disease. First, fetal hydrops usually develops when the fetal hematocrit is below 20%. Therefore ultrasound will detect only advanced degrees of fetal anemia. Second, in many patients the onset of fetal hydrops is rather sudden, and its detection by ultrasound will require frequent evaluations.

Amniotic fluid bilirubin determinations and cordocentesis can detect fetuses with moderate and severe hemolysis when ultrasound evaluation is still normal. Therefore only in special circumstances should ultrasound be used as the main criterion for judging the extension of the hemolytic process and the need for intervention.

Amniotic fluid analysis. In pregnancies affected by the presence of irregular antibodies capable of producing erythroblastosis fetalis, spectrophotometric analysis of the amniotic fluid is a reliable method for evaluating the severity of the fetal hemolytic process and for determining the optimal time for IUT or for delivery of the infant. Amniotic fluid analysis is mandatory in the management of the Rh-negative immunized gravida in all of her pregnancies except the first sensitized one, during which the patient can be assessed with antibody titers under the conditions described before. The follow-up with amniocentesis is of particular importance for those patients with histories of prior deliveries of infants with erythroblastosis.

The first amniocentesis traditionally is carried out at 26 weeks because this gestational age was the limit of viability before the development of modern neonatal intensive care and because the Liley graph,[10] used to evaluate severity of sensitization, starts at 27 weeks (Figure 6-3) and cannot be extrapolated into the second trimester.[11] More recently, normal amniotic fluid bilirubin values between 14 and 20 weeks have been reported[12] and found to be useful in predicting the severity of Rh disease.[13]

Amniocentesis may be performed at any time after 16 weeks in patients who start off with a high titer, have had a baby who was hydropic or died in uterus, or have had ultrasound evaluation demonstrating early signs of fetal hydrops. If the first amniocentesis fails because of a bloody tap, the procedure should be repeated after 1 week. If amniocentesis is successful, the decision about when to repeat the procedure will be dictated by the results of the amniotic fluid analysis (see Figure 6-4).

Before performing an amniocentesis, the best site for the procedure should be determined using real-time ultrasound. The use of ultrasound has increased the success rate in obtaining adequate samples for amniotic fluid analysis to nearly 100%. Ultrasound allows identification of the placenta and delineation of the placental edges, and in the majority of cases amniocentesis can be performed safely and without blood contamination. Ultrasound is also helpful in showing "pockets" of fluid in patients with little fluid or with difficult placental localizations and for measuring the distance from the skin to the pocket of fluid to determine the length of the needle to be used. More recently, color mapping has become invaluable for visualization of the umbilical cord and has given the operator almost absolute

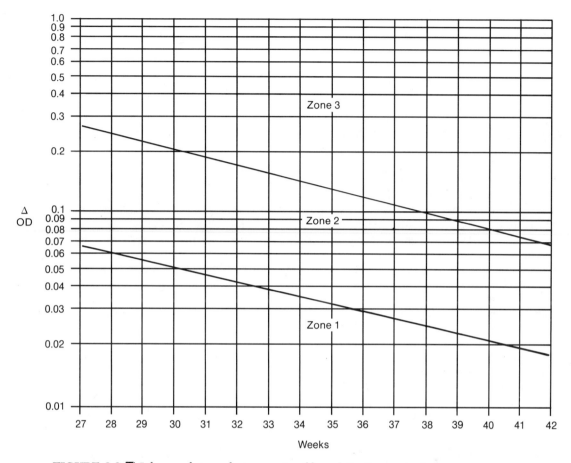

FIGURE 6-3 ◪ Liley graph to evaluate severity of hemolytic disease. (Redrawn from Liley AW: Liquor amnii analysis in management of pregnancy complicated by rhesus sensitization. *Am J Obstet Gynecol* 1961;82[6]:1359-1370.)

certainty that the pocket selected for amniocentesis does not contain loops of cord.

Once the tap site has been selected, the patient is instructed to empty her bladder, and the abdomen is prepared with aseptic technique using povidone-iodine (Betadine) solution. Local anesthetic infiltration of the skin may be used. Depending on the depth of the pocket, a 3½- to 7-inch long, 22-gauge disposable needle is inserted to the depth previously determined with a double thrust of the obstetrician's hand. With the first thrust, the needle goes through the skin and subcutaneous tissue only. Usually the anterior abdominal muscles contract involuntarily after the insertion of the needle through the skin, and it is necessary to wait for a few seconds until the muscles relax to advance the needle, with a second thrust, into the amniotic sac. Slow, hesitant thrusts usually result in either a tap failure or a bloody tap. The tip or the whole length of the needle should be visualized with ultrasound, and the needle should be advanced or withdrawn until it reaches the center of a pocket of fluid.

About 5 to 10 ml of amniotic fluid are required for spectrophotometric analysis. The fluid should be kept in a brown bottle to protect it from exposure to the sunlight, which destroys some of the bilirubin and causes false low readings. The fluid is centrifuged at 4000 rpm for 20 minutes, filtered through a Whatman 2 filter, and analyzed in the spectrophotometer.

When normal amniotic fluid is examined in a spectrophotometer using water as a blank, the optical density (OD) readings between 350 and 650 nm form an almost straight line. If the amniotic fluid contains bilirubin, the OD readings will show a peak at 450 nm, and the size of the peak will be proportional to the amount of pigment in the fluid. Rather than using continuous scanning between 350 and 650 nm, the majority of laboratories measure the OD at 375, 450, and 525 nm. The results are plotted on semilogarithmic paper, and a straight line is drawn between the readings at 375 and 525 nm. The difference between the point at which the line crosses the 450-nm mark (expected value) and the actual reading at this wavelength is the delta OD 450 that is used by the clinician for patient management purposes. When using amniotic fluid analysis in the management of sensitized Rh-negative patients, the obstetrician must keep a number of points in mind. These are discussed below.

Bilirubin content of normal amniotic fluid. Amniotic fluid bilirubin concentration increases from 10 to 17 weeks, remains stable until 26 weeks, and decreases thereafter to term.[11,14]

Premature labor. Mild contractions are usually the rule after amniocentesis, but they often subside after 30 to 40 minutes. In rare cases, contractions may continue and result in premature labor. Patients undergoing amniocentesis should be instructed to report to their physicians if the contractions continue and become stronger several hours after the procedure, and if such occurs, therapy with beta-mimetics is indicated.

Bloody taps. Even if an amniocentesis is atraumatic and yields clear amniotic fluid, a small button of red cells is frequently found after centrifugation. However, this is not a *bloody tap,* a term that is reserved for gross, visible contamination of the fluid with fetal or maternal blood. Bloody taps are less common now that amniocenteses are done under ultrasound guidance. In the large majority of cases, the blood is maternal in origin, but it may be a mixture of maternal and fetal cells, especially in cases of transplacental amniocentesis. If fluid grossly contaminated with blood comes out of the needle after amniocentesis, the best thing to do is to let the fluid escape to see if spontaneous clearing occurs. If the hematocrit value after clearing is more than 5%, the OD 450 reading will be distorted and should not be used for patient management purposes. If the fluid is grossly contaminated, the chances of adequate spontaneous clearing are

low, and the position of the needle must be assessed with ultrasound.

When amniocentesis is carried out in a patient who is already immunized, there is no value in administering D immunoglobulin after the tap. In contrast, administration of D immunoglobulin is indicated after amniocentesis in nonimmunized patients, especially if the tap is bloody.

Infection. Infection is a rare complication of amniocentesis. The resulting chorioamnionitis usually leads to preterm labor and results in preterm delivery. The treatment is evacuation of the uterus. Adherence to aseptic technique is the key to the prevention of this problem.

Fetal distress. Rarely, after amniocentesis there are marked changes in fetal heart rate. Electronic monitoring in the majority of these cases is characterized by the presence of wide oscillations in baseline heart frequency. These changes usually disappear spontaneously within 1 or 2 hours after the procedure. However, if the tap has been bloody and especially if a sinusoidal pattern is observed after amniocentesis, there are reasons for concern; this pattern is frequently an indicator of fetal anemia, and if a good proportion of the red cells obtained with the procedure are of fetal origin, the possibility of fetal hemorrhage should be strongly considered.

Aspiration of urine. The best way to avoid aspiration of urine is to instruct the patient to empty her bladder immediately before amniocentesis. If there is any doubt that the liquid obtained is urine, a drop of it should be placed on a glass slide, smeared with a cotton tip, and observed with the microscope for ferning. Amniotic fluid ferns; urine does not. Also, the fluid may be checked for protein using an Albustix strip: the amniotic fluid has protein; normal urine does not.

Meconium-stained fluid. The peak absorption of meconium in amniotic fluid is similar to the Soret band of hemoglobin (410 nm). As a consequence, meconium causes a marked rise in delta OD 450, and this change does not disappear after centrifugation. For this reason, delta OD 450 values from meconium-stained specimens should not be used for patient management.

Polyhydramnios. Excessive production and accumulation of amniotic fluid are complications of erythroblastosis fetalis, usually indicating deterioration of the fetal status. In this situation, the bilirubin content of the amniotic fluid becomes diluted, resulting in a falsely low delta OD 450 value that may be misleading when evaluating the severity of the disease. If polyhydramnios is suspected or diagnosed, the total volume of amniotic fluid should be determined using ^{51}Cr, Evans blue, or sodium paraaminohippurate, and the OD 450 value should be corrected for dilution. For example, a delta OD 450 value of 0.15 at 27 weeks of gestation (zone 2) in a patient with a total amniotic fluid volume of 2.5 L is equivalent to a delta OD 450 of 0.6 (zone 3) when corrected for excessive volume (normal fluid volume at 26 weeks equals 675 ml).

Multiple gestation. If the immunized Rh-negative mother has a multiple pregnancy, each fetus should be evaluated separately. In the case of twin pregnancy, both, neither, or only one of the twins may be affected, and each one of the amniotic sacs should be aspirated. In these cases, the help of ultrasound is invaluable. It allows visualization of the membrane separating the sacs and visualization of penetration by the needle if a single puncture is chosen as the procedure of choice. If each sac is to be entered using different puncture sites, 1 ml of indigo carmine may be injected into the sac entered first. The fluid obtained from the second sac must not contain any dye; if it does, the tip of the needle is probably still in the first sac.

Management based on delta OD 450 values. In patients with a poor obstetric history resulting from fetal hemolytic disease or who start off the pregnancy with titers above 1:1024, early assessment is desirable. In these situations, amniocentesis may be performed between 16 and 24 weeks, and an OD 450 greater than 0.15 will indicate severe immunization and the need for cordocentesis and early transfusion. Values below 0.09 indicate mild or no disease. Values between 0.09 and 1.5 will require further evaluation with cordocentesis. Depending on the situation, amniocentesis can be repeated every 1 to 3 weeks between 16 and 24 weeks. After 27 weeks the need for intervention can be determined using the Liley graph (see Figure 6-3).

In his original description, Liley[15] recorded the delta OD 450 of 101 immunized patients on semilogarithmic paper (gestational age in weeks on the ordinate, delta OD 450 values on the abscissa) and divided the graph into three zones (see Figure 6-3). The upper zone (3) corresponded to severely affected infants, the low zone (1) to nonaffected or mildly affected babies, and the middle zone (2) included both types of patients (severely and mildly affected).

If the amniotic fluid shows a delta OD 450 value in zone 1, there is no immediate danger of intrauterine fetal death, and the procedure should be repeated in 4 weeks. If the delta OD 450 values remain in zone 1 with amniocentesis carried out every 4 weeks, the patient should be delivered at term, and the birth of a nonaffected (Rh-negative) or a mildly affected baby should be anticipated.

If at any time during gestation the amniotic fluid shows a delta OD 450 value in zone 2, the procedure should be repeated in 1 week, since values in this zone may correspond to moderately or severely affected infants. If the following amniocentesis shows an OD 450 value in zone 1, there is no need for another tap before 4 weeks. If the following amniocentesis shows a smaller delta OD 450 value (decreasing trend) but still within zone 2, the amniocentesis should be repeated in 2 weeks. If the following amniocentesis shows a delta OD 450 value similar to the previous one but still within zone 2 (horizontal trend), the procedure should be repeated in another week, and if the horizontal trend continues, cordocentesis and evaluation of the fetal hematocrit are indicated with the exception of those patients who show adequate indexes of fetal lung maturity and are better managed by immediate delivery.

If the initial amniotic fluid examination shows a delta OD 450 in zone 3 or if any delta OD 450 value previously in zone 1 or 2 moves to zone 3 (rising trend), the infant may be in imminent danger of intrauterine death. In these cases, fetal blood sampling should be performed immediately, and intrauterine transfusion should be performed if the fetal hematocrit is less than 30%. Intrauterine transfusion may be avoided in fetuses with adequate indexes of lung maturation; delivery of these fetuses is the management of choice. A summary of the management protocol using Liley's zones is shown in Figure 6-4.

The method of Robertson[16] is similar to the one previously described and is used in many places around the world (Figure 6-5). It has the advantage over Liley's method of greater individualization of care by using amniocentesis intervals of 1, 2, 3, and 4 weeks, depending on the delta OD 450 value and the gestational age.

Another method of fetal evaluation in erythroblastosis is that of Freda,[3] which uses the net value (not the delta value) of the OD at 450 nm.

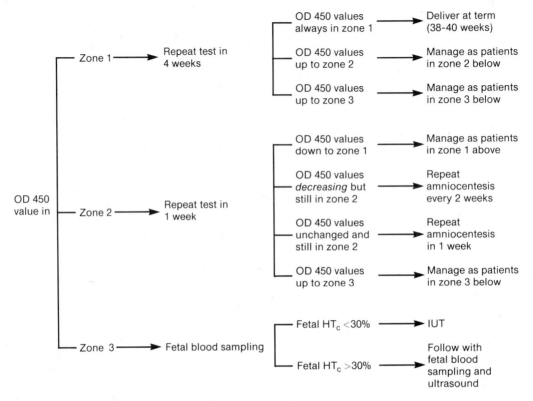

FIGURE 6-4 ◪ Management of the Rh-immunized patient after 24 weeks based on amniotic fluid analysis.

TABLE 6-4 ◪ Net value of amniotic fluid OD 450 and fetal status

Freda's grade	Net OD 450 value	Bilirubin in the fluid (mg/dl)	Fetal status
1+	0 to 0.20	0 to 0.28	Normal or possibly affected
2+	0.2 to 0.34	0.28 to 0.46	Affected but not in jeopardy
3+	0.35 to 0.70	0.47 to 0.95	Distressed, probably in failure
4+	More than 0.70	More than 0.95	Impending fetal death

From Freda VJ: *Am J Obstet Gynecol* 1965;93:321.

Freda correlated these absolute values with the bilirubin concentration in the fluid and the fetal status at birth (Table 6-4).

Cordocentesis. The introduction of cordocentesis by Daffos et al.[17,18] changed dramatically the management and therapy of Rh-sensitized patients. Blood sampling allows a precise measurement of the fetal hematocrit and hemoglobin concentration to determine the severity of the hemolytic process and the need for intrauterine transfusion. Also, the same technique may be used for direct intravascular transfusion to the fetus,[19,20] a technique that has allowed successful *in utero* treatment of hydropic fetuses unresponsive to transfusions into the peritoneal cavity.

For fetal blood sampling or transfusion, the site of the placental insertion of the umbilical

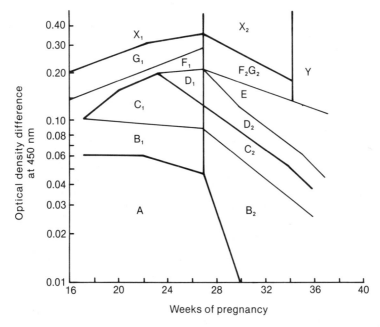

FIGURE 6–5 ◪ Management zones in Rh isoimmunization based on delta OD 450 values and gestational age, according to Robertson.[16] A, Repeat every 4 weeks and deliver at term; B1 and B2, repeat every 4 weeks and deliver at term; C1, repeat every 3 weeks; C2, repeat every 3 weeks and deliver at 39 weeks; D1 and D2, repeat every 2 weeks and deliver at 38 weeks; E, repeat every week or every 2 weeks and deliver between 36 and 38 weeks; F1, repeat every 2 weeks until delivery feasible; F2, G1, and G2, repeat every 2 weeks until delivery feasible or intrauterine transfusion mandatory; X1, intrauterine transfusion; X2, immediate delivery or intrauterine transfusion; Y, immediate delivery.

cord is found using high resolution ultrasound and color flow mapping. Then, under ultrasound guidance a needle is introduced into the umbilical vein, and fetal blood is drawn for determination of fetal blood group and Rh, direct Coomb's, hemoglobin, and hematocrit. A hematocrit of less than 30% is an indication for intrauterine transfusion. In competent hands the procedure has few serious complications. It does not require maternal sedation and is performed as an outpatient procedure.

The main indication for fetal blood sampling in the Rh-sensitized patient is the finding of amniotic fluid bilirubin values in the high middle zone or in zone 3 after 26 weeks of gestation. Others have proposed using cordocentesis instead of amniocentesis between 16 and 26 weeks in the evaluation of patients at high-risk for severe hemolytic disease. The proponents of this approach cite the lack of reliability of amniotic fluid analysis at this gestational age as the main

reason for the use of cordocentesis. Other investigators prefer to use amniocentesis or ultrasound as the primary test and argue that cordocentesis has a risk of fetal mortality of approximately 5% at this gestational age, that not every fetus at high risk for severe hemolytic disease becomes anemic before 26 weeks, and that routine cordocentesis in this group of patients will expose many healthy fetuses to unnecessary procedural risk.

We use cordocentesis before 26 weeks only in those fetuses at high risk for severe Rh disease that show ascites in ultrasound evaluation or have an OD 450 greater than 0.15. In this way we expose to the substantial risk of cordocentesis only those fetuses that have a clear indication of severe hemolytic disease early in pregnancy.

Some investigators[21] have proposed performing cordocentesis at 18 to 20 weeks in sensitized Rh-patients if the father's Rh genotype indicates a probability of less than 90% that the fetus has the D antigen. The apparent advantage of this approach is to avoid serial amniocentesis if the fetus is Rh negative. The disadvantage of this approach is that in the majority of patients, the risk of serial amniocentesis for mother and fetus is very low compared with the risk of fetal blood sampling.

In summary, cordocentesis provides precise information about the fetal situation because the blood type and Rh, hematocrit, direct Coombs, and reticulocyte count can be determined. It also provides access for direct intravascular transfusion. However, cordocentesis is not without problems. It frequently causes fetomaternal bleeding, massive increase in antibody concentration, and worsening of the hemolytic process. Also, bleeding from the sampling site, thrombosis of the umbilical vessels, and severe vasospasm with secondary fetal bradycardia are relatively frequent procedural complications. The risk of fetal death after cordocentesis is approximately 1.5% after 24 weeks, and it may be as high as 5% before 24 weeks.

Intrauterine transfusion. Since its introduction in 1963, IUT has been instrumental in saving hundreds of infants affected by erythroblastosis fetalis. IUT results are not uniform. They are modified by variables such as the experience and skills of the obstetrician performing the procedure, the severity of the fetal disease, the placental implantation site, the obesity of the mother, and the fetal lie, among many other factors.

There are two types of IUT: intraperitoneal and intravascular. In both methods the procedure is carried out under visual control with real-time ultrasound. In intraperitoneal IUT the blood is injected into the peritoneal cavity and transported by the lymphatic system into the fetal bloodstream. In intravascular transfusion, the blood is injected directly into the umbilical circulation.[4]

The two types of IUT are not mutually exclusive. They complement each other, and one or both of them may be used, depending on the circumstances, to obtain a good fetal outcome.[22,23] Although the direct intravascular approach is the procedure of choice, it is not without problems.[24] It is preferable to perform an intraperitoneal transfusion if the approach to the umbilical cord is difficult (posterior placenta, maternal obesity) or if a sample of fetal blood cannot be obtained after several attempts. The survival rate of fe-

tuses transfused intravascularly is 84.8%, 80.1% for hydropic and 89.5% for nonhydropic fetuses.

In the severely hydropic fetus, the intravascular approach offers the best possibility for successful fetal therapy.[25] In these cases, if the access to the umbilical cord near the placental insertion is difficult, it is possible to transfuse using the intrahepatic portion of the umbilical vein.[26] Another route of access to the intravascular compartment of the fetus when everything else fails is the right ventricle of the heart.[24]

Early delivery and use of glucocorticoids. The classic approach to the management of sensitized Rh-negative mothers was early delivery or IUT depending on the severity of the fetal hemolytic process. This has changed with the development of intrauterine transfusions and the availability of laboratory indexes to assess fetal lung maturation. Also, it is possible to use drugs that accelerate the maturation of the infant's lungs and decrease the occurrence of neonatal hyaline membrane disease (HMD).

Evaluation of the lecithin to sphingomyelin (L/S) ratio and the presence of phosphatidylglycerol (PG) should be a part of the amniotic fluid analysis whenever the delta OD 450 value is in zone 3 or upper zone 2 and the pregnancy is at 32 or more weeks. Under those circumstances, if the L/S ratio is greater than 2.2 or PG is present, the baby should be delivered. In these patients, the fetal mortality and morbidity caused by IUT is greater than that resulting from the delivery of the infant.

As discussed extensively in Chapter 4, maternal administration of glucocorticoids is effective in preventing the development of HMD in infants delivered before term, and this may be used advantageously in the management of Rh-sensitized pregnancies. All patients for whom the amniotic fluid analysis indicates the need for IUT or immediate delivery and who also have immature L/S ratio should receive glucocorticoids if IUT cannot be performed. We use betamethasone, 12 mg intramuscularly daily for 2 consecutive days, before delivery. We[27] found that glucocorticoid treatment has little immediate effect on the L/S ratio, and the studies by Caritis et al.[28] have shown that respiratory distress syndrome (RDS) prevention occurs even if corticosteroid-treated erythroblastotic infants are delivered when they still have immature L/S ratios. Corticosteroids cause a decrease in delta OD 450 values by a mechanism that may or may not be related to the hemolytic process. Therefore the obstetrician must avoid the false sense of security given by the drop in delta OD 450 values that occurs after glucocorticoid treatment and should deliver the infant 24 hours after the second dose of betamethasone.

◢ IMPORTANT POINTS ◣

1. In the majority of cases Rh isoimmunization results from the passage of fetal Rh-positive cells into the bloodstream of Rh-negative mothers at the time of delivery.

2. The distinction between homozygous and heterozygous Rh-negative fathers is complicated because there is no antiserum against the d antigen and it has to be made using genotype frequency tables based on allelic frequencies.

3. Some individuals have a gene that produces only a part of the D antigen. This varient is called *Du,* and it should be absent (Du negative) for a given individual to be considered Rh negative.

4. Some antigens frequently found in routine antepartum testing belong to the Lewis group. The Lewis antigens do not cause fetal hemolytic disease.

5. Usually there is an interval of several weeks between the time of the fetomaternal bleeding and the appearance of anti-Rh antibodies in the maternal serum. The administration of D immunoglobulin shortly after delivery inhibits this immune response.

6. In as many as 10% of the cases, postpartum administration of the usual dose of D immunoglobulin is ineffective in preventing the development of Rh isoimmunization. In most cases this is the consequence of a large fetomaternal transfusion and insufficient antigenic neutralization by the D immunoglobulin. A large fetomaternal transfusion should be suspected with the birth of a pale baby, a fetal hemoglobin of less than 10 g/dl, abruptio placentae, midforceps operations, and traumatic deliveries.

7. Maternal antibody titers are useful exclusively for the follow-up of patients in their first immunized pregnancy. They are not useful during subsequent pregnancies.

8. Traditionally, the first amniocentesis was carried out at 26 weeks because the Liley graph used to evaluate the severity of fetal hemolysis starts at this gestational age. At the present time evaluation of fetuses at high-risk for hemolytic disease before 26 weeks is performed using amniocentesis, ultrasound examinations, and cordocentesis.

9. The most important indication for cordocentesis is an amniotic fluid bilirubin in Liley's zone 3.

10. A good fetal outcome should be expected in approximately 85% of the fetuses that require intrauterine transfusion.

11. Direct intravascular intrauterine transfusion can reverse fetal hydrops and result in better than 80% good outcomes in these seriously compromised fetuses.

REFERENCES

1. Weinstein L: Irregular antibodies causing hemolytic disease of the newborn: A continuous problem. *Clin Obstet Gynecol* 1982;25:321.
2. Clayton EM Jr, Feldhaus W, Phythyon JM, et al: Transplacental passage of fetal erythrocytes during pregnancy. *Obstet Gynecol* 1966;28:194.
3. Freda VJ: The Rh problem in obstetrics and a new concept of its management using amniocentesis and spectrophotometric scanning of amniotic fluid. *Am J Obstet Gynecol* 1965;93:321.
4. Gorman JG: *The Role of the Laboratory in Hemolytic Disease of the Newborn.* Philadelphia, Lea & Febiger, 1975, pp 36 and 163-164.
5. Erlandson ME, Huber JM: Severe erythroblastosis fetalis in first immunized pregnancies. *Am J Obstet Gynecol* 1964;90:779.
6. Cohen F, Zueler WW: Identification of blood group antigens by immunofluorescence and its application to the detection of the transplacental passage of erythrocytes in mother and child. *Vox Sang* 1964;9:75.
7. Quennan JT: *Modern Management of the Rh Problem.* New York, Harper & Row Publishers Inc, 1977, pp 31-32.
8. Frigoletto FD, Greene MF, Benacerraf BR, et al: Ultrasonographic fetal surveillance in the management of the isoimmunized pregnancy. *N Engl J Med* 1986;315:430-432.
9. Reece EA, Cole SW, Romero R, et al: Ultrasonography versus amniotic fluid spectral analysis: Are they sensitive enough to predict neonatal complications associated with isoimmunization? *Obstet Gynecol* 1989;74:357-360.
10. Liley AW: Liquor amnii analysis in management of pregnancy complicated by Rhesus sensitization. *Am J Obstet Gynecol* 1961;82:1359-1370.
11. Nicolaides KH, Rodeck CH, Mibashan RS, et al: Have Liley charts outlived their usefulness? *Am J Obstet Gynecol* 1986;155:90.
12. Ananth U, Warsof SL, Coulihan JM, et al: Midtrimester amniotic fluid delta optical density at 450 nm in normal pregnancies. *Am J Obstet Gynecol* 1986;155:664-666.

13. Ananth U, Queenan JT: Does midtrimester delta OD 450 of amniotic fluid reflect severity of Rh disease? *Am J Obstet Gynecol* 1989;161:47-49.

14. Niswander KR: Spectrophotometric analysis of amniotic fluid early in gestation. *Am J Obstet Gynecol* 1970;108:1296.

15. Liley AW: Liquor amnii analysis in management of pregnancy complicated by rhesus sensitization. *Am J Obstet Gynecol* 1961;82:1359.

16. Robertson JG: Management of patients with Rh isoimmunization based on amniotic fluid analysis. *Am J Obstet Gynecol* 1969;103:713.

17. Daffos F, Capella-Pavlovsky M, Forrestier F: A new procedure for fetal blood sampling in utero: Preliminary result of fifty-three cases. *Am J Obstet Gynecol* 1983;146:985-987.

18. Daffos F, Capella-Pavlovsky M, Forrestier F: Fetal blood sampling during pregnancy with use of a needle guided by ultrasound: A study of 606 consecutive cases. *Am J Obstet Gynecol* 1985;153:655-660.

19. Poissonnier M-H, Brossard Y, Demedeiros N, et al: Two hundred intrauterine exchange transfusions in severe blood incompatibilities. *Am J Obstet Gynecol* 1989;161:709-713.

20. Berkowitz RL, Chitkara U, Goldberg JD, et al: Intrauterine intravascular transfusion for severe red blood cell isoimmunization: Ultrasound-guided percutaneous approach. *Am J Obstet Gynecol* 1986;155:574-581.

21. Reece EA, Copel JA, Scioscia AL, et al: Diagnostic fetal umbilical blood sampling in the management of isoimmunization. *Am J Obstet Gynecol* 1988;159:1057-1062.

22. Barss VA, Benacerraf BR, Frigoletto FD, et al: Management of isoimmunized pregnancies by use of intravascular techniques. *Am J Obstet Gynecol* 1988;159:932-937.

23. Gravenhorst JB, Kanhai HHH, Meerman RH, et al: Twenty-two years of intrauterine intraperitoneal transfusions. *Eur J Obstet Gynecol Reprod Biol* 1989;33:71-77.

24. Westgren M, Selbing A, Stangenberg M: Fetal intracardiac transfusions in patients with severe rhesus isoimmunization. *Br Med J* 1988;296:885-886.

25. Seeds JW, Bowes WA: Ultrasound-guided fetal intravascular transfusion in severe rhesus immunization. *Am J Obstet Gynecol* 1986;154:1105-1107.

26. Nicolini U, Santolaya J, Ojo O, et al: The fetal intrahepatic umbilical vein as an alternative to cord needling for prenatal diagnosis and therapy. *Prenat Diagn* 1988;8:655-671.

27. Arias F, Pineda J, Johnson LW: Changes in human amniotic fluid lecithin/sphyngomyelin ratio and dipalmitoyl/lecithin associated with maternal betamethasone therapy. *Am J Obstet Gynecol* 1979;133:894.

28. Caritis SN, Mueller-Heubach E, Edelstone DI: Effect of betamethasone on analysis of amniotic fluid in the rhesus-sensitized pregnancy. *Am J Obstet Gynecol* 1977;127:529.

7

MULTIFETAL GESTATION

Few topics in obstetrics have stimulated more interest and generated more literature than multiple gestation. Communications on twins are abundant and reflect the multidisciplinary approach followed in the study of this biologic phenomenon. Therefore, it is not surprising that serious efforts have been made to unify all kinds of contributions on twins into a new branch of science named *gemellology*. In this chapter the emphasis is on the management of problems associated with twin gestations and the reasons behind the proposed management, and only a small part is devoted to the study of gestations with higher fetal numbers. However, most of the problems associated with twin gestations may be applied to triplet and quadruplet gestations and to gestations with higher fetal numbers. Furthermore, the incidence of pregnancies with more than two infants is so low that there is no reason for a generous treatment of that subject in this book.

■ INCIDENCE

The frequency of twinning is highest among the black race and consistently lowest among Orientals. The white race is between these two extremes. For example, in China there are 3 twins per each 1000 live births; in Scotland, 12.3 per 1000; and in Nigeria, 57.2 per 1000. These differences in frequency are the result of varia-

tions in double-ovum twinning because the rate of monozygotic twins is apparently constant (3.5 per 1000) throughout the world.

Factors influencing the frequency of dizygotic twinning are maternal age, parity, and conception soon after cessation of oral contraceptives. In fact, it has been reported that the incidence of twin gestation increases with maternal age (up to 35 to 39 years) and parity. Also, studies show that if oral contraceptives have been used for more than 6 months and conception occurs within 1 month after discontinuation, the chances of a twin gestation double.

An important factor increasing the incidence of multiple gestations has been the development of ovulation induction in infertile couples. The incidence of multifetal pregnancies after induction of ovulation with clomiphene is between 6.8% and 17%. Following induction of ovulation with gonadotropins, the incidence of multifetal gestations is between 18% and 53%.[1] In patients treated with gonadotropins, the rate of multifetal pregnancies is highest in hypogonadotropic patients (50%) followed by normogonadotropic patients (32%), oligomenorrheic patients (18.4%), and then patients with corpus luteum deficiency (17.6%).[2] Unfortunately, there is a narrow margin between the amount of gonadotropin that is necessary to achieve ovulation in the infertile patient and the amount that will cause multiple follicle development and multifetal pregnancies.

With the development of ultrasonic techniques for the evaluation of pregnancy, it has become apparent that the incidence of multiple gestation in humans may be more common than previously indicated. In fact, the incidence of multiple gestation in a white population may be as high as 20 per 1000 pregnancies. Half of these fail to be recognized as twin gestations because one of the sacs either spontaneously aborts or spontaneously reabsorbs early in pregnancy. For example, in one study[3] 30 multiple pregnancies were found by first-trimester ultrasonic examination among 1500 pregnant patients (incidence of 20 per 1000). Only 14 of these patients, however, produced live multiple-birth infants (13 twins and one set of triplets). In seven of the 30 patients (23.3%), one of the sacs developed normally, and the other became smaller and showed no heart movements. Two of them aborted, and the remaining five delivered single babies. The other nine patients (30%) of the original 30 aborted, eight early in pregnancy and one at 24 weeks of gestation. This and other studies strongly suggest that the presence of a blighted ovum or the reabsorption of a gestational sac does not have any adverse effect on a coexisting normal pregnancy.

◢ CLASSIFICATION

There are two types of twins: (1) monozygotic, identical, uniovular, or single-egg twins and (2) dizygotic, fraternal, biovular, nonidentical, or two-egg twins. Monozygotic twins have identical genotypes and therefore are of the same sex. The similarity of their genetic composition is the result of the early division of an ovum fertilized by one sperm cell into two cell masses containing identical genetic information. In contrast, dizygotic twins are the result of the fertilization of two ova by different sperm, resulting in separate maternal and paternal genetic contributions to each infant. Approximately two thirds of all twin pregnancies are dizygotic, and one third are monozygotic.

Pregnancies with dizygotic twins have two placentas and two amniotic sacs. Therefore all dizygotic gestations are dichorionic-diamniotic. Placentation is more complex in monozygotic twins, and the number of chorions and amnions varies with the time from fertilization until the zygotic division. In about 30% of monozygotic twins, the zygotic division occurs within 72 hours of fertilization, and the placenta will be dichorionic-di-

amniotic, similar to that of dizygotic gestations. In approximately 65% of monozygotic twins, the zygotic division occurs 4 to 8 days after fertilization, and in these cases the twins will share a single placenta (monochorionic), but each will be in a separate amniotic sac (diamniotic). In approximately 5% of monozygotic twin gestations, the zygotic division occurs more than 8 days after fertilization, and they will share a single placenta and a single amniotic sac (monochorionic-monoamniotic). In very rare cases (1 in 50,000 deliveries), the zygotic division occurs more than 13 days after fertilization, and the result will be conjoined twins.

The method most frequently used to determine the zygosity of twins is examination of the placenta at birth.[4] However, because of the variations that exist in monozygotic placentation, this does not always permit determination of zygosity. The microscopic examination of a piece of the septum dividing the two fetal cavities is most important. In dichorionic-diamniotic placentas there is chorionic tissue present between the two amnions. In monochorionic-diamniotic placentas the septum consists of two amnion layers without interposing chorion. Examination of the placenta itself will also show, in the case of dichorionic-diamniotic placentas, whether the two placentas are fused or separated (Figure 7-1).

The finding of a monochorionic placenta is unequivocal proof of monozygosity. However, it is difficult in some cases to decide whether a single placenta is monochorionic-diamniotic or whether it is a fused dichorionic-diamniotic placenta. Also, the presence of a dichorionic-diamniotic placenta does not necessarily imply the existence of a dizygotic state, since up to 30% of monozygotic twins exhibit this type of placentation.

Several other methods have been used with varied success to determine twin zygosity. Among them, the study of blood groups and types (ABO, MNSs, Rh, Kell, Duffy, Kidd, etc.) is popular.[5] A technique used with increasing frequency to determine twin zygosity is genetic fingerprinting using DNA probes to identify similarities or differences in restriction fragment length polymorphisms present in highly polymorphic areas of the genome.[6]

◢ COMPLICATIONS

Maternal morbidity is increased 3 to 7 times in multiple gestations. The main causes of maternal morbidity are increased incidence of hyper-

DICHORIONIC DIAMNIOTIC

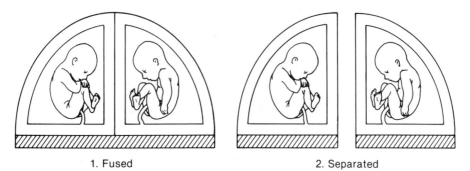

1. Fused   2. Separated

MONOCHORIONIC

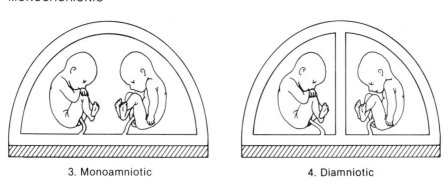

3. Monoamniotic   4. Diamniotic

FIGURE 7-1 ◪ Placental morphology in twin pregnancy.

tension during pregnancy (14% to 20% in twins versus 6% to 8% in singleton pregnancies), sepsis associated with premature rupture of the fetal membranes (3 times more frequent in twins), and excessive postpartum bleeding (about 20% of all twin pregnancies). Overall, antenatal complications occur in approximately 83% of twin pregnancies compared with an incidence of 32% in singleton gestations. The most common complications are preterm labor, hypertension, and fetal death.[7]

The main problems affecting the fetal and neonatal outcome are mortality, preterm labor, premature rupture of the membranes, twin-twin transfusion syndrome, fetal growth retardation, congenital abnormalities, umbilical cord problems, abruptio placentae, malpresentations, and other intrapartum complications.

Table 7-1 compares the most frequent causes of perinatal mortality in twins and singleton pregnancies as found in the Collaborative Perinatal Project of the National Institute of Neurological and Communicative Disorders and

TABLE 7-1 ◪ Causes of perinatal death in twins and singleton pregnancies in the United States

Cause	Perinatal deaths per 1000 births		
	Twins	Singleton	p
Amniotic fluid infection with intact membranes	22.6	5.9	<0.001
Premature rupture of membranes	15.9	3.5	<0.001
Fetal hypoxia of unknown cause	15.1	2.6	<0.001
Twin transfusion syndrome	11.7		
Congenital anomalies	10.1	3.2	<0.04
Large placental infarcts	10.9	2.1	<0.001
Hydramnios	8.3	0.1	<0.001
Overall perinatal mortality	138.7	33.4	<0.001

Data from the Collaborative Perinatal Project, in Naeye RL, et al: *Am J Obstet Gynecol* 1978;131:267.

Stroke.[8] Perinatal mortality in twins is on the average around 14.2%, and this is 3 to 11 times greater than in singleton pregnancies. A recent study found that the mortality is predominantly neonatal (51 per 1000) rather than fetal (28 per 1000).[9] Perinatal mortality varies with birth order and the type of placentation. Second twins do not do as well as first twins, with perinatal mortality approximately 9% for the first and 14% for the second twin. Also, monochorionic-monoamniotic twins have a poor prognosis, with perinatal mortality approximately 50%. Monochorionic-diamniotic twins have an approximate perinatal mortality of 26%. The best prognosis is for dichorionic twins, although their perinatal mortality is high, approximately 9%, when compared with singletons, approximately 2.9%. The most common causes of perinatal mortality in twins are prematurity, usually resulting from preterm labor or preterm rupture of membranes; abnormal development, such as twin-twin transfusion syndrome; congenital defects; placental insufficiency; and traumatic delivery.

Perinatal morbidity is high in multifetal pregnancies. The largest threat is preterm birth, which affects between 22% and 54% of all twin pregnancies. Cerebral palsy, microcephaly, porencephaly, and multicystic encephalomalacia occur more frequently in preterm twins than in preterm singletons.[10] Growth retardation affects 12% to 34% of twins. Trauma at delivery affects 5% to 10%, and cord prolapse occurs in 1% to 5% of twin deliveries.[11]

Hypertension

There is an increased frequency of hypertension during pregnancy in patients with multifetal gestations (12.9%).[12] In a large number of these patients, hypertension occurs without proteinuria (pregnancy-induced hypertension [PIH]). It is possible that hypertension and edema develop because of an excessive expansion of intravascular volume. In these cases, the glomerular filtration rate is increased, proteinuria is absent, and serial hematocrit determinations show expansion of plasma volume. With bed rest PIH improves markedly, and a pregnancy may be significantly prolonged.

Patients with multifetal gestations may also develop preeclampsia that may be extremely severe. In these cases, proteinuria is marked, and there is clinical and laboratory evidence of vasoconstriction and decreased intravascular volume.

Anemia

Maternal anemia is a common complication of twin pregnancy. It occurs in 9.4% of twin gestations, compared with 4.1% in singleton pregnancies.[12] This results from the large degree of intravascular volume expansion that occurs during multifetal gestations. Because the predominant element in the expansion is the plasma volume, the net result is a drop in hematocrit and hemoglobin levels, especially during the second trimester, although these patients have an active hematopoiesis and their total red cell volume is larger than at the beginning of pregnancy. Also, in many patients the large increase in red cell synthesis that occurs during a twin pregnancy may exhaust limited iron storages, and iron deficiency anemia may occur. For further discussion on the diagnosis and workup of anemia in pregnancy, see Chapter 13.

Postpartum bleeding

Severe postpartum bleeding after the delivery of twins is in most cases a consequence of uterine atony. Postpartum hemorrhage is more common in twin pregnancies delivered near term when the muscle fibers have been stretched to their maximum. This complication may be prevented by the aggressive use of oxytocic agents immediately after delivery of the placenta. If excessive bleeding occurs in spite of adequate use of oxytocin, the intramuscular administration of prostaglandins may be lifesaving. Many physicians are using prostaglandins as the primary oxytocic agent in these cases. Additional information about the management of postpartum hemorrhage may be found in Chapter 21.

Preterm birth

The single largest factor associated with fetal and neonatal mortality and morbidity in twin gestation is low birth weight. A review of 26 large series of twin pregnancies[13] shows that 55.85% of twins have birth weights under 2500 g. In most cases this results from preterm birth caused by preterm labor or preterm premature rupture of the membranes. However, in many cases preterm birth is the result of certain problems that are specific to this type of gestation.

The reason for the increased frequency of preterm labor in twins is not completely clarified. Some investigators believe that distention of the uterus is the main cause. This hypothesis originated from observations of length of gestation versus litter number and size, which demonstrated a direct correlation between uterine stretching and initiation of parturition. The observation of increased frequency of preterm labor in patients with polyhydramnios substantiates this hypothesis. However, more research in this area is necessary.

Another hypothesis is that intrauterine infection is an important cause of preterm labor in twins. Some of the original data in this respect came from the Collaborative Perinatal Project.[8] In this study autopsies were carried out on 171 twin and 1264 single-born infants, and the causes of death were analyzed. Amniotic fluid infection with intact membranes or with preterm rupture of the fetal membranes was the single leading cause of perinatal mortality in twins. It seems that the excessive growth of the uterus in twin gestation results in an early opening of the cervix and exposure of the fetal membranes to the bacterial flora of the vagina, leading to amnionitis with intact membranes and, in more severe cases, to amnionitis with ruptured membranes. Variations in the virulence of the vaginal pathogens would account for differences in the severity and natural history of the process. The data implying that infection is the most important cause of preterm birth in twin gestations need further corroborative evidence.

Discordant growth

One of the problems more frequently found in the antepartum care of patients with twin gestations is the occurrence of discordant growth, a problem that affects between 15% and 29% of these pregnancies.[14] Discordant growth causes a difference in the weight of the twins. This difference is expressed as a percentage of the larger twin's weight, and most authors consider significant a discrepancy of 20% or more. Some investigators classify discordant twins in two different categories depending on the magnitude of the weight difference. Grade I indicates a difference of 15% to 25%. Grade II is any discordancy greater than 25%. Discordant twins are also classified as discordant-first and discordant-second, indicating the birth order of the smaller twin.

The smaller twin is at high risk for perinatal complications. Many of them die as a result of congenital abnormalities or prematurity, and those who are born alive are often affected by neonatal morbidity with physical and intellectual sequelae. The frequency of complications is

greater and the prognosis is worse for second-discordant twins.[15]

Several ultrasound criteria have been used to diagnose discordant twin growth before birth. Initially, the diagnosis was based on the presence of a biparietal diameter difference of 6 mm or greater. Later, it was found that biparietal diameter measurements were inaccurate, and a difference of 5% or more in head circumference was recommended as the criterion for diagnosis of discordant growth. Even later, it was proposed that a difference of 20 mm in abdominal circumference should be used. In the last few years, the criterion most frequently used is a difference of 15% to 25% in estimated fetal weight.

Abnormal umbilical artery Doppler waveforms are associated with poor perinatal outcome in twin pregnancies[16] and have been proposed as a means of making the diagnosis of discordant growth. Unfortunately, the correlation of umbilical Doppler ultrasound with abnormal fetal growth is far from ideal.[17] The combination of a systolic to diastolic (S/D) ratio difference greater than 15% and an estimated fetal weight difference greater than 15% has been found to have a 73% positive and a 90% negative predictive value for the diagnosis of discordancy.[18]

The causes of discordant growth are unequal placental mass, genetic syndromes, and twin-twin transfusion syndrome. Discordant growth because of unequal placental mass occurs in both monochorionic and dichorionic twins but is more common in twins with dichorionic placentation.[19] This is a typical example of fetal growth retardation caused by a defect in the transfer of substrates from mother to infant. Characteristically, ultrasound measurements in these babies are asymmetric, with elevated head-to-abdomen and femur-to-abdomen ratios. In most patients the discordant growth is noticed after 24 weeks. If the placental insufficiency is severe enough, these babies show fetal heart rate monitoring signs of distress and may become acidotic.

Discordant growth because of genetic syndromes occurs in both monochorionic and dichorionic twins but is much more frequent in twins with monochorionic placentas. Usually the discordancy in growth can be detected by 16 to 20 weeks. Neural tube defects, cardiac abnormalities, and chromosomal defects are the most commonly found underlying problems. Ultrasound examination of these fetuses usually shows symmetric measurements without alterations in the head-to-abdomen and head-to-femur ratios. Similar to twins that are small because of placental insufficiency, genetically abnormal twins may show signs of fetal distress in monitoring tracings.

Growth discordancy because of twin-twin transfusion syndrome is limited to monochorionic twins. This phenomenon is discussed more extensively later in this chapter.

The management of twin pregnancies with growth discordancy differs depending on the cause of the problem. If the underlying reason is unequal placental mass, the well-being of the smaller twin should be assessed by means of frequent nonstress test and amniotic fluid volume. Treatment with weekly injections of betamethasone is desirable in anticipation of a preterm delivery. Delivery of both babies is usually the best management when signs of fetal distress arise. Elective delivery should be seriously considered when the pregnancy reaches 34 weeks and is definitely indicated at 36 weeks.

If the underlying problem causing the discordant growth is a genetic problem, the management will vary depending on the nature of the defect, its prognosis, and the possibilities for corrective therapy. If the growth discordancy is caused by a twin-twin transfusion syndrome, the best approach seems to be serial amniocentesis of the polyhydramniotic sac.

The route of delivery of discordant twins is an area of controversy. Some authors recommend delivery of all of these babies by cesarean section, regardless of gestational age and fetal presentation.[20] Others prefer a more selective approach to the problem and deliver vaginally if the cervix is ripe, the presentation is vertex/vertex, and the estimated weight of the discordant twin is greater than 1500 g.

Twin-twin transfusion syndrome

Twin-twin transfusion syndrome is a complication affecting 5% to 17% of monochorionic twin pregnancies. The problem is created by the existence of vascular communications between the infants causing a circulatory imbalance that results in anemia for one and polycythemia for the other. Vascular anastomoses in monochorionic placentation may be from artery to artery, artery to vein, and vein to vein. For the twin-twin transfusion syndrome to occur, it is necessary to have artery-to-vein vascular anastomosis. Compensation may occur if there is coexistent artery-to-artery anastomosis. Since there is wide variation in the number and size of the vascular anastomoses, the degree of hematologic imbalance between the twins may also vary greatly. The existence of vascular anastomosis in dichorionic placentas is so rare that, for all practical purposes, the possibility of twin-twin transfusion should be disregarded when this type of placentation is present.[21]

The criteria most commonly used for the diagnosis of twin-twin transfusion syndrome are a difference in hematocrit and birth weight greater than 20%. However, a recent study[22] shows that large differences in hemoglobin/hematocrit concentration may exist in the absence of twin-twin transfusion and that discordance in birth weight of 20% or more is as common in dichorionic as in monochorionic twins. The same study shows that most of the twins fulfilling the criteria for twin-to-twin transfusion are dichorionic.

The prenatal diagnosis of twin-twin transfusion is presumptive and requires that the following conditions be present:

1. Only one placenta is seen by ultrasound.
2. The twins are of the same sex.
3. There is a thin membrane between the twins (diamniotic placentation).
4. There is a 20% or larger discordancy in estimated fetal weight between the twins.
5. There is a significant discrepancy in the amniotic fluid volume surrounding each twin.
6. Fetal hydrops is present in one or both twins.
7. The umbilical cords differ in size.
8. Gestational age is less than 28 weeks.

The *stuck* twin is a term used to describe the sonographic appearance of an extreme form of twin-twin transfusion syndrome. In these cases the donor twin, markedly smaller in size and surrounded by little or no amniotic fluid, appears stuck against the uterine wall, in marked contrast with the large size and the polyhydramniotic sac of the recipient twin. The stuck twin mortality is approximately 80%, but it may decrease to 30% after treatment with serial amniocentesis.[23]

The value of Doppler ultrasound in the diagnosis of twin-twin transfusion is questionable. Some investigators have reported discordant umbilical waveforms,[24] whereas others have reported no significant differences[25] and no consistent patterns.[26] The latter finding seems more logical, and there is a wide range in the results of the umbilical artery Doppler analysis depending on the degree of anemia, the presence or absence of heart dysfunction, the coexistence of placental vascular changes, and the magnitude of the compensatory changes.

The twin-twin transfusion syndrome is a complication with very high perinatal mortality. In a recent study, Shah and Chaffin[27] found that the overall mortality for twin gestations delivered before 28 weeks was 55% to 80%. Before 26 weeks, the mortality is almost 100%. The overall mortality, irrespective of gestational age, is approximately 60% to 70%. These figures reflect the severe effects of the parabiotic circulation for both the donor and the recipient. The recipient, as a consequence of the maximally increased intravascular volume, often develops cardiomegaly and congestive heart failure. Recipients frequently die in utero and, when born alive, may develop respiratory distress and congestive heart failure. They also frequently develop hyperbilirubinemia. The donor twin usually has retarded somatic growth and will develop hydrops fetalis and high output heart failure if the anemia is severe. Polyhydramnios occurs frequently in the sac of the recipient twin, and oligohydramnios occurs in the donor.

The treatment of twin-twin transfusion consisted, until recently, of bed rest and preterm delivery. The results of this conventional therapy have been disappointing. Recently, better results have been reported with the use of serial amniocentesis.[28] The perinatal mortality of twin-twin transfusion syndrome, which was 100% in untreated pregnancies, decreased to 40% in the group treated with serial amniocentesis. Another approach to the treatment of this problem has been proposed by DeLia et al.[29] These investigators have occluded the vascular anastomosis between the twins using YAG laser coagulation through the fetoscope.

Preterm delivery is necessary in the overwhelming majority of twin-twin transfusion patients. Ideally, delivery should be effected after fetal lung maturation in both infants is documented by amniocentesis. However, this almost never occurs in practice, and in most cases it is necessary to deliver before lung maturity is achieved because of progressive, severe fetal deterioration. Because of the high probability of preterm delivery, glucocorticoids should be used to accelerate fetal lung maturity when the diagnosis of twin-twin transfusion is made. If amniocentesis is done to assess lung maturity, it is important to remember that the smaller, anemic twin usually has a more advanced degree of lung maturation than the plethoric twin. Therefore the amniocentesis should preferentially be performed in the large twin.

The incidence of cerebral palsy and neurologic abnormalities is greater in pregnancies affected by twin-twin transfusion. In one study, 55% of nine babies with twin-twin transfusion had white matter necrosis, whereas only 26% of twins with placental shunts but without twin-twin transfusion had brain damage.[10]

Monoamniotic twins

Monoamniotic twin pregnancies are relatively rare, occurring approximately once in every 12,500 births. They are of particular concern to the obstetrician because the associated perinatal mortality is approximately 50%, mostly caused by umbilical cord entanglement. Twin-twin transfusion, congenital abnormalities, and preterm delivery are also significant contributors to the poor outcomes.

The prenatal diagnosis of monoamniotic placentation is made when it is not possible to visualize the amniotic membrane separating the twins in at least three different examinations. Ideally, one of the attempts to visualize the membranes should be carried out between 20 and 26 weeks of gestation. Additional evidence supporting this diagnosis is the presence of twins of the same sex moving freely in an adequate amount of fluid and the presence of a single placenta.

Care of monoamniotic twins should be in tertiary centers equipped to handle preterm babies. Fetal surveillance with ultrasound examinations performed at least every 2 weeks is necessary once the diagnosis of monoamniotic twins is made. Color Doppler should be a part of the examination because of its value in determining umbilical cord entanglement. Also, fetal heart rate monitoring may show variable decelerations when cord entanglement is present.

There is controversy over the best time to deliver patients with monoamniotic twins. Some investigators[30] recommend early delivery, but others[31,32] argue that fetal survival does not decrease after 30 weeks and that early delivery is not necessary. The optimal route of delivery seems to be by cesarean section. Operative delivery will avoid umbilical cord problems and twin entanglement during parturition.

Single fetal demise in twins

The death of one twin occurs in approximately 3% to 4% of all twin pregnancies and generates difficult management problems for the obstetrician. Most of the single fetal demises occur in monochorionic twin pregnancies. The most significant problem is that the mortality and morbidity of the surviving twin are significantly increased. In fact, morbidity may affect as many as 46.2% of survivors, and approximately 20% of them will have neurologic damage.[33,34]

The effect of the death of one twin on the survivor varies depending on the gestational age at the time of death. A fetal demise before 14 weeks places no increased risk on the survivor. However, after 14 weeks, death or severe morbidity in the remaining twin may ensue. The most feared sequela is neurologic damage of the survivor. This probably results from transfer of thromboplastin from the dead twin, producing thrombotic arterial occlusions. These occlusions affect mainly the anterior and middle cerebral arteries, causing multicystic encephalomalacia.[35] Renal cortical necrosis may also occur.

The death of one twin may also have potential morbid effects on the mother. The most serious problem is disseminated intravascular coagulation (DIC). This complication usually occurs 3 or more weeks after the fetal demise, and since it may affect as many as 25% of the mothers, periodic monitoring of the hemostatic system is necessary in those patients who continue with the pregnancy.

The traditional approach to the demise of a twin has been to deliver the survivor to avoid embolization. This approach is unacceptable when the demise occurs before 24 weeks because the chance of extrauterine survival for the remaining twin is minimal. Between 24 and 30 weeks, the probability of survival is better, but neonatal morbidity may be substantial. After 30 weeks, the complications of preterm delivery on the survivor are probably less serious than those that may happen if intrauterine life continues, and delivery may be the best course of action.

The problem with the above plan of management is the inability to predict embolization. If it happens shortly after or simultaneously with fetal demise, then delivery of the survivor will not modify the neurologic outcome. Also, in most cases it is impossible to know how many days have passed since the fetal demise, and it is possible that brain damage has already occurred. It is preferable to deliver the survivor immediately only if it is known that the demise occurred 24 to 48 hours before it was discovered and the pregnancy is more than 28 weeks. It is also adequate to deliver the survivor when the pregnancy is 34 weeks or more, even if the interval between death and diagnosis is not known. Patients should be informed that delivery may not prevent neurologic damage in the surviving infant. In all other cases, expectant management should be adopted, and the parents should be informed of the 20% probability of neurologic damage and the inability to predict its occurrence. The surviving twin should be evaluated with ultrasound and with magnetic resonance imaging (MRI).[36] If no lesions are observed, the parents may be reassured. If damage is observed, they can be prepared for the disastrous outcome.

Congenital abnormalities

Congenital malformations occur more often in twins than in singleton pregnancies. This has been consistent in all studies, but there is some variation in the figures reported by different investigators. Hendricks,[37] in his review of 438 multiple pregnancies, found an incidence of congenital abnormalities of 10.6% for twins vs. 3.3% for all births. Guttmacher and Kohl,[38] in their analysis of 1327 twin deliveries, found 6.86% of twins and 3.98% of singletons to have abnormalities. In the material collected for the Collaborative Perinatal Project,[8] the malformation rate was 17.4% and 17.2%, respectively, in monochorionic and dichorionic twins. However, malformations among monochorionic twins were multiple or lethal, whereas those occurring in dichorionic infants were mostly minor. The congenital abnormalities affecting twin pregnancies are mostly multifactorial. The most common are cleft lip and palate, central nervous system defects, and cardiac defects.

Congenital abnormalities occur more frequently in twins of the same sex and in monochorionic twins. The spectrum of abnormalities is wide; however, they may not be unique to multiple gestations. The abnormalities that are unique to multiple gestations are conjoined twins and fetal acardia. Neural tube defects[39] and congenital heart disease[40] are abnormalities occurring more frequently in twins.

There are conflicting opinions in the medical literature concerning the frequency of chromosome abnormalities in twins. Several studies suggest that there is no increase in this type of abnormality, but other studies show the opposite. It is logical that because the majority of twins are dizygotic and each fetus has a risk of carrying a chromosomal abnormality, the likelihood that one will be affected is greater than one would expect for a singleton gestation. Some authors[41] have used formulas to calculate that risk and have concluded that the risk of chromosomal abnormalities for a 33-year-old patient with twins is similar to that of a 35-year-old woman with a singleton pregnancy.

Conjoined twins

An interesting anomaly unique to multiple pregnancy is conjoined twins. This is a rare disorder affecting 1 of every 200 monozygotic twin pregnancies, 1 of every 900 total twin pregnancies, and 1 of every 25,000 to 100,000 births. Conjoined twins are monoovular and have the same sex and karyotype. The phenomenon occurs predominantly in females (3:1 vs. males), and the cause is unknown. However, most investigators believe that it results from an incomplete fission of the embryonic inner cell mass rather than a partial fusion of two separate centers of growth. In any case, the phenomenon happens early in gestation, probably before the second week after fertilization.

Conjoined twins are classified according to the site of union. The different types include the following[42]:

Thoracopagus (40%), joined at the chest
Omphalopagus (35%), joined at the anterior abdominal wall
Pygopagus (18%), joined at the buttocks
Ischiopagus (6%), joined at the ischium
Craniopagus (2%), joined at the head

The antepartum diagnosis of conjoined twins is possible if an effort is made to rule out this condition in all monoamniotic twin gestations. In these cases ultrasound examination of the twins should include a careful inspection of the thorax and abdomen of the infants, especially if they are in the same position. The following ultrasound findings increase the probability that conjoined twins are present:

1. The twins face each other.
2. The heads are at the same level and plane.
3. The thoracic cages are in unusual proximity.
4. Both fetal heads are hyperextended.
5. There is no change in the relative position of the fetuses with movement, manipulation, or in repeat examination obtained hours or days later.

If the sonogram and fetogram are suggestive of conjoined twins, the diagnosis may be confirmed by introducing 40 ml of radiopaque material into the amniotic cavity. This technique, amniography, makes it possible to demonstrate the existence and location of the union between the fetuses. Repeated ultrasound examinations, computer tomography (CT), and MRI scanning are useful for antenatal determination of cardiac connections between the twins.

Once the diagnosis is made, plans should be made for delivery by cesarean section unless there are special circumstances indicating the possibility of a safe vaginal delivery. If allowed to labor, the majority will show abnormal patterns of cervical dilation and descent.

The outcome of conjoined twins is poor: approximately 40% of them will be stillborn, and another 35% will die within 1 day after delivery. The only hope of independent life is through surgical separation. The first successful surgical separation of conjoined twins was achieved in 1953. At the present time, with further advances in organ imaging, it is possible to obtain a better assessment of the characteristics of the union between conjoined twins and therefore determine more accurately the feasibility of separation. The absence of malformations, the lack of bone unions, and the existence of separate hearts are the most important indicators of the possibility of a successful surgical outcome.

Acardiac twinning

Acardia is another rare malformation that is unique to twin pregnancies. In this situation, one twin has no cardiac structures, and the circulation for both infants is maintained by the other twin's heart. The circulatory load may be so large that the normal twin eventually succumbs to high output heart failure. Mortality of the normal twin is approximately 50%.

The diagnosis of acardiac twinning is not always simple. The most frequent confusion is with anencephaly or with fetal demise of one twin. It is easy to erroneously diagnose fetal death in these cases because of the absence of cardiac motion and movement in the acardiac twin.

Management of this disorder is complex. Potential treatments include administration of cardiotonics to the mother or the fetus, serial amniocenteses, selective removal of the acardiac twin,[43] or insertion of a thrombogenic coil in the umbilical artery of the acardiac twin.[44]

Fetal malpresentations during labor

There is a high incidence of malpresentation at the time of delivery in twin gestations. In the review by Farooqui et al.,[45] the frequency of different fetal presentations was as follows:

Vertex-vertex	39.6%
Vertex-breech	27.7%
Vertex-transverse	7.2%
Breech-breech	9.0%
Breech-vertex	6.9%
Breech-transverse	3.6%
Other combinations	6.9%

A rare malpresentation occurring one time per every 1000 twins and per every 50,000 births is the *interlocking of twins.* The perinatal mortality of this complication is high (62% to 84%), probably because most cases are not recognized until late in the expulsive phase of labor. A typical case is a primipara with generous pelvic measurements and a breech-vertex presentation who is allowed to deliver vaginally. The labor proceeds smoothly until twin A is partially delivered and there is difficulty in delivering the infant head, which remains high in the pelvis. Manual examination at this time reveals the head of twin B interposed between the body and the head of twin A. In most cases, attempts to elevate twin B using various pelvic and abdominal maneuvers fail, and it is necessary to proceed with an emergency cesarean section. Death for twin A is an almost certain outcome.

To avoid this disastrous sequence of events, one must rule out interlocking twins in every case of breech-vertex presentation delivering vaginally. Interlocking of various body parts may also rarely happen in vertex-vertex, vertex-transverse, and breech-breech presentations. Perhaps the first indication of interlocking is an abnormal labor pattern, usually an arrest disorder. In these cases it is best to perform a cesarean section. Some investigators suggest obtaining anteropos-

terior and lateral x-ray films of the twins and repeating the films after 2 hours of active labor.[46] If the head of twin B is descending below the level of the head of twin A, suggesting collision of the twins, cesarean-section delivery is the best method of delivery.

Umbilical cord problems

Umbilical cord problems are more frequent in twins than in singleton pregnancies: a single umbilical artery is 3 to 4 times more frequent, and velamentous insertion of the cord occurs 6 to 9 times more frequently in twins. Cord prolapse, vasa previa, and torsion of the umbilical cord at its abdominal wall insertion because of focal absence of Wharton's gelatin also happen more frequently in twins. Umbilical cord entanglement is a common problem in monoamniotic twins.

Cerebral palsy

Cerebral palsy is 5 times more common in twins than in singleton pregnancies.[47] The main causes of this problem are the intrauterine death of a co-twin, severely discordant twins, twin-twin transfusion syndrome, and asphyxiated, intrauterine–growth retarded twins.

◪ DIAGNOSIS

One of the most important factors in the successful outcome of a twin pregnancy is early diagnosis. In fact, studies demonstrate that perinatal losses are significantly larger when the diagnosis is made after 28 weeks. With earlier diagnosis, measures important in the prevention of prematurity and a planned approach to the delivery can be implemented. Fortunately, in most developed countries ultrasound examination has become a part of routine obstetric practice, and the delivery of undiagnosed twins is rare.

The most important clinical finding suggesting the possibility of a multifetal pregnancy is the presence of a uterine size disproportionately large for the patient's dates. Other findings suggestive of the possibility of a twin pregnancy include conception through the use of fertility agents, family history of twins, auscultation of two fetal hearts, and abdominal palpation of three fetal poles.

The sonographic diagnosis of twin pregnancy can be made as early as 6 to 7 postmenstrual weeks with the use of a vaginal probe. Early in pregnancy, it is difficult to see the thin membrane separating the amniotic sacs when the placentation is monochorionic-diamniotic. However, when the placentation is dichorionic-diamniotic, it is easier to see the division.

The ultrasonic diagnosis of twin pregnancy should include an assessment of the placentation. This may require more than one examination and sometimes is impossible, particularly when the initial diagnosis of twins is made late in pregnancy. The first step is to determine whether the number of placentas is one or two and whether membranes are present. If two placentas and a thick membrane are seen, the pregnancy is dichorionic-diamniotic. If only one placenta is seen, the next step is to identify the sex of the babies. If they are of different sexes, the placentation is dichorionic-diamniotic. If the babies are of identical sex or it cannot be determined, the next step is to study the thickness of the membranes. For this purpose, it is best to look between 16 and 24 weeks near the placental insertion of the membranes. The membranes should be examined using the largest magnification allowed by the ultrasound equipment. In monochorionic placentation the membranes are difficult to see and have a paper-thin or hairlike appearance. In dichorionic placentation, the membranes are readily seen and have a thickness similar to that of one wall of the umbilical cord. According to D'Alton and Dudley,[48] if only two layers are seen, the placentation is monochorionic. If three or more layers are seen, the placentation is dichorionic. The predictive accuracy of this method is 100% for dichorionic and 94.4% for monochorionic placentas. Other authors[49] recommend measuring the thickness of the membrane and using a 2-mm cut-off for differentiating between monochorionic and dichorionic. According to these investigators, the thickness of the membrane in monochorionic placentation is 1.4 mm +/− 0.3 and in dichorionic placentation is 2.4 mm +/− 0.7. The accuracy of this method is 82% for monochorionic and 95% for dichorionic placentations.

Because it is difficult to visualize a thin membrane in the first trimester and because of the serious implications of a monoamniotic pregnancy, a repeat ultrasound between 20 and 26 weeks is necessary for confirmation of a single sac. Also, the umbilical cord of each twin can be seen with color Doppler. If the cords are entangled, the diagnosis of monoamniotic twin pregnancies can be made with confidence.

In some instances it is necessary to use invasive methods to diagnose monoamniotic twins. An x-ray film 24 hours after intraamniotic injection of 30 ml of iothalamate meglumine (Conray 40) will show the contrast medium in the gastrointestinal tract of both twins if the pregnancy is monoamniotic. If the patient suspected of monoamniotic pregnancy needs genetic amniocentesis, the test can be done at that time. For that purpose, 0.1 ml of air and 0.5 ml of indigo carmine are mixed with 5 ml of amniotic fluid, and this is injected into the amniotic cavity after a sample has been drawn for genetic studies. Ultrasound examination following the injection will demonstrate the microbubbles around one or both twins depending on the type of placentation.[50]

◢ ANTEPARTUM MANAGEMENT

Once the diagnosis of twin gestation and the type of placentation are made, the efforts of the obstetrician must be directed toward prevention of preterm birth, evaluation of fetal growth, and determination of the best mode of delivery. There are differences in the approach to these three problems depending on the type of placentation.

Prevention of preterm birth

The measures most commonly used for the prevention of preterm birth in twins are bed rest, administration of tocolytic agents, and ambulatory uterine contraction monitoring. Another method of treatment, the cervical cerclage, may be useful in certain cases, but its generalized use does not improve the outcome of twin pregnancies and should be discouraged.

Bed rest. Bed rest is widely used for the prevention of preterm labor in twins. The rationale behind its use is that with bed rest in the lateral position there is reduced pressure on the cervix and an increase in uteroplacental blood flow. The increase in blood flow in turn has a quieting effect on myometrial contractility. Despite this apparently solid idea, its use has been a highly controversial subject. However, recent studies[51,52] have clearly shown that bed rest decreases perinatal mortality and morbidity in twins.

It is clear that the worst morbidity and mortality caused by preterm delivery in twins occurs before 30 weeks of gestation. This point was clearly demonstrated in the study of Jeffrey et al.[53] at the University of Colorado. These investigators demonstrated that if deliveries of twins occurring before 30 weeks of gestation are excluded from consideration, bed rest does not significantly change perinatal mortality or length of gestation. Another study by Powers and Miller,[54] in agreement with the Colorado data, shows that twins are most vulnerable if born between 27 and 34 weeks. The conclusion is that bed rest should begin at approximately 24 weeks and finish at 34 weeks, when the chances of survival are almost 100%. These are general guidelines, and there is room for variation depending on the particular situation of each patient.

Prophylactic tocolysis. The purposes of administering drugs that inhibit uterine activity are to avoid preterm labor and prevent cervical changes that facilitate ascending infection or preterm rupture of the membranes. The medications most commonly used are beta-mimetic agents and calcium channel blockers (see Chapter 4).

Similar to bed rest, the usefulness of prophylactic tocolysis is controversial. In one study,[55] 42 patients with twin pregnancies were treated with salbutamol, and their outcome was compared with an equal number of matched twin pregnancies that were treated with bed rest alone. The treated patients received an amount of salbutamol that kept the maternal pulse above 100 beats per minute during weekly checks. The authors found a significant increase in the length of gestation and in the birth weight in the medicated group. Only four of the salbutamol-treated babies weighed less than 2000 g, and only one infant weighed less than 1500 g. It is not clear in this study, however, whether there was a significant difference between the groups in gestational age at the time of initiation of therapy. The results of other studies are not as supportive of prophylaxis. One randomized study of 200 women with multiple pregnancies[56] showed no difference with respect to duration of pregnancy and birth weight between treated and untreated patients.

It is clear that more research with careful control of confounding variables is necessary to define the potential usefulness of tocolytic prophylaxis in twin pregnancies. It is believed that until definitive research results are available, prophylactic tocolysis should be used selectively in those who have increased uterine activity.

Home uterine activity monitoring. A new subject of controversy in the management of twin pregnancies is that of home uterine monitoring. The patient at her home uses a tocodynamometer to monitor the frequency of her uterine contractions. The activity registered by the dynamometer is transmitted through a telephone line to a central station. The obstetrician and the patient are notified if the number of contractions per hour exceeds a certain threshold, usually four to six contractions per hour.

The proponents of this system believe that because approximately 35% of all patients with multiple pregnancies are not aware of their uterine contractions, detection of those contractions is important to institute adequate therapy and to avoid preterm delivery. Other investigators question the accuracy of a monitoring system that frequently identifies simple uterine irritability as contractions, and they point out its high cost. Most studies have shown beneficial effects of home monitoring for patients with multifetal pregnancies. However, more well-designed, prospective, randomized studies in this area are needed.

Infection surveillance and control. The data from the Collaborative Perinatal Project indicate that infection of the amniotic membranes, with or without ruptured membranes, is the most common pathologic finding underlying prematurity in twin gestations. More recently, Romero et al.[57] found positive amniotic fluid cultures in one or both sacs in 10.8% of a series of twin pregnancies admitted in preterm labor. The presenting sac was involved in all of their infected patients, a fact that supports the theory of ascending infection.

The increasing amount of information suggesting that a significant number of twin patients in preterm labor are infected, possibly through a mechanism of ascending infection, should be incorporated into the management of twin pregnancies. Infections of the urinary tract, the cervix, and the vagina in patients carrying twins must be treated aggressively.

Monitoring fetal growth

Alterations in fetal growth occur frequently in twin gestations, and in many instances they are the initial indication of fetal and neonatal distress and death. Thus monitoring of fetal growth has become an essential component of the antenatal management of twin pregnancies.

Not all of the alterations in twin growth result from pathologic influences. Recent investigations[58] have demonstrated that at delivery there is a difference in the birth weight of twins and singletons of the same gestational age. The growth of twins and singletons is similar between 24 and 35 weeks, but at 36, 37, and 38 weeks the mean difference in weight is 365, 327, and 362 g, respectively. At 39 weeks, the mean difference is 791 g, and at 40 weeks it is 757 g. This correlates with the ultrasound findings of Socol et al.[59] and Grumbach et al.,[60] as well as the data of Naeye et al.,[61] who all found that twin weight was similar to singleton weight until 33 weeks of gestation, and less thereafter. These findings suggest that the uteroplacental circulation is unable to supply nutrients for the full development of multiple pregnancies after 36 weeks.

In summary, every twin pregnancy should be followed with serial ultrasound measurements every 3 to 4 weeks after 16 weeks. If discordant growth is detected, an investigation of the underlying cause should be made. Depending on the findings, antepartum fetal surveillance, serial amniocentesis, and/or intervention and preterm delivery may be necessary.

Antepartum fetal surveillance. Because of the frequency of complications in multifetal pregnancies, there is a tendency among obstetricians and perinatologists to recommend antepartum fetal surveillance of all multifetal pregnancies using nonstress or biophysical profile testing. This is probably unnecessary before 36 weeks in dichorionic-diamniotic twins with concordant growth.

Amniocentesis and lung maturation. Because evaluation of fetal lung maturation is often required in the management of twin pregnancies, especially in cases of discordant fetal growth, the question arises of the need for amniotic fluid studies of each sac. The evidence collected to date indicates that lung maturation in normal twins occurs simultaneously and that results of biochemical analysis of one amniotic sac may be applied to the other. However, this general rule does not apply to twins with discordance. In these cases, the growth-retarded fetus usually has a more advanced degree of lung maturity than the other. Therefore the timing of premature delivery of discordant twins should be based on the testing of the amniotic fluid surrounding the larger twin.

Summary of antenatal management

In summary, once twins are diagnosed, the following rules should be observed:

1. The patient should be scheduled for office visits every 2 weeks, or more frequently if she develops complications. Attention should focus during those visits on evaluation of blood pressure, proteinuria, uterine fundal growth, and fetal movements.

2. The patient should be scheduled for an ultrasound every 3 to 4 weeks to evaluate fetal growth. It may be necessary to perform examinations at closer intervals if complications appear.

3. Vaginal and bladder infections should be recognized and treated promptly.

4. All patients with twins should stop working and rest in the lateral decubitus position for a minimum of 2 hours each morning and afternoon. They should sleep at least 10 hours each night, starting at 22 weeks of gestation. Bed rest may be necessary before 22 weeks in patients who develop polyhydramnios, an early increase in uterine activity, or early discordant growth.

5. Vaginal examinations should be done at every office visit beginning at 22 weeks of gestation. Patients who develop polyhydramnios or increased frequency and intensity of contractions before 22 weeks should have regular vaginal examinations after the onset of symptoms. During an examination, the obstetrician should avoid the introduction of the fingers through the cervix. This maneuver not only causes prostaglandin release, possibly producing contractions, but it also places a rather large inoculum of vaginal bacteria close to the amniotic membranes. The vaginal examination should assess only the lower uterine segment and the length of the cervix. The finding of a bulging lower segment and a cervix less than 0.5 cm is indicative of a high risk for preterm delivery. In these cases administration of tocolytic agents, bed rest at home or in the hospital, and uterine contractility monitoring should be initiated and continued until 36 weeks.

6. Administration of betamethasone, 12 mg intramuscularly daily for 2 consecutive days starting at 28 weeks of gestation, with repeated weekly treatments until the patient delivers or until she reaches 34 weeks, should be part of the management of every twin gestation for which preterm birth is a strong possibility. This includes patients showing discordant growth patterns, cervical changes, or poor compliance with bed rest and medications.

7. If discordant fetal growth is observed, an at-

tempt should be made to find the underlying cause. A search for congenital abnormalities, for the type of discordancy (symmetric or asymmetric), and for the presence of indicators of twin-twin transfusion is necessary. Genetic studies, cordocentesis, serial amniocentesis, and fetal surveillance may be required depending on the circumstances. Consultation with or referral to a perinatologist is advisable.

◢ MANAGEMENT OF LABOR AND DELIVERY

One of the most important questions in the intrapartum management of a twin gestation is the appropriate route of delivery. Ideally, this decision should be made before labor begins or when the patient is in the early stages of labor.

The most important element in the decision is fetal presentation at time of labor, best determined by an ultrasound examination when the patient presents in labor. Even if the patient has had a recent ultrasound examination, a sonogram should be obtained in all cases to avoid error.

Some investigators believe that twins should be delivered by cesarean section unless both are in vertex presentation. The supporters of this mode of delivery believe that the generous use of cesarean deliveries eliminates the difference in perinatal mortality and morbidity between first and second twins delivered vaginally.[62]

Others believe that if the first twin is in transverse lie or in a breech presentation, cesarean section is the best management, but that vertex/nonvertex presentations should be managed by the vaginal delivery of the first infant, followed by external version and vaginal delivery[63] or by vaginal breech delivery[64] of the second twin. When these approaches are followed, 71.2% of nonvertex second twins can be delivered vaginally without problems.

To perform an external version after the delivery of the first twin, the exact fetal position should be determined by ultrasound. The obstetrician, with the help of the linear transducer, gently attempts first a forward rotation, with frequent monitoring of the fetal heart rate. Fetal bradycardia requiring emergency cesarean delivery may occur in up to 15% of these cases. If there are no signs of fetal distress and the fetus does not move forward easily, a backward flip may be attempted. If the backward rotation fails,

a decision should be made to deliver the breech vaginally or perform a cesarean section on the second twin.

To be delivered vaginally, a breech second twin should have an estimated weight between 2000 g and 3000 g, have the head flexed, and should be of the same or smaller size than the first vaginally delivered twin. These limits are based on the fact that with an ultrasonic estimated weight of 2000 g, the actual weight will rarely be less than 1500 g and with an estimated fetal weight of 3000 g, the true weight will rarely be greater than 3500 g.

The main problem with breech presentation of a second twin is the high chance of cord prolapse. Singleton babies in frank breech presentation fill the low uterine segment and the vagina with the buttocks, usually preventing cord prolapse, but second twin breech infants are high within a uterus that remains large and flaccid after the birth of the first twin. They do not occlude the birth canal, and if the membranes rupture or if the gestation is monoamniotic, the probability of a cord prolapse is high (overall incidence of 4.2% in twins). For that reason, it is important not to artificially rupture the sac of the second twin until the baby has descended and the breech is well engaged. Another problem with second twin vaginal breech delivery is the use of manual and instrumental maneuvering by the obstetrician to shorten the delivery interval. Rayburn et al.[65] have demonstrated that with fetal heart rate monitoring the interval between delivery of twins is not a critical factor. As long as there are no signs of fetal distress, the obstetrician should wait for the presenting part to descend.

A transverse lie in the first twin is an indication for cesarean section, although it is not an indication in the second. A first twin in transverse lie rarely changes position during labor, but a second twin often changes to vertex or to breech. Few of these infants remain transverse requiring cesarean delivery.

A situation requiring cesarean delivery in twin pregnancies is a monoamniotic placentation. The fetal mortality in these pregnancies is greater than 50%, and the overwhelming cause is cord accidents such as cord prolapse or entanglement. Therefore, if a membrane separating the twins is not visualized by ultrasound, it must be assumed that a single sac is present, and the pregnancy should be delivered by cesarean section.

In the past it was thought that cesarean section was better than vaginal delivery if the twins were less than 1500 g. This theory has been refuted by the work of Morales et al.,[66] who found no advantage to cesarean vs. vaginal delivery in nondiscordant twins of less than 1500 g.

Vaginal delivery

There is no contraindication to the judicious use of oxytocin in patients with twins. Ideally, pain relief should be by epidural anesthesia. Electronic monitoring should include both twins, which can be done by coupling the intrauterine pressure transducer to two fetal heart monitoring instruments.[67] Also, modern fetal monitoring equipment allows simultaneous recording of one fetal heart rate by fetal scalp electrode and of the other by transabdominal Doppler ultrasound. Once the first twin is delivered, ultrasound examination and electronic monitoring of the second twin are necessary to evaluate fetal presentation and to detect signs of fetal distress. The delivery room must be prepared for emergency cesarean section, and the necessary personnel must be on standby until the second twin is delivered.

If after the first delivery the monitor tracing is normal and contractions have not resumed in 10 minutes, augmentation with oxytocin may begin. Once the second presenting part is engaged, the membranes are ruptured, and a scalp electrode for direct fetal heart rate monitoring is applied. As long as the monitor tracing remains normal, there is no reason to expedite delivery. If vaginal bleeding occurs suggesting abruptio placentae or if a sinusoidal rhythm, indicating fetal anemia, or a pattern of late decelerations with loss of beat-to-beat variability, indicating fetal distress, is detected, delivery should be immediate, by use of forceps, cesarean section, or breech extraction.

A second twin in transverse lie should be managed similarly to a second twin in breech presentation. The linear ultrasound transducer should be used to apply gentle pressure on the back and neck of the fetus and to attempt to change the presentation to vertex or breech. No intrauterine manipulations should be carried out to influence or determine a change in presentation. If the infant converts to a breech or a vertex spontaneously or with the help of external manipulation, the possibilities for a safe vaginal

delivery are excellent. If the infant remains in transverse lie, the pregnancy should be terminated by cesarean section.

Some obstetricians perform total breech extractions in cases of transverse lie or breech presentations. The expertise of the obstetrician in intrauterine manipulation is the most important factor in this decision. If that expertise does not exist, the safe management is a cesarean section.

After delivery of the second twin and the placenta, the attention of the obstetrician should be directed to the prevention of postpartum hemorrhage. The uterus should be massaged continuously, and intravenous oxytocin (30 U in 1000 ml of 5% dextrose in lactated Ringer's solution) should be administered simultaneously. Many obstetricians prefer to administer prostaglandins immediately after delivery of the placenta.

Cesarean section delivery

The ideal anesthesia for the cesarean delivery of twins is epidural because it allows a systematic, unhurried approach to the delivery of the infants without fetal hypoxia or depression caused by the transplacental passage of general anesthetics. Ideally, epidural anesthetic should be administered by an obstetric anesthesiologist aware of the peculiarities of twin pregnancy and able to prevent or treat the hemodynamic changes caused by the anesthetic blockade.

The best abdominal incision for the delivery of twins is vertical. It can be made quickly, the blood loss is less, it allows more room for manipulation of abnormal presentations,[68] and it allows a more thorough exploration of the abdominal cavity. Also, it is easier to close and easy to reopen when repeated cesarean section is necessary. The disadvantages are a higher incidence of dehiscence and a less acceptable aesthetic result than with transverse incision.

Most patients with twin pregnancies have a well-developed low uterine segment that favors transverse uterine incisions. Any vertical uterine incision predisposes the patient to future uterine rupture, and it forces repeated cesarean section. In contrast, the patient who receives a low transverse uterine incision and is allowed to labor in a subsequent normal pregnancy has a high chance of a vaginal delivery. Vertical incisions on the uterus are rarely needed if the twins are near term, if the precise fetal lies are known, and if the incision on the abdominal wall is vertical.

☑ MANAGEMENT OF GESTATIONS WITH HIGH FETAL NUMBER

Everything that has been said about twin pregnancies applies to gestations with greater fetal numbers. They are a rare event, however. Triplets occur once in every 6000 to 9000 deliveries in the United States, and quintuplets occur once in every 41 million births. Recently they have become more frequent as a result of the use of ovulation-inducing drugs in the management of infertility. In patients treated with gonadotropins, the occurrence of multiple pregnancies is 20%, of which 75% are twins and 25% are triplets or gestations of higher number. In patients treated with clomiphene, the occurrence of multiple pregnancy is 10%.

Fetal and neonatal morbidity and mortality are high in patients with high fetal numbers. Preterm delivery affects more than 85%, and the neonatal death rate is approximately 20%. Similar to twins, preterm delivery is the most important hazard for patients with high fetal numbers. The mean gestational age at delivery for triplets is 32 to 33 weeks, and for quadruplets it is 30 to 32 weeks. The incidence of fetal growth retardation is greater than 15%. Other frequent problems are antepartum anemia, postpartum bleeding, and preeclampsia.[69] Cesarean section is very common, mainly because of the difficulties in ensuring adequate monitoring of all babies during labor. The fetal mortality and morbidity is high and closely related to fetal weight, birth order, and fetal position. Small babies, those born last or close to last, and those in breech or transverse presentation have the worst outcomes. The complexity of the antepartum, intrapartum, and neonatal care of multiple pregnancies of high fetal number necessitates referral to tertiary care perinatal centers. With modern perinatal management, more than 80% of triplets, quadruplets, and quintuplets will survive, and 90% of survivors will not have major handicaps.[70]

In the last few years, selective reduction of high-order multifetal pregnancies has developed as an alternative to the large mortality and morbidity figures associated with this condition.[71,72] Patients undergoing this procedure usually have four or more fetuses. Between 9 and 12 weeks, under ultrasound guidance, the chosen fetuses receive intracardiac injection of potassium chloride. Usually, two fetuses are left undisturbed. The procedure is not completely free of complications. Technical failure, such as the development of uterine contractions and amnionitis, also may occur. The likelihood of losing all of the fetuses may be as high as 30%. When the figures about fetal survival in triplet, quadruplet, and quintuplet pregnancies[68] are contrasted with the risks associated with selective feticide, it becomes difficult to support a decision to reduce the number of fetuses in pregnancies with fewer than five fetuses.

☑   IMPORTANT POINTS   ◼

1. Approximately two thirds of all twin pregnancies are dizygotic, and one third are monozygotic. All dizygotic gestations are dichorionic-diamniotic. In about 30% of monozygotic twins, the zygotic division occurs within 72 hours of fertilization, and the placenta will also be dichorionic-diamniotic. In approximately 65% of them, the placenta will be monochorionic-diamniotic, and in approximately 5% it will be monochorionic-monoamniotic.

2. The diagnosis of chorionicity and amnionicity is one important objective of ultrasound examination of twin pregnancies. In monochorionic placentation, the thickness of the amniotic membrane is less than 2 mm, and it shows only two layers. In dichorionic placentation, thickness of the membranes is more than 2 mm, and three or more layers are seen.

3. The main causes of maternal morbidity in multifetal pregnancies are preeclampsia, sepsis, and postpartum bleeding.

4. The main causes of perinatal mortality in multifetal pregnancies are prematurity, twin-twin transfusion syndrome, congenital defects, placental insufficiency, and traumatic delivery.

5. The main causes of discordant twin growth are unequal placental mass, genetic syndromes, and twin-twin transfusion syndrome.

6. The criteria most commonly accepted for the diagnosis of twin-twin transfusion are a difference in hematocrit of 20% or more, a difference in birth weight of 20% or more, and signs of fetal hydrops in one or both twins.

7. After the death of a twin, morbidity may affect as many as 46% of survivors. The most

severe morbidity, affecting 20% of them, is neurologic damage caused by multicystic encephalomalacia.

8. Congenital malformations occur in approximately 17% of twins. Malformations among monochorionic twins are frequently multiple or lethal, whereas those occurring in dichorionic twins are mostly minor.

9. Several studies indicate that there is a difference in birth weight between twins and singletons of the same gestational age after 36 weeks.

10. Frequent office visits, ultrasound examinations every 3 to 4 weeks, frequent vaginal examinations after 20 weeks for cervical assessment, and fetal surveillance with nonstress test and fluid volume after 36 weeks are important components of the antepartum care of patients with twins.

11. If the first twin is in breech presentation or transverse lie, it is better to deliver by cesarean section. Vertex/nonvertex presentations should be managed by vaginal delivery of the first twin followed by external version or vaginal breech delivery of the second twin.

12. As long as fetal heart rate monitoring remains normal, there is no reason to shorten the delivery interval between twins.

13. Fetal and neonatal morbidity and mortality are high in patients with more than two fetuses. Preterm delivery affects more than 85%, and the neonatal death rate is approximately 20%.

REFERENCES

1. Schenker JG, Yarkoni S, Granat M: Multiple pregnancies following induction of ovulation. *Fertil Steril* 1981;35:105-123.
2. Caspi E, Ronen J, Schreyer P, et al: The outcome of pregnancy after gonadotropin therapy. *Br J Obstet Gynaecol* 1976;83:967-973.
3. Varma TR: Ultrasound evidence of early pregnancy failure in patients with multiple conceptions. *Br J Obstet Gynaecol* 1979;86:290-292.
4. Fujikura T, Froehlich LA: Twin placentation and zygosity. *Obstet Gynecol* 1971;37:34-43.
5. Wilson RS: Blood typing and twin zygosity. *Hum Hered* 1970;20:30.
6. Kovacs B, Shahbahrami B, Platt LD, et al: Molecular genetic prenatal determination of twin zygosity. *Obstet Gynecol* 1988;72:954-956.
7. Kovacs BW, Kirschbaum TH, Paul RH: Twin gestations. I. Antenatal care and complications. *Obstet Gynecol* 1989;74:313-317.

8. Naeye RL, Tafari N, Judge D, et al: Twins: Causes of perinatal death in 12 United States cities and one African city. *Am J Obstet Gynecol* 1978;131:267-272.
9. Kiely JL: The epidemiology of perinatal mortality in multiple births. *Bull NY Acad Med* 1990;66:618.
10. Bejar R, Vigliocco G, Gramajo H, et al: Antenatal origin of neurologic damage in newborn infants. II. Multiple gestation. *Am J Obstet Gynecol* 1990;162:1230-1236.
11. Newton ER, Cetrulo CL: Management of twin gestation, in Cetrulo CL, Sbarra AJ (eds): *The Problem-Oriented Medical Record for High-Risk Obstetrics.* New York, Plenum, 1984.
12. Spellacy WN, Handler A, Ferre CD: A case-control study of 1253 twin pregnancies from a 1982-1987 perinatal data base. *Obstet Gynecol* 1990;75:168-171.
13. Powers WF: Twin pregnancy: Complications and treatment. *Obstet Gynecol* 1973;42:795-808.
14. Erkkola R, Ala-Mello S, Piiroinen O, et al: Growth discordancy in twin pregnancies: A risk factor not detected by measurements of biparietal diameter. *Obstet Gynecol* 1985;66:203-206.
15. Blickstein I, Shoham-Schwartz Z, Lancet M, et al: Characterization of the growth-discordant twin. *Obstet Gynecol* 1987;70:11-15.
16. Gaziano EP, Knox GE, Bendel RP, et al: Is Doppler velocimetry useful in the management of multiple-gestation pregnancies? *Am J Obstet Gynecol* 1991;164:1426-1433.
17. Hastie SJ, Danskin F, Neilson JP, et al: Prediction of the small for gestational age twin fetus by Doppler umbilical artery waveform analysis. *Obstet Gynecol* 1989;74:730-733.
18. Divon MY, Girz BA, Sklar A, et al: Discordant twins—A prospective study of the diagnostic value of real-time ultrasonography combined with umbilical artery velocimetry. *Am J Obstet Gynecol* 1989;161:757-760.
19. Fakeye O: Twin birth weight discordancy in Nigeria. *Int J Gynaecol Obstet* 1986;24:235-238.
20. Hays PM, Smelter JS: Multiple gestation. *Clin Obstet Gynecol* 1986;29:264-285.
21. Robertson EG, Neer KJ: Placental injection studies in twin gestation. *Am J Obstet Gynecol* 1983;147:170-173.
22. Danskin FH, Neilson JP: Twin-to-twin transfusion syndrome: What are appropiate diagnostic criteria? *Am J Obstet Gynecol* 1989;161:365-369.
23. Mahony BS, Petty CN, Nyberg DA, et al: The "stuck twin" phenomenon: Ultrasonographic findings, pregnancy outcome, and management with serial amniocentesis. *Am J Obstet Gynecol* 1990;163:1513-1522.
24. Farmakides G, Schulman H, Saldana LR, et al: Surveillance of twin pregnancy with umbilical artery velocimetry. *Am J Obstet Gynecol* 1985;153:789-792.
25. Giles WB, Trudinger BJ, Cook CM, et al: Doppler umbilical artery studies in the twin-twin transfusion syndrome. *Obstet Gynecol* 1990;76:1097-1099.
26. Pretorious DH, Manchester D, Barkin S, et al: Doppler ultrasound of twin transfusion syndrome. *J Ultrasound Med* 1988;7:117-124.
27. Shah DM, Chaffin D: Perinatal outcome in very preterm births with twin-twin transfusion syndrome. *Am J Obstet Gynecol* 1989;161:1111-1113.
28. Urig MA, Clewell WH, Elliott JP: Twin-twin transfusion syndrome. *Am J Obstet Gynecol* 1990;163:1522-1526.

29. DeLia JE, Cruikshank DP, Keye WR: Fetoscopic neodymium: Yag laser occlusion of placental vessels in severe twin-twin transfusion syndrome. *Obstet Gynecol* 1990;75:1046-1053.

30. Rodis JF, Vintzileos AM, Campbell WA, et al: Antenatal diagnosis and management of monoamniotic twins. *Am J Obstet Gynecol* 1987;157:1255-1257.

31. Carr SR, Aronson MP, Coustan DR: Survival rates of monoamniotic twins do not decrease after 30 weeks' gestation. *Am J Obstet Gynecol* 1990;163:719-722.

32. Tessen JA, Zlatnik FJ: Monoamniotic twins: A retrospective controlled study. *Obstet Gynecol* 1991;77:832-834.

33. Enbom JA: Twin pregnancy with intrauterine death of one twin. *Am J Obstet Gynecol* 1985;152:424-429.

34. D'Alton ME, Newton ER, Cetrulo CL: Intrauterine fetal demise in multiple gestation. *Acta Genet Med Gemellol* 1984;33:43-49.

35. Yoshioka H, Kadomoto Y, Mino M, et al: Multicystic encephalomalacia in liveborn twin with a stillborn macerated co-twin. *J Pediatr* 1979;95:798-800.

36. McCarthy SM, Filly RA, Stark DD, et al: Obstetric magnetic resonance imaging: Fetal anatomy. *Radiology* 1985;154:427.

37. Hendricks CH: Twinning in relation to birth weight, mortality, and congenital anomalies. *Obstet Gynecol* 1966;27:47-53.

38. Guttmacher AF, Kohl S: The fetus of multiple gestations. *Obstet Gynecol* 1958;12:528-541.

39. Windham GC, Sever LE: Neural tube defects among twin births. *Am J Hum Genet* 1982;34:988-998.

40. Richards MR, Merritt KK, Samuels MH, et al: Congenital malformations of the cardiovascular system in a series of 6053 infants. *Pediatrics* 1955;12:12-32.

41. Rodis JF, Egan JFX, Craffey A, et al: Calculated risk of chromosomal abnormalities in twin gestations. *Obstet Gynecol* 1990;76:1037-1041.

42. Kling S, Johnston RJ, Michalyschyn B, et al: Successful separation of xiphopagus-conjoined twins. *J Pediatr Surg* 1975;10:267-271.

43. Robie GF, Payne GG, Morgan MA: Selective delivery of an acardiac acephalic twin. *N Engl J Med* 1989;320:512-513.

44. Porreco RP, Barton SM, Haverkamp AD: Occlusion of umbilical artery in acardiac, acephalic twin. *Lancet* 1991;337:326-327.

45. Farooqui MO, Grossman JH, Shannon RA: A review of twin pregnancy and perinatal mortality. *Obstet Gynecol Surv* 1973;28:144.

46. Fox RL, Nathanson HG, Tejani N, et al: Interlocking twins: Experience with four cases and suggested management. *Obstet Gynecol* 1975;46:53-57.

47. Durkin MV, Kaveggia EG, Pendleton E, et al: Analysis of etiologic factors in cerebral palsy with severe mental retardation. I. Analysis of gestational, parturitional, and neonatal data. *Eur J Pediatr* 1976;123:67-81.

48. D'Alton ME, Dudley DK: The ultrasonographic prediction of chorionicity in twin gestation. *Am J Obstet Gynecol* 1989;160:557-561.

49. Winn HN, Gabrielli S, Reece EA, et al: Ultrasonographic criteria for the prenatal diagnosis of placental chorionicity in twin gestations. *Am J Obstet Gynecol* 1989;161:1540-1542.

50. Tabsh K: Genetic amniocentesis in multiple gestation: A new technique to diagnose monoamniotic twins. *Obstet Gynecol* 1990;75:296-301.

51. Saunders MC, Dick JS, Brown IM: The effects of hospital admission for bed rest on the duration of twin pregnancy: A randomized trial. *Lancet* 1985;2:793-795.

52. Gilstrap LC, Hauth JC, Hankins GDV, et al: Twins: Prophylactic hospitalization and ward rest at early gestational age. *Obstet Gynecol* 1987;69:578-581.

53. Jeffrey RL, Bowes WA, Delaney JJ: Role of bed rest in twin gestations. *Obstet Gynecol* 1974;43:822-826.

54. Powers WF, Miller TC: Bed rest in twin pregnancy: Identification of a critical period and its cost implications. *Am J Obstet Gynecol* 1979;134:23-29.

55. TambyRaja RL, Atputharajah V, Salmon Y: Prevention of prematurity in twins. *Aust N Z J Obstet Gynecol* 1979;18:179-181.

56. Gummerus M, Halonen O: Prophylactic long-term oral tocolysis of multiple pregnancies. *Br J Obstet Gynaecol* 1987;94:249-251.

57. Romero R, Shamma F, Avila C, et al: Infection and labor. VI. Prevalence, microbiology, and clinical significance of intraamniotic infection in twin gestations with preterm labor. *Am J Obstet Gynecol* 1990;163:757-761.

58. Luke B, Feng T, Witter F, et al: Gestational age-specific birth weights of twins versus singletons. Abstract presented at the 1989 Clinical Meeting of the American College of Obstetricians and Gynecologists.

59. Socol ML, Tamura RK, Sabbagha RE, et al: Diminished biparietal diameter and abdominal circumference growth in twins. *Obstet Gynecol* 1984;64:235-238.

60. Grumbach K, Coleman B, Arges PH, et al: Twin and singleton growth patterns compared using ultrasound. *Radiology* 1986;158:237.

61. Naeye RL, Benirschke K, Hagstrom JWC, et al: Intrauterine growth of twins as estimated from live-born birth-weight data. *Pediatrics* 1977;37:409-422.

62. Cetrulo CL: The controversy of mode of delivery in twins: The intrapartum management of twin gestation. I. *Semin Perinatol* 1986;10:39.

63. Chervenak FA, Johnson RE, Berkowitz RL, et al: Intrapartum external version of the second twin. *Obstet Gynecol* 1983;62:160-165.

64. Gocke SE, Nageotte MP, Garite T, et al: Management of the nonvertex second twin: Primary cesarean section, external version, or primary breech extraction. *Am J Obstet Gynecol* 1989;161:111-114.

65. Rayburn WF, Lavin JP, Miodovnik M, et al: Multiple gestation: Time interval between delivery of the first and second twins. *Obstet Gynecol* 1984;63:502-506.

66. Morales WF, O'Brien WF, Knuppel RA, et al: The effect of mode delivery on the risk of intraventricular hemorrhage in nondiscordant twin gestations under 1500 g. *Obstet Gynecol* 1989;73:107-110.

67. Read JA, Miller FC: Technique of simultaneous direct intrauterine pressure recording for electronic monitoring of twin gestation in labor. *Am J Obstet Gynecol* 1977;129:228-230.

68. Pelosi MA, Apuzzio J, Fricchione D, et al: The "intraabdominal version technique" for delivery of transverse lie by low-segment cesarean section. *Am J Obstet Gynecol* 1979;135:1001-1011.

69. Syrop CH, Varner MW: Triplet gestation: Maternal and neonatal implications. *Acta Genet Med Gemellol* 1985;34:81-88.

70. Gonen R, Heyman E, Asztalos EV, et al: The outcome of triplet, quadruplet, and quintuplet pregnancies managed in a perinatal unit: Obstetric, neonatal and follow-up data. *Am J Obstet Gynecol* 1990;162:454-459.

71. Berkowitz RL, Lynch L, Chitkara U, et al: Selective reduction of multifetal pregnancies in the first trimester. *N Engl J Med* 1988;318:1043-1047.

72. Evans MI, Fletcher JC, Zador IE, et al: Selective first-trimester termination in octuplet and quadruplet pregnancies: Clinical and ethical issues. *Obstet Gynecol* 1988;71:289-296.

8

PROLONGED PREGNANCY

There is general consensus that perinatal mortality and morbidity are increased several fold when pregnancies are prolonged beyond 42 weeks.[1-3] Controversy is centered on the adequacy of different methods for detecting the fetus at risk, the time when testing should start, and the optimum time for delivery.

◢ DEFINITION

The best name to use for a pregnancy that advances beyond 42 weeks is *postterm*. This is consistent with the names given to other stages of pregnancy, that is, preterm and term. Other names commonly used are *postdatism* and *postmaturity*. The term *postdatism* is inadequate because there is no definition of the dates to which the term refers. Postmaturity is a specific syndrome of intrauterine growth retardation associated with a prolonged gestation. Some authors use the term *dysmaturity* to refer to postmature infants. In this chapter the term *prolonged* is used to refer to those pregnancies advancing beyond the expected date of delivery (EDD), and *postterm* is used to designate pregnancies that advance beyond 42 weeks.

◢ INCIDENCE

Studies performed years ago indicated that about 11% of all pregnancies end after 42 weeks.

However, when ultrasound is used to verify the accuracy of the gestational age, the incidence of postterm pregnancies is lower. Boyd et al.[4] found an incidence of postterm pregnancy of 7.5% when the diagnosis was based on menstrual dating. The incidence was 2.6% when dating was based on early ultrasound examination and 1.1% when the ultrasound and the menstrual history coincided. Prolongation of pregnancy beyond 40 weeks occurs more frequently, about 1 in every 10 pregnancies.

◢ PHYSIOLOGIC CHANGES ASSOCIATED WITH PROLONGED GESTATION

A series of changes occur in the amniotic fluid, placenta, and fetus with prolongation of pregnancy. Adequate understanding of them is essential for the management of these patients.

Amniotic fluid changes

There are quantitative and qualitative changes in the amniotic fluid with prolongation of pregnancy. The amniotic fluid volume reaches a peak of about 1000 ml at 38 weeks of gestation and decreases to about 800 ml at 40 weeks. This reduction in volume continues, and the amount of fluid is approximately 480, 250, and 160 ml at 42, 43, and 44 weeks, respectively.[5-7] An amniotic fluid volume under 400 ml at 40 or more weeks is associated with fetal complications. The mechanism of production of oligohydramnios in prolonged pregnancy seems to be diminished fetal urine production.[8]

In addition to changes in volume there are changes in the composition of the amniotic fluid with prolonged gestation. After 38 to 40 weeks, the fluid becomes milky and cloudy because of abundant flakes of vernix caseosa. The phospholipid composition changes because of the presence of a large number of lamellar bodies released from the fetal lungs, and the lecithin to sphingomyelin (L/S) ratio becomes 4:1 or greater. The color of the fluid has a green or yellow discoloration when the fetus passes meconium. The presence of meconium, particularly if it is "thick," increases the probability of a poor outcome.[9]

Placental changes

The postterm placenta shows a decrease in diameter and length of chorionic villae, fibrinoid necrosis, and accelerated atherosis of chorionic and decidual vessels. These changes occur simultaneously with or precede the appearance of hemorrhagic infarcts, which are the foci for calcium deposition and formation of white infarcts. Infarcts are present in 10% to 25% of term and 60% to 80% of postterm placentas, and they are more common at the placental borders.[7] Deposition of calcium in the postterm placenta reaches up to 10 g/100 g of dry tissue weight, whereas it is only 2 to 3 g/100 g at term.

The morphologic changes that occur with placental senecence can be observed by ultrasound and have been described by Grannum, Berkowitz, and Hobbins.[10] During the first part of gestation, the ultrasonic appearance of the placenta is homogeneous, without echogenic densities, and limited by a smooth chorionic plate (grade 0 placenta). With progression of pregnancy, the chorionic plate begins to acquire subtle undulations, and echogenic densities appear randomly dispersed throughout the organ but spare its basal layer (grade I placenta). Near term the indentations in the chorionic plate become more marked, echogenic densities appear in the basal layer, and commalike densities seem to extend from the chorionic plate into the substance of the placenta (grade II). Finally, when the pregnancy is at term or postterm, the indentations in the chorionic plate become more marked, giving

the appearance of cotyledons. This impression is reinforced by increased confluency of commalike densities that become the intercotyledonary septations. Also, characteristically, the central portion of the cotyledons become echo-free (fallout areas), and large irregular densities, capable of casting acoustic shadows, appear in the substance of the placenta (grade III placenta). The correlation between ultrasonic signs of placental senescence and the functional capacity of the placenta is poor. The correlation between grade III placenta and fetal pulmonary maturity is excellent in pregnancies near term.

Fetal changes

As many as 45% of the fetuses undelivered after their EDD continue to grow in utero. With each additional week, more babies have a birth weight greater than 4000 g, which is the most commonly used definition of fetal macrosomia. At 38 to 40 weeks the incidence of fetal macrosomia is 10%, and at 43 weeks it is 43%.[11] With increase in fetal size, there is a corresponding increase in traumatic deliveries.

Approximately 5% to 10% of fetuses undelivered after their EDD show wasting of their subcutaneous fat, characteristic of intrauterine malnutrition. Most of them are affected by inadequate nutrition and poor growth since early in gestation.

◪ FETAL PROBLEMS WITH PROLONGATION OF PREGNANCY

Several fetal problems may occur in prolonged pregnancies. The most frequent are described in the following paragraphs.

Intrapartum fetal distress

Aproximately 25% of prolonged pregnancies are delivered by cesarean section because of nonreassuring fetal heart rate patterns. The most common of them are moderate-to-severe variable decelerations with slow recovery and episodes of fetal bradycardia with loss of beat-to-beat variability. Less common are repetitive late decelerations.

There are two main reasons for the occurrence of nonreassuring fetal heart patterns in patients with prolonged pregnancies. In a majority of cases they result from umbilical cord compression caused by oligohydramnios.[12] In a minority of patients they are the result of placental insufficiency.[13]

Meconium aspiration

Meconium aspiration syndrome (MAS) is a severe complication of prolonged pregnancy. The problem occurs more frequently when thick meconium, fetal tachycardia, and absence of fetal heart rate accelerations are present.[14] However, not only thick meconium is of concern. Patients with thin meconium at the beginning of labor may have thick meconium and MAS at the time of birth.

Fetal trauma

Difficult vaginal deliveries with varied degrees of fetal trauma occur commonly in prolonged pregnancies, especially in those complicated by fetal macrosomia. Shoulder dystocia is one of the most feared complications because it may result in brachial plexus injury, fracture of the humerus or clavicle, or severe asphyxia with neurologic damage. Cephalic hematomas and skull fractures may also occur during the vaginal delivery of large babies.

Postmaturity syndrome

The postmaturity syndrome, also known as fetal dysmaturity, was one of the fetal complications associated with prolonged pregnancy described first in the medical literature.[1] For many years it was thought that postmaturity was the most frequent complication of prolonged pregnancy, when in reality, it occurs only in approximately 5% to 10% of the cases. Postmature fetuses have decreased amounts of subcutaneous fat and wrinkled skin because they have lost the vernix caseosa and are in direct contact with the amniotic fluid. They also have long hair and long fingernails. Their skin may have a greenish or yellowish staining if they have had prolonged exposure to meconium. Postmaturity is a complication that ideally should be discovered before labor because these fetuses are fragile, tolerate labor poorly, and frequently are acidotic at birth.

◪ ANTEPARTUM EVALUATION AND MANAGEMENT

Adequate antepartum management of patients with prolonged gestations requires the use of clinical and laboratory information. The most important elements used to determine management are discussed below.

Reliability of gestational age estimation

To determine the reliability of the patient's dates, it is necessary to review the information used to determine the EDD. The reliability of the EDD is excellent if the following conditions are met:

1. The patient was not using oral contraceptives, had three or more regular periods before the last one, and the last period was normal in duration and amount of flow.
2. The EDD calculated from the menstrual history was confirmed by an ultrasound examination performed between 12 and 20 weeks of gestation.

Other situations that allow classification of the patient's dates as excellent are:

1. The pregnancy was achieved during infertility treatment following the administration of clomiphene (Clomid), menotropin (Pergonal), or human chorionic gonadotropin (hCG), and the date of conception is known.
2. The EDD was established by means of an ultrasound estimation of the fetal crown-rump length between 7 and 11 weeks of gestation.
3. The EDD was established by means of two or more ultrasound examinations, 3 or 4 weeks apart, obtained between 12 and 28 weeks of gestation.
4. The EDD corresponds to 36 weeks since the patient had a positive serum or urine pregnancy test.
5. Fetal heart tones were documented 20 weeks before the EDD by nonelectronic fetoscope or 30 weeks before with Doppler.

Only patients that fulfill one or several of the conditions mentioned above have *reliable* dates. If none of those conditions are fulfilled, the dates are unreliable, and the diagnosis of prolonged pregnancy is questionable. This is very important because many of the conflicting reports in this subject result from the inclusion of patients with unreliable dates. In pregnancies with reliable EDD, the incidence of postterm pregnancies is less than 2%.[5]

Pelvic examination

Ripeness of the cervix is important in the management of prolonged pregnancies. To evaluate the cervix, it is better to use the Bishop score (Table 8-1). A score of 6 or less indicates poor inducibility.

Ultrasound evaluation

Good communication between the obstetrician and the individual performing the ultrasound examination is important to obtain adequate information. Patients with prolonged preg-

TABLE 8-1 ◪ Bishop score

Factor	0	1	2	3
Cervical dilation (cm)	Closed	1-2	3-4	5+
Cervical effacement (%)	0-30	40-50	60-70	80+
Fetal station	−3	−2	−1,0	+1,+2
Cervical consistency	Firm	Medium	Soft	
Cervical position	Posterior	Mid	Anterior	

From Bishop EH: Pelvic scoring for elective induction. *Obstet Gynecol* 1964;24:266.

nancies are frequently referred to the ultrasound laboratory with a request for estimation of gestational age. This is inadequate because ultrasound examination in patients with prolonged gestation is not to determine the EDD but to answer questions about amniotic fluid volume, fetal size, fetal malformations, and placental grade. Also, estimation of gestational age by means of ultrasound examinations performed at the end of the pregnancy is unreliable.

Amniotic fluid volume. The evaluation of amniotic fluid volume is of fundamental importance in prolonged pregnancies. Chamberlain et al.[15] have demonstrated that perinatal mortality increases dramatically with progressive severity of oligohydramnios. Leveno et al.[12] have demonstrated that umbilical cord compression caused by oligohydramnios is the most common cause of intrapartum fetal distress in these patients.

Ultrasound is a reliable technique for estimation of amniotic fluid volume. Experienced sonographers can make a precise qualitative assessment of the amount of fluid. Others have proposed that the absence of pools of amniotic fluid measuring less than 1 cm,[16] 2 cm,[13] or 3 cm[17] is indicative of oligohydramnios. However, the four-quadrant technique[18] has become the most popular method to effect this evaluation.

The four-quadrant technique consists of measuring the vertical diameter of the largest pocket of fluid found in each of the four quadrants of the uterus. The sum of the results is the amniotic fluid index (AFI). An AFI less than 5 cm indicates oligohydramnios. An AFI between 5 and 10 cm indicates a decreased fluid volume. An AFI between 10 and 15 cm is normal. An AFI

between 15 and 20 cm indicates increased fluid volume. Finally, an AFI greater than 25 cm is diagnostic of polyhydramnios.

Fetal size. Estimation of fetal size by ultrasound is another important component in the evaluation of a pregnancy that extends beyond the expected date of delivery. It has been shown that a significant part of the neonatal morbidity associated with prolongation of pregnancy is the result of fetal macrosomia.[10,19,20] The estimation of fetal size with ultrasound is not perfect, and the sensitivity and specificity of the method are low. An estimated fetal weight at term has a margin of error of approximately 1 lb, and in some instances the error is even larger. The error may be in either direction, and babies thought to be large by ultrasound may be of normal size, and more frequently, babies thought to be of normal size are macrosomic. However, ultrasound can confirm the clinical impression of fetal macrosomia and help the obstetrician in making decisions about the management of these patients.

The following considerations are important to maximize the accuracy of the ultrasonic evaluation:

1. The technical quality of the measurements is important. When oligohydramnios is present or the mother is obese, visualization of fetal structures is difficult, and measurements are inaccurate.
2. The abdominal circumference is the most important measurement in estimating fetal weight. There is a high probability that the baby is macrosomic even when the estimated fetal weight indicates a smaller size if this measurement is two or more standard deviations above the mean.
3. Measurement of the baby's subcutaneous fat may be useful in the evaluation of fetal size. The majority of macrosomic babies have a subcutaneous fat thickness, measured at the anterior abdominal wall, that exceeds 10 mm. Babies with less than 6 mm of subcutaneous fat rarely are macrosomic.

Fetal abnormalities. Before the generalized use of ultrasound, some major congenital defects, particularly neural tube defects, were a relatively frequent finding in patients with prolonged gestations. Today, most of these defects are found early, and these pregnancies do not become postterm. However, these defects should be sought in the rare patient with prolonged pregnancy who did not have an ultrasound examination early in gestation.

Placental grade. Approximately 35% of all patients at term have a grade III placenta. The presence of a grade III placenta does not indicate fetal distress. However, poor outcomes are more frequent in patients with advanced degrees of placental maturity than in patients of the same gestational age with less mature placentas.

Fetal surveillance

The old literature indicates that there is no need for fetal surveillance before 42 weeks. This concept has been questioned in the last years, and there are several studies[10,18,21,22] indicating that fetal danger is present before 42 weeks. At 40 weeks, 5.6% of the fetuses have complications, and 10.4% of them are macrosomic. Both fetal complications and macrosomia increase to 20% at 41 weeks. By 42 weeks, 28.5% of the fetuses have complications, and 34.0% are macrosomic. In view of these findings, it is clear that fetal assessment should start at 40 weeks and continue as long as the patient remains undelivered.

Traditionally, obstetricians have relied on the nonstress test (NST) for the evaluation of prolonged pregnancies. The NST was designed for the detection of placental insufficiency and is inadequate to diagnose oligohydramnios or predict fetal trauma. Therefore use of the NST as the only method of evaluating the fetus in prolonged pregnancy is not ideal, and some serious fetal complications may be undetected.[23,24]

Theoretically, the biophysical profile (BPP) should be better than the NST for assessing patients with prolonged pregnancy because in addition to the NST it also evaluates the amniotic fluid volume. There are, however, problems with the use of this test. One problem is that oligohydramnios is considered to be present only when the largest pocket of fluid found in the examination has a diameter less than 1 cm.[14] To obviate this problem the definition was changed to the absence of a pocket measuring 2 cm in diameter.[13] This still is not adequate, and patients with significantly decreased fluid will be classified as normal. Another problem is that the result of the BPP is expressed as a numeric score resulting from giving an equal number of points to the presence of breathing movements, fetal tone, fetal movements, normal amniotic fluid volume, and reactive NST. In prolonged pregnancies, a decreased amount of fluid, which is a variable of critical importance, will cause only a decrease of 2 in the total number of points, and the test may be falsely interpreted as normal. To avoid this problem, the authors of the test have recently decided that the test is abnormal when the amniotic fluid is decreased.[25] A third problem is that fetal movements, fetal tone, and fetal reactivity are variables affected by relatively advanced fetal hypoxemia, and an ideal test should detect early rather than late stages of fetal compromise. The problems associated with the use of the BPP have been the subject of a cogent review by Vintzileos et al.[26]

The contraction stress test (CST) combined with evaluation of the amniotic fluid volume is the best test for fetal surveillance in prolonged pregnancies. In the chain of events leading to fetal acidosis and hypoxia, late decelerations, demonstrable by the CST, are one of the first signs to appear. Also, the efficacy of the CST in postterm pregnancy has been clearly demonstrated.[27] Finally, the contractions induced during the CST will help to ripen the cervix.

An important consideration in patients with prolonged pregnancies is the appropiate time interval between fetal surveillance tests. The classic concept has been that a 1-week interval is adequate. However, the value of this concept is being questioned. There is evidence[28] that in prolonged pregnancies amniotic fluid may decrease from a normal volume to rather severe oligohydramnios in a 24-hour period. Also, there are case reports of fetal deaths occurring within 24 hours of a reactive NST.[21,22] The frequency of fetal surveillance must be related to the risk of fetal mortality and morbidity—risk that increases with gestational age. For that reason testing should be perfomed at 40 and 41 weeks and twice weekly after 41 weeks.

Amniotic fluid analysis

In the rare patient who still is pregnant after 42 weeks, amniocentesis may be carried out to determine if meconium is present. The presence of meconium in the amniotic fluid, specially if it is thick, is an indication for delivery and alerts the obstetrician to the need for amnioinfusion to dilute the meconium.[29] In these cases it is necessary to have present at the time of delivery personnel adequately trained in the management of meconium aspiration.

When amniocentesis is performed in patients with prolonged pregnancies, it is not unusual to find an L/S ratio of 4:1 or greater.[30] The elevated L/S ratio is an early sign of postmaturity, and these babies may show wrinkling of the skin and some other stigmata at the time of delivery.

The accuracy of the patient's dates is suspect when amniocentesis reveals clear fluid with immature L/S ratio. The possibility of an immature L/S ratio in a prolonged pregnancy is minimal.

Management

The information provided by the history and physical examination, the assessment of reliability of gestational age, ultrasound examination, fetal surveillance tests, and amniotic fluid analysis will allow identification of patients that need delivery because of ripe cervix, congenitally abnormal fetuses, decreased amniotic fluid, large fetal size, abnormal fetal surveillance tests, and meconium in the fluid. Patients with high-risk pregnancies, especially those with diabetes and hypertension, should also be delivered because prolongation of pregnancy will place their infants at increased risk.[31] Those left will be a group of patients who have unripe cervix, normal amount of fluid, normal-size babies, and normal CST or NST. These patients need frequent assessment of cervical ripening, fetal status, and amniotic fluid volume. Induction of labor will be the best choice if the cervix becomes ripe or the fluid decreases. Cesarean delivery is indicated if the oxytocin challenge test (OCT) is positive. These tests should be at 40 and 41 weeks and twice weekly after 41 weeks. At 41 weeks it is desirable to perform an amniocentesis to look for meconium. The indication for amniocentesis is stronger if ultrasound shows advanced maturity of the fetal gastrointestinal tract or the pregnancy reaches 42 weeks.

A decreased amount of amniotic fluid is a sign indicating the need for delivery.[13] The patient must be admitted to the hospital for induction of labor. An intrauterine pressure catheter (IUPC) should be placed in the amniotic cavity as soon as feasible, and amnioinfusion with 1000 ml of warm normal saline solution should be performed. The amnioinfusion will prevent cord compression and signs of fetal distress.

Patients with prolonged pregnancies and estimated fetal weight of 4500 g or larger should be counseled to have cesarean delivery because the possibility of traumatic vaginal delivery is substantial. Cesarean section should be offered also to those patients who have previously delivered infants with similar or larger birth weights be-

cause prior delivery of a large baby does not guarantee an easy delivery of another large baby.

Patients with estimated fetal weights between 4000 and 4500 g should be counseled to have cesarean section if they are insulin-dependent diabetics, gestational diabetics, or they had abnormal diabetic screening and normal glucose tolerance testing, or only one abnormal value in the glucose tolerance test. Infants of mothers with abnormalities in carbohydrate metabolism have large subcutaneous pads in the shoulders and develop shoulder dystocia more frequently than babies of similar weight from mothers without carbohydrate intolerance.[32]

The counseling of patients with estimated fetal weight between 4000 and 4500 g, unripe cervix, and no carbohydrate intolerance is difficult. Prolongation of pregnancy with further fetal weight gain will increase the possibilities of cesarean delivery. Induction of labor with an unripe cervix also will increase the possibilities of a cesarean delivery. In this situation other variables should be taken into consideration. One of those variables is parity; induction will have a greater chance of success if the patient is a multipara. Another is the frequency of uterine contractions; waiting for labor will be more advisable if the patient is having frequent contractions. The presence of other risk factors will make induction a preferable option. Availability of and experience in the use of prostaglandin (PG) preparations or extraamniotic saline for cervical ripening may also incline the balance in favor of induction.

The best approach for ripening the cervix and inducing labor is the use of PGE_2 gel. Unfortunately, there are no commercial gel preparations available in the United States. Instead of the gel, 20-mg PGE_2 vaginal suppositories may be divided into small fragments, or "chips," in an attempt to obtain pieces containing 2 mg. The chip is placed in the posterior fornix. The problem with this system is that the amount of medication given to the patient is unknown and hyperstimulation is common. Also, placement of the chip in the posterior fornix is not easy, and it frequently melts during placement.

There are other ways of preparing the PGE_2 vaginal suppositories. One method melts the suppository in a 38° C water bath, mixing it with 20 ml of fatty-based suppository transfer medium.[33] The mixture is dispensed in 2-ml aliquots into 2-ml individual, disposable supposi-

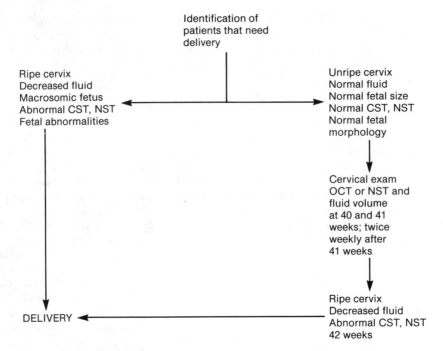

FIGURE 8-1 ◪ Management of prolonged pregnancy.

tory molds. After they become hard they are kept in the freezer until needed. Each one of the suppositories should contain 2 mg of PGE_2. One suppository is placed into the posterior vaginal fornix; the dose is repeated every 6 hours until the cervix is ripe. At this time conventional oxytocin induction may be started. However, the PG content of these suppositories varies and may be 50% less than the expected amount.

Another method of preparing PGE_2 vaginal suppositories for cervical ripening is grating them, using the smallest grater-hole size and mixing the product with a small amount of Surgilub until a uniform suspension, with the consistency of a heavy cream, is obtained. This suspension is progressively diluted with larger and larger amounts of Surgilub until a total volume of 100 ml is obtained. The concentration of the newly prepared gel will be 2 mg in 10 ml. Aliquots of 12 ml of this solution will be drawn into hypodermic syringes and kept in a freezer. The extra 2 ml in the syringe is to allow for the gel that will be left in the French catheter that will be used for dispensing the drug. The gel will thaw in about 20 to 30 minutes. At the time of application, the syringe is connected to a No. 16

French catheter, 4 inches long, that is inserted into the vagina, with the tip placed in the posterior fornix. More dilute solutions of the PGE_2 suppository can be prepared for intracervical use. The intracervical dose should not exceed 0.5 mg of PGE_2.

Another method of ripening the cervix is using a Foley catheter for extraamniotic instillation of saline solution.[34] A size 26 Foley catheter with a 30-ml balloon is inserted through the cervix, the baloon is inflated with saline or with air, and normal saline solution is infused into the extraamniotic space at 60 ml/hr. Low-dose intravenous oxytocin induction is initiated after the extraamniotic infusion is started. This is an excellent method for cervical ripening. Users of this methodology should be cautioned that the cervix frequently remains dilated 3 or 4 cm for several hours after the Foley catheter is passed, and this should not be interpreted as a failure to progress in labor. Continuation of the induction will lead to further effacement, dilation, and descent in the majority of cases.

Patients should be delivered at 42 weeks of gestation irrespective of the status of their cervix. The morbidity and mortality associated with prolonged pregnancy is substantial after 42 weeks, and delivery is the procedure of choice. In Dallas, perinatal mortality was reduced from 19 per 1000 to zero by induction of labor at 42 rather than 43 weeks.[35] The patient should be induced using PGE_2 if the cervix is not ripe and delivered by cesarean section if induction is unsuccessful. Inductions should not be prolonged for more than 2 days.

A summary of the antepartum management protocol for patients suspected of prolonged pregnancies is shown in Figure 8-1.

■ INTRAPARTUM MANAGEMENT OF THE PATIENT WITH PROLONGED GESTATION

Once it has been determined that a patient with prolonged gestation must be delivered, the obstetrician should be ready to face potentially serious problems during the intrapartum period.

Nonreassuring fetal heart rate monitoring patterns

It is not uncommon that nonreassuring fetal heart rate (FHR) patterns will develop during labor in patients with prolonged gestation. Variable decelerations and decreased beat-to-beat variability are most commonly observed. The presence of these signs must be followed by amnioinfusion with 500 ml of warmed saline solution. If amnioinfusion fails in correcting the abnormal FHR pattern, measurement of scalp pH is mandatory. Labor may continue in the presence of variable decelerations or decreased variability if the fetal scalp pH is normal. If the abnormal FHR pattern persists, fetal scalp pH sampling should be repeated every 15 to 30 minutes. Labor should be arrested with a tocolytic agent, and the pregnancy delivered by cesarean if the patient has a cervix that does not allow performance of scalp sampling.

In patients with prolonged gestation, decreased variability frequently is the only manifestation of fetal hypoxia. Also, decreased beat-to-beat variability may be the only sign preceding the onset of fetal bradycardia that frequently ends in intrapartum or neonatal death. It is important to remember that if the variability is decreased using external monitoring, it will be worse with direct FHR monitoring. Also, remember that the fetus at term and the healthy postterm fetus normally have *increased* variability. Cesarean delivery may be necessary in patients with decreased variability even if severe variable or late decelerations are not present. Fetal tachycardia (190 to 200 bpm) has also been reported preceding fetal death in postterm pregnancies.[36]

Fetal trauma

Labor in a patient with prolonged pregnancy must be preceded by an evaluation of fetal size. If fetal macrosomia is present, close attention must be given to the development of labor abnormalities, and cesarean section should be used liberally if arrest or protraction disorders occur. Traumatic vaginal delivery is 12 times more frequent in infants weighing 4500 g or more than in those with 3000 to 3999 g birth weight.[37] Unfortunately, in many cases labor proceeds without detectable abnormalities until the moment when the fetal head is delivered and shoulder dystocia becomes apparent. Fetal trauma is common after shoulder dystocia, but it may also occur in its absence, most commonly after the use of vaccuum or forceps. The use of these devices may cause cephalic hematomas and skull fractures.

Shoulder dystocia

The obstetrician should be aware of the possibility of shoulder dystocia in every delivery of patients with prolonged pregnancy or with macrosomic fetus, even if their labor is completely normal. When shoulder dystocia is anticipated, the obstetrician should mentally rehearse the sequence of steps necessary to treat this problem and be ready to act in a logical, step-by-step fashion. Lack of anticipation is the most common underlying reason for the confusion that occurs after the onset of this complication.

Dr. James O'Leary is the author of a mnemonic technique for anticipating the occurrence of shoulder dystocia. According to O'Leary and Leonetti,[38] every time an obstetrician provides care for a patient in labor, he or she should ask the question:

Is this patient a DOPE?

The word *DOPE* is a reminder of the most important risk factors associated with shoulder dystocia:

D is for diabetes
O is for obesity
P is for postterm (also for prior large baby)
E is for excessive weight gain during pregnancy

If the patient in labor is a DOPE, the obstetrician should mentally rehearse the following steps to manage the complication:

Step 1 (preparation)

A. Have the time noted when the problem is recognized, and have minutes counted off by a designated individual.

B. Call anesthesia and alert the operating room.

C. Call for somebody to help during the delivery.

D. Do not pull the baby's head.

E. Do not apply fundal pressure.

Step 2 (diagnosis)

A. Enlarge the episiotomy.

B. Explore manually behind the baby's head and find out whether the posterior shoulder of the baby is in the hollow of the sacrum.

If the posterior shoulder *is not* in the hollow of the sacrum, the diagnosis is **bilateral** shoulder dystocia (both shoulders are above the pelvic inlet), and the best thing to do is restitute the baby's head inside the vagina and perform a cesarean delivery (see step 6).

If the posterior shoulder *is* in the hollow of the sacrum, the problem is **unilateral** shoulder dystocia (only the anterior shoulder is above the inlet), and the chances of correcting the problem are good. Then the obstetrician should perform the McRoberts maneuver.

Step 3 (McRoberts maneuver)

A. Remove the mother's legs from stirups.

B. Abduct her legs and sharply flex them against her abdomen. This causes a cephalad rotation of the symphysis and often frees an impacted anterior shoulder without manipulation of the fetus.

C. Ask your assistant to apply firm **suprapubic** (not fundal) pressure directed laterally and inferiorly. This will help force the anterior shoulder under the pubic arch.

D. The operator should apply constant, moderate traction on the fetal head for a count of 30. Avoid intermittent pulling.

If the McRoberts maneuver and suprapubic pressure fail to solve the shoulder dystocia, attempts should be made to rotate the anterior shoulder into the oblique diameter of the pelvis.

Step 4 (oblique diameter)

A. Attempt to rotate the shoulder by applying pressure on the posterior aspect of the impacted anterior shoulder to move it from the anteroposterior to the oblique diameter of the inlet. Suprapubic pressure in the same direction should be applied simultaneously. If there is not enough room under the symphysis to perform the manuever or if it fails, try the corkscrew maneuver.

B. Apply pressure on the posterior aspect of the **posterior** shoulder, attempting to rotate it anteriorly under the symphysis (corkscrew maneuver of Woods). Suprapubic pressure in the opposite direction should be applied simultaneously.

If the prior steps have been unsuccessful in resolving the shoulder dystocia, the next thing to do is extract the posterior arm.

Step 5 (extraction of the posterior arm)

Slide your hand in the vagina behind the posterior shoulder and along the posterior humerus, and sweep the posterior arm of the fetus across the chest keeping the arm flexed at the elbow. Grasp the fetal hand and pull the hand and the arm along the fetal head delivering the posterior arm.

If extraction of the posterior arm is unsuccessful, proceed to step 6.

Step 6 (Zavanelli restitution)

To restitute the baby's head, it is necessary to do the following:

A. Turn the baby's head to the original position at the time of delivery (usually occipitoanterior).

B. Flex the baby's head and apply upward pressure. The fetal head should move easily up into the birth canal.

C. Move the patient to the operating room and perform a cesarean section.

The step-by-step application of different maneuvers to solve a shoulder dystocia should not take more than 5 minutes. The most serious risk to the fetus during those 5 minutes is that of trauma. If the problem persists unsolved, the next major potential risk is neurologic damage. The probability of serious fetal damage is minimized by this protocol because one of the first steps is the recognition of the most dangerous type of dystocia (bilateral dystocia) and the use in those cases of the Zavanelli restitution.

Meconium aspiration

One of the most frequent neonatal complications associated with prolonged pregnancy is meconium aspiration syndrome (MAS). Until recently this problem had a mortality up to 60%. Now, fortunately, with the use of amnioinfusion before delivery, nasopharyngeal aspiration before the first breath, and endotracheal aspiration immediately after birth,[8,39] the mortality and morbidity associated with MAS have substantially decreased.

In every delivery of patients with prolonged pregnancy, and especially when meconium has been detected, the obstetrician must be ready to prevent the occurrence of MAS. For this purpose a suction device must be ready at the time of delivery, and as soon as the fetal head appears on the maternal perineum, or in the open uterus in the case of cesarean section, and before the first fetal breathing effort, the nasopharynx should be aspirated completely. There is no difference in efficacy between rubber bulb and DeLee suction in clearing the meconium from the nasopharynx and oropharynx of neonates.[40] During this time, in the case of vaginal deliveries, the mother must be panting and avoiding expulsive efforts. Once the obstetrician feels certain that all or most of the meconium that was present in the oropharynx has been removed, the delivery is completed, and the infant is moved to an Ohio table where a qualified person should perform endotracheal aspiration. The largest endotracheal tube compatible with the baby's tracheal size must be inserted in the infant's trachea and then removed slowly under continuous aspiration with the mouth or with a suction machine.

The literature shows decreased neonatal mortality and morbidity with the combined use of aspiration of the oropharynx before the first breath followed by endotracheal aspiration.[33,41] This technique must be routine in the delivery room management of the meconium-stained infant.

◣ IMPORTANT POINTS ◥

1. The incidence of postterm pregnancy is 7.5% when the diagnosis is based on menstrual dating. It decreases to 2.6% when dating is based on early ultrasound examination and to 1.1% when the ultrasound and the menstrual history are in agreement. Therefore the best prophylaxis of postterm pregnancy is accurate dating.

2. The incidence of fetal macrosomia is approximately 10% for babies delivered between 38 and 40 weeks. It increases to 23% between 41 and 42 weeks and reaches 42% between 43 and 44 weeks.

3. The main fetal problems associated with prolongation of pregnancy beyond the EDD are a high incidence of intrapartum distress mostly caused by oligohydramnios, fetal trauma resulting from macrosomia, postmaturity syndrome, and meconium aspiration.

4. Evaluation of the amniotic fluid volume is of fundamental importance in patients with prolonged pregnancy. Umbilical cord compression caused by decreased fluid is the most common cause of fetal distress in these patients, and perinatal mortality increases directly with the severity of oligohydramnios.

5. The abdominal circumference is the most important measurement in the sonographic estimation of fetal weight. If this measurement is two or more standard deviations above the mean, there is a high probability of fetal macrosomia.

6. The CST, combined with evaluation of the amniotic fluid volume, is the best test for fetal surveillance in postterm pregnancies. In patients with contraindications, the CST may be substituted by the NST. Patients should be tested at 40 and 41 weeks and twice per week thereafter.

7. The presence of meconium in the amniotic fluid is an indication for amnioinfusion. In these cases it is necessary to have present at the time of delivery personnel trained in the management of meconium aspiration.

8. Patients with prolonged pregnancy that need to be delivered include those with ripe cervix, decreased amniotic fluid, large fetal size, abnormal fetal surveillance tests, and meconium in the fluid.

9. Patients with decreased amniotic fluid should be admitted to the hospital and receive amnioinfusion before induction of labor.

10. The best method to ripen the cervix is use of PGE$_2$ vaginal gel. The use of a Foley catheter for extraamniotic instillation of saline solution is equally effective.

11. Amnioinfusion is the preferred treatment for patients with prolonged pregnancies that develop variable decelerations during labor.

12. The obstetrician should be prepared to manage shoulder dystocia in every patient with DOPE (D for diabetes, O for obesity, P for postterm, and E for excessive weight gain during pregnancy).

13. In cases of unilateral shoulder dystocia, the following procedures should be performed sequentially: McRoberts maneuver, corkscrew maneuver, extraction of the posterior arm, and Zavanelli restitution.

14. With the use of amnioinfusion before delivery, nasopharyngeal aspiration before the first breath, and endotracheal aspiration immediately after birth, the morbidity and mortality associated with meconium aspiration has substantially decreased.

REFERENCES

1. Clifford SA: Postmaturity with placental dysfunction. *J Pediatr* 1954;44:1.
2. Field TM, Dabiri C, Hallock A, et al: Developmental effects of prolonged pregnancy and the postmaturity syndrome. *J Pediatr* 1977;90:836.
3. Zwerdling MA: Factors pertaining to prolonged pregnancy and its outcome. *Pediatrics* 1967;42:202.
4. Boyd ME, Usher RH, McLean FH, et al: Obstetric consequences of postmaturity. *Am J Obstet Gynecol* 1988;158:334.
5. Beisher NA, Evans JH, Townsend L: Studies in prolonged pregnancy. I. The incidence of prolonged pregnancy. *Am J Obstet Gynecol* 1969;103:476.
6. Hytten FE, Thomson AM: Maternal physiological adjustments, in Assali NS (ed): *Biology of Gestation.* New York, Academic Press Inc, 1968, vol 1, pp 449-479.
7. Vorherr H: Placental insufficiency in relation to postterm pregnancy and fetal postmaturity. *Am J Obstet Gynecol* 1975;123:67.
8. Trimmer KJ, Leveno KJ, Peters MT, et al: Observations on the cause of oligohydramnios in prolonged pregnancy. *Am J Obstet Gynecol* 1990;163:1900-1903.
9. Miller FC, Read JA: Intrapartum assessment of the postterm fetus. *Am J Obstet Gynecol* 1981;141:516.
10. Grannum PA, Berkowitz RL, Hobbins JC: The ultrasonic changes in the maturing placenta and their relation to fetal pulmonic maturity. *Am J Obstet Gynecol* 1979;133:915-922.
11. Arias F: Predictability of complications associated with prolongation of pregnancy. *Obstet Gynecol* 1987;70:101.
12. Leveno KJ, Quirk JG, Cunningham FG, et al: Prolonged pregnancy. I. Observations concerning the causes of fetal distress. *Am J Obstet Gynecol* 1984;150:465.
13. Silver RK, Dooley SL, MacGregor SN, et al: Fetal acidosis in prolonged pregnancy cannot be attributed to cord compression alone. *Am J Obstet Gynecol* 1988;159:666.
14. Rossi EM, Philipson EH, Williams TG, et al: Meconium aspiration syndrome: Intrapartum and neonatal attributes. *Am J Obstet Gynecol* 1989;161:1106-1110.
15. Chamberlain PE, Manning FA, Morrison I, et al: Ultrasound evaluation of amniotic fluid volume. I. The relationship of marginal and decreased amniotic fluid volume to perinatal outcome. *Am J Obstet Gynecol* 1984;150:245.
16. Manning FA, Platt LD, Sipos L: Antepartum fetal evaluation: Development of a fetal biophysical profile. *Am J Obstet Gynecol* 1980;136:787.
17. Crowley P, O'Herlihy P, Boylan P: The value of ultrasound measurement of amniotic fluid volume on the management of prolonged pregnancies. *Br J Obstet Gynaecol* 1984;91:444.
18. Phelan JP, Smith CV, Broussard P, et al: Amniotic fluid volume assessment with the four-quadrant technique at 36-42 weeks' gestation. *J Reprod Med* 1987;32:540.
19. Benedetti TJ, Gabbe SG: Shoulder dystocia: A complication of fetal macrosomia and prolonged second stage with mid-pelvic delivery. *Obstet Gynecol* 1978;52:526.
20. Grauz JP, Heimler R: Asphyxia and gestational age. *Obstet Gynecol* 1983;62:175.
21. Bochner CF, Williams J, Castro L, et al: The efficacy of starting postterm antenatal testing at 41 weeks as compared to 42 weeks of gestational age. *Am J Obstet Gynecol* 1988;159:550.
22. Guidetti DA, Divon MY, Langer O: Postdate fetal surveillance: Is 41 weeks too early? *Am J Obstet Gynecol* 1989;161:91.
23. Barrs VA, Frigoletto FD, Diamond F: Stillbirth after nonstress testing. *Obstet Gynecol* 1985;65:541.
24. Kiyazaki FS, Miyazaki BA: False reactive nonstress tests in postterm pregnancies. *Am J Obstet Gynecol* 1981;140:209.
25. Manning FA, Harman CR, Morrison I, et al: Fetal assessment based on fetal biophysical profile scoring. IV. An analysis of perinatal morbidity and mortality. *Am J Obstet Gynecol* 1990;162:703-709.
26. Vintzileos AM, Campbell WA, Nochimson DJ, et al: The use and misuse of the fetal biophysical profile. *Am J Obstet Gynecol* 1987;156:527.
27. Freeman RK, Garite TJ, Modanlow H, et al: Postdate pregnancy: Utilization of contraction stress test for primary fetal surveillance. *Am J Obstet Gynecol* 1981;140:128.
28. Clement D, Schifrin BS, Kates RB: Acute oligohydramnios in postdates pregnancies. *Am J Obstet Gynecol* 1987;157:884.
29. Sadovski J, Amon E, Bade M, et al: Prophylactic amnioinfusion during labor complicated by meconium: A preliminary report. *Am J Obstet Gynecol* 1989;161:613.
30. Gluck L, Kulovich MV, Borer RC, et al: The interpretation and significance of the lecithin/sphyngomyelin ratio in amniotic fluid. *Am J Obstet Gynecol* 1974;120:142.
31. Eden RD, Seifert LS, Winegar A, et al: Maternal risk status and postdate pregnancy outcome. *J Reprod Med* 1988;33:53-57.
32. Houchang D, Modanlou MD, Komatsu G, et al: Large-for-gestational-age neonates: Anthropometric reasons for shoulder dystocia. *Obstet Gynecol* 1982;60:417.
33. Chez RA: Prostaglandin E$_2$ for cervical ripening. *Contemp Ob Gyn,* November 1989, p 121.
34. Schraeyer P, Sherman DJ, Ariely S, et al: Ripening the highly unfavorable cervix with extraamniotic saline instillation or vaginal prostaglandin E$_2$ application. *Obstet Gynecol* 1989;73:938.
35. Pritchard JA, MacDonald PC, Gant NF: Preterm and postterm pregnancies and inappropriate fetal growth, in *Williams Obstetrics,* ed 17. Norwalk, Conn, Appleton & Lange, July-August 1985, suppl 1, p 7.
36. Ron M, Adoni A, Hechner-Celnikier D, et al: The significance of baseline tachycardia in the postterm fetus. *Int J Gynaecol Obstet* 1980;18:76.
37. Wikstrom I, Axelsson O, Bergstrom R, et al: Traumatic

injury in large-for-dates infants. *Acta Obstet Gynecol Scand* 1988;67:259.

38. O'Leary JA, Leonetti HB: Shoulder dystocia: Prevention and treatment. *Am J Obstet Gynecol* 1990;162:5-9.

39. Carson BS, Losey RW, Bowes WA, et al: Combined obstetric and pediatric approach to prevent meconium aspiration syndrome. *Am J Obstet Gynecol* 1976;126:712.

40. Locus P, Yeomans E, Crosby U: Efficacy of bulb versus DeLee suction at deliveries complicated by meconium stained amniotic fluid. *Am J Perinatol* 1990;7:87-91.

41. Ting P: Tracheal suction in meconium-aspiration. *Am J Obstet Gynecol* 1975;122:767.

9

THIRD-TRIMESTER BLEEDING

Vaginal bleeding at any stage of pregnancy constitutes a significant concern to the patient and her doctor. Severe vaginal bleeding is rare before 24 weeks of gestation, and when it happens, the mother's management is not markedly influenced by considerations for fetal survival. However, once the third trimester is reached, fetal survival becomes a significant probability. Indeed, in many tertiary centers, an uncompromised neonate at 26 weeks of gestation may have a greater than 75% chance of survival. This chapter analyzes some clinical aspects of patients with third-trimester vaginal bleeding and proposes plans for the management of the main causes of this problem.

◪ PLACENTA PREVIA
Definition and classification

According to the latest edition of *Williams Obstetrics,* there are four types or degrees of placenta previa:

1. *Total placenta previa,* in which the internal cervical os is completely covered by the placenta
2. *Partial placenta previa,* in which the internal cervical os is partially covered by the placenta
3. *Marginal placenta previa,* in which the edge of the placenta does not cover but is close to the internal cervical os

4. *Low-lying placenta previa,* in which the placental edge is not near the internal cervical os, but it may be palpated by a finger introduced through the cervix

These definitions of the different types of placenta previa are based on findings noted during vaginal examinations performed at the time of delivery or on the visual observation of the placenta/cervix relationship at the time of cesarean section. Despite the apparent precision of those definitions, prenatal and intrapartum differentiation between partial, marginal, and low-lying placenta previa is difficult. Today, with the use of endovaginal ultrasound, it is possible to define precisely the relation of the low border of the placenta to the internal cervical os. Symptomatic patients requiring cesarean delivery usually have total previa (the placenta completely covers the internal cervical os) or partial previa (the low placental border does not cover but is within 30 mm of the internal cervical os). When the placental border can be seen with the endovaginal probe but is more than 30 mm from the internal os, the placenta is classified as low-lying.

The classification of placenta previa with endovaginal probe ultrasound as total, partial, or low-lying has prognostic value: the probability of severe maternal and fetal complications is low when the placenta is low-lying.

Incidence

The incidence of placenta previa varies greatly from one series to another, ranging from 1 of 167[1] to 1 of 327[2] pregnancies beyond 24 weeks of gestation. The incidences of the different types are, approximately, the following:

Total placenta previa	23% to 31.3%
Partial placenta previa	20.6% to 33%
Low-lying placenta	37% to 54.9%

Etiology

No specific etiology can be found for most cases of low placental implantations. However, some investigators[3] have found that history of prior cesarean section and history of uterine curettage unrelated to pregnancy or following a spontaneous abortion are events occurring significantly more frequently in patients with placenta previa than in normal controls. This suggests that damage to the endometrium or myometrium may be the initial event causing the necessary conditions for abnormal placental implantation.

Abnormal fetal presentations and congenital malformations are strongly associated with placenta previa. Breech, shoulder, and compound presentations may be found in up to 30% of the cases. In addition, when patients with placenta previa have fetuses in vertex presentation, they are in persistent occiput posterior or transverse positions in as many as 15% of the cases. However, malpresentations are the result rather than the cause of low placental implantations.

Other associations include increasing maternal age, increasing parity, multiple gestations, anemia, closely spaced pregnancies, tumors distorting the contour of the uterus, and endometritis. Brenner et al.[1] have also suggested a sex predilection, with male fetuses predominant. Also, patients who have placenta previa have 12 times the usual risk of having placenta previa in a subsequent pregnancy.

The association of placenta previa with prior cesarean section is of particular importance in view of the increasing number of patients being delivered abdominally. The probability of placenta previa is 4 times greater in patients with prior cesareans than in patients without uterine scars.[4] The probability of placenta accreta and the need for cesarean hysterectomy are also greater in patients with prior cesareans and placenta previa than in patients with placenta previa

and no uterine scars.[5] Twenty-four percent of patients with placenta previa and one previous cesarean section have placenta accreta, and this incidence rises with the number of prior cesareans, reaching 67% for patients with placenta previa and four prior cesarean deliveries. Most of these problems occur when the placenta is implanted anteriorly, over the cesarean section scar.

Clinical presentation

The most common symptom associated with placenta previa is painless vaginal bleeding. The bleeding may occur as early as the second trimester. According to Crenshaw et al.,[2] approximately one third of patients with placenta previa have their first bleeding episode before 30 weeks of gestation, one third from 30 to 35 weeks, and one third after 36 or more weeks. The mean gestational age at the first bleeding episode is 29.6 weeks. Although dramatic in nature, the initial bleeding episode is not usually associated with maternal mortality and stops completely a few hours after its onset.

The earlier in pregnancy the first bleeding occurs, the worse is the outcome of the pregnancy. In fact, the incidence of preterm delivery, the number of bleeding episodes, the severity of the bleeding, and the number of units of blood required for transfusion are higher for patients who begin bleeding before 28 weeks.[6] The worst prognosis is for those patients with placenta previa who have had prior cesarean sections.

The severity of the bleeding and the need for blood transfusion usually increase with each bleeding episode. Fetal distress is unusual unless the hemorrhage is severe enough to cause maternal hypovolemic shock. Uterine contractions occur commonly in association with episodes of bleeding and may aggravate the bleeding tendency.

Major long-term complications of placenta previa are related to hemorrhagic shock and prolonged hypotension. Naturally, all complications inherent in cesarean section and emergency surgery pertain. Postpartum uterine atony and bleeding from the placenta implantation site are uncommon events. Disseminated intravascular coagulation (DIC) rarely occurs in connection with placenta previa.

Diagnosis

The antepartum diagnosis of placenta previa is made by transabdominal and endovaginal ultrasound examination of the patient with vaginal bleeding. The diagnosis may be confirmed by direct visual observation at the time of operative delivery. The diagnosis of placenta previa should not be made by digital vaginal examination. In fact, there is no justification for vaginal digital examination in patients with painless vaginal bleeding. The prohibition of vaginal examinations in these patients may appear, particularly to an inexperienced resident, to be an unjustified holdover from less sophisticated days. However, even when the pelvic examination is cautious and gentle, 1 of every 16 examinations produces a major hemorrhage, and 1 of every 25 examinations results in hypovolemic shock.[7] Also, the accuracy of digital pelvic examination in the diagnosis of placenta previa is only 69%. A gentle speculum examination is not associated with increased risk of hemorrhage and probably is necessary, although the vaginal and cervical causes of significant third-trimester bleeding are rare.

Attempts to diagnose placenta previa without digital vaginal examination have included methods such as listening for the placental souffle, soft tissue x-ray films, ^{125}I-labeled albumin scans, technetium scans, and magnetic resonance imaging. The placental scanning techniques have approximately 85% accuracy, but they have the drawback of fetal and maternal irradiation. Placental localization with ultrasound has superseded all previous techniques, since to date, it is associated with no known risks or dangerous sequelae and is painless, efficient, and relatively simple. The accuracy of transabdominal ultrasound in the diagnosis of placenta previa is excellent, with false-positive and false-negative rates of 7% and 8%, respectively.[8] This accuracy is even higher when a vaginal probe is used for evaluation of the patient with vaginal bleeding during pregnancy.[9] Endovaginal ultrasound (Figure 9-1) has a positive predictive value of 93.3% and a negative predictive value of 97.6%.[10] Both transabdominal and endovaginal ultrasound are safe techniques with minimal or no risks for mother and fetus.

An understanding of the evolution of uterine anatomy throughout pregnancy is necessary for an appropriate interpretation of ultrasonic findings with respect to the placental localization. In many patients, early in pregnancy the placenta appears to cover the internal cervical os, but as the uterus enlarges and the lower uterine segment develops, the placenta appears to move cephalad, away from the internal os. This move-

ment is referred to as *migration*. Therefore, before 24 weeks of gestation, only a cautionary significance should be attributed to the finding of a placental position close to the internal cervical os, particularly in asymptomatic patients. In 97% of these patients, the placenta has moved away from the cervical os by term.[11] Therefore all diagnoses of placenta previa in asymptomatic patients based on ultrasonic examinations performed during the first and second trimesters of pregnancy must be confirmed during the third trimester. If both the transabdominal and endovaginal examinations show that the bulk of the placenta is centered over the internal os after 24 weeks of gestation, it is much less likely for the placenta to be away from the cervix at term.

In the past the so-called *double set-up* examination was necessary in a small percentage of symptomatic patients in whom transabdominal ultrasound was not capable of accurately diagnosing placenta previa. This situation typically occurred in patients with vaginal bleeding after 36 weeks, with posterior placentas extending below the fetal presenting part and with the presenting part impeding adequate visualization of the relation between the low border of the placenta and the cervix. In some patients this problem could be solved by manual elevation of the presenting part, but in a few cases the double set-up was necessary for diagnosis.

In the performance of a double set-up, the patient is taken to the operating room, and after all the necessary personnel and equipment are ready for cesarean delivery, the patient is prepared and draped, and a vaginal digital examination is performed to determine the placental localization. If vaginal bleeding occurs as a result of the examination, a cesarean section is performed immediately. If no placenta previa is found and there is no bleeding with the digital examination, the patient is allowed to labor and to deliver vaginally. The diagnosis of placenta previa by double set-up examination is not absolutely accurate, and confusion may occur because of the presence of blood clots at the level of the internal os, which can mimic placental tissue, or the existence of a thick *decidual reaction*, which can appear like a very thin placenta. Fortunately, with the advent of endovaginal ultrasound, the double set-up examination belongs to the history of medicine.

In most patients the vaginal blood is maternal in origin. However, a fetal component could be significant if some disruption of the villi occurs.

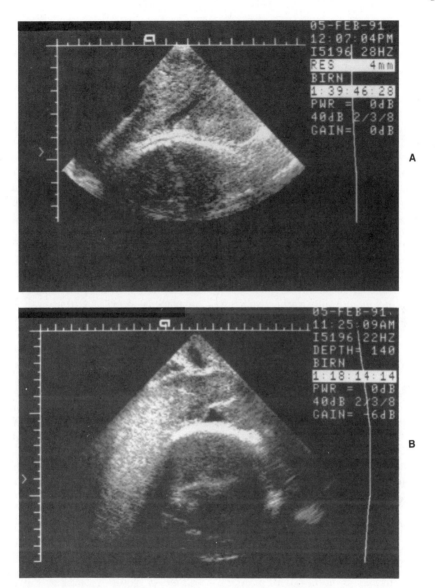

FIGURE 9-1 ◪ Diagnosis of placenta previa with endovaginal ultrasound. **A,** Endovaginal ultrasound of a normal patient: the endocervical canal is clearly seen, as well as part of the fetal head. There is no placenta previa. **B,** Endovaginal ultrasound of a patient with a total placenta previa: the placenta is posterior, and its low border covers completely the internal cervical os.

Certainly, if a portion of the vaginal blood is fetal, the pregnancy is at higher risk for fetal and neonatal mortality and morbidity than if the blood is all maternal. The possibility of fetal blood loss may be suspected by the occurrence of fetal tachycardia, decreased variability, sinusoidal rhythm, or episodes of bradycardia in the fetal heart rate monitor tracing.

There are several tests available to determine the presence of fetal blood, but they are unreliable or difficult to perform in an emergency situation. A simple test to distinguish fetal from maternal blood consists of placing 5 ml of tap water into each of two small test tubes and adding 6 drops of 10% potassium hydroxide (KOH). To one of the tubes add 3 drops of vaginal blood and to the other 3 drops of maternal blood. The tube with maternal blood will turn green yellowish brown after 2 minutes. If the vaginal blood contains fetal red cells, the KOH solution will be pink.[12]

Outcome

A placenta previa is destined to bleed unless the pregnancy is interrupted by cesarean section. The amount of blood loss does correlate with the degree of previa. With total, partial, and marginal placenta previa, the number of units of blood replaced per patient were, respectively, 4.7, 3.6, and 2.5 in Crenshaw et al.'s series.[2]

There is a significant correlation between the gestational age at which the first bleeding episode occurs and preterm delivery. Perinatal mortality is high when the first bleeding episode occurs before 28 weeks of gestation, but there is a progressive decline in mortality with advancing gestational age. The number of bleeding episodes does not correlate with the total amount of blood loss or with perinatal mortality.

All types of placenta previa, whatever the gestational age at the first bleeding episode or the amount of bleeding, are associated with high perinatal mortality. However, the perinatal mortality is greater with earlier bleeding, with a larger amount of bleeding, and with a greater extent of placenta previa. The main reason for the perinatal mortality in placenta previa is preterm birth. When Crenshaw et al.'s data[2] are broken down according to gestational age and fetal weight, the predominance of preterm fetuses is evident. Most authors suggest that if preterm delivery could be avoided, the perinatal mortality problem would disappear. However, there are other factors in addition to preterm birth that compromise the infants of mothers with placenta previa. In fact, for babies born after 28 weeks of gestation, there is a greater neonatal mortality associated with placenta previa than there is for babies born at a similar gestational age because of other reasons. This is also evident if the data are broken down by fetal weights. For fetal weights above 1000 g and under 3000 g, there is a greater neonatal mortality if the pregnancy was affected by placenta previa. Fetal and neonatal hypovolemia and fetal asphyxia are the logical explanations for these findings.

Beyond hemorrhage, the single most common cause for preterm delivery in patients with placenta previa is preterm labor, which occurs in approximately 30% of these patients. Many patients who have increased bleeding also have spontaneous uterine contractions, which may contribute to the excessive bleeding. Another reason for preterm delivery is preterm rupture of the membranes, which may occur even in patients with total previa.

The risk of fetal congenital malformations is increased 2 to 4 times in patients with placenta previa. It is a sobering experience to manage expectantly a patient with previa and to maintain her pregnancy for several weeks only to deliver an infant with no capacity for extrauterine life. There are no abnormalities specifically associated with placenta previa.

Management

Three fundamental areas of concern must be evaluated quickly and efficiently when dealing with a patient who is bleeding as a consequence of placenta previa: (1) the mother's condition as primarily evidenced by the degree of obstetric hemorrhage; (2) the fetal condition including, in particular, gestational age estimation; and (3) the ability of the neonatal unit to handle an infant of that gestational age.

A massive hemorrhage threatening maternal life requires termination of the pregnancy without regard to the maturity of the fetus. A mild-to-moderate bleeding episode in a patient at term should be managed similarly by operative delivery. However, if the patient is preterm and the bleeding is not an immediate threat to the mother's life, a more conservative approach is appropriate.

With respect to the fetus, no single issue is as important in the management of placenta previa as gestational dating. In fact, the risk of neonatal mortality and morbidity if the pregnancy is interrupted is closely related to the gestational age and should be balanced against the risk of increased maternal morbidity if the pregnancy is allowed to continue.

Finally, the ability of pediatricians to handle preterm infants must also be strongly considered. Intervention on behalf of a fetus at 26 weeks is inappropriate when a neonate at 30 weeks of gestation has a great deal of difficulty surviving in the same hospital. If neonatal facilities are limited, the mother should be transported to a perinatal center where obstetric intervention on behalf of 26-week fetuses is relatively common and produces a high proportion of normal outcomes. The transport after birth of these high-risk preterm infants to a tertiary center does not produce the same good outcome found when the infant is delivered at the tertiary hospital.

Evaluation of severity of bleeding. Evaluation of the severity of the bleeding is the initial and decisive step in the management of patients with placenta previa. However, making an adequate evaluation of the severity of a bleeding episode is difficult. Visual inspection of the patient and her blood-stained clothes is notoriously inaccurate. Blood pressure and pulse may remain within normal ranges despite considerable blood loss because of the unusual tolerance for bleeding of the hypervolemic pregnant woman. Hematocrit and hemoglobin determinations during or shortly after a bleeding episode may be within normal ranges because of compensatory vasoconstriction. Measurements of blood volume are usually inaccurate during bleeding and may be normal in spite of significant blood loss. Finally, the absolute amount of bleeding should always be evaluated in relation to the clinical status before the bleeding episode: an anemic patient may lose 1 U of blood and show signs of profound hypovolemia, whereas a normal patient may handle this loss without any significant change in vital signs.

The following clinical criteria are used to classify the severity of a bleeding episode:

Mild bleeding (the patient has lost less than 15% of her intravascular volume)
No change in vital signs
No postural hypotension
  No peripheral evidence of circulatory volume deficit
  Normal urinary output

Moderate bleeding (the patient has lost between 15% and 30% of her blood volume)
  Postural changes in pulse rate (increase of 10 to 20 bpm when changing from the supine to the upright position) and in diastolic blood pressure (drop of 10 mm Hg or more)
  Evidence of inadequate circulatory volume (dyspnea, thirst, pallor, tachycardia, clammy extremities); mental status changes may also be present (apathy or agitation)

Severe bleeding (the patient has lost 30% to 40% of her blood volume)
  Patient in shock with decreased or unrecordable blood pressure
  Persistent loss of fresh blood from the vagina

The fetus may be dead or showing signs of distress
Oliguria or anuria

Management of patients with severe bleeding. In patients with severe, acute third-trimester bleeding, little emphasis should be placed on finding the etiology of the hemorrhage. It should be assumed that a catastrophic event is present and that the patient could exsanguinate in a matter of minutes. In these situations an efficient management plan including life-support measures and immediate operative intervention are the only hopes of avoiding a maternal death. Management includes constant observation and monitoring, administration of intravenous fluids, transfusion therapy, assessment of renal function and intravascular status, assessment of the fetus, and delivery.

Intensive observation and monitoring. Pregnant patients with severe bleeding should never be left alone. Frequent monitoring of vital signs, precise measurement of the fluid input and the urinary output, recording the amount of vaginal bleeding, and keeping complete records of what has transpired are essential for a positive outcome. Retrospective reconstruction of what went on in an emergency is, at best, inadequate. One health professional must be in charge of directly executing the physician's orders without leaving the room.

When the intravenous lines are being established, samples of blood should be obtained for evaluating complete blood count; type and crossmatch of at least 4 U; electrolytes, glucose, creatinine, or blood urea nitrogen levels; and DIC profile. Although the hemoglobin and hematocrit values have been the basis for evaluation of blood loss for decades, acute and dramatic changes can often remain hidden in a constant blood cell level, only to be fully revealed a few days later after complete vascular equilibration. On the other hand, rapid fluid infusion can expand the intravascular space and produce a decrease in erythrocyte level that a few days later will also reequilibrate, only at a higher value. The electrolyte, glucose, and creatinine levels are baseline, primarily in preparation for anesthesia, and also serve as a crude screening for major problems. The DIC profile is essential for identifying the rare patient with previa who develops disseminated intravascular coagulation and requires more sophisticated management.

Intravenous fluids. A large-bore cannula, at least 18 gauge, should be inserted for the administration of a balanced electrolyte solution such as lactated Ringer's. If the patient is in shock, two intravenous administration lines should be started because if a second line is necessary, it may be exceedingly difficult to initiate. The patient's response to the initial fluid administration provides a rough index of the severity of the bleeding. In fact, if the blood pressure becomes normal and the pulse rate decreases with less than 3 L of intravenous fluids, the blood volume loss is probably less than 50%.

Transfusion therapy. Blood transfusion is an essential component in the treatment of obstetric hemorrhage, and the support of a good blood bank is vital to any obstetric service. Blood transfusions, however, are not without danger. Blood cell transfusion reactions, transmission of infection, and volume overload are some of the most frequent complications associated with transfusion therapy.

The most severe transfusion reaction is acute intravascular hemolysis, occurring at a frequency of 1 in every 6000 U transfused and usually resulting from incorrect identification of the donor or the recipient. Most severe transfusion reactions are the consequence of clerical errors. To avoid these errors, it is necessary to identify carefully the patient and the blood product that is going to be administered before the transfusion starts.

One of the dangers of transfusion therapy is the possibility of infecting the recipient with some microorganism present in the donor's blood. Hepatitis C and B, human immunodeficiency virus (HIV), and cytomegalovirus (CMV) are some of the microorganisms that may be transmitted with the administration of blood products. Fortunately, the probability of infection with transfusion therapy is small. The risk of acquiring hepatitis C is approximately 1% for any unit of blood or blood products. The risk of infection with HIV virus in the United States following transfusion with volunteer donor blood is 1 in 400,000 to 1 in 1,000,000. Despite this small risk, the fear of acquiring HIV infection has caused a considerable increase in request for autologous blood transfusions.

Autologous blood donation during pregnancy is safe,[13] but is limited by the mother's hemoglobin concentration and by the potential effects on the fetus and on uterine activity caused by sudden changes in intravascular volume. Autologous blood donation for routine vaginal delivery or routine cesarean section should be discouraged. The likelihood of requiring transfusion during these procedures is low,[14] and it is difficult to predict which patients will require transfusion.[15] Only 0.3% to 1.6% of patients receive transfusion after vaginal delivery, and 4.6% to 7.3% receive transfusion after cesarean section. Also, special arrangements and procedures are necessary for the collection of the blood (Box 9-1), and this places a burden on the obstetrician and the blood bank.

In the majority of situations, before the initiation of transfusion therapy, it is necessary to know the recipient's blood type and whether irregular antibodies are present. This is accomplished by means of a procedure named *type and screen*. With this information the blood bank can rapidly select units of donor red blood cells (RBCs) that are most compatible with the recipient. A given unit of RBCs may be compatible and selected for potential use by several recipients. Because all the anticipated transfusions do not actually result in patients being transfused,

---

BOX 9-1

Procedure for Autologous Blood Donation During Pregnancy

1. The patient's gestational age should be greater than 20 and less than 35 weeks.
2. Patient's hemoglobin and hematocrit the day of blood drawing should be greater than 11 g/dl and 35%, respectively.
3. Patients with preeclampsia, fetal growth retardation, and chronic hypertension are excluded.
4. Normal fetal heart rate (FHR) and uterine contraction monitoring should be observed for 30 minutes before drawing blood.
5. Start IV with D_5LR. Administer 250 ml in 1 hour.
6. Draw 1 U of blood.
7. Infuse 300 ml of IV fluids 1 hour after the blood is drawn. Maintain FHR monitoring.
8. Decrease the rate of administration of IV fluids to 100 ml/hr. Continue FHR and contractions monitoring.
9. If contractions do not develop or if they subside quickly with IV fluids, the patient may have some light food, the IV fluids may be discontinued, and the patient may be discharged.

the type and screen procedure allows a more efficient use of resources and a more rapid response of the blood bank. Also, the typing and screening procedure is more likely to detect significant antibodies than is the crossmatch test.

In the past, to select blood for a potential transfusion, a *type and crossmatch* was ordered. In this procedure the patient's *serum* is tested for antibodies against the donor's RBCs, and if no antibodies are detected, 1 or more units of blood are set aside for eventual use in that particular patient only. It is obvious that the type and crossmatch procedure limits the use of the blood bank's resources and should not be used to select blood when the transfusion is only probable.

The units of stored blood that are determined to be compatible with the recipient's RBCs by means of the typing and screening procedure should be crossmatched only when the transfusion becomes necessary. For this procedure the recipient's serum and the donor's RBCs are mixed and incubated at 37° C for at least 10 minutes. The probabilities of finding an unrecognized significant antigen in the crossmatch are less than 0.05% if the recipient's antibody screening was negative and the ABO typing was adequate.

Most patients receiving blood transfusions will receive packed RBCs. Transfusion of whole blood is unnecessary in most cases and is a waste of useful products. A similar comment can be made about transfusion of *fresh blood* when a patient is bleeding and in need of clotting factors. These factors can be replaced much better by transfusion of specific blood components.

In most cases of severe obstetric bleeding, the blood bank can type and screen the patient's blood while she is receiving crystalloid solutions. However, if there is no time to wait for type-specific blood, the patient should be given type O Rh-negative packed RBCs. Type O Rh-positive packed RBCs can be used if type O Rh-negative blood is not available. The potential problem with type O Rh-positive blood is the possibility of Rh isoimmunization if the patient is Rh negative. However, this consideration should not be an obstacle to transfusing the patient with massive obstetric hemorrhage. The next step is to use type-specific blood, which requires 15 to 30 minutes for its preparation. A complete crossmatch usually requires 45 to 60 minutes if no major antibodies are found. Transfusion of type O or type-specific, noncrossmatched blood requires physician's release and is justified only in situations of extreme emergency. The military experience has demonstrated the safety of administering type-specific noncrossmatched blood in severe emergencies.

As blood is used for patients with severe obstetric hemorrhage, more units need to be crossmatched so as to constantly have 4 U available. The need for massive blood transfusion (10 U or more within 24 hours) occurs occasionally in obstetrics, mostly in patients with placenta previa and accretta, abruptio placentae, and severe postpartum bleeding. There are multiple problems associated with massive transfusions, but the most common is platelet depletion caused by the replacement with platelet-poor blood. If this problem appears, the patient should receive a platelet transfusion. If the patient becomes deficient in clotting factors, 1 U of fresh frozen plasma should be administered for every 4 U of packed RBCs. The routine use of fresh blood or whole blood for the purpose of avoiding coagulopathy is a waste of resources.

Assessment of renal function. Most longterm complications from severe hemorrhage are related to shock. Particularly, acute tubular and cortical necroses are associated with anuria or oliguria resulting from hypovolemic shock. Thus urine output observation is critical for appropriate management. A patient with severe hemorrhage needs a Foley catheter and aggressive therapy for decreased urine output. The initial treatment should consist of expansion of the intravascular volume. Maintenance of a urine output of 30 ml/hr should protect the kidney from permanent damage. Furosemide in an intravenous bolus of 20 to 40 mg is usually sufficient to reestablish urinary output once adequate hydration and blood replacement have been obtained.

Central venous pressure. A patient in critical condition needs accurate monitoring of her intravascular status. Hemoglobin, pulse, and blood pressure can all be misleading, particularly in the presence of a decreased urine output. A peripherally inserted central venous pressure line, especially if there is coagulopathy, or a more centrally inserted line, internal jugular, will provide the necessary information for safe and rapid expansion of the intravascular space. A femoral arterial line may be necessary in patients with shock or when noninvasive monitoring of the patient's blood pressure is inadequate.

Fetal evaluation. Initially, the objectives of the treatment are to restore the maternal intravascular volume, to improve her oxygen-carrying capacity, and to prepare for pregnancy termination. During these critical minutes, no time is usually available for an in-depth fetal evaluation. However, fetal heart rate monitoring should begin shortly after the patient is admitted to the hospital. Also, as soon as it is feasible, an ultrasound examination should be performed to determine fetal number, fetal position, and estimated fetal weight. The ultrasound will also be useful for determining the placenta localization, and in patients with abruption, the examination occasionally reveals the presence of a subplacental hematoma.

Speculum examination. There is no indication in the acutely bleeding patient for a digital vaginal examination. However, once the patient's vital signs become stable after the infusion of packed red cells and crystalloids and after preparations are complete for operative delivery, a speculum examination may be performed. Visual inspection of the vagina and the cervix will confirm the intrauterine origin of the hemorrhage and rule out the rare vaginal or cervical causes of bleeding.

Delivery. Patients with placenta previa and severe bleeding should be delivered by cesarean section irrespective of the type of placenta previa. The anesthesia of choice for the patient who is hemorrhaging or who may hemorrhage (i.e., patient with previa and prior cesarean section scar) is general anesthesia with endotracheal intubation. Systemic maternal disease must be quickly evaluated in preparation for surgery. A history of hypertension, diabetes, renal disease, and so forth may alter management and the choice of anesthesia. Diabetic patients should receive less glucose, and those with renal disease should have strict electrolyte and fluid management.

The uterus customarily is entered through a low transverse incision, regardless of the placental location or fetal lie. However, effective delivery of a transverse lie or a preterm infant through a low transverse incision may be difficult. This type of incision is appropriate if the presenting part is easily accessible and the lower uterine segment has developed enough to allow a generous incision. Also, a low vertical incision provides greater flexibility in the approach to delivery and perhaps somewhat less trauma to the fetus. If the placenta previa is anterior, it is necessary to cut through the placenta to access the fetus, a maneuver that occasionally produces varied degrees of fetal anemia.

Management of patients with moderate bleeding. In a patient with moderate bleeding, knowledge of the gestational age and evaluation of fetal pulmonary maturity dictate the plan of management. Delivery by cesarean section should be performed if the pregnancy is 36 weeks or more. If the pregnancy is between 32 and 36 weeks, it is necessary to evaluate the fetal pulmonary maturity as soon as the acute bleeding episode subsides and the patient's condition is stabilized.

In the majority of patients under 36 weeks of gestation, the rapid tests for fetal pulmonary maturity, TD_x-FLM test and phosphatidylglycerol (PG), show fetal immaturity. Therefore the management of patients with moderate bleeding who are between 32 and 36 weeks should be based on the result of the lecithin to sphingomyelin (L/S) ratio. If the L/S ratio is mature, greater than 2.0 in most laboratories, the fetus should be delivered. Delivery should not be delayed in patients with mature L/S ratios and immature PG or TD_x-FLM determinations. Under these circumstances, the probability that neonatal respiratory distress syndrome (RDS) will occur is less than 5%, and if it occurs, it will be mild. Obviously, the dangers of continuation of pregnancy are greater than the dangers of delivery.

If the fetal lungs are immature, the patient with placenta previa and moderate bleeding should remain under intensive monitoring in the labor and delivery unit for a period of 24 to 48 hours. A hemoglobin level of roughly 11 g/dl should be maintained by transfusion. The uterus should be kept quiescent with the use of calcium channel blockers or beta-adrenergic agents. Steroids should be administered to induce lung maturation at a dose of 12 mg betamethasone intramuscularly, to be repeated in 24 hours. If the patient's condition remains unstable, with steady blood loss in moderate amounts, and she requires 2 or more units of blood daily for several days to compensate for losses, she should be delivered in spite of the early gestational age or lack of fetal lung maturation. The pediatrician should be alerted to the imminent delivery of a baby at risk for developing RDS. If the patient's condition becomes stable and remains stable for 24 to 48 hours, she becomes a candidate for expectant management, as is described later.

Most patients with placenta previa and moderate bleeding stop bleeding and return to a stable condition shortly after admission, thereby becoming candidates for expectant management. However, in some cases the presence of complicating factors such as premature rupture of the membranes, other maternal medical conditions, or fetal distress may make continuation of the pregnancy inappropriate.

Attempts have been made to identify patients at high risk for life-threatening hemorrhage so as to preclude their being included in an expectant management protocol. For example, if the initial bleeding episode results in hemorrhage of more than 600 ml or if the placenta previa is total, immediate termination of pregnancy has been recommended. However, objective evaluation of published series on placenta previa does not substantiate these caveats. If the patient is stable, conservative management is the plan of choice, since even a few days of delay in delivery may radically improve the neonatal outcome.

Management of patients with mild bleeding. As with moderate bleeding, fetal pulmonary maturity dictates the management of patients with mild bleeding. Immediate delivery of mature fetuses is the appropriate course, regardless of the minor degree of bleeding. Each published series on placenta previa recounts term infants dying while awaiting cesarean section. If the fetal lungs are immature or gestational age is less than 36 weeks, the patient with mild bleeding and placenta previa becomes a candidate for expectant management.

The objective of the conservative or expectant management of placenta previa is to reduce the high fetal mortality associated with early delivery. Before 1920, when the risk of abdominal delivery was high because of the lack of availability of blood transfusion, maternal mortality was approximately 10% and fetal mortality as high as 70%. When cesarean section became safe and practical, it was common to deliver patients with placenta previa immediately after a bleeding episode, regardless of the fetal age. With this aggressive approach, maternal mortality was drastically reduced, but perinatal mortality, mostly the result of prematurity, remained high. Approximately 25 years later, a reevaluation of the aggressive surgical approach was initiated because it was thought that maintenance of the pregnancy under close supervision might decrease perinatal mortality. However, not all patients with placenta previa are eligible for expectant

management. Noneligible patients include those at term, with excessive bleeding, with ruptured membranes, and so forth. In individual cases, one must assess the risk of pregnancy maintenance in terms of the chance that massive hemorrhage will result in fetal demise against the chance of complications of preterm delivery. In modern obstetrics, however, a delay of delivery for even a few days may significantly alter the neonatal outcome.

The following discussion outlines some characteristics of our expectant management regimen.

Patient selection. The importance of proper selection of patients cannot be overemphasized. Only hemodynamically stable patients between 32 and 36 weeks of gestation with proven fetal pulmonary immaturity or patients of less than 32 weeks should be managed expectantly. Patients with unstable vital signs or bleeding in moderate amounts should remain in Labor and Delivery until bleeding stops and vital signs become stable.

Hospitalization. Because of the potential financial burden, attempts have been made to isolate a "safe" group of patients who could be managed at home with constant supervision.[16] The selection criteria for outpatient management of patients with previa are shown in Box 9-2. Although the financial implications are appreciated, continued hospitalization is the best management plan that can be offered to these patients.[17]

BOX 9-2

Criteria for Outpatient Management of Patients with Placenta Previa

1. Inpatient observation for 72 hours without vaginal bleeding
2. Stable serial hematocrit ≥35%
3. Reactive nonstress test at the time of discharge
4. Telephone-available 24-hour transportation between home and hospital
5. Bed rest compliance at home
6. Patient's and family's comprehension of potential complications
7. Weekly clinical follow-up until delivery including serial hemoglobin levels and repeat sonography

From Silver R, Depp R, Saggagha RE, et al: *Am J Obstet Gynecol* 1984;150:15-22.

Prevention of labor. Uterine contractions are common in patients with placenta previa admitted to the hospital because of vaginal bleeding. Since uterine contractions have the potential to develop the lower uterine segment, disrupting the placental attachment and aggravating the bleeding, most investigators favor the use of tocolytic agents in the expectant management of patients with placenta previa. Once the patient's condition is stabilized, the use of nifedipine, 10 mg orally every 4 to 6 hours, is strongly recommended. In patients with placenta previa, terbutaline and ritodrine are not the drugs of choice because they cause tachycardia and make the assessment of the patient's pulse rate unreliable. Indomethacin (Indocin), another powerful tocolytic agent, is not the first-choice drug for uterine activity inhibition in patients with placenta previa because it causes inhibition of the platelet cyclooxygenase system and prolongs the bleeding time. Also, it has fetal cardiovascular side effects. If terbutaline or ritodrine is used, the patient should not be actively bleeding, and her vital signs should be in the normal range. The patients should continue on tocolytic agents until they deliver.[18]

Acceleration of fetal lung maturation. The objective of expectant management in the patient with placenta previa is to achieve fetal lung maturity. Once this is reached, the baby should be delivered. Therefore it becomes important to periodically determine the stage of fetal lung maturity and to pharmacologically accelerate this process.

To determine fetal lung maturity, amniocentesis for TD_x-FLM, PG, and L/S ratio is necessary every week or two depending on the gestational age, the frequency and severity of the bleeding episodes, and the prior treatment with glucocorticoids. As mentioned, the most important test in this situation is the L/S ratio. The obstetrician should have no trepidation in interrupting the pregnancy once a mature L/S ratio is obtained, even if the other tests are negative. The risk of significant neonatal RDS after a mature L/S ratio is significantly smaller than the risk of an obstetric catastrophe if pregnancy is not interrupted.

Multiple studies have shown about a 50% reduction in the incidence of hyaline membrane disease (HMD) in preterm infants born after the mother received glucocorticoids. The time necessary for this effect to occur can be as little as 24 hours or as much as 72 hours. In the clinical situation of placenta previa and preterm gestation, glucocorticoids may be lifesaving for the baby. Under 32 weeks of gestation, it should be assumed that the fetal lungs are immature, and the medication should be given empirically without first evaluating the amniotic fluid L/S ratio. Between 32 and 36 weeks of gestation, however, a mature L/S ratio is more likely to occur, and amniocentesis is recommended. If immediate access to an amniotic fluid test is not available, steroid treatment should be given without hesitation. The known risks of HMD far outweigh the unknown risks of brief fetal exposure to steroids, which have been used extensively in pregnancy without fetal side effects.

It is important to note that the significant reduction in HMD found in the original study by Liggins and Howie[19] was restricted to preterm babies delivered 1 to 7 days after maternal glucocorticoid treatment. After 7 days, they found no difference between glucocorticoid and placebo groups, and there was a rebound effect in the treated group that was not statistically significant. Thus it is possible that if pulmonary maturation is obtained with glucocorticoids at an early gestation, it may not persist if more than 1 week intervenes before delivery. For this reason, give glucocorticoids (two 12-mg doses of betamethasone, 24 hours apart) every week as long as the patient remains undelivered or until 36 weeks of gestation are reached.

Other measures. Bed rest is an essential component of expectant management. Limited bathroom privileges are usually allowed after the patient has been asymptomatic for a number of days.

Although the clinician is acutely aware of the danger of vaginal manipulation, the patient may not appreciate the significance of the problem. Intercourse, douching, and vaginal suppositories are contraindicated. In addition, stool softeners are appropriate to avoid straining at defecation.

The antenatal use of vitamin K and phenobarbital for the prevention of intraventricular bleeding in the neonate is controversial. However, the potential advantages of giving those medications clearly outweigh the minimal risks associated with their administration.

Cervical cerclage. In 1959, Lovset[20] presented evidence, obtained through uncontrolled observations, of the beneficial effect of cervical cerclage for patients with placenta previa. This

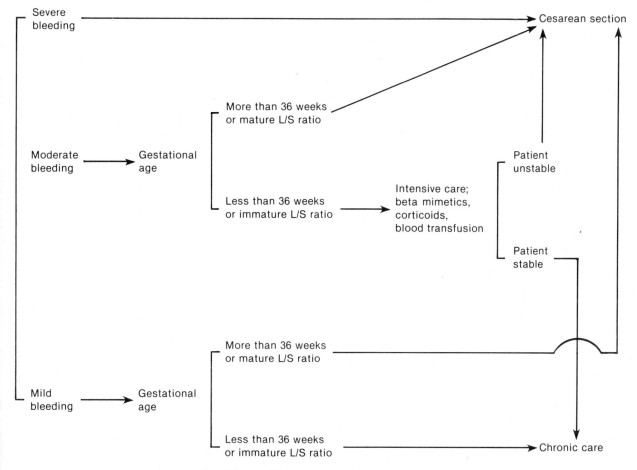

FIGURE 9-2 ◪ Management of placenta previa.

observation was further extended by von Frie-sen.[21,22] The rationale behind this temporizing approach is that a cervical cerclage limits the de-velopment of the low uterine segment brought about by advancing gestation and the effect of uterine contractions. This, in turn, avoids the partial detachment of the placenta from the low uterine segment that most likely is the cause of bleeding in these patients.

We have used a cervical cerclage as a tempo-rary measure in those patients with placenta pre-via who start bleeding early in pregnancy and who have significant probabilities of requiring early delivery. Results have been excellent: pa-tients undergoing cerclage have reached more advanced gestational ages and larger birth weights and have had fewer neonatal complica-tions than patients treated with expectant man-agement alone.[23]

A distinct advantage of the cervical cerclage treatment is that patients may go home after the operation and thus avoid extended, expensive hospitalizations. We use a simple McDonald pro-cedure with a single purse-string suture of 0 prolene. Antibiotic prophylaxis is used and toco-lysis is maintained before, during, and after the procedure.

When to deliver. Controversy exists concern-ing the advantages and disadvantages of deliver-ing fetuses at less than 36 weeks in those pa-tients with fetal lung maturation demonstrated by amniocentesis. The question is whether or not the non-RDS-related neonatal complications are frequent and severe enough at less than 36 weeks to warrant continuation of the pregnancy despite the risk of maternal bleeding. No clear answers are available at this time. Delivery be-fore 36 weeks of gestation should be mainly for maternal reasons. After reaching this gestational age, the pregnancy should be terminated if the fetal lungs are mature, even if there are no maternal complications. Therefore in pregnancies remote from term, give an initial course of glucocorticoids at the time the patient is admitted to the hospital, prescribe nifedipine and bed rest, and continue to give glucocorticoids weekly as long as the patient remains undelivered. If there is no maternal indication for delivery, weekly amniocentesis for L/S ratio is initiated at 36 weeks, and the patient is delivered when lung maturity is documented.

Following is a summary of the main points in the expectant management of patients with placenta previa:

1. Selection criteria:
   Only patients in stable conditions and remote from term should be managed expectantly. Patients actively bleeding or with unstable vital signs should remain in Labor and Delivery and should be monitored frequently.
2. Duration of hospitalization:
   The patient should stay in the hospital for the duration of her pregnancy unless she undergoes cervical cerclage or meets the criteria shown in Box 9-2.
3. Medications:
   a. Nifedipine, 10 to 20 mg orally every 4 to 6 hours.
   b. Betamethasone, 12 mg IM every 24 hours, for two doses. Repeat treatment every week as long as the patient remains undelivered or until mature L/S ratio is obtained.
   c. FeSO$_4$, 325 mg orally 3 times daily.
   d. Stool softeners, high residue diet.
4. Laboratory tests:
   Test blood count weekly. Maintain hemoglobin level above 11 g/dl using blood transfusion if necessary.
5. Criteria for delivery:
   a. Before 36 weeks indications for delivery are mostly maternal, especially continuous or recurrent bleeding.
   b. After 36 weeks, if there is no maternal indication for delivery, terminate pregnancy as soon as a mature L/S ratio is obtained.

A flow chart for the management of patients with placenta previa is shown in Figure 9-2.

◼ ABRUPTIO PLACENTAE
Definition and incidence

Abruptio placentae is the separation of the placenta from its implantation site before the birth of the fetus. The initial event in abruption is bleeding into the decidua basalis. The hematoma formed separates the placenta from the maternal vascular system, causing an impairment in fetal oxygenation and nutrition.

Abruptio placentae occurs in approximately 1% of all deliveries. Knab[24] reviewed a large number of articles on this subject and found a range of 0.52% to 1.29%. This wide range probably reflects true differences in the incidence of abruptio between disparate socioeconomic groups. The incidence of abruptio placentae increases with gestational age, and more than 90% of the fetuses involved weighed more than 1500 g at birth.

The majority of serious maternal complications in abruptio placentae are the consequence of hypovolemia. The most common consequence of hypovolemia is acute renal failure, a topic that is extensively discussed in Chapter 14. Coagulopathy can aggravate hemorrhagic problems, but this complication resolves quickly after delivery of the placenta and becomes significant only if operative treatment is necessary. Postpartum uterine atony and Couvelaire uterus can occur with abruptio placentae. Amniotic fluid embolization, having increasing frequency with abruption, is a catastrophic complication that cannot be anticipated. Also, it is important to remember that the Rh-negative mother with abruptio placentae may have had massive fetomaternal transfusion requiring a larger than usual Rh$_o$(D) immunoglobulin (RhoGAM) dosage to avoid isoimmunization.

With respect to the fetus, the majority of complications result from prematurity and hypoxia. Hypovolemic shock of the newborn is rare but may be associated with any maternal antepartum hemorrhage. A fetal and neonatal coagulopathy has been suggested in connection with abruption but is very infrequent.

Etiology

External trauma, cocaine abuse, acute decompression of polyhydramnios, and preterm rupture of the fetal membranes are known to cause abruptio placentae. More controversial is the role of chronic or acute hypertension during pregnancy in the origin of this obstetric problem. Pritchard et al.[25] found that 45% of their patients with abruption severe enough to kill the fetus had elevated blood pressure. This association between hypertension and abruptio was confirmed by Abdella et al.[26] However, both of these studies were performed in patients with severe abruptio, and it seems that the association between hypertension and abruptio is not strong in patients with lesser degrees of placental separation.

Naeye[27] found a strong association between abruption and poor weight gain during pregnancy. He also demonstrated that maternal smoking is a significant factor contributing to the development of placental infarcts and abruption. He found increased frequency of thrombosed arteries and necrosis of the decidua basalis, supporting the possibility that a vascular factor is the underlying cause.

Several studies have shown an association between high parity and abruption, but its strongest association is with a previous history of the problem. The risk of recurrence is approximately 17% for patients with one abruption and as high as 25% for patients who have had more than one episode.[28] Advanced maternal age, short umbilical cord, uterine anomalies, inferior vena cava occlusion, and dietary folate deficiency do not appear to be significant etiologic factors.

Clinical presentation

The predominant sign of placental abruption is vaginal bleeding, present in 78% of the patients. Uterine tenderness and back pain are present in 66% of the patients. Uterine hypertonicity and frequent contractions are exhibited by approximately 17% of the patients. Fetal demise occurs before admission to the hospital in 25% to 35% of the patients. The classic clinical presentation involving all of these signs—vaginal bleeding, uterine tenderness, hypertonic uterus, fetal demise—does not occur frequently. The majority of patients with abruptio have at least one of these signs, but occasionally none of them will be present. Indeed, no vaginal bleeding will be observed in 25% to 35% of patients. These patients with concealed bleeding usually exhibit severe forms of the disease. DIC is a complication in approximately 13% of patients with abruptio, and it is usually limited to patients with severe separation and fetal demise.

The natural history of abruptio placentae is controversial. Some investigators believe that the magnitude of the placental separation is determined at its onset and no further enlargement occurs. Others believe that abruptio causes progressive placental separation. There is no way to measure the dimensions of the initial separation and the frequency and severity of further separations if they occur.

Examination with ultrasound rarely helps in the diagnosis of placental abruptio. However, ultrasound is useful for assessing fetal presentation, fetal size, and fetal well-being.

Classification

Sher,[29] in a review of clinical material from the Groote Schur Hospital in Cape Town, South Africa, proposed the following clinical grading system for placental abruption:

Grade I corresponds to those cases in which the diagnosis of abruptio placentae is made retrospectively. Most of these patients had a retroplacental clot volume of approximately 150 ml, and none were more than 500 ml. With this small degree of abruption, fetuses are usually not at risk, and a favorable perinatal outcome is usually achieved.

Grade II corresponds to those cases in which antepartum hemorrhage is accompanied by the classic features of abruptio placentae and the fetus is alive. The retroplacental clot volume in these patients is usually 150 to 500 ml, with approximately 27% of them having a clot larger than 500 ml. Of patients in this category, 92% have abnormal fetal heart patterns, and perinatal mortality is high, especially if patients are delivered vaginally. It appears that the presence of a palpable rigid uterus represents a significant high-risk situation for the fetus.

Grade III incorporates the features of grade II, but fetal demise is confirmed. It is further subdivided based on (1) the presence or (2) the absence of coagulopathy. Virtually all maternal mortalities in association with abruptio placentae occur in grade III patients. Meticulous attention to the cardiovascular and renal status of these patients is necessary to ensure a good maternal outcome.

Management of severe abruption causing fetal demise

The question of fetal viability in abruptio placentae is particularly important because it provides an index for evaluating the severity of the disease, the size of the retroplacental clot, and the probability of coagulopathy. With fetal demise, the placental detachment is usually greater than 50%, and approximately 30% of the patients will show evidence of coagulopathy. Therefore any case of abruptio with fetal death should be classified as severe.

The management of such patients, obviously, should focus on decreasing maternal morbidity and mortality. To achieve this objective, delivery is necessary. However, it is necessary to evaluate the mother carefully before delivery to obtain information useful for the successful management of this obstetric catastrophe.

Evaluation and replacement of blood loss. Pritchard[30] has demonstrated that if abruptio placentae is severe enough to kill the fetus, the average intrapartum blood loss, mostly retroplacental, is about 2500 ml. Therefore all patients with severe abruptio placentae have had significant blood loss and require aggressive measures to avoid progressive impairment in organ perfusion. Immediate transfusion of at least 2 U of packed red cells should be instituted regardless of the initial vital signs. Transfusion should not be withheld because the patient exhibits a normal blood pressure, because if the patient was previously hypertensive, she may be close to shock. The pulse in these patients may also be normal until appropriate hydration produces a tachycardia. In patients with concealed hemorrhage, a vast underestimation of blood loss frequently occurs, and when the vital signs deteriorate, hypovolemia is so severe that adequate replacement is difficult. Caution should also be used in the interpretation of hemoglobin and hematocrit values in patients with severe abruption. Very frequently blood counts are within the normal range as a consequence of intense reactive vasoconstriction. Therefore the patient with abruptio placentae severe enough to cause fetal demise should be transfused despite normal hematocrit/hemoglobin values or normal vital signs.

Packed red cells will improve the patient's oxygen-carrying capacity. The intravascular volume should be expanded simultaneously using normal saline or lactated Ringer's solution. After transfusion of every fourth unit of packed red cells, the clotting mechanism should be evaluated, particularly the platelet count, since hemodilution can create a coagulopathy itself. It is recommended that 1 U of fresh frozen plasma be administered after every 4 U of packed red cells. Platelets should be given to the bleeding patient when the count is less than 40,000. It may take up to 60 minutes to prepare blood components

for use; therefore the blood bank should be notified of the clinical condition of the patient and the probability that blood components will be required.

The guidelines for the administration of red blood cells and intravenous fluids have been established by Pritchard. To maintain adequate organ perfusion in the patient with severe abruptio placentae, it is necessary to keep a hematocrit of at least 30% and a urinary output of at least 30 ml/hr. These two criteria are of fundamental importance. By keeping the hematocrit at 30% or more, the patient's oxygen-carrying capacity is sustained. By maintaining the urinary output at 30 ml/hr or more, one can be relatively confident that the effective intravascular volume is being preserved and that acute tubular necrosis or bilateral cortical necrosis, the most common causes of death for patients with abruptio placentae, will be avoided.

Internal jugular vein catheterization. In cases of severe abruption, one should anticipate the need for large amounts of intravenous fluids, and a central venous pressure catheter should be inserted to monitor their administration.

Management of coagulopathy. According to Pritchard and Brekken,[31] 38% of patients with severe abruptio placentae have plasma fibrinogen concentrations below 150 mg/dl, and in 28% of patients the fibrinogen level is less than 100 mg/dl as a result of acute DIC. Simultaneous with the drop in fibrinogen, patients with DIC may also show prolonged partial thromboplastin time (PTT) and prothrombin time (PT), increased D-dimer concentration, and low platelet count.

DIC has many causes, including sepsis, giant hemangiomas, and malignancies. The syndrome occurs rather frequently in obstetric conditions such as abruptio placentae, amniotic fluid embolization, and prolonged fetal death in utero. In the case of abruption, DIC seems to result from a massive release of thromboplastin into the circulation, causing intravascular formation of fibrin, consumption of coagulation factors, and subsequent activation of the fibrinolytic system.

For evaluation of the hemostatic system in patients with abruptio placentae, most laboratories use a DIC profile. This is a battery of laboratory tests, including PT, PTT, D-dimer, quantitative fibrinogen determination, and platelet count. Normal values for the DIC profile are shown in Box 9-3.

In the past the test for the evaluation of he-

BOX 9-3

Normal Values for DIC Profile

Test	Normal results
Fibrinogen	150 to 600 mg/dl
PT	11 to 16 seconds
PTT	22 to 37 seconds
Platelet count	120,000 to 350,000/mm^3
D-dimer	<0.5 mg/L
FDP	<10 µg/dl

---

mostasis in patients with abruptio placentae was the direct observation of clot retraction and lysis. Clot retraction depends on adequate functioning of intact platelets and the presence of divalent cations. The degree of retraction does not correlate well with the platelet count, and the test may give normal results with platelet counts as low as 20,000/mm^3. The clot lysis test is a gross way of observing the fibrinolytic system. The increased amount of plasmin in patients with DIC should result in dissolution of a clot, whereas a normal clot should remain intact for at least 48 hours. If the clot dissolves within 24 hours, fibrinolysis is increased. If fibrinolysis is very active, the clot may be dissolved within 1 hour. This test can be misleading, since clot lysis must be differentiated from clot retraction, and fragmentation of a friable clot may be mistaken for lysis.

The DIC profile is useful for evaluating and following the patient's coagulopathy, but abnormal results are not necessarily an indication for therapy. In fact, without clinical evidence of excessive bleeding, no therapy is warranted. Vaginal delivery can be managed in the presence of extremely low clotting components if episiotomy and unusual trauma are avoided. However, to minimize excessive blood loss at the time of delivery, it is safer to replace critically depleted coagulation factors, particularly platelets and fibrinogen.

Postpartum the coagulopathy will resolve within hours with appropriate blood replacement and preservation of the intravascular volume. However, the uterus is occasionally a source of excessive bleeding. Sher[32] has proposed that high levels of fibrin degradation products (FDP) inhibit myometrial contractility. Fortunately, there are extremely effective measures to combat postpartum uterine atony.

The use of heparin for the treatment of DIC complicating abruption should be strongly condemned. DIC in the patient with abruption originates in the premature separation of the placenta, and its treatment is delivery of the fetus and the placenta. The use of heparin in these patients often causes additional blood loss and increases the need for further transfusions. Another unfounded caveat is that the presence of DIC in a patient with abruptio placentae is an indication for immediate cesarean section. In reality, in the presence of a generalized hemostatic defect, any type of operative intervention should be avoided if at all possible.

Evaluation of fetal presentation and size. The basic obstetric assessment of fetal position and size is frequently forgotten when dealing with this extreme emergency. Because of the rigidity of the uterine wall and the presence of a closed, uneffaced cervix, it is often difficult to clinically evaluate the fetal presentation and size. Therefore a sonogram should be obtained in every case of abruptio placentae in which there is the slightest doubt about the fetal presentation. If a malpresentation is detected, pregnancy should be terminated by cesarean section, with the exception of infants less than 800 g, which may be delivered vaginally even if in a transverse lie. A failure to properly evaluate the fetal presentation may result in uterine rupture after oxytocin stimulation. External version should not be attempted in patients with abruptio and rigid uterus.

Delivery. Unless there is a malpresentation, every effort should be made to deliver the patient with a fetal death vaginally. Amniotomy should be carried out as soon as possible, followed by the insertion of an intrauterine pressure catheter. Oxytocin infusion should be used regardless of maternal age and parity unless there is clear evidence of active spontaneous labor. The rigidity of the uterus or the presence of a high intrauterine resting pressure should not deter the use of oxytocin. In patients with fetal death and unripe cervix, prostaglandin E$_2$ vaginal gel or chips containing 2.5 to 5.0 mg or high-dose oxytocin, 50 to 100 mU/min, may be used.

The clinical pattern and the monitoring characteristics of spontaneous or induced labor in patients with severe abruptio placentae are different from those observed in normal pregnancies at term. In these patients the uterus remains rigid at all times, and there is constant pain superimposed on the cyclic and intermittent pain of labor. The resting pressure measured with an intrauterine pressure catheter is very high, usually around 40 mm Hg, and contractions are seen as small waves on top of the resting pressure recording. Despite the meager clinical and monitoring signs of cyclic uterine activity, the cervix starts to change, and after complete effacement, dilation is usually rapid.

Pritchard[30] has demonstrated that there is no time limit for obtaining a vaginal delivery in patients with abruptio placentae and fetal death. In the past there was a dictum that these patients should be delivered in 4 to 6 hours. Today we know that with appropriate maintenance of the maternal status, the time for obtaining vaginal delivery may be extended safely up to 24 hours. If there is an abnormal fetal presentation or if cephalopelvic disproportion is suspected, the patient should be delivered by cesarean section.

Patients with fibrinogen concentrations of less than 100 mg/dl will benefit from the administration of 10 to 20 U of cryoprecipitate immediately before and during cesarean delivery. This amount of cryoprecipitate contains enough fibrinogen to secure adequate hemostasis during surgery and to prevent additional blood loss. Platelet transfusions are indicated in a bleeding patient with a count below 40,000/mm and in patients with a count of 20,000, even if abnormal bleeding is absent.

Following is a summary of measures to be taken in the initial management of the patient with abruptio placentae causing fetal demise:

1. Initiate transfusion of packed red cells regardless of the initial vital signs and the initial hemoglobin concentration and hematocrit.
2. Give enough blood and crystalloid solutions to maintain a hematocrit of at least 30% and a urinary output of at least 30 ml/hr.
3. Obtain a sonogram to confirm fetal death and assess fetal presentation. If there is no fetal malpresentation, start an intravenous infusion of oxytocin. Remember that high doses of oxytocin may be required, that monitoring of uterine activity is unreliable, and that the best index of progress in labor is cervical change.
4. Obtain a DIC profile. Patients with consumption coagulopathy most likely will re-

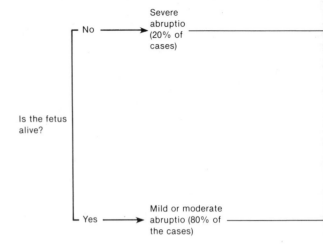

FIGURE 9-3 Management of abruptio placentae.

quire administration of fresh frozen plasma or cryoprecipitate if cesarean section or episiotomy is carried out.

Some caveats in the management of pregnancy complicated by abruption and DIC are:

1. Do not give heparin. There is no place for heparin in the management of obstetric bleeding. Heparin use in abruptio placentae is dangerous and contraindicated.
2. Do not perform a cesarean section unless there is a clear indication for the procedure. Remember that DIC by itself **is not** an indication for cesarean section, but rather a strong contraindication. Surgical procedures should be avoided if at all possible in the presence of existing or impending generalized hemostatic defect.
3. The presence of a long, hard cervix **is not** an indication for cesarean section. In most patients the cervix will efface and dilate rapidly after oxytocin induction or vaginal prostaglandin administration.

Management of abruptio placentae with a live fetus

The complexity of the management of a patient with abruptio placentae increases if the fe-

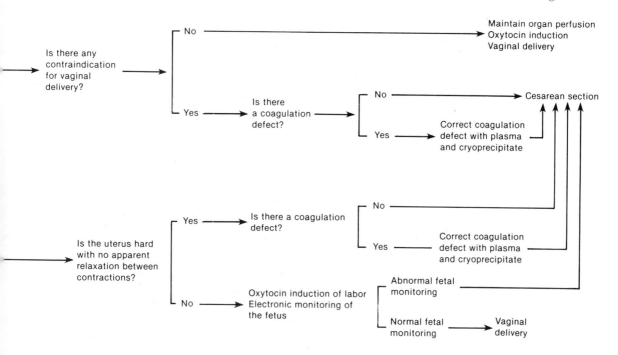

tus is alive when the patient is admitted. Both the mother and the fetus are at risk for loss of life. There are two main subgroups of patients: those with palpably hypertonic uteri and those with palpably soft uteri.

If the infant is alive and the uterus is rigid, the abruption is probably large but under 50%, and the chances of fetal distress are more than 90%. In this case the patient should be prepared for an immediate cesarean section unless there are very special circumstances that preclude surgical intervention (e.g., maternal shock, previable fetus). The preparations for cesarean section should include evaluation of the patient's hemostatic profile and preparation for transfusion. Overt coagulopathy with abruption not associated with fetal demise is extremely rare. However, coagulopathy and bleeding may develop during or immediately after the surgical intervention.

If the uterus is soft and the clinical history strongly suggests abruptio placentae, the pregnancy should be terminated by induction of labor. If an abruption is present, it probably will not be greater than 25%, the chances of significant coagulopathy are extremely low, and the prospects for a vaginal delivery with a favorable outcome is excellent. If the uterus becomes hypertonic during labor or if fetal distress appears,

it must be assumed that abruption has extended and cesarean section should be done. In the absence of uterine rigidity, fetal distress, or obstetric contraindication for vaginal delivery, the large majority of patients should have uneventful courses.

Figure 9-3 summarizes the overall plan of management for patients with abruptio placentae.

Prognosis

Patients who have abruptio placentae have a higher incidence of complications in future pregnancies. Approximately 14% of future pregnancies will end in spontaneous abortion, and 9.3% of the patients will have repeated abruption. It has also been suggested that the risk of repetition after two consecutive pregnancies with abruptio placentae is 25%.

Delivery before term has been recommended for patients with prior abruptio because of the significant risk of recurrence and because a repeat abruption may be more severe. However, there are no data to substantiate this recommendation. Most likely, corrections of factors such as poor nutrition, low weight gain, and smoking would have a far greater effect on reducing the incidence of recurrence than would early delivery with its potential for fetal morbidity.

◪ OTHER CAUSES OF THIRD-TRIMESTER BLEEDING

After excluding placenta previa and abruptio placentae from the differential diagnosis of third-trimester bleeding, the tendency is to ascribe the problem to marginal placental separation or marginal sinus bleeding. However, this group of patients with third-trimester bleeding of unknown origin has a higher than normal incidence of preterm labor (17%) and perinatal mortality (14.2%). Although these risks are less than those associated with abruptio and previa, caution and appropriate monitoring of these patients should be exercised.

Other causes of antepartum bleeding are as follows:

Cervicitis
Cervical erosions
Endocervical polyps
Cancer of the cervix
Vaginal, vulvar, and cervical varicosities
Vaginal infections
Foreign bodies
Genital lacerations
Bloody show
Degenerating uterine myomata
Vasa previa
Marginal placental separation

This list confirms that at one point in the management of third-trimester bleeding there is a need for a direct cervical examination with a speculum. Except for vasa previa and marginal placental separation, these complications usually pose a minimal risk to the fetus.

Vasa previa

Vasa previa is an anomaly in which the umbilical vessels have a velamentous insertion on a low-lying placenta and traverse the membranes in the lower uterine segment in front of the fetal presenting part. The vessels may be lacerated at the time of membrane rupture causing fetal exsanguination. Because of the absence of the protective Wharton's gelatin, the vessels may bleed before rupture of the membranes occurs. Fetal hypoxia and death may be caused when the vessels are compressed by the fetal presenting part, particularly during uterine contractions. With all these possibilities, it is not surprising that fetal mortality in vasa previa approaches 75% to 100%. There is little, if any, increase in maternal complications. Fortunately, vasa previa is a rare condition (1 of 2000 to 3000 deliveries).

The diagnosis of vasa previa should be considered in all cases of third-trimester bleeding associated with a fetal tracing suggestive of distress or cord compression.[33] In these cases vaginal blood should be examined for fetal hemoglobin as previously described in the discusssion of placenta previa (p. 165). Emergency delivery should be effected if there is evidence of fetal bleeding. Since vasa previa occurs more frequently in patients with twins, careful fetal monitoring is necessary in these situations.

Marginal placental separation

Most patients with third-trimester vaginal bleeding, negative findings on speculum examination, and no evidence of placenta previa or abruption receive the diagnosis of marginal placental separation or marginal sinus bleeding. In some cases placental examination postpartum shows old clots attached to the border, but in the majority no explanation is found for the antepartum bleeding.

Little is known about the natural history of marginal sinus separation. Usually bleeding stops after a few days, and the pregnancy proceeds uneventfully until term. Other patients have repetitive episodes of mild bleeding. A minority of patients continue to bleed and become anemic, requiring preterm delivery. Preterm labor, preterm rupture of membranes, and chorioamnionitis occur frequently in patients who bleed chronically.

The diagnosis of marginal placental separation can rarely be confirmed before birth by ultrasound visualization of retromembranous dissection or retroplacental clot. The majority of patients with marginal placental separation have normal ultrasound findings.

The management of these patients is expectant. However, the obstetrician should be aware of the possibility of complications and should follow these patients at frequent intervals. There are suggestions in the literature that administration of tocolytic agents to these patients prolongs gestation without increasing the frequency of abnormal outcomes.[34]

◪   IMPORTANT POINTS   ◫

1. Classification of a placenta previa as total, partial, or low-lying has little value for patient management. This classification, however, has prognostic value because the frequency and severity of complications are greatest with total placenta previa.

2. The incidence of placenta previa is 4 times greater in patients with prior cesarean than in patients without uterine scars. Placenta accreta occurs more frequently when implantation occurs on the uterine scar.

3. The incidence of preterm delivery, the number of bleeding episodes, the severity of bleeding, and the number of units of blood transfused are significantly greater for patients with previa that initially have bleeding before 28 weeks.

4. There is no justification for vaginal digital examination in patients with painless vaginal bleeding in the third trimester.

5. An accurate diagnosis of placenta previa often requires examination with endovaginal ultrasound.

6. Before 24 weeks only a cautionary significance should be given to the finding of placenta previa in routine ultrasound examination of asymptomatic patients. In 97% of these patients the placenta has moved away from the cervix by term.

7. Pregnant patients that have acutely lost between 15% and 30% of their blood volume in the third trimester exhibit orthostatic changes in pulse rate and diastolic blood pressure.

8. The probability of acquiring infection with transfusion therapy is small. The risk of acquiring hepatitis C is 1% and will decrease when screening for this virus is available. The risk of infection with HIV is 1 in 400,000 to 1 in 1,000,000.

9. Autologous blood donation for routine vaginal delivery or elective cesarean section should be discouraged, since the likelihood of requiring transfusion during these procedures is low.

10. Typing and screening should be the first test ordered in anticipation of blood transfusion. It allows a more efficient use of resources and a more rapid response of the blood bank than does the type and crossmatch procedure.

11. Patients with placenta previa selected for expectant management should be hemodynamically stable, less than 32 weeks, or between 32 and 36 weeks with proven fetal pulmonary immaturity.

12. Cervical cerclage may be used as a temporary measure for patients with placenta previa that start bleeding early in gestation and have significant potential for premature delivery.

13. In patients with previa, delivery before 36 weeks is mainly for maternal reasons. After 36 weeks the pregnancy should be terminated when a mature L/S ratio is obtained.

14. Examination with ultrasound rarely helps in the diagnosis of abruptio placenta.

15. If an abruption is severe enough to cause fetal demise, the average blood loss, mostly retroplacental, is 2500 ml. For this reason transfusion of packed red cells should be instituted in these patients shortly after admission, regardless of their initial vital signs.

16. To maintain adequate organ perfusion in a patient with severe abruption, it is necessary to keep a hematocrit of at least 30% and a urinary output of at least 30 ml/hr.

17. With appropriate maintenance of the maternal status, vaginal delivery in patients with abruptio placentae and fetal death may be safely delayed up to 24 hours.

18. Patients with abruptio placenta, a live fetus, and soft uterus likely have a separation of less than 25%, and the probability of vaginal delivery is excellent.

19. There are no data to substantiate early delivery as appropriate for patients with a history of abruptio.

REFERENCES

1. Brenner WE, Edelman DA, Hendricks CH: Characteristics of patients with placenta previa and results of expectant management. *Am J Obstet Gynecol* 1978;132:180-189.
2. Crenshaw C, Jones DED, Parker RT: Placenta previa: A survey of twenty years experience with improved perinatal survival by expectant therapy and cesarean delivery. *Obstet Gynecol Surv* 1973;28:461-470.
3. Rose GL, Chapman MG: Aetiological factors in placenta praevia—A case-controlled study. *Br J Obstet Gynaecol* 1986;93:586-588.
4. Nielsen TF, Hagberg H, Ljungblad U: Placenta previa and antepartum hemorrhage after previous cesarean section. *Gynecol Obstet Invest* 1989;27:88-90.
5. Clark SL, Koonings PP, Phelan JP: Placenta previa/accreta and prior cesarean section. *Obstet Gynecol* 1985;66:89-92.
6. McShane PM, Heyl PS, and Epstein MF: Maternal and perinatal morbidity resulting from placenta previa. *Obstet Gynecol* 1985;65:176-182.

7. Hibbard LT: Placenta previa. *Am J Obstet Gynecol* 1969;104:172-182.

8. Bowie JD, Rochester D, Cadkin AV, et al: Accuracy of placental localization by ultrasound. *Radiology* 1978;128:177-180.

9. Farine D, Fox HE, Jakobson S, et al: Vaginal ultrasound for diagnosis of placenta previa. *Am J Obstet Gynecol* 1988;159:566-569.

10. Leerentveld RA, Gilberts ECAM, Arnold MJCWJ, et al: Accuracy and safety of transvaginal sonographic placental localization. *Obstet Gynecol* 1990;76:759-762.

11. Kurjak A, Barsic B: Changes of placental site diagnosed by repeated ultrasound examination. *Acta Obstet Gynecol Scand* 1977;56:161-165.

12. Loendersloot EW: Vasa previa. *Am J Obstet Gynecol* 1979;135:702-703.

13. McVay PA, Hoag RW, Hoag MS, et al: Safety and use of autologous blood donation during the third trimester of pregnancy. *Am J Obstet Gynecol* 1989;160:1479-1488.

14. Kamani AA, McMorland GH, Wadsworth LD: Utilization of red blood cell transfusion in an obstetric setting. *Am J Obstet Gynecol* 1988;159:1177-1181.

15. Andres RL, Piacquadio KM, Resnik R: A reappraisal of the need for autologous blood donation in the obstetric patient. *Am J Obstet Gynecol* 1990;163:1551-1553.

16. Silver R, Depp R, Sabbagha RE, et al: Placenta previa: Aggressive expectant management. *Am J Obstet Gynecol* 1984;150:15-22.

17. D'Angelo LJ, Irwin LF: Conservative management of placenta previa: A cost-benefit analysis. *Am J Obstet Gynecol* 1984;149:320-323.

18. Tomich PG: Prolonged use of tocolytic agents in the expectant management of placenta previa. *J Reprod Med* 1985;30:745-748.

19. Liggins GC, Howie RN: A controlled trial of antepartum glucocorticoid treatment for prevention of the respiratory distress syndrome in premature infants. *Pediatrics* 1972;50:515-525.

20. Lovset J: Preventive treatment of severe bleeding in placenta previa. *Acta Obstet Gynaecol Scand* 1959;38:551-554.

21. von Friesen B: Encircling suture of the cervix in placenta previa. *Acta Obstet Gynaecol Scand* 1964;43:122-128.

22. von Friesen B: Encircling suture of the cervix in placenta previa: Ten years' experience. *Acta Obstet Gynaecol Scand* 1972;51:183-186.

23. Arias F: Cervical cerclage for the temporary treatment of patients with placenta previa. *Obstet Gynecol* 1988;71:545-548.

24. Knab DR: Abruptio placentae: An assessment of the time and method of delivery. *Obstet Gynecol* 1978;52:625-629.

25. Pritchard JA, Mason R, Corley M, et al: Genesis of severe placental abruption. *Am J Obstet Gynecol* 1970;108:22-27.

26. Abdella TN, Sibai BM, Hays JM, et al: Relationship of hypertensive disease to abruptio placentae. *Obstet Gynecol* 1984;63:365-370.

27. Naeye RL: Placental infarction leading to fetal or neonatal death: A prospective study. *Obstet Gynecol* 1977;50:583-588.

28. Hibbard BM, Jeffcoate TNA: Abruptio placentae. *Obstet Gynecol* 1966;27:155-167.

29. Sher G: A rational basis for the management of abruptio placentae. *J Reprod Med* 1978;21:123-129.

30. Pritchard JA: Haematological problems associated with delivery, placental abruption, retained dead fetus, and amniotic fluid embolism. *Clin Haematol* 1973;2:563-586.

31. Pritchard JA, Brekken AL: Clinical and laboratory studies on severe abruptio placentae. *Am J Obstet Gynecol* 1967;97:681-695.

32. Sher G: Pathogenesis and management of uterine inertia complicating abruptio placentae with consumption coagulopathy. *Am J Obstet Gynecol* 1977;129:164-170.

33. Dougall A, Baird CH: Vasa praevia—Report of three cases and review of literature. *Br J Obstet Gynaecol* 1987;94:712-715.

34. Sholl JS: Abruptio placentae: Clinical management in nonacute cases. *Am J Obstet Gynecol* 1987;156:40-51.

10

PREECLAMPSIA AND ECLAMPSIA

Compared with normotensive gravidas, patients with elevated blood pressure have significantly greater maternal and fetal mortality and morbidity.[1] Although maternal hypertension is diagnosed in approximately only 7% of all deliveries, 1.5% in private hospitals and up to 15% in university hospitals, it is associated with as much as 22% of all perinatal deaths and 30% of all maternal deaths in the United States.

Pregnancy may induce hypertension in women who are normotensive before pregnancy and may aggravate hypertension in those that are hypertensive before pregnancy. The clinical and laboratory characteristics of hypertension associated with pregnancy are difficult to differentiate from those of hypertension independent of pregnancy. As a consequence, severe pregnancy-induced or pregnancy-aggravated hypertension is frequently confused with other disease processes such as thrombotic thrombocytopenic purpura (TTP), acute glomerulonephritis, and chronic essential hypertension occurring during pregnancy. As a result, a dangerous delay in appropriate treatment may occur. Also, diseases causing hypertension, such as brain tumors, pheochromocytoma, systemic lupus erythematosus, and renovascular hypertension, may not be diagnosed during pregnancy because their symptoms are similar to those of pregnancy-induced or pregnancy-aggravated hypertension.

◼ DEFINITIONS
American College of Obstetricians and Gynecologists (ACOG)

According to the ACOG, the diagnosis of hypertension in pregnancy is made by any one of the following criteria:

1. A rise of 30 mm Hg or more in systolic blood pressure
2. A rise of 15 mm Hg or more in diastolic blood pressure
3. A systolic blood pressure of 140 mm Hg or more
4. A diastolic blood pressure of 90 mm Hg or more

These alterations in blood pressure should be observed on at least two different occasions at least 6 hours apart.

Hypertension in pregnancy is classified into the following groups:

1. Pregnancy-induced hypertension
   a. Preeclampsia
   b. Eclampsia

2. Chronic hypertension of whatever cause, but independent of pregnancy
3. Preeclampsia or eclampsia superimposed on chronic hypertension
4. Transient hypertension
5. Unclassified hypertensive disorders

Each of these forms of hypertension are defined by ACOG as follows:

preeclampsia   Hypertension associated with proteinuria, greater than 0.3 g/L in a 24-hour urine collection or greater than 1 g/L in a random sample; generalized edema, greater than 1^+ pitting edema after 12 hours of rest in bed or a weight gain of 5 lb or more in 1 week; or both after 20 weeks of gestation.

eclampsia   Convulsions occurring in a patient with preeclampsia.

chronic hypertension   The presence of sustained blood pressures of 140/90 mm Hg or higher before pregnancy or before 20 weeks.

preeclampsia or eclampsia superimposed on chronic hypertension   The occurrence of preeclampsia or eclampsia in women with chronic hypertension. To make this diagnosis it is necessary to document a rise of 30 mm Hg or more in diastolic blood pressure, associated with proteinuria, generalized edema, or both.

transient hypertension   The development of hypertension during pregnancy or the early puerperium in a previously normotensive woman whose pressure normalizes within 10 days postpartum. There must be no evidence of preeclampsia.

unclassified hypertensive disorders   Those in whom there is not enough information for classification.

Most authors recognize that preeclampsia may be mild or severe, but some also describe a *moderate* subgroup. We accept three degrees of severity according to the criteria shown in Table 10-1. The most important criterion for differentiation is the magnitude of the blood pressure elevation.

International Society for the Study of Hypertension in Pregnancy (ISSHP)

The diagnosis of hypertension in pregnancy, according to ISSHP, is made by either of the following criteria:

1. One measurement of diastolic blood pressure equal to or greater than 110 mm Hg
2. Two consecutive measurements of diastolic blood pressure equal to or greater than 90 mm Hg, 4 or more hours apart

These criteria[2] do not have the deficiencies of those proposed by the Committee on Terminology of ACOG that uses rises in systolic and diastolic pressures, as well as absolute levels in both pressures, as diagnostic criteria. The ACOG definition is imprecise because of the natural tendency of blood pressure to rise during the third trimester and the variability of systolic pressure values during normal pregnancy.

TABLE 10-1 ◪ Severity classification of preeclampsia-eclampsia

Variable	Mild	Moderate	Severe
Diastolic blood pressure	90-100 mm Hg	100-110 mm Hg	> 110 mm Hg
Convulsions	Absent	Absent	Present
Blindness	Absent	Absent	Present
Headaches	Minimal	Mild	Marked, persistent
Visual symptoms	Minimal	Mild	Marked, persistent
Oliguria	Absent	Absent	Present
Upper abdominal pain	Absent	Absent	Present
Fetal distress	Absent	Absent	Present
Fetal growth retardation	Absent	Absent	Present
Intravascular hemolysis	Absent	Absent	Present
Thrombocytopenia	Absent	Absent	Present
Blood urea nitrogen (BUN), creatinine, uric acid levels	Normal	Mildly elevated	Markedly elevated
Serum glutamic-oxaloacetic transaminase (SGOT), serum glutamic-pyruvic transaminase (SGPT), lactate dehydrogenase (LDH)	Normal	Mildly elevated	Markedly elevated

According to the ISSHP, Korotkoff's IV sound, the point at which the sound becomes muffled, should be used when measuring the diastolic blood pressure. The ISSHP recommends obtaining blood pressure measurements with the patient in the lateral decubitus position with the cuff placed on her right arm at the level of the heart. In this position both systolic and diastolic pressures are usually lower than the actual values by 10 to 20 mm. For this reason, Sibai[3] believes that measurements should be taken with the woman sitting with the right arm in a roughly horizontal position at heart level, supported on a table or desk.

The ISSHP has proposed the following classification for hypertensive disorders in pregnancy:

gestational hypertension and/or proteinuria   Hypertension and/or proteinuria developing during pregnancy, labor, or the puerperium in a previously normotensive nonproteinuric woman. This group of patients is subdivided into:

1. Gestational hypertension (without proteinuria)
   a. Developing antenatally
   b. Developing for the first time in labor
   c. Developing for the first time in the puerperium
2. Gestational proteinuria (without hypertension)
   a. Developing antenatally
   b. Developing for the first time in labor
   c. Developing for the first time in the puerperium
3. Gestational proteinuric hypertension (preeclampsia)
   a. Developing antenatally
   b. Developing for the first time in labor
   c. Developing for the first time in the puerperium

chronic hypertension and chronic renal disease   Hypertension and/or proteinuria in pregnancy in a woman with chronic hypertension or chronic renal disease diagnosed before, during, or after pregnancy. This group is subdivided into:

1. Chronic hypertension (without proteinuria)
2. Chronic renal disease (proteinuria with or without hypertension)
3. Chronic hypertension with superimposed preeclampsia: proteinuria developing for first time during pregnancy in a woman with known chronic hypertension

unclassified hypertension and/or proteinuria   Hypertension and/or proteinuria found either (1) at first examination after twentieth week of pregnancy (140 days) in a woman with known chronic hypertension or chronic renal disease or (2) during pregnancy, labor, or the puerperium, in a case in which information is insufficient to permit classification. This category is subdivided into:

1. Unclassified hypertension (without proteinuria)
2. Unclassified proteinuria (without hypertension)
3. Unclassified proteinuria hypertension

According to this classification:

A. Hypertension and/or proteinuria at the first visit before the twentieth week of pregnancy, in the absence of trophoblastic disease, is presumed to be caused by either:
   1. Chronic hypertension (hypertension only)
   2. Chronic renal disease (proteinuria with or without hypertension)
B. Unclassified hypertension and/or proteinuria may be reclassified after delivery:
   1. If the hypertension and proteinuria disappear, into:
      a. Gestational hypertension (without proteinuria)
      b. Gestational proteinuria (without hypertension)
      c. Gestational proteinuric hypertension (preeclampsia)
   2. If the hypertension and/or proteinuria persists after delivery or other tests confirm the diagnosis, into:
      a. Chronic hypertension (without proteinuria)
      b. Chronic renal disease (proteinuria with or without hypertension)
      c. Chronic hypertension with superimposed preeclampsia
C. Gestational proteinuric hypertension is synonymous with *preeclampsia*, and gestational hypertension without proteinuria is the same as *pregnancy-induced hypertension* (PIH).

The definition of gestational proteinuria is more than 300 mg in a 24-hour urine sample. However, in practice proteinuria is detected by the use of reagent strips. A diluted (<1010 sp.gr.) or concentrated (>1030 sp.gr.) urine or an alkaline specimen (pH >8.0) may produce false results when tested with the reagent strips. Also, the frequency of false positives may be as high as 25% in trace reactions and as high as 6% when the result is 1+. If one considers a value of 2+ as the lower limit of significance, false-positive results will be eliminated.

The ISSHP does not consider degrees of severity for hypertension in pregnancy. However, it has been suggested that severe hypertension occurs when:

1. A diastolic blood pressure equal to or greater than 120 mm Hg is present on any one occasion
2. A diastolic blood pressure equal to or greater than 110 mm Hg is present on two or more consecutive occasions 4 hours apart

The ISSHP classification has not been universally accepted. Many consider that it is cumbersome and has little clinical value.

◪ PATHOGENESIS

The exact nature of the primary event causing preeclampsia is not known. However, evidence accumulated in the past 20 years indicates that abnormal placentation is one of the initial events in this disease. The main feature of abnormal placentation is inadequate trophoblastic invasion of the maternal spiral arterioles. In normal pregnancy the wall of the spiral arteries is invaded by trophoblastic cells and transformed into large, tortuous channels that carry a large amount of blood to the intervillous space and are resistant to the effects of vasomotor agents. These physiologic changes are restricted in patients with preeclampsia[4,5] with resulting decreased uteroplacental perfusion.[6] The anatomic and physiologic disruption of normal placentation is thought to lead to altered endothelial cell function[7,8] and multiple organ damage by a mechanism that is unknown at the present time.

The evidence indicating that endothelial cell dysfunction is responsible for the most significant biochemical changes and the wide spectrum of clinical presentations that characterize preeclampsia is increasing rapidly.[9-12] A search for the factor(s) released by the inadequately perfused trophoblast and responsible for endothelial cell damage and trials of medications potentially capable of modifying endothelial cell dysfunction probably will dominate the research in this subject in the next few years.

◪ PATHOPHYSIOLOGY

There are several important pathophysiologic changes in preeclampsia. They are discussed below.

Hyperdynamic circulation

Recent studies suggest that an increase in maternal cardiac output, rather than increased peripheral vascular resistance, is the most common hemodynamic feature of preeclampsia. The work of Easterling et al.[13] demonstrated that cardiac output values significantly higher than those found in normotensive gravidas are a common feature in preeclamptic patients. This elevation in cardiac output is already apparent at 11 weeks and remains in the puerperium despite resolution of the hypertension. These investigators also found that the systemic vascular resistance of preeclamptic patients was always less than that of normotensive patients and remained lower in the postpartum period. Clark et al.[14] found that normotensive primigravidas in the last trimester of pregnancy have peripheral vascular resistance in the range previously described for patients with severe preeclampsia (Box 10-1). However, these patients do not have the hyperdynamic cardiac activity consistently found in patients with preeclampsia.

The findings of hyperdynamic left ventricular function and decreased peripheral vascular resistance in preeclampsia may have important consequences in selecting the best approach to the treatment of severe hypertension in these patients. Beta-adrenergic blockers, rather than vasodilators, may be the drugs of choice. Also, these observations open the possibility of screening patients at risk for developing preeclampsia by measuring the cardiac output early in gestation.

Changes in intravascular volume

It is known that the increase in intravascular volume that normally occurs during pregnancy is minimal or completely absent in patients with preeclampsia. This limited blood volume expansion is probably the result of generalized constriction of the capacitance vessels.[15] However, it is also possible that the decrease in capacitance may be a result rather than the cause of the decreased intravascular volume. The reduced volume is predominantly of plasma, and as a result, hemoconcentration results as the disease progresses. After delivery the plasma volume increases, and the hemoglobin and hematocrit values will decrease. Postpartum, a significant drop in hematocrit almost always results from decreased vasospasm, excessive blood loss during delivery, or mobilization

---

BOX 10-1

Normal Hemodynamic Changes in Pregnancy

	Nonpregnant	Pregnant
Cardiac output (L/min)	4.3 ± 0.9	6.2 ± 1.0
Heart rate (bpm)	71 ± 10	83 ± 10
Systemic vascular resistance (dyne.cm.sec^{-5})	1530 ± 520	1210 ± 266
Pulmonary vascular resistance (dyne.cm.sec^{-5})	119 ± 47	78 ± 22
Mean arterial pressure (mm Hg)	86.4 ± 7.5	90.3 ± 5.8
Pulmonary capillary wedge pressure (mm Hg)	6.3 ± 2.1	7.5 ± 1.8
Central venous pressure (mm Hg)	3.7 ± 2.6	3.6 ± 2.5
Left ventricular stroke work index (g.m.m^{-2})	41 ± 8	48 ± 6

From Clark SL, Cotton DB, Lee W, et al: *Am J Obstet Gynecol* 1989;160:678.

---

of extracellular fluids or from a combination of all of these phenomena.

Loss of resistance to angiotensin II and catecholamines

Women who remain normotensive during pregnancy show a progressive resistance to the pressor effect of catecholamines and angiotensin II throughout gestation. In contrast, patients destined to develop preeclampsia show a progressive loss of resistance to the pressor effects of these agents.[16] For example, at 24 to 26 weeks' gestation a woman that remains normotensive will require an infusion of 12 to 14 ng/kg/min of angiotensin II to raise the diastolic pressure by 20 mm Hg. At the same gestational age, a patient likely to develop preeclampsia will need less than 8 to 9 ng/kg/min to have a similar pressure response.[17] A pattern of decreased vascular resistance to the pressor effects of angiotensin II also exists in patients with chronic hypertension destined to develop superimposed preeclampsia.[18]

Coagulation abnormalities

The work of Pritchard et al.[19] demonstrated that overt coagulation abnormalities exist in only a minority of patients with severe preeclampsia. The most serious hematologic complication of preeclampsia has become well known since its designation as the HELLP syndrome (hemolytic anemia, elevated liver enzymes, low platelet count). This name was used first by Weinstein[20] to distinguish those patients with severe pre-

eclampsia that have alterations in coagulation and fibrinolysis, thrombocytopenia, hemolytic anemia, and an elevation in liver enzymes. The prognosis of this complicated form of preeclampsia is guarded, and these patients would be best cared for in tertiary centers.

◢ MORPHOLOGIC CHANGES

The kidney has been the most studied organ in women with preeclampsia. The distinctive renal lesion in preeclampsia has been called *glomerular endotheliosis*,[21] and when evaluated by light microscopy, it is indistinguishable from acute membranous glomerulonephritis. However, under the electron microscope it is apparent that the capillary lumen is not narrowed by swelling of the basal membrane but as the result of deposits of osmophilic material between the basal membrane and the endothelial cells and an increase in the cytoplasm of the endothelial and intercapillary cells. There is no change in the epithelial cells or foot processes, no proliferation of intercapillary cells, and no alteration in the architecture of the renal medulla. The nature of the osmophilic deposits has been elucidated with the help of immunofluorescent techniques. It has been found that these deposits correspond to a material that reacts with antibodies against fibrinogen and fibrin. We have found a similar material in immunofluorescent studies of liver biopsies from patients with preeclampsia.[22]

When nulliparous patients with hypertension during pregnancy are submitted to kidney biopsy studies, only 75% of them show glomerular endotheliosis, 16.3% have chronic renal lesions, and 7.6% of them have both preeclampsia and chronic renal disease. When the same study is carried out in multiparous patients with hypertension in pregnancy, the characteristic histologic lesion of preeclampsia will be found in only 23%, chronic renal disease will be present in 51%, renal lesion plus preeclampsia will be found in 13%, and normal histology in 11%.[23] Another study, performed with women who developed preeclampsia before 37 weeks, found histologic evidence of renal disease, mostly mesangial IgA nephropathy, in 67% of primiparas and 63% of multiparas.[24]

There are some practical implications in these facts about the histology of preeclampsia and eclampsia. First, the difficulties and complications associated with kidney biopsy during pregnancy make tissue diagnosis of the disease far from routine. Second, it is difficult to rigorously interpret information obtained from populations selected on the basis of clinical criteria. Third, a tissue diagnosis of preeclampsia is positive in only 1 of every 10 multiparous patients. Therefore chronic renal disease must be strongly considered in every multiparous patient developing preeclampsia, and she must receive proper workup.

◾ PREDICTION

Several tests have been proposed to identify women at risk of developing preeclampsia. Some of these tests, such as the cold pressor test, the isometric hand grip exercise, and the roll-over test, depend on the presence of some pathophysiologic changes that occur in preeclampsia. Other tests, such as the measurement of urinary calcium or plasma fibronectin, are based on the presence of biochemical alterations peculiar to this disease.

Angiotensin sensitivity test

Since the abnormal vascular reactivity of patients destined to develop preeclampsia may be detected several weeks before the development of clinical signs and symptoms, the degree of sensitivity to angiotensin II may be used as a screening test to identify patients at risk for the disease. Unfortunately, this test has a high incidence of false-negative and false-positive results and is not ready for the routine evaluation of pregnant women. Also, no angiotensin II preparations for human use are available in the United States.

Roll-over test

The roll-over test was originally described as a noninvasive office procedure having excellent correlation with the angiotensin sensitivity test and as an excellent predictor of the development of preeclampsia.[25] A positive test is an elevation of 20 mm Hg or more in blood pressure when the patient rolls over from the lateral decubitus to the supine position. Unfortunately, the test has poor sensitivity and poor specificity and is of limited clinical value.

Second-trimester mean arterial pressure

Page and Christianson[26] have emphasized the importance of the mean arterial pressure (MAP) during the second trimester as a predictor of the development of preeclampsia. These findings have been contradicted by Chesley and Sibai[27] who found, in an analysis of 39,876 patients with preeclampsia and 207 patients with eclampsia, that second-trimester MAP has low sensitivity and low positive predictive value as an indicator of the future development of preeclampsia.

Urinary calcium

Several recent studies[28-30] have demonstrated that preeclampsia is associated with hypocalciuria. A urinary calcium concentration equal to or less than 12 mg/dl in a 24-hour collection has positive and negative predictive values of 85% and 91%, respectively, for the diagnosis of preeclampsia. Determination of the calcium/creatinine ratio in a randomly obtained single voided urine sample seems to be as accurate as 24-hour collections. Another study[31] indicates that this phenomenon occurs early and persists throughout gestation, being potentially useful for the early identification of patients at risk.

Fibronectin

Patients with preeclampsia have elevated levels of plasma fibronectin, a glycoprotein that has an important role in cellular adhesions and is a component of connective tissue and basement membranes. There are studies[12] indicating that increased plasma levels of endothelium-originated fibronectin precede the clinical signs of preeclampsia and may be useful for prediction of the disease.

Doppler ultrasound

Some investigators[32] have suggested that Doppler velocimetry may be useful at early gestational age, 18 to 24 weeks, to detect those patients destined to develop preeclampsia. Unfortunately, abnormal Doppler waveforms at this gestational age have a low sensitivity and low positive predictive value.

DIAGNOSIS
Blood pressure elevation

Hypertension is the most important sign of preeclampsia because it reflects the severity of the disease. Unfortunately, mistakes are frequently made because of lack of consistency in the measurement of blood pressure. One common error is taking the blood pressure of an obese patient with a regular-size cuff. This causes abnormally high readings and generates unnecessary alarm, testing, and consultation. Another common error is not using the same maternal position when taking repeated measurements.

A common mistake is that if an abnormally high reading is obtained, the measurement is repeated with the patient in the lateral recumbent position. In the majority of patients, the second blood pressure reading will be lower because in the pregnant woman the lateral recumbent values are always lower than those taken in the sitting position. The initial high blood pressure value is then considered spurious and disregarded, thus delaying proper diagnosis and treatment. To avoid this error, repeated blood pressure measurement should be taken with the patient in the sitting position.

A third error is the use of different end points to measure the diastolic blood pressure. In the United States the cessation of sound is most frequently used as the indicator for diastolic blood pressure. The experts in the field, as well as multiple professional organizations, recommend that the Korotkoff IV sound, the point of muffling, is the best marker of the diastolic pressure and should always be used.

Proteinuria

Proteinuria is a sign of preeclampsia that usually follows, or appears simultaneously with, hypertension. The proteinuria of preeclampsia is *nonselective*, corresponding to a mixture of several proteins of different molecular weights.

The proteinuria of preeclampsia characteristically occurs in the absence of either a nephritic (red cells, red cell casts) or a nephrotic (birefringent lipids, wax casts) urinary sediment. The urinary sediment in preeclampsia is usually unrevealing and in most cases shows an abundance of fine and coarse granular casts. The presence of a nephritic or nephrotic type of sediment must alert the clinician to the possibility of an underlying renal disease.

Proteinuria is extremely valuable as a prognostic sign in preeclampsia. Frequent monitoring of the amount of protein excreted in the urine must be a part of the evaluation of these patients. A significant increase in proteinuria indicates that the disease has worsened.

Vasospasm

Clinical evidence of vasospasm may be obtained by ophthalmologic examination, which must be a part of the initial evaluation of the patient with preeclampsia. The most common findings in patients with moderate or severe preeclampsia are an increase in the vein-to-artery ratio (normal is 4:3) and segmental vasospasm. Patients with *mild* preeclampsia usually have a normal funduscopic examination.

Examinations of the optic fundi in patients with gestational hypertension without proteinuria is also important because it may suggest the presence of chronic hypertensive disease independent of pregnancy. The presence of hemorrhages, exudates, or extensive arteriolar changes will signify chronic hypertension. Papilledema is not a common finding in preeclampsia, and it suggests the possibility of a brain tumor causing increases in intracranial pressure and secondary hypertension. The presence of microaneurysms will indicate diabetes.

Excessive body weight gain and edema

Excessive weight gain and edema are no longer considered signs of preeclampsia. Large increases in body weight as well as edema of hands, face, or both are common in normal pregnancy, and the incidence of preeclampsia is similar in patients with or without generalized edema. There is no evidence to indicate that measures limiting weight gain during pregnancy, such as the use of low-salt diet or diuretics, prevents the development of preeclampsia.

Other signs and symptoms of preeclampsia

Headaches are usually present in moderate-to-severe forms of preeclampsia. They also may appear before other indications of overt disease.

The pain may be frontal or occipital, may be pulsatile or dull, may occur simultaneously with visual symptoms, and may frequently be intense, especially when preceding the onset of convulsions.

Epigastric or right upper quadrant pain is also common in patients with severe forms of the disease but may also occur before the onset of obvious signs or symptoms of preeclampsia. This complaint is frequently attributed to indigestion or to gallbladder disease and is treated with antacids and antispasmodics. When such pain appears in patients with severe hypertension, it is frequently a harbinger of convulsions and is often accompanied by marked alterations in serum glutamic-oxaloacetic transaminase (SGOT), serum glutamic-pyruvic transaminase (SGPT), and lactic dehydrogenase (LDH) values.

The most common visual symptom appearing in patients who are going to develop preeclampsia is scotoma, a transient perception of bright or black spots. This may progress to sudden inability to focus, to blurred vision, and in severe cases, to complete blindness. In most patients who complain of visual symptoms, ophthalmologic examination reveals only vasospasm. This indicates that the abnormality originates in the occipital cortex rather than in the retina. Patients with severe preeclampsia who suffer from cortical blindness quickly recover their vision after delivery.

Brisk deep tendon reflexes are also common and result from central nervous system irritability. In some cases clonus and twitching of digits may also occur. Seizures rarely occur in preeclamptic patients without the patients first showing signs of excessive nervous system irritability.

Laboratory findings in preeclampsia

The laboratory values are usually unrevealing in cases of mild preeclampsia, but there are multiple findings in severe forms of the disease.[33] The laboratory changes reflect the effects of the disease on the kidney, liver, fetoplacental unit, and in some cases, the hematologic elements.

Altered renal function. In severe preeclampsia there are elevations in serum creatinine, blood urea nitrogen (BUN), and uric acid levels, as well as decreases in creatinine clearance, proteinuria, and changes in the urinary sediment. The serum creatinine almost never exceeds 1.3 to 1.4 mg/dl (the upper limit of normal during pregnancy is 0.8 mg/dl) and the BUN

rarely exceeds 20 to 25 mg/dl (the upper limit of normal in pregnancy is 15 mg/dl) unless there are unusual complications. The creatinine clearance is usually at the normal, nonpregnant level. It is important to remember that a creatinine clearance of 100 ml/min is abnormal during gestation when the lower limit of normal is 130 ml/min.

Many investigators have postulated that serum uric acid elevation is a specific laboratory finding in preeclampsia. However, there is a high degree of overlap among the values found in normal pregnancy, mild preeclampsia, severe preeclampsia, and eclampsia.[34] Serum uric acid levels normally decrease at the beginning of pregnancy, remain low during the second trimester, and slowly increase during the third trimester, nearly reaching nonpregnant levels at term. In most cases of mild or moderate preeclampsia, serum uric levels are indistinguishable from those obtained in normotensive patients at term. Marked elevation of uric acid, BUN, and creatinine only occur with severe preeclampsia.

Changes in liver function tests. Patients with mild preeclampsia show little or no alteration in hepatic enzyme levels, but in severe preeclampsia marked increases in SGPT, SGOT, and LDH are commonly found. The raised total LDH is usually reflected in elevations of isoenzyme 5 (LD_5, liver). If hemolytic anemia is also present, the electrophoretic pattern will show elevation of isoenzymes 1, 2, and 5. After delivery, SGPT and SGOT levels rapidly decrease and, in most cases, reach normal levels by the fifth postpartum day. LDH falls more slowly, and normal values are reached by postpartum day eight to ten.

Hematologic abnormalities. The only hematologic change that may be observed in patients with mild preeclampsia is an elevation of hemoglobin and hematocrit caused by the characteristic decrease in plasma volume. With more severe disease other hematologic abnormalities, commonly thrombocytopenia, may be present. Pritchard et al.[35] found 26% of 91 eclamptic patients to have platelet counts below 150,000; 17% had platelet counts below 100,000; and 3% had platelet counts below 50,000. The plasma fibrinogen concentration is usually normal or slightly increased, and it is unusual to find a fibrinogen level below 200 mg/dl unless the clinical course is complicated by abruptio placentae.

The thrombin time may also be altered in preeclamptic patients, and it is likely to be prolonged in about 50% of those patients with severe forms of preeclampsia. This change is peculiar because it may occur in patients with normal fibrinogen concentration and normal levels of fibrinogen-split products.

Determination of D-dimer, a peptide derived specifically from the degradation of fibrin, has recently become available. The initial information[36] suggests that preeclamptic patients with positive D-dimer (> 0.5 mg/dl) have a more severe form of the disease than those with a negative test.

Abnormal fetoplacental function. A common finding in women with moderate or severe preeclampsia is fetal measurements showing growth of 2 to 4 weeks less than expected for their gestational age, suggesting the presence of intrauterine growth retardation. The head-to-abdomen and femur-to-abdomen ratios frequently are abnormally elevated in these cases.

The nonstress test (NST) and contraction stress test (CST) are useful when a quick evaluation of the fetal status is necessary. However, the use of these tests of fetal well-being in patients with preeclampsia may be limited. In fact, the commonly accepted 8-day safety interval after a negative NST or CST, the time at which fetal demise is highly improbable, has little or no validity when there is an unstable or rapidly deteriorating maternal situation.

According to Ducey et al.,[37] hypertensive pregnant patients with normal umbilical and uterine velocimetry have fetal outcomes that are similar to those of normotensive patients. In contrast, patients with abnormal umbilical and uterine Doppler waveforms have poor outcomes: 51% deliver small-for–gestational age infants, 62% require cesarean section for fetal distress, 89% are admitted to neonatal intensive care units, and 84% are delivered preterm. However, association between abnormal umbilical Doppler waveforms and poor fetal outcomes does not mean that the test is useful in the management of patients with preeclampsia. Doppler studies of the umbilical and uterine arteries have a limited value in the management of patients with preeclampsia.

Diagnostic difficulties

There are few diagnostic difficulties in cases of mild preeclampsia. The usual problem in these cases is the reluctance of the physician to accept the diagnosis and establish an appropriate plan of management of the disease.

Unfortunately, most diagnostic problems are found in patients with severe preeclampsia. Mistakes are made because conditions such as systemic lupus erythematosus, kidney diseases, hepatitis, gallbladder disease, idiopathic hemolytic anemia, thrombotic thrombocytopenic purpura, or epilepsy may mimic the signs and symptoms of preeclampsia. There are no simple rules to follow to avoid mistakes in the diagnosis of preeclampsia, but the following suggestions may be helpful:

1. Severe preeclampsia is not common in multiparous patients. Multiparous patients with severe hypertension must be suspected of having underlying chronic hypertension or chronic renal disease and must have a minimal workup, including antinuclear antibody (ANA) titer, anticardiolipin antibodies, and potassium determination in plasma and, if low, in the urine. Some of these patients should have a rapid sequence intravenous pyelogram (IVP) postpartum.

2. The earlier in gestation severe hypertension occurs, the greater the possibility of its being caused by a condition independent of pregnancy.

3. If pregnancy is terminated by cesarean section in a patient with severe hypertension, the surgeon may carefully palpate the kidneys, adrenal glands, and periaortic region during the procedure in an attempt to discover underlying problems that may explain the clinical picture of the patient. During such explorations it is possible to find large renal tumors, lymphatic cysts compressing the aorta just above its bifurcation, adrenal tumors, and more frequently, small, scarred kidneys of chronic pyelonephritis indicating causes of hypertension other than preeclampsia.

4. Hypertension is the key element in the differential diagnosis of preeclampsia. Hepatitis, gallstones, idiopathic thrombocytopenic purpura (ITP), epilepsy, and many other diseases that may appear during pregnancy do not have hypertension as a manifestation. In contrast, when a bizarre clinical condition appears during pregnancy, preeclampsia must be suspect if hypertension is present.

◪ MANAGEMENT

Once a diagnosis of preeclampsia is established, the patient must be admitted to the hospital. Preeclampsia should not be treated on an outpatient basis. However, patients with gestational hypertension without proteinuria (PIH) may be managed as outpatients after careful evaluation.

When confronted with the management of a patient with preeclampsia, the clinician must first determine the severity of the disease.

Severe cases

If the patient has severe preeclampsia, the management will consist of (1) prevention of seizures, (2) control of hypertension, and (3) delivery.

Prevention of seizures

Magnesium sulfate. Magnesium sulfate is the most commonly used medication in the United States for the treatment or prevention of seizure activity in patients with preeclampsia and eclampsia. There is a great deal of controversy over the mechanism of seizure control by magnesium sulfate. The evidence in the literature, however, indicates that magnesium sulfate is the ideal anticonvulsant in preeclampsia.[38] For some investigators the effect of magnesium sulfate on the central nervous system does not account for its anticonvulsive effect. They argue that the cerebrospinal fluid Mg^{++} concentration is independent of and significantly higher (2.4 mEq/L) than the plasma concentration and increases very slowly despite therapeutic plasma levels. Accordingly, they believe that Mg^{++} is a peripheral anticonvulsant because of its ability to block neuromuscular transmission by decreasing the acetylcholine release in response to nerve action potentials. Other investigators argue that the magnesium levels reached during treatment of eclamptic seizures are never high enough to cause peripheral muscular paralysis, and therefore the anticonvulsant action of the medication should be explained through a central effect.

There are no prospective controlled studies demonstrating that treatment of preeclampsia and eclampsia with magnesium sulfate is better than other treatments or better than no treatment. However, in noncontrolled studies the best maternal and fetal outcomes have been obtained through regimens using magnesium sulfate.[39,40] Other protocols using different types of anticonvulsants require comparison with magnesium sulfate before they may claim superiority and are adopted for routine clinical use.

An intravenous dose of 4 g of magnesium sulfate causes an immediate elevation of the normal Mg^{++} level, 1.6 to 2.1 mEq/L, to about 7 to 9 mEq/L.[41] Intracellular transfer of the ion and elimination by the kidney will cause a drop in plasma concentration to 4 to 5 mEq/L 1 hour after injection. At this elevated plasma level, about one third of the Mg^{++} is protein bound, and its renal clearance is very similar to the glomerular filtration rate. Most centers administer magnesium sulfate by continuous intravenous infusion following the protocol described by Anderson and Sibai (Box 10-2). In other medical centers intramuscular administration is preferred (Box 10-3). In most cases of eclampsia, the initial loading dose of magnesium sulfate is enough to arrest convulsions. Rarely, a patient will convulse again after the loading dose. In these cases 100 to 150 mg of phenobarbital sodium should be injected very slowly intravenously.

Magnesium sulfate is not an innocuous drug. It is necessary to monitor those patients who are receiving the medication to prevent serious side effects. The clinical variables to monitor are urinary output, patellar reflex, and respiratory rate. Because Mg^{++} is eliminated by the kidneys, monitoring of the urinary output is extremely important. Urine production is frequently decreased in patients with severe preeclampsia. This may lead to an abnormally high Mg^{++} level, resulting in respiratory or cardiac arrest. A urinary output of at least 30 ml/hr is necessary for the continuous administration of magnesium sulfate.

Disappearance of the patellar reflex is important because it is the first sign of impending toxicity. The patellar reflex is usually lost when plasma Mg^{++} concentration reaches 8 to 10 mEq/L. In this case the drug must be discontinued until the reflex returns. Otherwise, the plasma level will continue to increase until a level is reached, usually more than 12 mEq/L, at which respiratory depression and respiratory paralysis may ensue. Pritchard[42] has observed that administration of diuretics to a preeclamptic patient with impaired renal function did not prevent excessive Mg^{++} accumulation to toxic levels despite the increase in urine output. Obviously, the increase in urinary output was not equivalent to improved renal function or to improved magnesium excretion.

<hr>

BOX 10-2

University of Tennessee Guidelines for Intravenous Magnesium Sulfate Administration

Loading dose

Give 30 ml of 20% magnesium sulfate solution (6 g) in 100 ml of 5% dextrose over 10- to 15-minute period.

Maintenance dose

Add 20 g of magnesium sulfate (four 10-ml ampules of 50% solution) to 1000 ml of D_5W and give intravenously at a rate of 100 ml/hr (2.0 g/hr). Obtain a serum magnesium level 4 to 6 hours later and adjust the rate of infusion to keep serum magnesium between 4.8 and 9.6 mg/dl.

If serum magnesium levels are not available, the dose is adjusted according to the patellar reflex and the urine output in the previous 4-hour period.

Monitoring for magnesium toxicity

Urine output should be at least 30 ml/hr. Deep tendon reflexes should be present. Respiration rate should exceed 14/min.

Any decrease in these indexes makes it necessary to reevaluate the rate of magnesium sulfate administration.

<hr>

Modified from Anderson GD, Sibai BM: Hypertension in pregnancy, in Gabbe SG, Niebyl JR, Simpson JL (eds): *Obstetrics: Normal and Problem Pregnancies.* New York, Churchill Livingston, 1986, p 832.

<hr>

BOX 10-3

Pritchard's Guidelines for Intramuscular Magnesium Sulfate Administration to Patients with Preeclampsia

Intravenous loading dose (only for patients with eclampsia)

Dilute 8 ml of 50% magnesium sulfate solution (4 g) with 12 ml of sterile water or use 20 ml of a 20% solution (4 g) and give intravenously in a 3- to 5-minute period.

Intramuscular loading dose

Administer 10 ml of 50% magnesium sulfate solution (5 g) deeply in the outer quadrant of *each* buttock, using a 3-inch, 20-gauge needle. The intramuscular (IM) dose should immediately follow the intravenous dose in patients with convulsions. *Patients without convulsions receive only the intramuscular loading dose.*

Maintenance dose

Give 5 g (10 ml of 50% solution) deep by IM injection in alternate buttocks every 4 hours if (1) the patellar reflex is present, (2) the urine output has been at least 100 ml during the preceding 4 hours, and (3) the respiration rate is normal (at least 14/min). Continue maintenance dose until 24 hours postpartum.

<hr>

From Pritchard JA, Cunningham FG, Pritchard SA: The Parkland Memorial Hospital protocol for treatment of eclampsia. *Am J Obstet Gynecol* 1984;148:951.

<hr>

An excess of Ca^{++} will increase the amount of acetylcholine liberated by the action potentials at the neuromuscular junction. Thus, if respiratory depression is induced by hypermagnesemia, intravenous calcium gluconate, 10 ml of a 10% solution, given over 3 minutes, is the logical antidote.

Magnesium sulfate may also be harmful to the fetus. Maternal levels rapidly equilibrate with fetal plasma, and the concentration in both compartments is similar. Respiratory depression and hyporeflexia have been observed in newborns delivered to mothers undergoing intravenous magnesium sulfate therapy. For unknown reasons, this problem does not occur or is significantly less frequent if the drug is given intramuscularly.

Magnesium sulfate decreases beat-to-beat variability as seen by electronic monitoring of the fetal heart rate (FHR). It is important to remember that the effect of Mg^{++} on variability is not marked. Therefore, in patients with preeclampsia who are receiving magnesium sulfate treatment, decreased or absent FHR variability is a sign of potential fetal compromise.

Magnesium sulfate acts synergistically with the muscle relaxants used for general anesthesia. Obstetric anesthesiologists are aware of this fact and prescribe a smaller dosage of such medication when giving general anesthetics to patients on magnesium sulfate therapy.

Phenytoin. Phenytoin has been successfully used for the treatment and prophylaxis of eclamptic seizures. The medication is well tolerated and has few side effects. Phenytoin acts by inhibiting the spread of abnormal activity from the seizure foci to the motor cortex. Unfortunately, the experience with phenytoin treatment in preeclamptic women is limited, and there is a need for trials comparing its effectiveness with that of magnesium sulfate.

For the treatment of eclampsia, the loading dose of phenytoin is 15 to 25 mg/kg depending on the patient's weight. The medication should be given slowly intravenously, never exceeding a rate of 25 mg/min.[42a] This will avoid cardiovascular toxicity and central nervous system depression. The loading dose should be followed by a second dose of 500 mg IV 12 hours after the end of the initial infusion, depending on the serum phenytoin levels in those patients who need continued anticonvulsive prophylaxis.

For prophylaxis, phenytoin should be given in a 100-mg dosage IV or IM every 4 hours. Oral administration should continue for several days in the postpartum period.

Antihypertensive treatment. The objective of antihypertensive treatment is to prevent intracranial bleeding and left ventricular failure. Also, some investigators believe that antihypertensive treatment may be useful in avoiding the selective cerebral arterial vasospasm that causes eclamptic seizures.[43] According to this theory, cerebral perfusion is maintained at a level of about 55 ml/min/100 g of tissue despite variations in mean arterial pressure and in blood composition. With worsening hypertension, the upper level of autoregulation may be reached, producing a reactive vasospasm designed to limit this increased tissue perfusion. This vasospasm may disrupt the endothelial capillary cell junctions, causing extravasation of blood into the perivascular space. These pericapillary hemorrhages are the foci of abnormal electrical discharges, which may spread, producing seizures.

According to this theory, the upper limit of cerebral perfusion pressure varies among individuals. Patients with chronic hypertension, for example, are capable of tolerating higher MAPs than others. This explains why a young preeclamptic patient may convulse with systemic blood pressure values of 140/95 mm Hg, whereas a patient with chronic hypertension and superimposed preeclampsia may tolerate pressures as high as 220/150 mm Hg or more without convulsions. In the former, an MAP of 110 mm Hg exceeded the limit of autoregulation of brain perfusion pressure, whereas in the second patient, an MAP of 173 mm Hg was not high enough to reach that limit, which had become higher than usual through the years of exposure to elevated pressure.

The majority of investigators believe that factors other than vasospasm are important in the genesis of eclamptic seizures. Microvascular thrombosis, cerebral edema, and endothelial damage are components of the eclamptic brain lesions and probably play an important role in the production of seizures. However, until the mechanism of eclamptic seizures is completely clarified, a potential pathogenic role of blood pressure elevation cannot be completely disregarded.

Hydralazine. Hydralazine is commonly used for the treatment of elevated blood pressure in obstetrics. This diminishes the likelihood of cerebral hemorrhage and left ventricular failure and may also be a contributing factor in seizure prevention. Hydralazine acts directly on arteriolar smooth muscle to reduce peripheral vascular resistance. The blood pressure response is almost immediate, although it is less dramatic than that with diazoxide. Hydralazine is used in repeated intravenous boluses. The most frequent side effects of hydralazine administration are decreased uteroplacental perfusion and hyperdynamic circulation. The first is indicated by late decelerations that may be observed after hydralazine injection in patients who previously had a normal fetal tracing. Recovery from this abnormal pattern can be seen after the drug is discontinued and the blood pressure rises. This complication occurs more often if there is a precipitous drop in the diastolic pressure, usually below 80 mm Hg. For this reason, fetal electronic monitoring is mandatory when IV hydralazine is used. The amount and frequency of repeated hydralazine doses must be based on both the maternal and the fetal response. Hyperdynamic circulation after hydralazine administration is a result of its positive inotropic effect and is manifested by tachycardia.

Labetalol. Labetalol is a combined alpha- and beta-adrenergic blocker. The ratio of alpha to beta blockade is approximately 1:3 for the oral form and 1:7 for the intravenous form. Labetalol is effective in the treatment of severe hypertension and can be given by continuous or intermittent intravenous infusion.

For continuous intravenous use, labetalol

should be started at a rate of 2 mg/min. This may be adjusted according to the blood pressure response. For intermittent dosing, 20 mg should be given over a 2-minute period. Additional doses of 20 to 40 mg may be given at 10-minute intervals. The maximum effect of IV labetalol is usually reached 5 minutes after injection.

Nifedipine. Nifedipine is a calcium channel blocker used mainly for the prevention of coronary artery spasm. The medication is also an excellent peripheral vasodilator and a good tocolytic agent. Nifedipine lowers the blood pressure by decreasing the cardiac afterload. The medication is absorbed rapidly after oral administration and reaches peak levels 30 minutes after ingestion. The plasma half-life of nifedipine is approximately 2 hours.

The initial dose of nifedipine is 10 mg orally. If no side effects occur, the medication may be given in a 10- or 20-mg dosage every 4 to 6 hours according to the blood pressure response. Dosage above 120 mg/day is rarely necessary.

Verapamil. Verapamil is another calcium channel blocker that may be useful in the treatment of elevated blood pressure. It is used mainly in the postpartum period when the hypertension persists. The starting dosage is 80 mg orally, 3 times per day, to which most patients respond.

Other antihypertensive agents. Other antihypertensive agents have disadvantages. Methyldopa, an excellent drug for chronic hypertension, is inadequate because of its delayed onset of action and prolonged response. Reserpine may cause nasal stuffiness in newborns, which is a rather serious problem because of their obligatory nasal breathing. Diazoxide may cause a rapid, dramatic hypotensive response. At least one maternal death has been reported in a preeclamptic patient who developed profound, irreversible shock after diazoxide administration.[44] Diazoxide may also cause fetal and maternal hyperglycemia, inhibition of uterine contractions, and sodium and water retention. Sodium nitroprusside is an excellent medication for gradually decreasing elevated blood pressure. However, because cyanide is its metabolite, significant fetal toxicity may occur.

Delivery. The decision to deliver a patient with severe preeclampsia is relatively simple when the pregnancy is 36 weeks or older. The decision is more difficult when the patient is less than 36 weeks and particularly arduous when she is less than 30 weeks. The problem is to balance the maternal risks associated with prolongation of pregnancy with the fetal risks associated with early delivery.

Sibai et al.[45] in 1985 reported the first large series on the conservative management of 60 patients with severe preeclampsia between 18 and 27 weeks of gestation. He found serious maternal complications including eclampsia in 16.7%, HELLP syndrome in 16.7%, acute tubular necrosis in 5%, and individual cases of hypertensive encephalopathy, intracerebral hemorrhage, and liver hematoma. With respect to the fetus, the overall perinatal mortality was 87%. Twenty-three of 31 pregnancies (74%) with severe preeclampsia developing before 25 weeks ended in fetal death, whereas the incidence of fetal death was 28% when severe preeclampsia developed after 25 weeks. The conclusion of this study was that the poor fetal prognosis and the high incidence of severe maternal complications justifies conservative management of severe preeclampsia in the second trimester only in a limited number of situations. Odendaal et al.[46] confirmed Sibai's observations and reported 100% and 75% perinatal mortality when expectant management was adopted for patients delivering fetuses with birth weights less than 750 g and less than 1000 g, respectively.

The authors of further studies[47,48] have clearly demonstrated that conservative management for severe preeclampsia developing before 24 weeks is not adequate. Maternal morbidity is severe and perinatal survival is less than 10%. Therefore these patients should be delivered to reduce maternal risk and avoid prolonged hospitalization and intensive therapy that offers little chance of success.

In selected patients with severe preeclampsia developing between 24 and 34 weeks, prolongation of pregnancy is advantageous for the fetus.[49] Before their assignment to a conservative management plan, patients should remain in Labor and Delivery for a minimum of 24 hours. They should be observed carefully and delivered if they exhibit one or more of the conditions shown in Box 10-4. Patients found not in need of immediate delivery may be transferred to an antepartum area for high-risk patients for intensive fetal and maternal monitoring. The main aspects of conservative management are shown in Box 10-5.

An important point is the use and interpreta-

BOX 10-4

Criteria for Delivering Patients with Severe Preeclampsia

Blood pressure persistently 160/100 or greater despite treatment
Urine output < 400 ml in 24 hours
Platelet count < 50,000/mm^3
Progressive increase in serum creatinine
LDH > 1000 IU/L
Repetitive late decelerations with poor variability
Severe IUGR with oligohydramnios
Decreased fetal movement
Reversed umbilical diastolic blood flow

BOX 10-5

Expectant Management of Severe Preeclampsia Less Than 36 Weeks

Bed rest
Daily weight
Antihypertensive treatment (methyldopa [Aldomet], labetalol, nifedipine)
Weekly betamethasone
Liver, renal, hematologic, and D-dimer evaluation daily or every other day
Daily questioning about headaches, visual disturbances, epigastric pain, and fetal movement
Daily NST
Daily fetal movement count
Fluid volume every week
Ultrasound for growth every 2 weeks

The criteria for delivering patients with severe preeclampsia managed expectantly are shown in Box 10-4. These patients need meticulous attention, and the desirability of expectancy vs. the need to deliver should be determined daily. The obstetrician should always remember that immediate delivery is the only measure that interrupts the progression of this disease. In a study in Los Angeles, reluctance in terminating a pregnancy, usually because of prematurity, was one of the most common errors resulting in maternal mortality.[50] This study found that other common errors in the management of preeclampsia-eclampsia were:

1. Underestimation of the severity of the disease
2. Mistaking the masking of symptoms with medications for improvement in the disease process
3. Failure to use antihypertensive drugs to combat extreme elevations of blood pressure

In most cases of severe preeclampsia, pregnancy may be terminated by oxytocin induction. This procedure is frequently successful even when the cervix appears firm and closed. Because fetal distress is common in these patients, labor should be carefully monitored. Fetal distress or failure of induction requires cesarean section.

The management of severe preeclampsia using medications for seizure prophylaxis, antihypertensive treatment, and delivery involves a series of positive actions, as well as continuous adherence to some other basic principles (Box 10-6).

The overall management plan for severe preeclampsia is shown in Figure 10-1.

Moderate cases

If the patient under consideration has moderate preeclampsia, the next step should be the assessment of gestational age and fetal lung maturation. There are several methods to assess gestational age (see Chapter 1). If the pregnancy is determined to be 36 or more weeks, steps should be taken for delivery. There is no benefit in continuing the pregnancy when the infant and mother have nearly a 100% chance of a good outcome if delivery is accomplished.

If the pregnancy is at less than 36 weeks of gestation, the chances for a good fetal outcome

tion of fetal well-being tests in these patients. Acceleration of the heart rate associated with movement or in response to vibroacoustic stimulation, which are the main criteria for determining *reactivity* in the NST, is not present in the second-trimester fetus. Therefore the elements for assessing fetal health will be the presence of short- and long-term variability and the absence of decelerations. With respect to the biophysical profile, only fetal movement, fetal tone, and amount of fluid can be assessed because the NST is nonreactive and respiratory movements are not present in the second-trimester fetus. Consequently, the maximum obtainable score is 6.

BOX 10-6

What Not to Do in the Management of Patients with Severe Preeclampsia or Eclampsia

Do not give diuretics

In the majority of cases severe oliguria and anuria are indications for prompt pregnancy termination or invasive hemodynamic monitoring and not for diuretics.

Do not give diazepam to stop a convulsion

Rapid administration of diazepam may produce apnea and facilitate aspiration. Furthermore, diazepam accumulates in the fetus, causing respiratory depression at birth.

Do not push the padded tongue blade to the back of the throat in the patient with seizures

The padded tongue blade is used to prevent the patient from biting her tongue. This blade should not be pushed to the back of the throat because the gag reflex will then be stimulated and cause vomiting and danger of aspiration.

Do not give heparin

Intracranial bleeding is a significant risk in the setup of severe hypertension and anticoagulation. There is no evidence that heparin improves the outcome of patients with severe preeclampsia.

Do not attempt to manage expectantly patients with severe preeclampsia unless you are in a tertiary care center

---

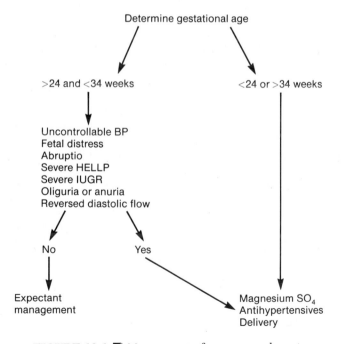

FIGURE 10-1 ◢ Management of severe preeclampsia.

decrease in proportion to the prematurity because of the rising incidence of respiratory distress syndrome and other illnesses associated with early gestation. However, preeclampsia is one obstetric condition that causes fetal stress and accelerated fetal lung maturation. Accordingly, some preterm infants born to mothers with preeclampsia have few of these problems. However, the chances of having sufficient lung maturation decrease precipitously at gestational ages less than 36 weeks.

Management of the patient with moderate preeclampsia at less than 36 weeks depends on clinical and laboratory observations during the 24 to 48 hours following admission. This period of observation is best handled in an intensive care area such as Labor and Delivery. An NST, followed by a CST if necessary, is performed. Simultaneously, maternal laboratory evaluation, including tests for serum creatinine, BUN, uric acid, SGOT, LDH, platelet count, and D-dimer, is done. These data will determine severity. Blood pressure, urinary output, qualitative proteinuria, and neurologic signs and symptoms should be measured frequently. If at any time during the period of observation the clinical and laboratory studies indicate that the patient's condition is deteriorating, or not improving, she must be delivered without consideration of the gestational age or fetal lung maturation.

Fortunately, most patients admitted with moderate preeclampsia at less than 36 weeks improve quickly with hospital bed rest. Diastolic blood pressure decreases to the mild range of 90 to 100 mm Hg. There is an increase in urinary output, as well as amelioration of headaches, visual symptoms, and nervous system irritability. If this occurs, the patient's classification changes to mild preeclampsia, and she should be entered into an expectant management program, as is described later.

Mild cases

If the patient has mild preeclampsia, as with moderate disease, an assessment of the gestational age and the lung maturity of the fetus should be done. For patients with mild preeclampsia, management is determined by the gestational age. If the pregnancy is 36 or more weeks, there is no reason for its prolongation. However, in mild cases there is not the same sense of urgency for delivery as with severe or moderate preeclampsia. In mild cases induction of labor by means of intravenous oxytocin ad-

ministration may be repeated on alternate days unless the disease worsens. Amniotomy should not be performed early in the induction process unless the cervix is ripe and the probability of success is high.

Patients with mild preeclampsia and less than 36 weeks should have amniocentesis to evaluate fetal pulmonary maturity. If the fetal lungs are mature, labor should be induced and the patient delivered. If the fetal lungs are immature, expectant management is the best alternative. It is necessary to remember that phosphatidylglycerol (PG) appears late in the process of fetal lung maturity, and therefore most patients less than 36 weeks will have negative PG. Under these circumstances the decision to deliver or to opt for conservative management should be based on the lecithin to sphingomyelin (L/S) ratio.

The patient with mild preeclampsia and proven fetal lung immaturity should be entered into an expectant management program. In-hospital limitation of her activity is effective in slowing the progression of the disease and may allow the time to achieve fetal maturity.

For expectant management to succeed, strict patient selection criteria and meticulous monitoring for signs and symptoms of aggravation of the disease are necessary. Proper selection of patients has been discussed (see Table 10-1). Maternal monitoring consists of the following:

1. Measurement of blood pressure at least 4 times per day
2. Measurement of body weight every other day
3. Measurement of qualitative urinary protein excretion with a reagent strip test (Albustix) in the first urine specimen every morning
4. Measurement of creatinine clearance every week
5. Measurement of biochemical profile (SMA-18) twice per week
6. Daily questioning about fetal movements, development of scotomas or headaches, and presence of epigastric or right upper quadrant pain

Fetal monitoring consists of:
1. Fetal biometry (biparietal diameter, head circumference, abdominal circumference, femur length) on admission to the hospital and every 3 weeks thereafter; evaluation of amniotic fluid volume twice weekly
2. NSTs at least every week (If the mother complains of decreased fetal movement or

if there is a clinical or sonographic suggestion of retarded fetal growth, NSTs may be done more frequently.)

3. Determining the L/S ratio when the pregnancy reaches 36 weeks (Before this gestational age, amniocentesis for lung maturity is rarely necessary because the decision to deliver usually results from maternal or fetal deterioration rather than lung maturity measurements.)

During the expectant management program:

1. The patient should not receive any medication other than vitamin and iron supplements. It must be emphasized that no diuretics or antihypertensives should be given. If the blood pressure of a preeclamptic patient during expectant management rises to a point at which treatment is necessary, the patient needs to be delivered.
2. There should be no dietary sodium restriction. Patients should eat the regular hospital diet.
3. Strict bed rest is unnecessary. In-hospital activity is much less than outpatient activity, and most patients will spend a majority of their time resting.
4. The preeclamptic patient under expectant management should remain in the hospital until delivered.

Elevation of the blood pressure to a moderate range, between 100 and 110 mm Hg diastolic, is the most common indication for delivery. Unfortunately, antihypertensive medications are sometimes given to try to prolong the pregnancy. However, these medications should be given to preeclamptic patients only in the labor room, simultaneously with magnesium sulfate, while preparing for delivery. Trying to deal with a deteriorating condition using antihypertensive drugs and avoiding delivery is an invitation for disaster.

Excessive weight gain; elevation of BUN, creatinine, or uric acid levels; and decreased creatinine clearance are not indications for delivery unless they occur simultaneously with elevated diastolic blood pressure. Proteinuria is an important sign of deteriorating renal function and is second only to hypertension as an index of worsening of the disease.

The limited intravascular volume expansion of the patient with preeclampsia leads to management problems with diuretics, blood loss and regional anesthesia, and use of plasma volume expanders.

Diuretics. Diuretics have been used and continue to be used in the treatment of patients with preeclampsia. These medications will further diminish intravascular volume and aggravate the deficient uteroplacental perfusion present in preeclamptic patients. The deleterious effect of diuretics on the placental blood flow has been demonstrated by experiments showing that they decrease the placental clearance of dehydroepiandrosterone sulfate.[51]

Some patients with preeclampsia have insidious sodium losses or are in negative sodium balance because of dietary manipulations. In these cases administration of diuretics may cause severe hyponatremia, which may be aggravated by the intrapartum administration of oxytocin and water. Also, diuretics may cause neonatal thrombocytopenia, as well as renal and auditory dysfunction.

Diuretics should not be used in the therapy of preeclampsia and eclampsia except under uncommon circumstances.

Blood loss and regional anesthesia. Hemorrhage in the preeclamptic patient is poorly tolerated because of limited intravascular volume. This is exemplified by the patient with severe preeclampsia who has profound shock after an average blood loss during cesarean delivery. The average blood loss of 1000 ml during a cesarean section corresponds to approximately 35% to 40% of the blood volume of a pregnant woman with severe preeclampsia.

Regional anesthesia in patients with severe preeclampsia may result in shock. The sympathetic blockade produced causes venous dilation, significant blood pooling, and a reduced preload. These hemodynamic effects may be avoided by administration of intravenous fluids, elevating the lower extremities, and assumption of the lateral decubitus position improving venous return.

In the hands of a competent obstetric anesthesiologist, epidural anesthesia is safe for the preeclamptic patient. It may have favorable hemodynamic effects and make blood pressure control easier. The main contraindication to epidural anesthesia in these patients is thrombocytopenia.

Use of plasma volume expanders. Some literature suggests that administration of plasma volume expanders such as dextran or albumin may be valuable in preeclampsia. This treatment attempts to correct the decreased intravascular

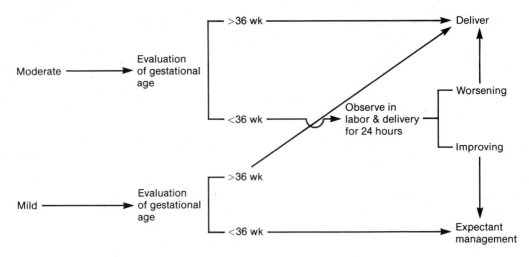

FIGURE 10-2 ◪ Management of moderate and mild cases of preeclampsia.

volume, which is important in the multiorgan perfusion defect exhibited by these patients. This therapy should be avoided because patients with severe preeclampsia or eclampsia have large capillary leaks allowing large–molecular weight molecules to pass into the pulmonary interstitial space causing pulmonary edema.

A summary of the overall plan of management for patients with moderate and mild preeclampsia is shown in Figure 10-2.

Complicated forms of preeclampsia

Eclampsia. Eclampsia is an extremely severe form of preeclampsia. Eclampsia is characterized by the onset of generalized tonic-clonic seizures in women with preeclampsia. This condition affects between 0.5% and 0.2% of all deliveries and may complicate as many as 1.5% of twin pregnancies. Eclampsia occurs antepartum in 46.3%, intrapartum in 16.4%, and postpartum in 37.3% of the cases, respectively.[52]

The pathogenesis of eclampsia remains unknown. It is possible that severe arterial vasospasm causes rupture of the vascular endothelium and pericapillary hemorrhage with the development of foci of abnormal electrical discharges that may generalize and cause convulsions. The rapid reversal of symptoms of an eclamptic patient with relentless neurologic deterioration treated with the selective cerebral vasodilator nimodipine[53] supports such a mechanism.

Eclampsia is associated with elevated maternal and fetal morbidity and mortality. The most common causes of maternal death are intracranial bleeding and acute renal failure caused by abruptio placentae.[50] The most common causes of fetal death are prematurity and fetal asphyxia and acidosis.[54] Eclampsia is a major obstetric emergency that requires mobilization of efforts and adequate management to avoid catastrophic events.

Alterations of the hemostatic system are infrequent in patients with eclampsia.[4,19] Only 16% have low platelet counts, and only 8% have low fibrinogen concentration. LDH is elevated in 74% of these patients.

The management of antepartum eclampsia is similar to that of other severe forms of preeclampsia, and treatment consists of magnesium sulfate to control the convulsive state, antihypertensive medications to control severe hypertension, and delivery. Treatment with magnesium sulfate should continue for at least 24 hours after delivery to avoid postpartum eclampsia.

Sibai et al.[55] has demonstrated that in 31.3% of the cases eclampsia is not preventable despite adequate prenatal care and admission to the hospital. However, 69.7% of the cases are preventable. The most common problems affecting the efficacy of preventive measures are physician errors in 36.3% and inadequate administration of magnesium sulfate in 12.8% of the cases.

The seizures characteristic of eclampsia are

acute and transient, and long-term neurologic deficits are rare in patients adequately treated.[56] However, 34.5% of patients who develop eclampsia will have preeclampsia in a subsequent pregnancy.[56]

HELLP syndrome. When a platelet count less than 100,000/mm^3 is seen in a severely preeclamptic patient, it is important to look at the blood smear for red cell fragmentation and obtain a serum haptoglobin, as well as a liver enzymes determination. If fragmented erythrocytes are seen in the smear, the haptoglobin is absent or markedly decreased, and the liver enzymes are elevated, the patient has preeclampsia with hematologic complications. Hemolysis in these cases results from cell passage through small vessels partially obliterated with fibrin deposits. This complication of preeclampsia has become known by the acronym HELLP (*H*emolytic anemia, *E*levated *L*iver enzymes, *L*ow *P*latelet count) proposed by Weinstein[20] to describe the condition. The criteria for the diagnosis of HELLP syndrome have been defined by Sibai[57] and are shown in Box 10-7.

It is difficult to differentiate between this disorder and thrombotic thrombocytopenic purpura (TTP) because their clinical, laboratory, and histologic characteristics are similar. However, severe preeclampsia occurs rather frequently, whereas TTP is a rare condition. Occasionally, the obstetrician and the internal medicine consultant fall into the trap of diagnosing TTP and then start a course of medical therapy that delays delivery, a dangerous procrastination. Every hypertensive pregnant patient with hematologic complications must be managed as if the process were induced by pregnancy. This implies delivery, and in most cases the patient will improve rapidly postpartum. If TTP is present, however, hemolysis and neurologic symptoms will not change with delivery. The plan of management for patients with HELLP syndrome includes the following:

1. Oxytocin induction must be initiated immediately unless there is a contraindication for vaginal delivery. Changes in the cervix should be observed shortly after initiation of induction. If vaginal delivery is not foreseen within 12 hours after the onset of induction, delivery by cesarean section is preferred.

2. Platelets are not given unless the platelet count is below 20,000/mm^3 or below 40,000 and the patient shows signs of altered hemostasis. If a platelet transfusion is necessary, each unit will raise the count by about 10,000/mm^3. Since the objective is to raise the count to about 50,000/mm^3, the transfusion of 10 U of platelets will usually suffice. The survival time of the transfused platelets in a presumably nonimmunized recipient will depend on the severity of the disease. After delivery the platelet count remains low initially but will rapidly increase after the third postpartum day. Platelet counts greater than 600,000/mm^3 are not uncommon by the seventh or eighth day. An upward trend in platelet count and a downward trend in LDH should be apparent by the fourth postpartum day in patients recovering without complications.[58]

   Packed red cells are transfused if the hematocrit drops below 30%. This occurs frequently in early postpartum, mostly as a result of vasodilation, hemodilution, and blood loss during delivery, rather than further hemolysis.

3. These patients are often oliguric, and a central venous pressure (CVP) line is frequently necessary to properly monitor the administration of intravenous fluids. Subclavian lines are contraindicated in the preeclamptic patient with thrombocytopenia because of the high risk of internal bleeding and hemomediastinum. If a CVP line is inserted, it should be through an internal jugular or a peripheral vein.

BOX 10-7

Criteria for the Diagnosis of HELLP Syndrome

Hemolysis
Schistiocytes in the blood smear
Bilirubin $\geq$ 1.2 ml/dl
Absent plasma haptoglobin

Elevated liver enzymes
SGOT > 72 IU/L
LDH > 600 IU/L

Low platelet count
Platelets < 100 $\times$ 10^3/mm^3

4. For those patients who follow a relentless course of deterioration despite conventional therapy, plasmapheresis may be a life-saving measure.[59] Plasmapheresis has a dramatic effect on the course of the disease and accelerates the recovery period. The main risk of plasmapheresis is the potential for viral hepatitis.

Preeclampsia complicated by pulmonary edema. Pulmonary edema is a rather common complication of severe preeclampsia and eclampsia affecting approximately 3% of these patients.[60] Most new cases are the result of aggressive use of crystalloid solutions for intravascular volume expansion. In the Los Angeles County study,[50] pulmonary edema was the cause of death in 3 of 67 eclamptic patients. Usually death occurs in the postpartum period and is characterized by profound respiratory distress, severe hypoxemia, and diffuse rales on auscultation.

There are clinical differences between the pulmonary edema of organic heart disease and that of preeclampsia. Most cases of patients with preeclampsia occur in young women without previous histories of heart disease, with normal electrocardiograms, and without cardiomegaly on chest x-ray films or echocardiogram. Also, the course of the disease in the preeclamptic patient is characterized by its slow response to therapy. In most preeclamptic patients, pulmonary edema results from fluid overload and left ventricular failure. Pulse oximetry is valuable for monitoring preeclamptic patients with oliguria who are receiving large amounts of intravenous fluids because it may detect changes in oxygen saturation before the development of overt pulmonary edema.

To best understand the altered hemodynamics of pulmonary edema in preeclamptic patients, it is necessary to use a Swan-Ganz catheter. Benedetti et al.[61] found in 10 preeclamptic patients with pulmonary edema that 5 had elevated pulmonary wedge pressure and reduced plasma colloid osmotic pressure, 3 had capillary leak, and 2 had left ventricular failure. Therefore, if available, catheter insertion should be the first step in the management of these patients. If it is not feasible to insert a Swan-Ganz catheter, a CVP line should be used. However, CVP measurements are not as reliable as the pulmonary capillary wedge pressure (PCWP). The Swan-Ganz or CVP measurements will also be valuable in monitoring the effects of therapy.

If the PCWP is more than 20 mm Hg, pump failure and fluid overload are the major causes. In this case rapid digitalization and intravenous furosemide will be the cornerstones of treatment. If the PCWP is normal or below normal, capillary leakage of high-protein fluid into the alveoli is the cause of the problem. In this case the therapeutic priority should be to provide adequate respiratory support.

Antepartum pulmonary edema in preeclamptic patients is an indication for delivery. In the case of a patient with capillary leakage, the chances of maternal survival will depend primarily on the effect of delivery on the basic disease process. Delivery should be performed after hemodynamic stabilization to avoid the deleterious effects of the acute hemodynamic changes that occur during and after parturition.

Preeclampsia complicated by electrolyte imbalance. Electrolyte disturbances in the preeclamptic patient almost always result from salt restriction and concomitant use of diuretics. Hyponatremia and hyperkalemia are the alterations most commonly found.

Hyponatremia rarely becomes symptomatic or falls below 110 mEq/L in preeclamptic patients. However, the sodium deficit should be corrected, even if asymptomatic, to prevent postpartum circulatory collapse. To correct hyponatremia, the approximate total sodium deficit, usually around 300 to 500 mEq, can be calculated as in the following example:

Normal sodium concentration	140 mEq/L
Patient's sodium concentration	−129 mEq/L
CONCENTRATION DEFICIT	11 mEq/L
Total body water (approximately 60% of body weight in kilograms)	45 L
TOTAL SODIUM DEFICIT (45 × 11)	495 mEq

We usually administer enough sodium, in the form of 3% NaCl solution, to compensate for about 50% of the total deficit. Full correction should not be attempted. In the hypothetical case above, 500 ml of 3% NaCl, containing 256 mEq of sodium, will be given at a rate of 100 ml/hr. If the plasma sodium measured after the infusion is 135 mEq/L or more, there is no need for further hypertonic saline administration.

Hyperkalemia in these cases is usually not severe and rarely exceeds 5.5 mEq/L. In most cases it can be corrected by administration of 45 mEq of sodium bicarbonate in 1000 ml of D_5NS. This solution should be given parallel to and in a different IV line from the 3% NaCl solution, over a period of 3 to 4 hours.

Fear of circulatory overload with the use of 3% NaCl frequently leads the obstetrician to attempt sodium deficit correction using normal saline. This is inadequate to rapidly achieve electrolyte balance.

Preeclampsia complicated by postpartum circulatory collapse. Occasionally, patients with severe preeclampsia develop profound shock after vaginal delivery or, more commonly, after cesarean section. If this is not rapidly corrected, it may lead to acute tubular necrosis, panhypopituitarism (Sheehan's syndrome), and maternal death.

Postpartum circulatory collapse usually occurs within the first hour after cesarean section, but it may happen any time within the first 24 hours postpartum.[62] The patient with moderate or severe hypertension who was agitated and hyperactive before delivery becomes hypotensive, tachycardic, clammy, and pale, and her urinary output is minimal. There is a rapid respiratory rate, and the chest x-ray film may show diffuse bilateral infiltrates. Unfortunately, there is no adequate explanation for the events leading to this postpartum circulatory collapse. Electrolyte disturbances, particularly hyponatremia, was found in eight cases and hyperkalemia in two cases.[62] These findings are the basis for the recommendation of sodium and potassium level normalization in patients with severe preeclampsia before delivery.

Hypovolemia is another component of postpartum circulatory collapse. Patients with severe preeclampsia that have a normal hematocrit before delivery may develop postpartum hypovolemia despite a normal estimated blood loss intrapartum. The explanation for this is a combination of the following facts:

1. Antepartum hemoglobin and hematocrit in the preeclamptic patient are frequently normal as a result of hemoconcentration resulting from decreased plasma volume.
2. Since the total intravascular volume is markedly decreased in severe preeclampsia, the average blood loss during delivery corresponds to a significant proportion of the patient's blood volume.
3. In preeclamptic patients with a normal preoperative hematocrit and hemoglobin, operative blood loss is usually replaced with crystalloid solution, causing further hemodilution.

4. Some of the vasospasm existing before delivery subsides postpartum, making more intravascular space available for fluid mobilization causing further hemodilution.

The combination of these factors means that a preeclamptic patient with, for example, a preoperative hematocrit of 35% may have a postpartum hematocrit of 18% with signs and symptoms of cardiovascular collapse. It is also possible that other factors, such as pump failure and adrenal insufficiency, may play a role in the genesis of this problem.

The management of the preeclamptic patient who develops postpartum circulatory collapse is similar to the management of any obstetric patient in hypovolemic shock, which is described in detail in Chapter 9.

Preeclampsia complicated by acute renal failure. Oliguria is not uncommon in patients with moderate or severe preeclampsia. In most cases oliguria resolves after delivery, but in a few instances it may progress to anuria, acute tubular necrosis, bilateral cortical necrosis, and maternal death. In fact, 7 of the 67 maternal deaths related to toxemia in the Los Angeles County study were caused by renal failure.[50]

Renal complications are more common in preeclamptic patients with abruptio placentae.[63] Patients with preeclampsia frequently develop oliguria, but rarely develop severe renal damage. In contrast, severe renal disease is the predominant cause of maternal death in patients with abruption.

The most common situation occurs when patients with moderate or severe preeclampsia show decreased urinary output, less than 30 ml/hr intrapartum. Usually this can be corrected, at least temporarily, by increasing the rate of intravenous fluid administration. Occasionally, however, patients do not respond to this treatment, and the oliguria becomes more marked. If the patient seems to be remote from delivery, pregnancy should be terminated by cesarean section. Operative delivery is usually quickly followed by improvement of the urinary output, most likely a result of decreased vasospasm and increased renal blood flow after loss of the placental circulation and redistribution of the cardiac output. If the patient is close to vaginal delivery, we maintain intravenous fluids at approximately 150 ml/hr and give 10 to 20 mg of furosemide. This usually results in adequate urinary output for 2 or 3 hours, which often is enough time for the patient to deliver vaginally. Once the patient delivers, urinary output usually continues within normal limits without additional diuretic therapy.

Making the decision of whether to proceed with cesarean section or to treat with intravenous fluids and diuretics when managing these patients is not easy. Both treatments have potential for fetal and maternal problems. However, reestablishment of adequate urinary output is an important priority. The longer the low output persists, the greater the possibility that the patient will develop severe or irreversible renal damage. We prefer furosemide to mannitol because the capillary damage in the severe preeclamptic patient negates the intravascular osmotic effect of mannitol, thus making its response unpredictable.

Clark et al.[64] have described three hemodynamic subsets in preeclamptic patients with acute oliguria. The first and largest group has low pulmonary capillary wedge pressure and moderately elevated systemic vascular resistance. These patients respond to volume expansion. The second group has normal wedge pressure and elevated systemic vascular resistance and requires treatment with vasodilators. The third subset is made of patients with elevated wedge pressure and decreased cardiac output. These patients require volume restriction to avoid pulmonary edema and aggressive afterload reduction.

The management of the patient with preeclampsia complicated by abruptio placentae and anuria is identical to the management of the obstetric patient in acute renal failure, as described in Chapter 14.

The remote prognosis of properly managed acute renal failure in patients with preeclampsia is good, and most patients have normal renal function on long-term follow-up.[63]

Preeclampsia complicated by hepatic rupture. The liver is involved in the multiple organ failure that characterizes severe preeclampsia.[48] In the majority of cases, this involvement is shown by elevations of SGOT, SGPT, and LDH. There are a few cases, however, with hepatic disorder that culminate in hepatic rupture. In the Los Angeles County series, hepatic involvement was the cause of death in 10 of 67 maternal deaths related to eclampsia.[50]

The majority of preeclamptic patients with hepatic involvement complain of epigastric or right upper quadrant pain several days before the onset of more serious symptoms. The pain is frequently disregarded or is confused with a minor gastrointestinal ailment. Some patients develop mild jaundice and are frequently diagnosed as having hepatitis or gallstones until worsening of the disease clearly demonstrates the presence of preeclampsia.

Hepatic rupture may occur antepartum or postpartum, and in both cases the signs and symptoms are those of profound circulatory collapse. The signs of peritoneal irritation and the progressive hypovolemia will point to intraabdominal bleeding as the cause of the problem. If the patient has not delivered, the pregnancy must be terminated immediately. At the time of the laparotomy, the laceration is almost always found on the diaphragmatic aspect of the right lobe. It frequently coexists with subcapsular petechiae and subcapsular hematomas.

The prognosis for preeclamptic patients with liver rupture is ominous. Attempts at surgical repair or excision are usually followed by extension of the laceration, more bleeding, consumption coagulopathy, and ultimately death. In these cases the least manipulation of the hepatic tissue will be rewarded with the best results. The bleeding hepatic surface should be covered with microfibrillar collagen hemostat (Avitene), oxidized cellulose (Oxycel), or absorbable gelatin (Gelfoam) and then packed with surgical sponges placed above the hemostatic agent. One of the sponges is brought outside throughout the abdominal incision to facilitate removal on the second or third postoperative day.

The success of this simple treatment has to do with the nature of the lesion causing the hepatic rupture. In traumatic liver rupture, the parenchyma is healthy, and surgical approximation of the tear may be carried out without provoking additional bleeding. However, in preeclampsia, as illustrated by Sheehan and Lynch,[65] the hepatic tissue is diffusely affected by a hemorrhagic process starting as periportal bleeding, continuing with the formation of hematomas, and terminating as capsular rupture. Any suture placed on this friable tissue will cause further bleeding and disruption.

Preeclampsia complicated by abruptio placentae. About 7% of all patients with eclampsia will have premature separation of the placenta. Abruption is often an unexpected finding at the time of delivery. The management of abruptio placentae in preeclamptic patients is no different than that under other circumstances and is described in Chapter 9.

Preeclampsia complicated by cerebral hemorrhage. Intracranial bleeding is the leading cause of death in patients with preeclampsia. In the Los Angeles County series, 21 of 67 (31%) maternal deaths related to eclampsia were caused by cerebral hemorrhage.[50] Underestimation of the severity of the disease, extended treatment as outpatients, failure to use antihypertensive drugs to treat extreme elevations of blood pressure, and discharge from the hospital before obtaining adequate control of the hypertension were the most frequent errors found in the analysis of those deaths.

In the majority of cases, the preeclamptic patient with intracranial bleeding is admitted to the hospital in coma after the onset of headaches and convulsions at home. The diagnosis is suggested by deepening stupor and sensorimotor deficits and becomes highly probable if focal neurologic signs, such as unilateral pupil dilation, are present. The diagnosis is confirmed by computerized axial tomography (CAT) scan. The prognosis is very poor, and recovery is the exception rather than the rule. In most cases coma becomes more profound, respiratory paralysis appears, and finally, the electroencephalogram shows loss of electrical activity.

Severe occipital and temporal headaches are important symptoms in pregnant patients because they are frequently harbingers of convulsions. These headaches are usually caused by inadequate blood pressure control, and they are an indication for aggressive treatment with hypotensive agents.

Preeclampsia complicated by visual disturbances. Blindness may occur in patients with severe preeclampsia and eclampsia and may persist for several days, although quick recovery after delivery is the rule. In most cases examination of the eyegrounds does not show severe retinopathy, since the problem usually is caused by multiple microhemorrhages and microinfarcts occurring in the occipital lobes. Cortical blindness is equivalent to a seizure, and patients with this symptom should be treated as having eclampsia.

The funduscopic examination of patients with preeclampsia usually does not reveal more than focal or generalized vasospasm and, in some cases, retinal edema, which frequently is missed in the examination because it begins in the periphery of the retina. Papilledema in these patients is highly unusual and demands a reevaluation to rule out the possibility of an intracranial tumor or bleeding. Diplopia is a symptom that may occur and is caused by functional impairment of the sixth cranial nerve pair. In some rare cases it is possible to find sixth nerve paralysis. This finding requires a CAT scan to rule out a tumor in the brainstem area. Like most lesions caused by preeclampsia, sixth nerve paralysis improves after delivery and eventually disappears several weeks later.

◼ LONG-TERM PROGNOSIS OF PREECLAMPSIA AND ECLAMPSIA

Frequently, preeclamptic patients ask about the prognosis for future pregnancies, about the possibility of developing chronic hypertension, and about the risk of developing hypertension if oral contraceptives are used for family planning.

When counseling primiparous women who have had preeclampsia, the obstetrician commonly is reassuring and tells the patients that preeclampsia is a disease of the first pregnancy that rarely recurs in future gestations. This counseling, based on old literature on the subject, is incorrect. In fact, data collected by Sibai[65a] show that the probability of recurrence in a future pregnancy is approximately 30% and that the probability changes according to the gestational age at which the patient developed the disease. If the patient had it at term, the chance of recurrence in a future pregnancy will be 25%. If the onset was between 30 and 37 weeks, the recurrence rate is 40%, but if preeclampsia developed before 30 weeks of gestation, the chances of recurrence are approximately 65%.

According to Sibai,[65a] the risk of developing mild preeclampsia in a second pregnancy when the first pregnancy was complicated by eclampsia is 19.5%, the chance of developing severe preeclampsia is 25.9%, and the risk of recurrence of eclampsia is 1.4%. Chesley[66] has periodically reexamined women with eclampsia for periods up to 44 years and compared their subsequent reproductive performance and their development of chronic hypertension with control women matched by race and age. He found that 33.8% of 151 women having eclampsia as nulliparas developed hypertension in later pregnancies. In about 40% of these cases, hypertension was mild. He also found that 50% of women with preeclampsia as multiparas developed hypertension in later pregnancies.

Chesley also found some factors useful in predicting the probability of recurrence of pre-eclampsia in nulliparous patients who had eclampsia:

1. If hypertension is still present on the tenth postpartum day, the probability of recurrence is 59%, compared to 21% in women whose blood pressures are back to normal at that time (p < 0.001).
2. If the weight of the patient in pounds divided by the height in inches is 2.2 or greater 6 weeks after delivery, the recurrence rate of preeclampsia will be 70%, compared with 27% for thinner women (p < 0.01).
3. If the onset of eclampsia was before 36 weeks, the chances of recurrence are 56%, compared with 27% if eclampsia was of late onset (p < 0.01).
4. If the average systolic pressure was greater than 160 mm Hg during eclampsia, the probability of recurrence is 46%, compared with 27% in patients with lower pressures (p < 0.01).

Chesley also found that the likelihood of recurrence of preeclampsia increases with the number of adverse factors. The chances of recurrence will be 25% for patients with one factor, 56% for patients with two factors, and 78% for patients with three or four factors.

With respect to the ultimate development of chronic hypertension, Chesley demonstrated that women who have eclampsia as nulliparas do not develop chronic hypertension more frequently than do normal control subjects. In contrast, women who have eclampsia as multiparas will have a higher prevalence of hypertension later in life than will normotensive control subjects. He found that multiparous patients who develop eclampsia have a higher incidence of hypertension in later life, an increased annual death rate, and a greater proportion of cardiovascular deaths than nulliparous patients with eclampsia.

The question about the risk of developing hypertension when oral contraceptives are used by women who had preeclampsia was answered by Pritchard and Pritchard.[67] They compared the incidence of hypertension in 200 nulligravid women and in 180 primiparous women who recently had preeclampsia while they were taking mestranol, 50 μg, plus norethindrone, 1 mg, for family planning purposes. He found that nine of the prior preeclamptic women and five of the control group developed diastolic blood pressures exceeding 90 mm Hg during the initial 3 months of oral contraceptive use. After the first 3 months, the incidence of diastolic blood pressure elevation was similar for both groups. Interestingly enough, the absence of hypertension while using oral contraceptives did not preclude the subsequent development of hypertension during pregnancy in women from both groups. These results suggest that if hypertension occurs during the first pregnancy and reappears during the first 3 months of oral contraceptive use, the patient most likely has chronic vascular disease. These investigators also concluded that the frequency and severity of oral contraceptive hypertension are not large enough to preclude the use of this medication in women who have had preeclampsia during their first pregnancies.

◢ PREVENTION OF PREECLAMPSIA
Low-dose aspirin

There is substantial evidence indicating that an imbalance in the production of thromboxane A_2 and prostacyclin is an essential feature in the pathophysiology of preeclampsia.[68] Thromboxane A_2 is produced primarily by the platelets and is a powerful vasoconstrictor and promoter of platelet aggregation. Prostacyclin is produced in the vascular endothelium, is a powerful vasodilator, and inhibits platelet aggregation. In preeclamptic patients prostacyclin synthesis is decreased, and thromboxane production is increased, leading to vasoconstriction and platelet aggregation.

Prostacyclin and thromboxane are products of arachidonic acid metabolism by the enzyme cyclooxygenase, which is irreversibly inhibited by aspirin. Selective inhibition of platelet cyclooxygenase should decrease thromboxane production and restore the balance between these antagonistic substances. Platelets cannot synthesize proteins *de novo*, and restoration of their cyclooxygenase activity after treatment with aspirin requires the production of new cells by the bone marrow. In contrast, endothelial cells can rapidly regenerate cyclooxygenase activity after aspirin treatment. Therefore the net effect of low-dose aspirin is a selective inhibition of platelet thromboxane production. This mechanism is the basis for attempts to prevent the development of preeclampsia with low-dose aspirin.

Six randomized trials of low-dose aspirin to prevent preeclampsia have been published.[69-74] A seventh trial had as end point the prevention of growth retardation.[75] All these trials have demonstrated that low-dose aspirin reduces the risk of preeclampsia and results in longer gestations and increased birth weights, without major side effects in the mother or newborn. A recent metaanalysis of the first six controlled trials[76] reached a similar conclusion. Unless larger randomized trials now in progress produce different results, low-dose aspirin (60 to 150 mg daily) seems to be effective in preventing preeclampsia and should be used in patients at risk for this disease.

Calcium

The literature suggests that dietary calcium supplementation may be effective in preventing the development of preeclampsia. In one study normal pregnant women receiving 2 g of calcium daily after 15 weeks of gestation had significantly lower blood pressure values than control subjects.[77] In another study daily administration of 600 mg of calcium decreased vascular sensitivity and reduced the incidence of preeclampsia from 21.2% in nonsupplemented patients to 4.5% in those patients who took calcium.[78] Other investigators have found similar decreases in the incidence of preeclampsia, from 28.2% in the placebo group to 6.5% in the calcium-supplemented group, using 2 g of calcium daily beginning at 24 weeks.[79] These results are encouraging, and more investigation in this area is necessary.

◪ IMPORTANT POINTS ◪

1. According to the ISSHP, the diagnosis of hypertension in pregnancy is made by either of the following criteria: (1) one measurement of diastolic blood pressure equal to or greater than 110 mm Hg or (2) two consecutive measurements of diastolic blood pressure equal to or greater than 90 mm Hg, 4 or more hours apart.

2. Korotkoff's sound IV, the point of muffling, should be used when measuring blood pressure during pregnancy. Measurements should be taken with the woman sitting with the right arm supported on a table or desk in a roughly horizontal position at heart level.

3. The exact nature of the primary event causing preeclampsia is not known. However, evidence indicates that abnormal placentation is one of the initial events in this disease. Abnormal placentation eventually will cause altered endothelial cell function and multiple organ damage.

4. Recent studies suggest that an increase in maternal cardiac output rather than increased peripheral vascular resistance is the most frequent hemodynamic finding in preeclampsia. The elevation in cardiac output in patients with preeclampsia may start as early as 11 weeks and remain in the puerperium despite resolution of the hypertension.

5. Only 75% of nulliparous patients with hypertension in pregnancy show typical lesions of preeclampsia in kidney biopsy specimens. Chronic renal lesions are found in 16%, and 7.6% show both preeclampsia and chronic renal disease. The same study in multiparous women shows chronic renal disease in 51%, preeclampsia in 23%, renal disease plus preeclampsia in 13%, and normal histology in 11%.

6. Endothelium-originated plasma fibronectin and urinary calcium creatinine ratio may be useful in predicting the development of preeclampsia.

7. Preeclamptic patients with positive D-dimer, a peptide derived specifically from degradation of fibrin, have a more severe form of the disease than those with a negative test.

8. Labetalol, nifedipine, and verapamil are three antihypertensive agents useful in the treatment of patients with preeclampsia.

9. Maternal morbidity is severe, and perinatal mortality is greater than 90% when conservative management is adopted for patients with severe preeclampsia developing before 24 weeks. In these patients expectancy is not justified, and delivery is the treatment of choice.

10. In selected patients with severe preeclampsia between 24 and 34 weeks, prolongation of pregnancy is advantageous for the fetus and not extremely dangerous for the mother. This plan of management should be undertaken exclusively in tertiary centers.

11. Fetal surveillance in the second trimester is difficult. The NST is nonreactive, and fetal breathing movements are not present. Fetal health is demonstrated by the presence of variability and the absence of FHR decelerations. The maximum possible biophysical profile score is 6.

12. Eclampsia is associated with elevated maternal and fetal mortality and morbidity. The most common causes of maternal death are intracranial bleeding and acute renal failure. The most common causes of fetal death are prematurity and fetal asphyxia.

13. Eclampsia is not preventable by adequate prenatal care in more than 30% of the cases.

14. Plasmapheresis may be life-saving for those preeclamptic patients with HELLP syndrome that follow a relentless course of deterioration after delivery.

15. Pulse oximetry is valuable in the monitoring of preeclamptic patients with oliguria receiving large amounts of intravenous fluids because it may detect changes in oxygen saturation that occur before the development of overt pulmonary edema.

16. Invasive hemodynamic monitoring is valuable in the management of preeclamptic patients with severe oliguria because it may differentiate three subsets of patients requiring different therapies.

17. Intracranial bleeding is the leading cause of maternal death in preeclampsia. Underestimation of the severity of the disease, extended treatment as outpatients, failure to use antihypertensive drugs, and discharge from the hospital before obtaining adequate control of the hypertension are frequent errors in the management of these patients.

18. Six randomized trials have reached similar conclusions: Low-dose aspirin reduces the risk of preeclampsia, prolongs gestation, and increases birth weight without major side effects in the mother and newborn.

19. Dietary supplementation with 2 g of calcium daily after 15 weeks of gestation has been shown to decrease the incidence of preeclampsia.

REFERENCES

1. Chesley LC: *Hypertensive Disorders in Pregnancy.* New York, Appleton-Century Crofts, 1978, p 2.
2. Davey DA, MacGillivray I: The classification and definition of the hypertensive disorders of pregnancy. *Am J Obstet Gynecol* 1988;158:892-898.
3. Sibai BM: Pitfalls in diagnosis and management of preeclampsia. *Am J Obstet Gynecol* 1988;159:1-5.
4. Brosens IA: Morphologic changes in the uteroplacental bed in pregnancy hypertension. *Clin Obstet Gynecol* 1977;77:573-593.
5. Robertson WB, Khong TY, Brosens IA, et al: The placental bed biopsy: review from three European centers. *Am J Obstet Gynecol* 1986;155:401-412.
6. Kaar K, Joupplia P, Kuikka J, et al: Intervillous blood flow in normal and complicated late pregnancy measured by means of an intravenous Xe method. *Acta Obstet Gynecol Scand* 1980;59:7-11.
7. Roberts JM, Taylor RN, Musci TJ, et al: Preeclampsia: An endothelial cell disorder. *Am J Obstet Gynecol* 1989;161:1200-1204.
8. Shanklin DR, Sibai BM: Ultrastructural aspects of preeclampsia. I. Placental bed and uterine boundary vessels. *Am J Obstet Gynecol* 1989;161:735-741.
9. Rodgers GM, Taylor RN, Roberts JM: Preeclampsia is associated with a serum factor cytotoxic to human endothelial cells. *Am J Obstet Gynecol* 1988;159:908-914.
10. Taylor RN, Heilbron DC, Roberts JM: Growth factor activity in the blood of women in whom preeclampsia is elevated from early pregnancy. *Am J Obstet Gynecol* 1990;163:1839-1844.
11. Stubbs TM, Lazarchick J, Horger EO: Plasma fibronectin levels in preeclampsia: A possible biochemical marker for vascular endothelial damage. *Am J Obstet Gynecol* 1984;150:885-887.
12. Lockwood CJ, Peters JH: Increased plasma levels of EDI$^+$ cellular fibronectin precede the clinical signs of preeclampsia. *Am J Obstet Gynecol* 1990;162:358-362.
13. Easterling TR, Benedetti TJ, Schmucker BC et al: Maternal hemodynamics in normal and preeclamptic pregnancies: A longitudinal study. *Obstet Gynecol* 1990;76:1061'1069.
14. Clark SL, Cotton DB, Lee W, et al: Central hemodynamic assessment of normal term pregnancy. *Am J Obstet Gynecol* 1989;161:1439-1442.
15. Pickles CJ, Brinkman CR, Stainer K, et al: Changes in peripheral venous tone before the onset of hypertension in women with gestational hypertension. *Am J Obstet Gynecol* 1989;160:678.
16. Talledo OE, Chesley LC, Zuspan FP: Renin-angiotensin system in normal and toxemic pregnancies. III. Differential sensitivity to angiotensin II and norepinephrine in toxemia of pregnancy. *Am J Obstet Gynecol* 1969;100:218.
17. Gant NF, Daley GL, Chand S: A study of angiotensin II pressor response throughout primigravid pregnancy. *J Clin Invest* 1973;52:2684.
18. Gant NF, Whalley P, Chand S, et al: A prospective study of angiotensin II pressor responsiveness in pregnancies complicated by chronic essential hypertension. *Am J Obstet Gynecol* 1977;127:369.

19. Pritchard JA, Cunningham FG, Mason RA: Coagulation changes in eclampsia: Their frequency and pathogenesis. *Am J Obstet Gynecol* 1976;124:855.
20. Weinstein L: Syndrome of hemolysis, elevated liver enzymes, and low platelet count: A severe consequence of hypertension in pregnancy. *Am J Obstet Gynecol* 1982;142:159-167.
21. Spargo B, McCartney CP, Winemiller R: Glomerular capillary endotheliosis in toxemia of pregnancy. *Arch Pathol* 1959;68:593.
22. Arias F, Mancilla-Jimenez R: Hepatic fibrinogen deposits in preeclampsia: Immunofluorescent evidence. *N Engl J Med* 1986;295:578.
23. Fisher KA, Luger A, Spargo BH, et al: A biopsy study of hypertension in pregnancy, in Bonnar J, McGillivray I, Symmonds EM (eds): *Pregnancy Hypertension*. Baltimore, University Park Press, 1980, pp 333-336.
24. Ihle BU, Long P, Oats J: Early onset preeclampsia: recognition of underlying renal disease. *Br Med J* 1987;294:79-81.
25. Gant NF, Chand S, Whorley RJ, et al: A clinical test useful for predicting the development of acute hypertension in pregnancy. *Am J Obstet Gynecol* 1974;120:1.
26. Page EW, Christianson R: The importance of mean arterial pressure in the middle trimester upon the outcome of pregnancy. *Am J Obstet Gynecol* 1976;125:740.
27. Chesley LC, Sibai MB: Clinical significance of elevated blood arterial pressure in the second trimester. *Am J Obstet Gynecol* 1988;159:275-279.
28. Taufield PA, Ales KL, Resnick LM, et al: Hypocalciuria in preeclampsia. *N Engl J Med* 1987;316:715-718.
29. Huikeshoven FJM, Quijderhoudt FMJ: Hypocalciuria in hypertensive disorder in pregnancy and how to measure it. *Eur J Obstet Gynecol Reprod Biol* 1990;36:81-85.
30. Sanchez-Ramos L, Sandioni S, Andren FJ, et al: Calcium excretion in preeclampsia. *Obstet Gynecol* 1991;77:510-513.
31. Sanchez-Ramos L, Jones DC, Cullen MT: Urinary calcium as an early marker for preeclampsia. *Obstet Gynecol* 1991;77:685-688.
32. Campbell S, Pearce JMF, Hackett G, et al: Qualitative assessment of uteroplacental blood flow: Early screening test for high-risk pregnancies. *Obstet Gynecol* 1986;68:649.
33. Sibai BM, Anderson GD, McCubbin JH: Eclampsia: II. Clinical significance of laboratory findings. *Obstet Gynecol* 1982;59:163.
34. Hill LM: Metabolism of uric acid in normal and toxemic pregnancy. *Mayo Clin Proc* 1978;53:743.
35. Pritchard JA, Cunningham FG, Mason RA: Coagulation changes in eclampsia: Their frequency and pathogenesis. *Am J Obstet Gynecol* 1976;124:855.
36. Trofatter KF, Howell ML, Greenberg CS, et al: The use of the fibrin D-dimer in screening for coagulation abnormalities in preeclampsia. *Obstet Gynecol* 1989;73:435.
37. Ducey J, Schulman H, Farmakides G, et al: A classification of hypertension in pregnancy based on Doppler velocimetry. *Am J Obstet Gynecol* 1987;157:680.
38. Sibai BM: Magnesium sulfate is the ideal anticonvulsant in preeclampsia-eclampsia. *Am J Obstet Gynecol* 1990;162:1141-1145.
39. Pritchard JA, Pritchard SA: Standardized treatment of 154 consecutive cases of eclampsia. *Am J Obstet Gynecol* 1975;123:543.
40. Zuspan FP, Ward MC: Improved fetal salvage in eclampsia. *Obstet Gynecol* 1965;26:893.
41. Sibai BM, Graham JM, McCubbin JH: A comparison of intravenous and intramuscular magnesium sulfate regimens in preeclampsia. *Am J Obstet Gynecol* 1984;150:728-733.
42. Pritchard JA: Management of severe preeclampsia and eclampsia. *Semin Perinatol* 1978;2:83.
42a. Slater RM, Wilcox FL, Smith WD, et al: Phenytoin infusion in severe pre-eclampsia. *Lancet* 1987;1:1417-1421.
43. Donaldson JO: *Neurology of Pregnancy*. Philadelphia, WB Saunders Co, 1987, p 216.
44. Henrich WL, Cronin R, Miller PD, et al: Hypotensive sequelae of diazoxide and hydralazine therapy. *JAMA* 1977;237:264.
45. Sibai BM, Taslimi M, Abdella TN, et al: Maternal and perinatal outcome of conservative management of severe preeclampsia in midtrimester. *Am J Obstet Gynecol* 1985;152:32-37.
46. Odendaal HJ, Pattinson RC, DeToit R: Fetal and neonatal outcome in patients with severe pre-eclampsia before 34 weeks. *S Afr Med J* 1987;71:555-558.
47. Pattinson RC, Odendaal HJ, DuToit R: Conservative management of severe proteinuric hypertension before 28 weeks' gestation. *S Afr Med J* 1988;73:516-518.
48. Sibai BM, Akl Sherif, Fairlie F, et al: A protocol for managing severe preeclampsia in the second trimester. *Am J Obstet Gynecol* 1990;163:733-738.
49. Odendaal HJ, Pattinson RC, Bam R, et al: Aggressive or expectant management for patients with severe preeclampsia between 28-34 weeks' gestation: A randomized controlled trial. *Obstet Gynecol* 1990;76:1070-1075.
50. Hibbard LT: Maternal mortality due to acute toxemia. *Obstet Gynecol* 1983;42:263.
51. Gant NF, Madden JD, Siiteri PK, et al: The metabolic clearance rate of dehydroisoandrosterone sulfate. *Am J Obstet Gynecol* 1985;123:159.
52. Sibai BM, McCubbin JA, Anderson GD, et al: Eclampsia: I. Observations from 67 recent cases. *Obstet Gynecol* 1981;58:609.
53. Horn EH, Filshie M, Kerslake RW, et al: Widespread cerebral ischemia treated with nimodipine in a patient with eclampsia. *Br Med J* 1990;301:794.
54. Sibai BM, Anderson GD, Abdella TN, et al: Eclampsia: III. Neonatal outcome, growth and development. *Am J Obstet Gynecol* 1983;146:307.
55. Sibai BM, Abdella TN, Spinnato JA, et al: Eclampsia: IV. The incidence of nonpreventable eclampsia. *Am J Obstet Gynecol* 1986;154:581-586.
56. Sibai BM, Spinnato JA, Watson DL, et al: Eclampsia: IV. Neurologic findings and future outcome. *Am J Obstet Gynecol* 1985;152:184-192.
57. Sibai BM: The HELLP syndrome (hemolysis, elevated liver enzymes, and low platelets): Much ado about nothing? *Am J Obstet Gynecol* 1990;162:311-316.
58. Martin JN, Blake PG, Perry KG, et al: The natural history of HELLP syndrome: Patterns of disease progression and regression. *Am J Obstet Gynecol* 1991;164:1500-1513.
59. Martin JN, Files JC, Blake PG, et al: Plasma exchange for preeclampsia: I. Postpartum use for persistently severe preeclampsia-eclampsia with HELLP syndrome. *Am J Obstet Gynecol* 1990;152:126-137.

60. Sibai BM, Mabie BC, Harvey CJ, et al: Pulmonary edema in severe preeclampsia-eclampsia: Analysis of thirty-seven consecutive cases. *Am J Obstet Gynecol* 1987;156:1174-1179.

61. Benedetti TJ, Kates R, Williams V: Hemodynamic observations in severe preeclampsia complicated by pulmonary edema. *Am J Obstet Gynecol* 1985;152:330-334.

62. Tatum HJ, Mule JG: Puerperal vasomotor collapse in patients with toxemia of pregnancy: A new concept of the etiology and a rational plan of treatment. *Am J Obstet Gynecol* 1956;71:492.

63. Sibai BM, Villar MA, Mabie BC: Acute renal failure in hypertensive disorders of pregnancy: Pregnancy outcome and remote prognosis in thirty-one consecutive cases. *Am J Obstet Gynecol* 1990;162:777-783.

64. Clark SL, Greenspoon JS, Aldahl D, et al: Severe preeclampsia with persistent oliguria: Management of hemodynamic subsets. *Am J Obstet Gynecol* 1986;154:490-494.

65. Sheehan HL, Lynch JB: *Pathology of Toxemia in Pregnancy.* Edinburgh, Churchill Livingstone, 1973, pp 328-490.

65a. Sibai BM, Mercer B, Sarinoglu C: Severe preeclampsia in the second trimester: Recurrence risk and long-term prognosis. *Am J Obstet Gynecol* 1991;165:1408-1412.

66. Chesley LC: Eclampsia: The remote prognosis. *Semin Perinatol* 1978;2:99.

67. Pritchard JA, Pritchard SA: Blood pressure response to estrogen-progestin oral contraceptive after pregnancy-induced hypertension. *Am J Obstet Gynecol* 1977;129:733.

68. Walsh WS: Preeclampsia: An imbalance in placental prostacyclin and thromboxane production. *Am J Obstet Gynecol* 1985;152:335-340.

69. Beaufils M, Uzan S, Donsimoni R, et al: Prevention of preeclampsia by early antiplatelet therapy. *Lancet* 1985;1:840-842.

70. Wallenburg HCS, Dekker GA, Makovitz JW, et al: Low-dose aspirin prevents pregnancy-induced hypertension and preeclampsia in angiotensin-sensitive primigravidae. *Lancet* 1986;1:1-3.

71. Schiff E, Peleg E, Goldenberg M, et al: The use of aspirin to prevent pregnancy-induced hypertension and lower the ratio of thromboxane A_2 to prostacyclin in relatively high-risk pregnancy. *N Engl J Med* 1989;321:351-356.

72. Benigni A, Gregorini G, Frasca T, et al: Effect of low-dose aspirin in fetal and maternal generation of thromboxane by platelets in women at risk for pregnancy-induced hypertension. *N Engl J Med* 1989;321:357-362.

73. McFarland P, Pearce JM, Chamberlain GVP: Doppler ultrasound and aspirin recognition and prevention of pregnancy-induced hypertension. *Lancet* 1990;335:1522-1555.

74. Sureau C: Prevention of perinatal consequences of preeclampsia with low-dose aspirin: Results of the Epreda trial. *Eur J Obstet Gynecol Reprod Biol* 1991;41:71-73.

75. Wallenburg HC, Rotmans N: Prevention of recurrent idiopathic fetal growth retardation by low-dose aspirin and dipyridamole. *Am J Obstet Gynecol* 1987;157:1230-1235.

76. Imperials TF, Petrulis AS: A meta-analysis of low-dose aspirin for the prevention of pregnancy-induced hypertensive disease. *JAMA* 1991;266:261-265.

77. Belizan JM, Villar J, Zalazar A, et al: Preliminary evidence of the effect of calcium supplementation on blood pressure in normal pregnant women. *Am J Obstet Gynecol* 1985;153:576-582.

78. Kawasaki N, Matsui K, Ito M, et al: Effects of calcium supplementation on the vascular sensitivity to angiotensin II in pregnant women. *Am J Obstet Gynecol* 1985;153:576-582.

79. Lopez-Jaramillo P, Narvaez M, Yepes R: Letter to the editors: Effect of calcium supplementation on the vascular sensitivity to angiotensin II in pregnant women. *Am J Obstet Gynecol* 1987;156:261-262.

PART THREE

Medical Disorders Affecting Pregnancy

11

CARDIAC DISEASE AND PREGNANCY

In the United States pregnancy complicated by maternal cardiac disease is relatively rare. This is largely because of a significant decrease in the occurrence of rheumatic fever and rheumatic heart disease in the last 40 years.[1,2] The overall incidence is about 1%, with figures ranging from 0.2% to 3.7% in the literature.[3,4]

For all practical purposes, the medical management of the pregnant cardiac patient is controlled by the cardiologist or the internist. The obstetrician, however, should have adequate information about cardiac diseases during pregnancy so that he or she can function effectively as a member of the team that will be taking care of the patient. Also, the obstetrician should be able to diagnose and in many cases initiate the management of some of the medical complications that may affect the pregnant patient with heart disease. Finally, the obstetrician should be able to recognize some of the cardiac problems that may occur during an otherwise uncomplicated pregnancy before consultation with the internist or cardiologist. To accomplish these functions, one should be familiar with the following topics that are discussed in this chapter:

1. Hemodynamic changes occurring during pregnancy

2. Effects of pregnancy on maternal cardiac disease
3. Effects of maternal cardiac disease on pregnancy
4. General measures for the care of pregnant patients with heart disease
5. Management of acute congestive heart failure during pregnancy
6. Management of acute pulmonary edema during pregnancy
7. Maternal cardiac arrhythmias during pregnancy
8. Mitral valve prolapse during pregnancy
9. Peripartum cardiomyopathy
10. Other cardiac problems of significance during pregnancy

◪ HEMODYNAMIC CHANGES DURING PREGNANCY

Pregnancy causes significant changes in cardiovascular physiology. One of the most important studies describing the normal hemodynamic changes of pregnancy is that of Clark et al.[5] They studied 10 healthy, primiparous patients between 36 and 38 weeks of gestation and between 11 and 13 weeks postpartum using pulmonary artery catheterization. They found that the

TABLE 11-1 ◪ Hemodynamic changes in normal pregnancy

	Nonpregnant	Pregnant
Cardiac output (L/min)	4.3 ± 0.9	6.2 ± 1.0
Heart rate (bpm)	71 ± 10.0	83 ± 10.0
Systemic vascular resistance (dyne - cm - sec^{-5})	1530 ± 520	1210 ± 266
Pulmonary vascular resistance (dyne - cm - sec^{-5})	119 ± 47.0	78 ± 22
Colloid oncotic pressure (mm Hg)	20.8 ± 1.0	18.0 ± 1.5
Colloid oncotic pressure–pulmonary capillary wedge pressure (mm Hg)	14.5 ± 2.5	10.5 ± 2.7
Mean arterial pressure (mm Hg)	86.4 ± 7.5	90.3 ± 5.8
Pulmonary capillary wedge pressure (mm Hg)	6.3 ± 2.1	7.5 ± 1.8
Central venous pressure (mm Hg)	3.7 ± 2.6	3.6 ± 2.5
Left ventricular stroke	41 ± 8	48 ± 6

From Clark SL, Cotton DB, Lee W, et al: *Am J Obstet Gynecol* 1989;161:1439-1442.

main changes in the pregnant status were (1) decreased peripheral vascular resistance, (2) decreased pulmonary vascular resistance, (3) decreased colloid oncotic pressure, (4) increased cardiac output, and (5) increased pulse rate (Table 11-1). The most important points to remember are that in normal pregnant patients circulation is hyperdynamic and that a high cardiac output is present.

The increase in cardiac output starts about 10 weeks into the pregnancy, reaches a maximum at about 24 to 28 weeks, and remains elevated until parturition (Figure 11-1). The rise in cardiac output is initially determined by an increase in stroke volume. Later, as pregnancy advances, there is an increase in heart rate of 10 to 15 beats per minute (bpm) that will contribute to this change.

The cardiac output during pregnancy is markedly sensitive to maternal positional changes.[6] Both echocardiographic and hemodynamic studies have demonstrated a significant decrease in cardiac output when the mother lies in the supine position. This phenomenon, which is usually observed after 24 weeks, is caused by compression of the vena cava by the pregnant uterus and a decrease in the venous return to the heart.

An increase in intravascular volume is one of the main determinants of the increased cardiac output of pregnancy. There is an increase in both red cell volume and plasma volume.[7] This increase starts at about 8 weeks of gestation and reaches a maximum at 32 to 36 weeks. In the third trimester the intravascular volume (IV vol-

ume) has increased by approximately 50% in a singleton pregnancy, reaching a mean value of approximately 85 ml/kg. The increase in IV volume is even greater in multifetal gestations. The plasma volume increases first, and then, to a lesser degree, the red cell volume increases causing a *physiologic hemodilution* during the midtrimester of pregnancy (Figure 11-1).

A good clinical marker of the presence of an expanded IV volume during pregnancy is the presence of a grade 2/6 systolic ejection murmur on auscultation of the heart. This physiologic murmur appears at about 10 to 12 weeks into the pregnancy and disappears in the beginning of the postpartum period. Patients who do not expand their IV volumes during pregnancy (i.e., some patients with hypertension and pregnancy) do not have this murmur.

The increase in IV volume fulfills the needs of the developing uteroplacental circulation and protects the mother against the potentially harmful effects of the blood loss that occurs at parturition. The increase in blood volume of pregnancy does not alter the central venous pressure (CVP), which is the same as in the nonpregnant situation.

Another important hemodynamic change in pregnancy is decreased peripheral vascular resistance (PVR). PVR decreases during pregnancy on the arterial side and the venous side of the circulation. The cause of this change is not well understood, but it is most likely a direct effect of placental hormones or vasodilator prostaglandins (prostacyclin) on the blood vessels.

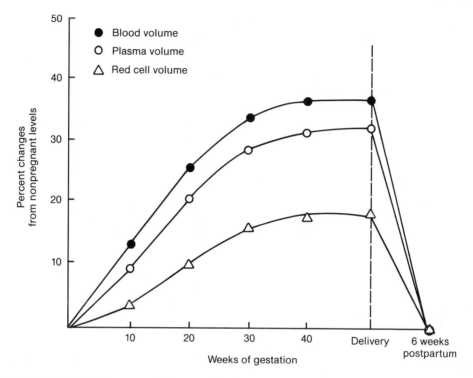

FIGURE 11-1 ◪ Expansion of plasma and red cell volume and increase in cardiac output during normal pregnancy. (Redrawn from Peck TM, Arias F: Hematologic changes associated with pregnancy. *Clin Obstet Gynecol* 1979;22:785. By permission of Harper & Row Publishers.)

The decreased PVR is manifested clinically by a decrease in both mean and diastolic blood pressures. This decrease is clearly observed during the second trimester, when the mean average blood pressure is 10 to 15 mm Hg lower than in the nonpregnant state. In patients with chronic hypertension, this drop in blood pressure may confuse the diagnosis if the patients are first observed during the midtrimester.

Because most of the IV volume is contained in the capacitance vessels, the decrease in venous resistance represents the adaptation of the vascular tree to blood volume expansion. If this adaptation does not occur, the IV volume will not expand, thereby seriously compromising the uteroplacental circulation.

Another physiologic change that is important, particularly for pregnant patients with Marfan's syndrome, is the increase in size and compliance of the aortic root. This tendency may facilitate aortic dissection for Marfan's patients, especially

those who have dilated aortic roots before they get pregnant.

◪ **EFFECTS OF PREGNANCY ON MATERNAL CARDIAC DISEASE**

The hemodynamic changes that occur during pregnancy have a profound effect on the patient with cardiac disease. Each one of these changes increases cardiac work, and their combined effect may exceed the limited functional capacity of an ailing heart. When this happens, sudden death or, more commonly, congestive heart failure (CHF) and pulmonary edema (PE) will occur. As a result of the deleterious effects of pregnancy on cardiac disease, maternal mortality may be as high as 10% for all cardiac patients, although it varies widely with the severity of the cardiac problem.

There are several periods during pregnancy when the danger of cardiac decompensation is especially great. The first is between 12 and 32 weeks of gestation, a time during which the hemodynamic changes of pregnancy develop. The most critical period is between 28 and 32 weeks of gestation, when the hemodynamic changes of pregnancy peak and cardiac demands are maximum. About 50% of those patients who develop CHF at this stage of pregnancy are in class I or II of the New York Heart Association (NYHA) classification earlier in gestation.

The second dangerous time for pregnant cardiac patients is during labor and delivery. During labor, every uterine contraction injects blood from the uteroplacental circulation into the maternal bloodstream increasing cardiac output by approximately 15% to 20%. This continuous demand on the heart may trigger congestive heart failure. During the second stage of labor, maternal pushing further compromises the venous return to the heart causing a decrease in cardiac output that may be critical for some cardiac patients. Immediately after delivery of the baby and placental separation, the obstructive effect of the pregnant uterus on the return circulation to the heart disappears. There is a sudden transfusion of blood from the lower extremities and the uteroplacental vascular tree to the systemic circulation. This large and abrupt increase in blood volume is more than many pregnant cardiac patients can tolerate, and CHF occurs frequently at this time.

The final dangerous time for the pregnant cardiac patient is 4 to 5 days after delivery. Patients with primary pulmonary hypertension, Eisenmenger's syndrome, aortic stenosis, and cyanotic heart disease may be able to go through pregnancy and labor and delivery without major complications. However, sudden death in the early postpartum period may occur. Decreased peripheral resistance with right-to-left shunting and pulmonary embolization from silent iliofemoral thrombus are two of the problems occurring at this time.

◼ EFFECTS OF MATERNAL CARDIAC DISEASE ON PREGNANCY

Pregnancy outcome is compromised by the presence of cardiac disease. Fetal death is usually caused by severe, chronic, or acute maternal deterioration. Fetal morbidity is usually caused by preterm delivery and fetal growth retardation. Also, if the mother has congenital heart disease, there is an increased incidence (4.5% vs. 0.6% in the overall population) of fetal congenital cardiovascular anomalies.[8,9]

Not long ago, the overall perinatal mortality for pregnant patients with cardiac disease was as high as 20%. This poor fetal outcome related to maternal cardiac disease has been drastically modified with adequate prenatal care, prolonged hospitalization, and intensive care when decompensation occurs. However, fetal death still occurs in pregnant cardiac patients, mostly in mothers with cyanotic heart conditions. In these cases the poor outcome is related to the degree of maternal polycythemia, which in turn is a result of chronic hypoxemia. Fetal death also occurs occasionally in the patient with Marfan's syndrome who has an acute aortic dissection and in cardiac patients who have significant functional impairment (classes III and IV, NYHA classification).

Fetal growth retardation and preterm labor are common in pregnant patients with heart disease. This is probably the result of their inability to maintain an adequate uteroplacental circulation. The frequency of these problems is related to the severity of the functional impairment of the heart and the severity of the chronic tissue hypoxia.

◼ GENERAL MEASURES FOR THE CARE OF PREGNANT PATIENTS WITH HEART DISEASE

To prevent the occurrence of serious complications, the obstetrician and the internist taking care of the pregnant cardiac patient should be prepared to:

1. Monitor cardiac function during pregnancy to determine whether the physiologic changes elicited by pregnancy are exceeding the functional capacity of the heart
2. Limit the extent of some of these physiologic changes

Monitoring cardiac function during pregnancy

Evaluation of the cardiac response of the patient with heart disease to the normal hemodynamic changes of pregnancy is done predominantly by clinical observation. Easy fatigability, shortness of breath, orthopnea, and pulmonary congestion are symptoms and signs characteristic of left-sided heart failure. Weight gain, dependent edema, hepatomegaly, and increased jugular venous pressure are symptoms and signs suggestive of right-sided heart failure. However, history and physical examination may be misleading because these signs and symptoms also occur in normal pregnant patients. Regardless of this in the pregnant patient with known heart disease these findings are always important and require careful evaluation.

Shortness of breath is one of the most common complaints of pregnant women. This "thirst for air" that occurs during pregnancy usually is not severe enough to limit the patient's activity, and normal pregnant women continue their activities despite shortness of breath. The dyspnea of left heart failure is different in that the patient is clearly limited in her level of activity, and often she will complain of orthopnea and orthopneic cough. Some patients with left heart failure develop bronchospasm and wheezing after a few hours of sleep, that is, *paroxysmal nocturnal dyspnea,* or *cardiac asthma.*

In the initial phases of left-sided heart failure, tachycardia and an S_3 gallop may be present on auscultation. However, the most important sign of left-sided failure is the presence of bibasilar rales.

The characteristic signs and symptoms of right heart failure are the products of systemic venous congestion. The main manifestations are increased jugular venous pressure, hepatomegaly, and dependent edema. The first two of these signs are not present in normal pregnancy, but the last is normally present.

Patients may exhibit varying degrees of biventricular failure, or symptoms and signs of one or the other may predominate, depending on the defect causing the congestive heart failure. Patients with mitral stenosis predominantly have signs of left ventricular failure, whereas patients with peripartum cardiomyopathy have symptoms and signs of biventricular failure.

At every prenatal visit, the obstetricians taking care of pregnant cardiac patients should search for clinical evidence suggesting the onset of congestive heart failure. Meticulous interrogation and examination of the patient are necessary. A sudden increase in body weight, orthopnea, tachycardia, hepatomegaly, and the presence of pulmonary rales are important findings potentially suggesting congestive heart failure and demanding further evaluation. A chest x-ray examination showing vascular redistribution with distention of the pulmonary veins in the upper lobes will provide additional evidence of pulmonary congestion. In such cases the patient should be admitted to the hospital for further assessment and treatment. Evaluation with electrocardiography is rarely necessary because it is insensitive to the changes directly caused by congestive heart failure.

Measures to decrease the effects on the heart of the hemodynamic changes elicited by pregnancy

Antepartum. The most important measure for attenuating the impact of pregnancy on a diseased heart is *bed rest.* Bed rest increases the venous return to the heart, improves renal perfusion, induces diuresis, and promotes elimination of water. Also, since bed rest reduces the metabolic needs of several organs, especially the muscle, the blood flow to these organs at rest decreases markedly, ameliorating the work load on the heart.

Dietary salt restriction is a measure that helps prevent excessive retention of sodium and water. Most pregnant cardiac patients tolerate a moderate sodium dietary restriction (4 to 6 g daily).

Diuretics should be given to the cardiac pregnant patient if a moderate restriction in sodium intake is insufficient to limit the normal intravascular volume expansion that occurs during gestation. The diuretic most commonly used is chlorothiazide. This drug acts by inhibiting sodium reabsorption in the distal tubule. For the most part, thiazides are benign drugs, and their most common side effect is hypokalemia, which can be avoided by the concurrent administration of a potassium-retaining agent or by increasing the dietary ingestion of potassium. Another problem with this diuretic during pregnancy is the occasional occurrence of neonatal thrombocytopenia.

The most important concern with the use of diuretics during pregnancy is that they may decrease the plasma volume to the point that placental perfusion and fetal growth are compromised. In fact, there is evidence indicating that a decrease in intravascular volume during pregnancy is associated with fetal growth retardation and that the severity of the fetal growth impairment is directly related to the magnitude of the intravascular volume depletion.[10] Unfortunately, one cannot accurately measure the intravascular volume contraction caused by diuretics in pregnant women, and there is no information addressing the degree of volume restriction that is compatible with adequate fetal growth. In these patients serial hematocrit determinations may prove helpful. The dosage of the diuretic may be adjusted to keep the hematocrit value equal to or slightly above that obtained before initiation of therapy.

Prophylactic digitalization is commonly used in pregnant patients with severe heart disease who are not in overt congestive heart failure. The objectives are to improve the contractility of the heart and to relieve symptoms such as easy fatigability, orthopnea, and weakness. A secondary benefit is avoiding the production of ventricular tachycardia in those patients who have a tendency to develop rapid atrial rhythms.

During labor and delivery. During labor it is possible to decrease the impact of the hemodynamic adaptions of pregnancy on an ailing heart by adopting some of the following measures.

The pregnant cardiac patient should always labor and deliver in the lateral supine position to avoid the hemodynamic impairment caused by the dorsal decubitus position. She should have effective pain relief during labor. During early stages, small doses of intravenous morphine (2 to 4 mg) may be used. Later, if the patient is not anticoagulated, the anesthesia of choice is epidural blockade administered by an experienced obstetric anesthesiologist.

Cardiac patients in labor should be continuously monitored with pulse oximetry. Mild degrees of desaturation may be corrected by oxygen administration via a rebreathing mask. The occurrence of desaturation in labor not corrected by oxygen suggests the development of pulmonary edema and indicates inability of the patient to tolerate labor.

Many cardiac pregnant patients will benefit from a double catheter epidural anesthesia technique. This method limits the extent of the sympathetic blockade and its effect on intravascular volume pooling and blood pressure. Also, it is better to administer an epidural narcotic (morphine, fentanyl) than epidural anesthetics. In fact, because of their inability to cause sympathetic blockade, epidural narcotics may be given in situations in which there is a relative contraindication to the epidural administration of local anesthetics, such as in patients with aortic stenosis, mitral stenosis, aortic coarctation, Marfan's syndrome with dilated aortic root, or hypertrophic subaortic stenosis.

An important aspect of the intrapartum care of the pregnant cardiac patient is the control of the rate of intravenous fluid administration. Al-most all cardiac patients in labor should be kept on the "dry" side, and intravenous fluids should be restricted to no more than 75 ml/hr.

Patients with congenital or acquired heart lesions and with artificial valve prostheses should have antibiotic prophylaxis at the time of delivery to avoid the possibility of subacute bacterial endocarditis. The antibiotic treatments recommended by the American Heart Association are shown in Box 11-1.

Pregnant cardiac patients who are not anticoagulated tend to develop thromboembolization in the postpartum period. Relative immobilization, pooling of blood in the lower extremities, and alterations in coagulation and fibrinolysis that occur peripartum combine to produce an environment conducive to the formation of thrombi in the lower extremities. The risk of thromboembolization is approximately 2% for patients with rheumatic heart disease. To avoid this serious complication, one can initiate ambulation shortly after delivery, use pneumatic compression of the lower extremities, and give prophylactic low-dose heparin during labor, delivery, and the immediate postpartum period.

As mentioned before, immediately after delivery the uterus decreases markedly in size and ceases to obstruct the return circulation to the heart. At the same time, most of the blood contained in the uterine vessels is suddenly infused into the systemic circulation. These two physiologic phenomena combine to increase preload and in the cardiac patient may exceed the pumping ability of the heart resulting in acute pulmonary edema. Patients with mitral stenosis and fixed cardiac output are especially at risk for this problem. To avoid it, these patients should be placed in the sitting position after delivery. Sitting will increase venous pooling in the lower extremities and decrease the venous return to the heart, and a more gradual adaptation to the postpartum hemodynamic will occur. Also, if the patient is under epidural anesthesia, the anesthesiologist may raise the level of anesthesia and the sympathetic blockade. Finally, tourniquets may be used in the lower extremities.

At the time of delivery, oxytocin is usually given to make the uterus contract, thereby avoiding intrapartum and postpartum bleeding. In the cardiac patient, it is important not to administer the medication as an intravenous bolus because it may cause a sudden drop in peripheral vascular resistance. The subsequent hypo-

---

BOX 11-1

Suggested Antibiotic Regimens for the Prevention of Bacterial Endocarditis in Patients with Heart Disease Who Have Genitourinary and Gastrointestinal Instrumentation or Surgery

Antibiotic dosages*

Aqueous crystalline penicillin G (2 million U IM or IV) *or*
Ampicillin (1.0 g IM or IV) *plus*
Gentamicin (1.5 mg/kg [not to exceed 80 mg] IM or IV) *or*
Streptomycin (1.0 g IM)

Give initial doses 30 minutes to 1 hour before the procedure. If gentamicin is used, give a similar dosage of gentamicin and penicillin (or ampicillin) every 8 hours for two additional dosages. If streptomycin is used, give a similar dosage of streptomycin and penicillin (or ampicillin) every 12 hours for two additional dosages.†

For those patients who are allergic to penicillin*

Vancomycin (1.0 gram IV given over 30 minutes to 1 hour) *plus* streptomycin (1.0 gram IM).

A single dose of these antibiotics given 30 minutes to 1 hour before the procedure is probably sufficient, but the same dose may be repeated in 12 hours.

---

*In patients with significantly compromised renal function it may be necessary to modify the dosage of antibiotics used. Some of these dosages may exceed the manufacturer's recommendations for a 24-hour period. However, since in most cases they are only recommended for a single 24-hour period, it is unlikely that toxicity will occur.
†During prolonged procedures or in the case of delayed healing, it may be necessary to provide additional dosages of antibiotics. For brief outpatient procedures such as uncomplicated catheterization of the bladder, one dose may be sufficient.

BOX 11-2

General Measures for the Cardiac Patient in Labor

1. Labor and delivery in lateral decubitus position
2. Pulse oximetry
3. Adequate pain relief (epidural narcotics, double catheter epidural)
4. Restrict IV fluids to 75 ml/hr
5. Oxygen by rebreathing mask
6. Avoid bolus oxytocin and ergot compounds
7. Antibiotic prophylaxis
8. Thrombosis prophylaxis
9. Prevention of postpartum pulmonary edema

---

tension may be difficult to tolerate for some patients. Also, cardiac patients should not receive ergot alkaloids for prophylaxis or treatment of postpartum uterine atony because these agents cause significant vasoconstriction and elevation of blood pressure, which can be deleterious as well. A summary of the measures to take in the management of the cardiac patient in labor is shown in Box 11-2.

◪ TREATMENT OF ACUTE CONGESTIVE HEART FAILURE DURING PREGNANCY

The majority of patients know of their heart disease before pregnancy. Occasionally, however, one will see a patient with a previously undiagnosed cardiac disorder who has congestive heart failure (CHF) during pregnancy. In this situation, it is necessary to define the cause of the problem because in many cases the primary defect is amenable to surgical correction. An example would be a patient with mitral or aortic stenosis undiagnosed before pregnancy. Timely operative intervention may be lifesaving in such a situation.

One must also consider other factors that may be contributing to the precipitation of CHF in these patients. Anemia, infections, arrhythmias, noncompliance with medications or salt restriction, excessive physical activity, and administration of salt-retaining medications are the factors most frequently associated with acute CHF in the pregnant cardiac patient.

Once the potentially correctable precipitating factors have been ruled out, the management of the pregnant patient in CHF consists of:

1. Reducing the cardiac work with bed rest
2. Decreasing the preload with diuretics
3. Improving cardiac contractility with digitalis or other agents (dopamine, dobutamine)
4. Reducing the afterload with vasodilators

Bed rest is an essential component of the treatment of pregnant patients with CHF. The pregnant patient in CHF should be placed on bed rest so as to reduce her metabolic rate and her heart work. Unfortunately, venous thrombosis and pulmonary embolization, the most common harmful effects of bed rest, occur more frequently in pregnant than in nonpregnant patients because of the decreased fibrinolytic activity and hypercoagulability that exist during gestation. Therefore passive leg exercises, prophylactic heparin (5000 U subcutaneously every 12 hours) and compression stockings should be used to avoid thromboembolic complications in these patients.

Diuretics should be used with caution in the pregnant patient with CHF. One should begin treatment with a mild diuretic, such as chlorothiazide, 25 to 50 mg daily, and advance to more potent agents, such as furosemide, only if it is absolutely necessary. Diuretic therapy should be monitored with daily weight checks, as well as serial measurements of hematocrit, electrolytes, and creatinine. A rapid decrease in weight concomitant with a rise in hematocrit results from a rapid constriction of the intravascular volume, which may be hazardous. The appearance of a low potassium value or a high serum creatinine also indicates the need for therapeutic adjustment.

Digoxin, as any other digitalis drug, can be used safely during pregnancy. However, the expanded intravascular volume associated with pregnancy results in a lower serum level of drug compared with a nongravid patient given the same dose. Placental transfer of digoxin is poor in early pregnancy but improves with advancing gestational age. Fetal toxicity has never been described with therapeutic maternal levels.

Digitalis therapy is an important aspect of the drug treatment of patients with CHF. The digitalis preparation most commonly used is digoxin because it can be given orally, has a rapid onset of action, and a relatively short life. It is usually started with a loading dose of 1.0 to 1.5 mg in a 24-hour period. Maintenance dosage is usually 0.25 mg daily (0.125 to 0.375 mg). Therapy is adjusted according to the patient's clinical response, the serum levels, and the electrocardiographic changes. The therapeutic serum level of digoxin is 1.0 to 1.5 ng/ml.

The most serious side effect of digitalis therapy is arrythmia. This can be recognized by an electrocardiogram and requires rapid treatment. Discontinuation of the medication, use of antiarrhythmic medications, and correction of hypokalemia usually suffice. However, severe intoxication may require the use of digoxin-specific antibodies (digoxin immune FAB, Digibind).

Vasodilator therapy has become an important part of the treatment of patients with CHF. The principle behind vasodilator therapy in patients with CHF is to reduce cardiac work by lowering peripheral vascular resistance. Several drugs may be used for this purpose. In emergency situations, the drugs most commonly used are hydralazine, nitroglycerin, and sodium nitroprusside. For maintenance therapy, hydralazine or a calcium channel blocker is the drug of choice.

Hydralazine, in oral or intravenous forms, has been used for many years in patients with preeclampsia and eclampsia. Hydralazine is primarily an arterial vasodilator. It is a drug that is relatively safe to use during pregnancy; it is accepted by obstetricians, and therefore it is frequently used in the treatment of hypertension during pregnancy. When hydralazine is used in large doses, a marked decrease in blood pressure may cause an alteration in placental perfusion, and subsequent signs of fetal distress will appear in fetal heart tracings.

Nitrates reduce both preload and afterload, but their predominant effect is on the capacitance vessels. They decrease the venous return to the heart and are particularly useful in reducing pulmonary congestion in doses that do not markedly affect systemic blood pressure. Both nitroglycerin and sodium nitroprusside are powerful antihypertensive agents that, similar to hydralazine, may cause maternal hypotension, decreased uteroplacental perfusion, and fetal distress. The effect of peripheral vasodilators is more pronounced when the pregnant patient is supine and the weight of the uterus interferes with the venous return.

The angiotensin-converting enzyme (ACE) inhibitors decrease peripheral vascular resistance, pulmonary capillary wedge pressure, and heart size, and they increase stroke index and exercise tolerance time. They also reduce preload by impairing the retention of sodium and water caused by aldosterone, reduce the vasoconstriction caused by angiotensin, and block the increase in sympathetic tone mediated by the renin-angiotensin-aldosterone system. These pharmacologic properties make them ideal agents in the treatment of CHF. However, the use of these drugs during pregnancy is contraindicated. Fetal growth retardation and fetal malformations have been described in pregnant patients taking these medications. ACE inhibitors cross the placental barrier and are classified in category C (adverse effects of the fetus in animal studies, no adequate studies in humans; the benefits from the drug may be acceptable despite its potential risks).

In acute cardiac emergencies, nitroglycerin is the vasodilator of choice for pregnant women, since nitroprusside may have undesirable fetal side effects. Also, in cardiac emergencies, dopamine and dobutamine can be used without fear of fetal side effects.

◪ MANAGEMENT OF ACUTE PULMONARY EDEMA DURING PREGNANCY

Treatment of acute pulmonary edema during pregnancy should preferably be given in an intensive care unit. Invasive hemodynamic monitoring using Swan-Ganz catheterization is usually necessary to adequately assess the severity of the process and the response to therapy.

Pulmonary edema is a life-threatening situation that occurs fairly frequently during pregnancy making it necessary for the obstetrician to be familiar with its diagnosis and treatment. The basic problem in acute pulmonary edema is the mobilization of fluid from the pulmonary interstitium into the alveolar space. Gas exchange is inhibited causing oxygen desaturation and retention of CO_2. If the condition remains uncorrected, generalized tissue hypoxia, acidosis, and death may ensue.

Pulmonary edema may be produced by alterations in any of the forces that govern the movement of fluid in the pulmonary alveoli. Increased pulmonary capillary pressure usually caused by fluid overload or congestive heart failure and al-

tered capillary permeability resulting from endothelial cell injury are the most common mechanisms. Alterations in capillary pressure or permeability are aggravated by the decrease in plasma colloid oncotic pressure that normally occurs during pregnancy.

The great majority of cases of pulmonary edema during pregnancy are caused by the following underlying problems:

1. Administration of beta-adrenergic agents
2. Preeclampsia and eclampsia
3. Congestive heart failure

The mechanism of pulmonary edema operating in each condition is different, and as a consequence, the management of the problem is also different.

The most common form of pulmonary edema seen by the obstetrician is that associated with the administration of beta-adrenergic agents for the treatment of preterm labor. This occurs in patients receiving continuous intravenous infusions, but it may also happen in patients taking the oral form. The physiology of the pulmonary edema in patients receiving such drugs is a matter of controversy, but in the majority of patients, fluid overload or altered capillary permeability can be found to be the cause. Patients with multifetal pregnancies, exaggerated intravascular volume expansion, or chorioamnionitis are more predisposed to develop pulmonary edema when treated with beta-mimetic agents.

Most pregnant patients who develop pulmonary edema in association with the administration of beta-adrenergic drugs respond to the following treatment:

1. Discontinuation of the offending drug
2. Administration of furosemide (20 mg IV push initially, followed by 20 mg IV in one or more additional doses every 30 to 60 minutes, depending on the response to the initial dose)
3. Administration of oxygen by mask

Pulmonary edema in severe preeclampsia results from endothelial cell injury, altered capillary permeability, and decreased plasma colloid oncotic pressure. In some patients, left ventricular failure caused by a marked increase in peripheral vascular resistance and fluid overload are contributory factors. Treatment of preeclamptic patients in pulmonary edema is difficult, and the outcome may be poor despite the use of sophisticated hemodynamic monitoring techniques. The main problem is the inability to modify with therapy the endothelial cell injury and capillary permeability problems. In this subset of patients, supportive therapy and expectant management are favored.

In pregnant patients with cardiac disease, acute pulmonary edema usually results from the inability of the diseased heart to compensate for acute or chronic increases in intravascular volume. This may occur antenatally because of the physiologic expansion in plasma volume, but it is also common after the autotransfusion following delivery of the fetus and the placenta. Patients with stenotic valvular lesions and fixed cardiac outputs are at high risk for this complication. Treatment of acute pulmonary edema in the context of chronic heart disease requires aggressive measures aimed at decreasing preload (fluid restriction, diuretics, tourniquets), increasing the contractility of the heart (digitalis, dobutamine), and decreasing afterload resistance (e.g., nitroglycerin,).

◼ MATERNAL CARDIAC ARRHYTHMIAS DURING PREGNANCY

Significant maternal arrythmias are rare. However, minor transient arrhythmic episodes frequently occur, but they are harmless and require no therapy. The cause of the increased frequency of minor arrythmias during pregnancy, usually premature beats, may be related to the adaptation of the heart to normal hemodynamic alterations.

One of the arrhythmias that the obstetrician occasionally observes is paroxysmal supraventricular tachycardia (PST). PST is characterized by a rate between 150 and 250 bpm, usually below 200 bpm. The patient is often aware of her tachycardia and may sense palpitations or feel anxious, short of breath, and lightheaded. An ECG will show narrow QRS complexes. In 90% of the cases the cause of the PST is atrioventricular node reentry. In these cases the ventricle and the atria are simultaneously activated, and no p wave is seen.

The first maneuver in converting a hemodynamically stable patient with PST to a normal sinus rhythm is carotid sinus massage. The patient should be supine with intravenous fluids running and should be continuously monitored with ECG. The right carotid sinus should be massaged first for about 10 seconds. If there is no response, try the left side for 10 seconds. The two sinuses should never be massaged simultaneously. The patient may attempt a Valsalva's maneuver during the carotid massage to increase the effectiveness of the procedure. If there is no response to this combination, the treatment of choice is 5 to 10 mg of intravenous verapamil administered as a bolus in 1 to 3 minutes. This dose may be repeated 15 minutes later if there is no response. The main side effect is hypotension, which is transient and responds easily to intravenous fluids. Adenosine is a recently available drug that is quickly replacing verapamil as the agent of choice in the treatment of supraventricular arrythmias.[11] Cardioversion is rarely necessary, but it can be used if there is no underlying cardiac lesion and no evidence of hemodynamic instability. Digitalis and quinidine are commonly used for prophylaxis and chronic maintenance therapy.

In patients with CHF, the treatment of choice for PST is digoxin rather than verapamil. The management of this situation should be left to the cardiologist.

Atrial flutter, atrial fibrillation, and ventricular tachycardia are rarely seen during pregnancy. These arrhythmias should be diagnosed and treated by the cardiologist. The drugs used for these conditions, as well as electrocardioversion, are innocuous for the fetus.

◼ MITRAL VALVE PROLAPSE DURING PREGNANCY

Mitral valve prolapse (MVP) is the most common maternal cardiac disease seen in obstetrics and it affects approximately 6% to 8% of all women of reproductive age. One reason MVP is diagnosed frequently during pregnancy is that the incidence of arrhythmias and palpitations during normal pregnancy is high. As a result, MVP is incidentally found during echocardiography performed to investigate these common cardiovascular complaints.

In patients with MVP, the leaflets and the chordae of the mitral valve stretch and bulge into the left atrium during systole. This is caused by a defect in collagen synthesis in the valve. This defect in collagen synthesis is most likely the result of a genetic disorder.

The main symptoms of MVP are chest pain and cardiac arrhythmias described by the patient as palpitations or skipped beats. Anxiety and even panic attacks may occur simultaneously with the onset of these symptoms.

On physical examination, it is sometimes possible to find a midsystolic click muffled by the physiologic holosystolic murmur appearing at the end of the first trimester. The diagnosis of MVP is made by two-dimensional echocardiography, which will show systolic displacement of the mitral leaflets into the left atrium. In severe cases, Doppler will demonstrate some degree of regurgitation.

The increase in intravascular volume and the decrease in peripheral vascular resistance that occur during normal pregnancy will increase the left ventricular end-diastolic volume and, theoretically, should alleviate the signs and symptoms of MVP. This has been corroborated by clinical observations and also by echocardiographic studies.[12]

The course and the outcome of pregnancy in patients with MVP are similar to that of patients who do not have this defect.[13] However, there are a few reported complications such as thromboembolism and endocarditis.

Most pregnant patients with MVP do not require treatment for their symptoms. Patients with recurrent, severe arrhythmias need treatment with propranolol. Most patients do well with dosages between 10 to 40 mg 4 times daily. Propranolol is safe for both mother and fetus.

The need for antibiotic prophylaxis at the time of delivery for patients with MVP is a matter of controversy. The risk of bacterial endocarditis after delivery in these patients is unknown but probably very low. Everybody agrees that patients who have frequent or severe symptoms, and especially those who have mitral regurgitation, should receive antibiotics at the time of delivery. Controversy centers on the need for prophylaxis in the asymptomatic patient with a mild lesion. We believe that, since in the majority of pregnant patients with MVP the obstetrician lacks adequate information to determine the severity of the MVP, it is best to give antibiotic prophylaxis to all of these patients. The recommended antibiotics and their dosages are shown in Box 11-1.

◪ PERIPARTUM CARDIOMYOPATHY

Every obstetrician should be familiarized with peripartum cardiomyopathy (PPCM), a rare form of congestive cardiac failure that is intimately related to pregnancy. This disease appears in 1 of every 4000 to 5000 live births.

The initial description of the syndrome suggested that it appears after parturition and for this reason it was named *postpartum cardiomyopathy* or *puerperal heart failure*. Today we know that the signs and symptoms of this disease may appear at any time in the last month of pregnancy and up to 5 months after delivery, and for this reason the name *peripartum cardiomyopathy* is being used more frequently.

The majority of patients with peripartum cardiomyopathy are 20 to 35 years of age and seek treatment in the second or third postpartum month for weakness, shortness of breath, orthopnea, cough, paroxysmal nocturnal dyspnea, and palpitations. Physical examination will reveal tachycardia, cardiac arrhythmias, pulmonary rales, and peripheral edema. Chest x-ray examination will show an enlarged heart and pulmonary vascular redistribution. Echocardiography and right heart catheterization will demonstrate enlargement of all chambers of the heart, predominantly the left ventricle. Ventricular wall motion, ejection fraction, and cardiac output are decreased, and pulmonary wedge pressure is increased. Some patients with PPCM will develop deep vein thrombosis and pulmonary embolization.

Bed rest, digitalis, diuretics, and anticoagulant therapy are the most important interventions in the management of patients with PPCM. The prognosis for these patients is guarded and is especially poor in patients with low left ventricular ejection fraction.[14] Patients who have dilated hearts 6 months after the onset of symptoms have very high mortality. Patients who have normal-sized hearts 6 months after the initiation of therapy usually have good prognoses. Also important in the prognosis is the time from the onset of symptoms to the initiation of therapy. In Burch's series,[15] when therapy was delayed more than 6 months from the initiation of symptoms, the prognosis was poor.

Women who recover from PPCM are at high risk for recurrence in subsequent pregnancies. This risk seems to be greater in patients with persistently dilated hearts.

Many investigators doubt that PPCM is a distinct clinical entity and consider it to be a form of the same dilated cardiomyopathy that is prevalent in older patients. This position is supported by the similarity in pathologic findings, clinical expression, and hemodynamic changes among patients with PPCM and patients with dilated cardiomyopathy. It is the exception, however, to observe dilated cardiomyopathy unrelated to childbearing in young women. Also, the disease tends to recur in subsequent pregnancies. These facts suggest that PPCM is a unique form of idiopathic myocardiopathy. This hypothesis is supported by work from two different institutions[16,17] where it has been found that a high number of patients with PPCM show evidence of myocarditis in biopsy specimens. Other authors disagree, and Cunningham et al.[18] found that 21 (75%) of 28 patients had associated cardiovascular diseases that could be the underlying etiology of their PPCM.

■ OTHER CARDIAC PROBLEMS OF SIGNIFICANCE DURING PREGNANCY

The ability of a patient with heart disease to tolerate pregnancy is proportional to the degree of functional impairment and the specific nature of the cardiac lesion. The method most commonly used to assess the degree of functional impairment is the New York Heart Association (NYHA) classification (Box 11-3). With respect to the nature of the cardiac lesion, it is well known that some heart conditions are very well tolerated during pregnancy, whereas others are not (Box 11-4). This section briefly describes some aspects of those specific conditions that are poorly tolerated during pregnancy and that present significant problems for the cardiologist as well as the obstetrician.

It is necessary to remember that termination of pregnancy is a valid legal and medical option for patients who have cardiac lesions with guarded maternal prognosis. Patients should be informed of the possibility of termination as an option for avoiding the potential serious problems associated with their pregnancies.

Mitral stenosis

Mitral stenosis is the most common rheumatic heart lesion and one of the most dangerous for pregnant women. In patients with mitral stenosis, an obstruction to the blood flow from the left atrium into the left ventricle makes it necessary to increase the left atrial pressure to maintain the cardiac output. With progressive narrowing of the mitral orifice, left atrial pressure increases, and the pressure is transmitted to the pulmonary veins and capillaries. Eventually the pulmonary capillary pressure may reach a value, usually above 25 mm Hg, at which the homeostatic balance of fluid in the lung cannot be maintained, resulting in pulmonary edema. This sequence of events is accelerated by the physio-

---

BOX 11-4

Maternal Tolerance to Specific Heart Conditions

Well-tolerated
Pulmonary stenosis
Aortic insufficiency
Mitral insufficiency
Congenital heart block

Well-tolerated if pulmonary hypertension is not present
Atrial septal defects
Ventricular septal defects
Patent ductus

Variable tolerance depending on the functional capacity of the heart
Uncomplicated aortic coarctation
Aortic stenosis
Mitral regurgitation
Aortic regurgitation

Poorly tolerated and source of significant problems during pregnancy
Mitral stenosis
Peripartum cardiomyopathy
Primary pulmonary hypertension
Eisenmenger's syndrome
Marfan's syndrome with dilated aortic root
Metallic valve prosthesis
Congenital cyanotic heart disease
Conditions listed in group C if pulmonary hypertension is present
Any class III or IV lesion (NYHA classification)

BOX 11-3

New York Heart Association Classification of Heart Disease During Pregnancy

Class I   Asymptomatic
Class II   Symptomatic with heavy exercise
Class III   Symptomatic with light exercise
Class IV   Symptomatic at rest

logic hemodynamic changes produced by pregnancy. The increase in intravascular volume of pregnancy results in more blood coming to the left atrium to be pumped through the restricted outlet. The increase in heart rate that occurs during pregnancy decreases the time available for ventricular filling. The result of these two influences, increased blood volume and increased heart rate, is increased left atrial and pulmonary capillary pressures, with a higher risk for pulmonary edema than in the nonpregnant state. It is not surprising that patients with mitral stenosis who are relatively asymptomatic (class I or II, NYHA classification) at the beginning of pregnancy may develop pulmonary edema when the pregnancy advances and the hemodynamic changes become more apparent. The general incidence of pulmonary edema in pregnant patients with mitral stenosis is approximately 23%.[19]

Successful management of pregnant patients with mitral stenosis requires meticulous application of the measures indicated under the heading "General management of cardiac patients during pregnancy." Bed rest, diuretics, and digitalization are the main elements of the therapy. If cardiac decompensation and pulmonary edema occur, the patient should be managed as outlined under the heading "Pulmonary edema during pregnancy." During labor, the essentials of management include adequate pain relief, laboring and delivering in the lateral supine position, and adoption of measures to minimize the effects of the autotransfusion that follows delivery.

Pregnant patients with mitral stenosis who respond poorly to medical treatment, and especially those with recurrent episodes of pulmonary edema, are candidates for cardiac surgery. The intervention of choice in most cases is closed mitral valvotomy. Open heart surgery and valve replacement have a very high fetal loss rate.[20]

Aortic stenosis

Most cases of aortic stenosis are congenital. However, in some patients the aortic valve is narrowed as a result of rheumatic heart disease. Pregnant patients with aortic stenosis have poor prognoses, maternal mortality is approximately 17.4%, and the fetal loss rate is approximately 31.6%.[21] Sudden death and irreversible heart failure are the most common causes of maternal death.

Patients with aortic stenosis develop left ventricular hypertrophy to generate the increased pressure necessary to pump blood through nonpliant valvular leaflets. Hemodynamically, these patients have fixed stroke volumes and increased left ventricular end-diastolic pressures. Eventually the left ventricular function fails to overcome the resistance to flow, and the patient develops CHF. Angina and syncope frequently occur with the onset of CHF.

The cornerstone of management of these patients is bed rest. Because of a fixed stroke volume, any activity will cause an increase in heart rate and a greater demand on the left ventricle. During labor, epidural anesthesia should be avoided because it will cause a decrease in peripheral vascular resistance, and this will increase the pressure gradient across the narrow valve. Epidural narcotics produce no sympathetic blockade and can be used in these patients. In contrast to most pregnant cardiac patients, the patient with aortic stenosis should not be restricted to 75 ml/hr of IV fluids during labor. A rate of IV fluids administration of 125 to 150 ml/hr is more adequate.

Eisenmenger's syndrome

Patients with Eisenmenger's syndrome have pulmonary hypertension with right-to-left or bidirectional shunt through an open ductus, an atrial or a ventricular septal defect. In these patients, increases in pulmonary pressures or decreases in peripheral vascular resistance, as occurs during normal pregnancy, may cause right-to-left shunting and arterial blood oxygen desaturation.

The outcome of pregnancy in patients with Eisenmenger's syndrome is very poor. Maternal mortality is approximately 52%, and total fetal wastage approximates 41.7%.[17] Despite the best medical and obstetric care, these patients often die in the postpartum period from irreversible cardiovascular collapse. Because of this poor prognosis, every pregnant patient with significant ventricular, atrial, or ductus defects should have cardiac catheterization to determine the status of her pulmonary pressure.

In addition to the general measures for pregnant cardiac patients described above, anticoagulation with heparin to avoid the formation of microthrombi in the pulmonary circulation should be used for Eisenmenger's syndrome. Epidural narcotics can be used for pain relief during labor. To maintain peripheral vascular resistance above that of the pulmonary artery and to avoid right-to-left shunting, it may be necessary to use intravenous fluids and peripheral vasoconstrictors during delivery and the puerperium.

Primary pulmonary hypertension

Primary pulmonary hypertension, an uncommon abnormality, is characterized by an increase in thickness of the pulmonary arterioles. The development of intimal fibrosis and fibroelastosis, as well as the production of a typical "onion skin" configuration of the vessels, can be seen on microscopic examination. The consequence of this lesion is a marked increase in pulmonary vascular resistance that results in pulmonary hypertension. There is dilation of the right-side chambers of the heart and a low, probably fixed, cardiac output. The cause of this disease is unknown.

Pregnancy is deleterious to patients with primary pulmonary hypertension. The maternal mortality is approximately 40%, and the fetal outcome is also poor, with frequent spontaneous abortions and fetal demises resulting from maternal deaths. Most maternal deaths occur in the last trimester and in the postpartum period as a result of sudden cardiac collapse.

Pregnant patients with primary pulmonary hypertension should be on hospital bed rest once they reach 20 weeks of gestation. At this time anticoagulation with heparin should be instituted. Also, vasodilator therapy with hydralazine (75 to 150 mg daily) may be beneficial for these patients. Epidural anesthesia may be used for pain control during labor.

Marfan's syndrome

Patients with Marfan's syndrome have defective connective tissue caused by an alteration in protein metabolism that affects mainly the collagen and elastic tissues. The abnormality is manifested in alterations of the skeletal tissues, the heart, and the eye. The main sites of cardiac involvement are the mitral valve and the ascending aorta. Most of these patients have mitral valve prolapse, and in some, mitral regurgitation is present. Dilation of the aortic root sinuses is often seen as well.

Marfan's syndrome is inherited as an autosomal dominant condition, and mothers should be informed of the 50% risk of transmission to their offspring. In addition, there is the risk that pregnant patients with Marfan's syndrome may develop serious cardiovascular complications during pregnancy. The most important of these complications is acute aortic dissection. In the old literature this was considered to occur in approximately 50% of all pregnant patients with Marfan's. In more recent reviews it has become apparent that pregnancy is relatively safe for these patients unless they have marked dilation of the aortic root or other severe cardiac problems.

Ideally, a patient with Marfan's syndrome contemplating pregnancy should have a preconceptional echocardiogram to determine the diameter of her aortic root. If it is greater than 4.0 cm, she is at significant risk for aortic dissection, and she should be offered surgery. If the patient is in early pregnancy, she should be informed that termination of pregnancy is an option. Once the pregnancy is advanced, the probability of a favorable outcome will depend on her response to bed rest and to beta-adrenergic blockade.

Aortic dissection is initiated by an intimal tear. This is followed by a separation of the medial layer of the vessel by the blood that is being propelled from the left ventricle. The dissection advances a variable distance, following the course of the blood flow. Since the outer wall is made up mainly of the adventitial layer of the vessel, the frequency of rupture is very high, resulting in extravasation of blood into the pericardial space or the mediastinum. It is widely accepted that hormonal influences on the connective tissue during pregnancy weaken the medial layer of the aorta and worsen the potential of Marfan's patients for aortic dissection.

The main symptom of aortic dissection is severe, excruciating precordial or interscapular pain that radiates to the back, shoulders, or abdomen. Characteristically, the blood pressure is normal despite the shocklike state of the patient. Symptoms of pericardial tamponade or internal bleeding may also be present if the adventitia is ruptured. Other symptoms occur if there is obstruction of one or more of the aortic branches and may include stroke, myocardial infarction, and paralysis or ischemia of the upper limbs. Chest x-ray films usually show widening of the mediastinal area and left pleural effusion. Thoracic aortography is the gold standard for diagnosis.

Patients with aortic dissection should be

treated and stabilized in an intensive care unit before corrective surgery. Pharmacologic treatment is directed toward decreasing peripheral vascular resistance and left ventricular ejection velocity with beta-blockers and vasodilators to avoid progression of the dissection. Surgical treatment varies depending on the extension of the dissection and the presence of complicating factors. In all cases the objective is to graft the ascending aorta obliterating the entry and, if present, the outflow of the dissecting channel. The operative mortality rate for acute proximal dissection is approximately 7% to 8%.

Patients with prosthetic heart valves

Prosthetic heart valves have been used for many years in the treatment of congenital and acquired disorders. For this reason, pregnancy in women with artificial heart valves is not rare. The pregnancy outcome in these patients will depend on the type of valve (mechanical, porcine, human allograft), the site and the number of valves that were replaced, and the functional capacity of the heart after surgery. In general these patients suffer from thromboembolization, complications derived from their anticoagulant regimen, valve dysfunction, endocarditis, and heart failure.

The type of valve is important in that porcine and human allograft valves do not require anticoagulation, in contrast to patients with metallic valves.[22] The site of valve replacement is important because patients with prosthetic mitral and tricuspid valves have a fixed cardiac output, whereas patients with aortic valves can respond to the physiologic needs of pregnancy with increases in cardiac output. Finally, prognosis is better if only one valve is abnormal and if the patient belongs to NYHA class I or II.

The most frequent complications in patients with prosthetic valves result from anticoagulation therapy. Outside of pregnancy these patients are anticoagulated with warfarin sodium (Coumadin) and have relatively few problems. During pregnancy warfarin sodium is no longer the medication of choice, and the patient should switch to heparin. The same dilemma occurs for other pregnant patients who need anticoagulation for conditions such as mitral stenosis, atrial fibrillation, deep vein thrombosis, pulmonary embolization within 3 months of pregnancy, and peripartum cardiomyopathy in the third trimester.

Warfarin sodium has well-known teratogenic effects when it is administered early in pregnancy. However, it is also associated with spontaneous fetal intracranial bleeding and fetal death when it is taken in the second or third trimesters of pregnancy. Its use in the early first trimester may produce nasal hypoplasia, hypertelorism, prominence of the frontal bone, short stature, abnormalities of the central nervous system, mental retardation, and stippling of the epiphyses of long bones (chondrodysplasia punctata). The most common of these defects are nasal hypoplasia, stippled epiphyses, which occur in approximately 4.6% of the patients, and abnormalities of the central nervous system, which occur in 2.6% of the cases.[23]

In view of the adverse effects of warfarin sodium, many authorities recommend switching to heparin therapy. Heparin must be administered subcutaneously every 8 to 12 hours. The frequency and discomfort of injections are reasons for noncompliance, inadequate anticoagulation, and subsequent thromboembolization. These problems may be obviated with the use of a heparin lock for self intravenous administration, but this method requires close attention for the possibility of infection. The new calcium salt of heparin causes significantly less discomfort and fewer hematomas at the injection sites.

Another potential side effect of heparin is that it may cause osteoporosis, a complication that occurs mainly in patients who receive 20,000 or more units per day for more than 6 months. Heparin-induced thrombocytopenia may also occur. Usually the platelet count remains above $100,00/mm^3$. Finally, heparin, even at therapeutic levels, is not as effective as warfarin sodium for clot prevention on the artificial valves.

Some investigators recommend that patients with prosthetic valves be given heparin during the first 12 and the last 4 weeks of pregnancy and that warfarin sodium be given in the interim months.[24] However, there is no adequate evidence to support this. Also, at labor and delivery, anticoagulation must be reversed. The patient on heparin will have normal clotting 4 to 6 hours after discontinuing the medication. Maternal effects of warfarin sodium can be reversed easily with the administration of fresh frozen plasma, but the fetus needs 1 to 2 weeks after discontinuing warfarin sodium to reverse anticoagulation. This is why patients on this drug should be switched to heparin several weeks before the anticipated delivery time.

◤ IMPORTANT POINTS ◣

1. In normal pregnancy circulation is hyperdynamic. There is a high cardiac output and decreased peripheral and pulmonary vascular resistance.

2. The increase in intravascular volume that occurs during normal pregnancy fulfills the need of the developing uteroplacental circulation and protects the mother from the potentially harmful effects of the blood loss that occurs at parturition.

3. The hemodynamic changes that occur during normal pregnancy increase the cardiac work. This effect may exceed the functional capacity of an ailing heart.

4. The danger of cardiac decompensation during pregnancy is greatest between 28 and 32 weeks, when the hemodynamic chances of pregnancy peak, but also is increased during labor and delivery.

5. Immediately after placental separation, the obstructive effect of the pregnant uterus on venous return disappears, and there is a sudden transfusion of blood from the lower extremities and the uteroplacental circulation into the systemic circulation. A patient with heart disease may not tolerate this increase in blood volume.

6. The pregnant cardiac patient should have effective pain relief during labor and deliver in the lateral supine position. In the majority of cases the anesthesia of choice is epidural blockade administered by an experienced obstetric anesthesiologist.

7. The most frequent fetal complications in patients with heart disease are preterm birth and growth retardation.

8. Almost all cardiac patients in labor should be kept "dry" and their IV fluids restricted to no more than 75 ml/hr. An exception to this rule is the patient with aortic stenosis.

9. The principal measures in the management of the pregnant patient in congestive heart failure are (1) decrease the cardiac work with bed rest, (2) decrease the preload with diuretics, (3) improve the cardiac contractility with digitalis, and (4) reduce the afterload with vasodilators.

10. The prognosis for a patient with peripartum cardiomyopathy is poor if she has significantly reduced left ventricular ejection fraction and if her heart remains dilated 6 months after initiation of therapy.

11. Patients with Marfan's syndrome contemplating pregnancy should have an echocardiogram to assess the diameter of the aortic root, and if it is greater than 4.0 cm, there is a high risk for aortic dissection.

REFERENCES

1. Land MA, Bisno AL: Acute rheumatic fever: A vanishing disease in suburbia. *JAMA* 1983;249:895.
2. Krause RM: The influence of infection in the geography of heart disease. *Circulation* 1979;60:972.
3. McFaul PB, Dornan JC, Lamki H, et al: Pregnancy complicated by maternal heart disease: A review of 519 women. *Br J Obstet Gynaecol* 1988;95:861-867.
4. Ueland K: Cardiovascular diseases complicating pregnancies. *Clin Obstet Gynecol* 1978;21:49.
5. Clark SL, Cotton DB, Lee W, et al: Central hemodynamic assessment of normal term pregnancy. *Am J Obstet Gynecol* 1989;161:1439-1442.
6. Lees HM, Taylor SH, Scotte BD, et al: The circulatory effect of recumbent postural change in late pregnancy. *Clin Sci* 1967;32:453-465.
7. Longo LD: Maternal blood volume and cardiac output during pregnancy: A hypothesis of endocrinologic control. *Am J Physiol* 1983;245:R720-R729.
8. Bitsch M, Johansen C, Wennevold A, et al: Maternal heart disease: A survey of a decade in a Danish University Hospital. *Acta Obstet Gynecol Scand* 1989;68:119-124.
9. Nora JJ: Etiologic factors in congenital heart disease. *Pediatr Clin North Am* 1971;18:1059.
10. Arias F: Expansion of intravascular volume and fetal outcome in patients with chronic hypertension and pregnancy. *Am J Obstet Gynecol* 1975;123:610.
11. DiMarco JP, Miles W, Akhtar M, et al: Adenosine for paroxysmal supraventricular tachycardia: Dose ranging and comparison with verapamil. *Ann Intern Med* 1990;113:104-110.
12. Rayburn WF, LeMire MS, Bird JL, et al: Mitral valve prolapse: Echocardiographic changes during pregnancy. *J Reprod Med* 1987;32:185-189.
13. Tank LCH, Chan SYW, Wong VCW, et al: Pregnancy in patients with mitral valve prolapse. *Br J Gynaecol Obstet* 1985;23:217-221.
14. Carvallo A, Brandao A, Martinez EE, et al: Prognosis in peripartum cardiomyopathy. *Am J Cardiol* 1989;64:540-542.
15. Burch GE, McDonald CD, Walsh JJ: The effect of prolonged bed rest on postpartal cardiomyopathy. *Am Heart J* 1971;81:186.
16. O'Connell JB, Costanzo-Nordin MR, Subramanian R, et al: Peripartum cardiomyopathy: Clinical, hemodynamic,

histologic and prognostic characteristics. *J Am Coll Cardiol* 1986;8:52-56.

17. Midei MG, DeMent SH, Feldman AM, et al: Peripartum myocarditis and cardiomyopathy. *Circulation* 1990;81:922-928.

18. Cunningham FG, Pritchard JA, Hankins JDV, et al: Peripartum heart failure: Idiopathic cardiomyopathy or compounding cardiovascular events. *Obstet Gynecol* 1986;67:157.

19. Szekely P, Snaith L: *Heart Disease and Pregnancy.* Edinburgh, Churchill-Livingstone, 1974, pp 21-79.

20. Arias F, Pineda J: Aortic stenosis and pregnancy. *J Reprod Med* 1978;20:229.

21. Gleicher M, Midwall J, Hochberger D, et al: Eisenmenger's syndrome and pregnancy. *Obstet Gynecol Surv* 1979;34:721.

22. Sareli P, England MJ, Berk MR, et al: Maternal and fetal sequelae of anticoagulation during pregnancy in patients with mechanical heart valve prosthesis. *Am J Cardiol* 1989;63:1462-1465.

23. Ginsberg JS, Hirsch J: Use of anticoagulants during pregnancy. *Chest* 1989;95:156S.

24. Iturbe-Alessio I, Fonseca MDC, Matchim KO, et al: Risk of anticoagulant therapy in pregnant women with artificial heart valves. *N Engl J Med* 1986;1390-1393.

12

CHRONIC HYPERTENSION AND PREGNANCY

Chronic hypertension complicates between 1% and 3% of all pregnancies and corresponds with 25% to 50% of all cases of hypertension during pregnancy. Other patients with hypertension during pregnancy have pregnancy-induced hypertension, or preeclampsia.

◢ DEFINITION

According to the American College of Obstetricians and Gynecologists (ACOG), to establish a diagnosis of chronic hypertension during pregnancy, it is necessary to have documented elevated blood pressure—140/90 mm Hg or above in repeated measurements several hours apart—before pregnancy or to discover the hypertension before 20 weeks of gestation.

The main problem with this definition is that in many patients it is not possible to document hypertension outside of pregnancy. Also, a significant number of women with undiagnosed chronic hypertension start their prenatal care after 20 weeks of gestation. To complicate the situation further, these patients frequently are normotensive in the second trimester, thereby obscuring the differential diagnosis.

The International Society for the Study of Hypertension in Pregnancy (ISSHP) recognizes two groups and six subgroups of patients with chronic hypertension during pregnancy:

A. *Chronic hypertension and chronic renal disease*

These are women with chronic hypertension or chronic renal disease (diagnosed before, during, or after pregnancy) who have hypertension and/or proteinuria during pregnancy.

These patients are subdivided into:

1. Chronic hypertension without proteinuria
2. Chronic renal disease (proteinuria with or without hypertension)
3. Chronic hypertension with superimposed preeclampsia (proteinuria developing for first time during pregnancy in a woman with known chronic hypertension)

B. *Unclassified hypertension and/or proteinuria*

Patients in this group have hypertension and/or proteinuria in either of the following situations:

• At first examination after twentieth week of gestation (140 days) in a woman without known chronic hypertension or chronic renal disease

- During pregnancy, labor, or the puerperium in cases in which information is insufficient to permit classification

Unclassified hypertension and/or proteinuria is subdivided into:
1. Unclassified hypertension without proteinuria
2. Unclassified proteinuria without hypertension
3. Unclassified proteinuric hypertension

Unclassified hypertension and/or proteinuria may be reclassified after delivery into:
1. Gestational hypertension without proteinuria
2. Gestational proteinuria without hypertension
3. Gestational proteinuric hypertension
4. Chronic hypertension without proteinuria
5. Chronic renal disease
6. Chronic hypertension with superimposed preeclampsia

The ISSHP classification is complex and contains too many subgroups. One of its merits is that it reflects the difficulties that frequently exist in classifying pregnant patients with chronic hypertension when they come to the obstetrician for medical treatment. The ACOG classification is prefered by most clinicians and investigators.

◪ ETIOLOGY

The majority of pregnant women with chronic hypertension have essential hypertension.[1] Rarely, the hypertension results from chronic renal disease, renal artery stenosis, pheochromocytoma, hyperaldosteronism, or other causes (Box 12-1).

◪ PATHOPHYSIOLOGY

Blood pressure elevation in patients with chronic hypertension is a symptom resulting from an imbalance in the complex mechanisms that normally regulate blood pressure. The most important determinants of blood pressure are the cardiac output (CO) and the peripheral vascular resistance (PVR). These hemodynamic parameters are, in turn, the result of multiple influences. PVR is affected by humoral factors such as angiotensin and catecholamines, nervous sympathetic activity, and local factors such as en-

---

> **BOX 12-1**
>
> ### Etiology of Chronic Hypertension during Pregnancy
>
> 1. Essential hypertension
> 2. Secondary hypertension
>   Renal
>   Renal parenchymal disease
>   Renovascular hypertension
>   Endocrine
>   Pheochromocytoma
>   Primary aldosteronism
>   Cushing's syndrome
>   Neurogenic
>   Increased intracranial pressure
>   Vascular
>   Aortic coarctation
> 3. Systolic hypertension
>   Thyrotoxicosis
>   Hyperkinetic circulation

---

dothelin and nitrous oxide. CO depends on cardiac contractility and the status of the intravascular volume. Elevated blood pressure may result from alterations in one or several of these factors.

For reasons unknown at the present time, essential hypertension starts with increased CO and normal PVR. This phase is followed by a gradual increase in PVR and a decrease in CO. Eventually the hypertension becomes established, accelerates the arteriosclerotic process, and produces damage to the heart, brain, kidneys, and other target organs. This process takes 30 or more years from beginning to end except in a few patients who develop accelerated hypertension. The large majority of pregnant women with chronic essential hypertension are in the early stages of this process and rarely exhibit funduscopic, cardiac, or renal alterations.

Since most pregnant women with chronic hypertension are in an early phase of this spectrum of hypertension, they usually show elevated CO and normal or mildly elevated PVR. However, a normal PVR in the presence of elevated CO is abnormal because the physiologic response to an increase in CO is a decrease in PVR. During the first 20 weeks of gestation, the predominant effect of pregnancy in both normotensive and hypertensive patients will be a decrease in PVR. This will compensate for the lack of antepartum regulatory response to the increased CO, and the result will be a decrease in blood pressure. This beneficial effect of pregnancy does not last too long. Pregnancy causes an increase in intravascular volume and cardiac output that starts at the end of the first trimester and peaks at about 28 or 30 weeks of gestation. Some chronic hypertensive pregnant patients will have difficulties compensating for the additional increase in CO with further decreases in PVR, and the blood pressure will start to rise. This phenomenon has been named *pregnancy-aggravated hypertension* and differs from preeclampsia because of the absence of proteinuria or other evidence of multiorgan endothelial injury.

◢ DIAGNOSIS

The diagnosis of chronic hypertension in pregnancy is established when an abnormal blood pressure (140/90 mm Hg or above) is found before 20 weeks of gestation or when there is evidence of hypertension before pregnancy. In many cases these conditions are not fulfilled, and the diagnosis cannot be made despite strong clinical suspicions.

It is possible to make false-positive and false-negative diagnoses of chronic hypertension in pregnancy as a result of inadequate technique for blood pressure measuring. The most common error is to measure the blood pressure in obese patients with a small cuff. Another common source of error is variation in the use of Korotkoff's sounds for determination of diastolic pressure. Although the use of Korotkoff V (point of disappearance of sounds) is recommended in nongravid patients, it is common in pregnancy to hear sounds even with no pressure in the cuff. Therefore it is better to use Korotkoff IV (point of muffling of the sounds). Patient posture is also important, and measurements of blood pressure during pregnancy should be obtained with the patient in the sitting position with the arm elevated at the level of the heart. When the patient lies on her left side and the blood pressure is taken on her right arm, the blood pressure is falsely low by as much as 15 mm Hg. Some guidelines for measurement of blood pressure in pregnancy are shown in Box 12-2.

◢ MATERNAL AND FETAL RISKS

The most important risks confronting pregnant patients with chronic hypertension are the

---

BOX 12-2

Guidelines for Measuring Blood Pressure during Pregnancy

1. Patient conditions

   For measurements taken in the office, the patient should be in the sitting position with her right arm supported in horizontal position at the level of her heart.

   For measurements taken in the hospital, the woman should be in semirecumbent position with the arm roughly at heart level.

2. Equipment

   The cuff should encircle and cover two thirds of the length of the arm. A large cuff should be used for obese patients.

   Aneroid manometers should be calibrated every 6 months against a mercury manometer.

3. Technique

   Inflate the cuff 20 mm above the systolic pressure, as recognized by disappearance of the radial pulse.

   Use Korotkoff IV (muffling of the sound) to determine diastolic blood pressure.

---

development of superimposed preeclampsia, fetal malnutrition, preterm labor, and abruptio placentae.

Superimposed preeclampsia

The risk of developing superimposed preeclampsia is approximately 30%. In patients with chronic hypertension, preeclampsia usually is severe, occurs early in pregnancy, and responds poorly to bed rest.

In some patients the differential diagnosis between superimposed preeclampsia and aggravation of chronic hypertension is difficult. Proteinuria is useful in making this distinction, but cannot be used in patients with chronic renal disease. In these patients it is necessary to search for other signs of end-organ damage indicating the presence of preeclampsia.

A laboratory test that may help in making the differential diagnosis between superimposed preeclampsia and aggravation of chronic hypertension is the determination of urinary calcium. Taufield et al.[2] found that the mean urinary calcium excretion in patients with preeclampsia or with chronic hypertension with superimposed preeclampsia was lower (42 ± 29 and 78 ± 49 mg/24 hr, respectively) than in women with chronic hypertension alone (223 ± 41 mg/24 hr). Other studies[3] have found that measurement of the calcium/creatinine ratio in a randomly obtained specimen of urine may be as useful as a 24-hour urine collection in the assessment of calciuria in patients with hypertension during pregnancy.

Fetal growth retardation

Fetal malnutrition, manifested as poor fetal growth, affects 15% to 25% of pregnancies with chronic hypertension.[4,5] In patients with growth-retarded fetuses, preterm labor, abruptio placentae, and intrapartum hypoxia and acidosis are more common than in patients with chronic hypertension and normal fetal growth.

Preterm labor

Preterm labor occurs in approximately 15.3% of patients with chronic hypertension.[4,5] Patients with fetal growth retardation and small, fibrotic, infarcted placentas are particularly prone to this complication. In these patients, preterm labor is a mechanism of fetal protection against a hostile intrauterine environment. The majority of infants born early because of preterm labor caused by placental insufficiency are vigorous at birth and require little or no ventilatory support.

Abruptio placentae

Abruptio placentae occurs in approximately 5% to 9% of chronically hypertensive pregnant patients. This is, unfortunately, an unpredictable event that occurs more frequently when superimposed preeclampsia or severe chronic hypertension is present. The fetal outcome in patients with severe abruptio is poor.

◼ MANAGEMENT

Ideally, the obstetric management of chronic hypertensive patients should start before conception. Prepregnancy evaluation will permit the physician to determine the severity and the hemodynamic characteristics of the hypertension and collect evidence about the presence of end-organ damage. Unfortunately, the majority of these patients are seen after conception, and in that case the first step is to take a careful history and perform a meticulous physical examination.

The history and physical examination should be focused on determining whether there are signs or symptoms suggestive of secondary hypertension or end-organ damage. Also, patients with chronic hypertension frequently have undiagnosed medical problems such as parenchymal renal disease, diabetes, or connective tissue disorders. For these reasons the history should be meticulous, and the physical examination should include measurement of blood pressure in both upper and lower extremities, auscultation of the flanks in search of a renal bruit, and examination of the optic fundi.

The majority of these women do not require extensive laboratory testing. Usually the workup can be limited to an ECG, a serum biochemical profile (SMA-18), and a urine culture for the detection of asymptomatic bacteriuria. A creatinine clearance is ordered only if the serum creatinine concentration is above 0.8 mg/dl, the upper limit of normal for pregnancy. Quantitative urinary protein and analysis of the urinary sediment are ordered if the patient shows 2+ or more albumin on spot checks. Antinuclear antibody (ANA) titers are important if the patient's history or examination suggests the possibility of autoimmune disease. Measurement of urinary electrolytes is needed only if there is an abnormality in serum electrolyte levels. Doppler analysis of umbilical and uterine artery waveforms has limited value in the initial assessment of these patients.

If the hypertension is severe or there are signs and symptoms suggesting a secondary cause of the hypertension (see Box 12-1), the patient may require determination of urinary vinyl mandelic acid and metanephrines, measurement of plasma renin activity, rapid-sequence intravenous pyelogram, chest x-ray film, and renal arteriogram or renal biopsy.

Severity assessment

Assessment of severity is based on the magnitude of the blood pressure elevation. Traditionally, 160 mm Hg systolic and 110 mm Hg diastolic blood pressure have been accepted as the limits differentiating mild from severe hypertension.

Determination of the severity of the hypertension is important for establishing a prognosis. Most clinicians and some data[6] agree that the more severe the hypertension, the worse the prognosis and the greater the potential for com-

---

BOX 12-3

Conditions That Place Patients with Mild Chronic Hypertension during Pregnancy at High Risk for Complications and Poor Outcome

1. Diastolic blood pressure 85 mm Hg or greater or mean arterial pressure 95 mm Hg or greater in repeated observations at least 6 hours apart, after 12 weeks of gestation
2. History of severe hypertension in previous pregnancies
3. History of abruptio placentae
4. History of stillbirth or unexplained neonatal death
5. History of previous deliveries of small-for-gestational-age babies
6. Older than 35 years of age or more than 15 years of hypertension
7. Marked obesity
8. Secondary hypertension

---

plications. Severity assessment is also useful for determining the necessity for medications. If the patient is classified as severe, the need for treatment is clear. If the patient has mild disease, the need for antihypertensives will depend on the presence of high-risk factors.

The large majority of pregnant patients with chronic hypertension have mild disease, and factors other than the level of the blood pressure should be taken into account in determining their prognosis. Patients with mild hypertension are at high risk for obstetric complications if one or several of the conditions listed in Box 12-3 is present.

Hemodynamic assessment

The majority of pregnant patients with mild chronic hypertension have increased CO and "normal" PVR. The PVR decreases during the second trimester as a result of physiologic vasodilation, and the blood pressure becomes normal. However, in some patients the increase in CO caused by pregnancy is not adequately compensated by further decreases in PVR, and the blood pressure rises again, usually at the end of the second trimester. This elevation of blood pressure is usually within the mild range.

Other chronic hypertensive patients have hyperkinetic circulation during gestation. This is characterized by increased CO caused by increased heart rate. The abnormal myocardial contractility most likely is the result of increased sympathetic activity. In addition to tachycardia, these patients have predominantly systolic hypertension. The hemodynamic changes induced by pregnancy will accentuate these characteristics.

Patients with more advanced hypertensive disease start pregnancy with normal CO and increased PVR. Characteristically, they do not show a significant decrease in diastolic blood pressure during the second trimester of pregnancy and have little or no increase in plasma volume.

In summary, the hemodynamic characteristics of patients with chronic hypertension are different and are therefore modified differently by the physiologic changes of pregnancy. The therapeutic implications of these hemodynamic peculiarities are described later (p. 239).

Self-monitoring of blood pressure during pregnancy

Self-monitoring of the blood pressure is of fundamental importance in the management of the pregnant patient with chronic hypertension because measurements taken in the office every 2 to 4 weeks provide very little information about this dynamic process. Therefore such measurements are inadequate for determining the need for treatment or for assessing the therapeutic response. Also, it has been recognized for many years that the medical office setting can provoke anxiety, temporarily raising the patient's blood pressure. This phenomenon, *white coat hypertension,* further demonstrates the frequent inaccuracy of office blood pressure measurements and supports the use of self-monitoring in the management of blood pressure disorders.

Normally blood pressure has a circadian rhythm with a nadir between 2 and 4 AM. This is followed by a rapid rise that reaches a peak between 6 and 8 AM. The blood pressure remains stable during the day and falls progressively in the evening and during the night. This pattern has multiple influences, especially stressful conditions. Therefore several measurements throughout a 24-hour period provide a better understanding of an individual need of or a response to treatment.

Patient self-monitoring of the blood pressure gives the obstetrician more reliable information on which better management decisions can be made. The method also supplies the patient with information that may enhance compliance.[7]

Electronic and mechanical devices for self-monitoring of blood pressure are sold at most pharmacies and drug stores. These devices are reliable, and because of their slow deflation rates (2 mm/sec), the measurements obtained with them are often more accurate than those obtained by the clinician. The digital devices are also simple to use because they do not require a stethoscope.

All pregnant patients with chronic hypertension should obtain a digital device for daily blood pressure monitoring and use it in the morning and the afternoon. They should bring their device to the obstetrician's office and be instructed in its correct use. They should maintain a daily record of their measurements as well. The majority of chronic hypertensive patients have lower blood pressure at home than at the office.[8] The reverse situation is very rare, and when the blood pressure rises at home, it will usually be elevated at the office.

Nonpharmacologic therapy

Bed rest. Bed rest has been used for many years as an adjunct in the management of pregnant patients with chronic hypertension. Blood pressure in the lateral recumbent position is approximately 10 mm Hg lower than in the sitting or standing position. Bed rest increases the venous return that is impaired because of compression by the pregnant uterus, and this permits mobilization of fluids, diuresis, decreased edema, and improved placental perfusion.

There are no controlled, randomized studies comparing the efficacy of bed rest to other treatment modalities in pregnancy. However, Curet and Olson[9] found that patients having 4 hours of bed rest daily had a decrease in perinatal mortality compared with prior pregnancies.

Despite the scarce scientific support, bed rest for the pregnant patient with chronic hypertension makes sense. These patients should be advised to rest 1 hour twice daily at the beginning of pregnancy. The bed rest periods should be increased to 2, 3, or 4 hours twice daily depending on the gestational age, the levels of blood pressure, and the accumulation of edema.

Salt restriction. The sodium content of the American diet is very high, 150 to 200 mEq/day (6 to 10 g of salt/day). A reduction in blood pressure of approximately 10 mm Hg can be achieved in the nonpregnant status by lowering the sodium intake to 90 mEq/day (4 g of salt/day). This decrease in sodium intake is not dangerous to the pregnant woman or her fetus, and it still provides enough sodium to allow adequate plasma volume expansion. Pregnant patients with chronic hypertension should be instructed to avoid processed foods, to minimize consumption of milk products, to scrutinize food labels for sodium content, and to resist adding salt to their food.

Coffee. Large amounts of caffeine may raise the blood pressure by sympathetic stimulation. Pregnant patients with chronic hypertension, particularly those with hyperkinetic circulation, should be advised not to drink coffee during pregnancy.

Weight and exercise. Excessive weight is frequently associated with hypertension, particularly among blacks, and weight reduction usually causes a decrease in blood pressure. However, obese hypertensive women should not lose weight during pregnancy. Rather, they should avoid a large weight gain by limiting caloric intake to only that necessary to cover their needs.

Exercise has a beneficial effect on blood pressure in nonpregnant patients. Pregnant hypertensive patients should avoid starting new exercise activities during pregnancy. However, they should continue any exercise program initiated before pregnancy.

Antihypertensive therapy

Pharmacologic treatment of chronic hypertension during pregnancy is indicated if it will decrease the severity of the associated complications. This stipulation is fulfilled in gravidas with severe hypertension,[10,11] and there is universal agreement that treatment of these patients decreases the frequency of maternal cardiac and cerebrovascular complications.[12]

The controversy over pharmacologic treatment concerns patients with mild chronic hypertension. In these patients the most common maternal complications are superimposed preeclampsia and abruptio placentae. The fetus may be affected by growth retardation, antepartum and intrapartum hypoxia and acidosis, preterm labor, and preterm delivery. Proponents of universal treatment believe that the risk of accelerated hypertension, preeclampsia, and perinatal mortality and morbidity will be significantly reduced by treatment with antihypertensive drugs. Those who favor not treating pregnant women with mild hypertension believe that most of these complications cannot be prevented by medication, that the risk of therapy is greater than the benefit, and that most of these patients have good perinatal outcome without treatment.

The results of controlled trials have given contradictory results.[4,13-15] The problem with these studies is that most of them have a small number of patients and a heterogenous population with respect to gestational age at the time of initiation of treatment, type of treatment, type of hypertension, and presence of high-risk factors.

Rather than adopting a universal policy of treatment or no treatment, it is better to individualize and use pharmacologic therapy for mild chronic hypertensive patients at high risk for maternal or fetal complications (see Box 12-3). This approach is logical, avoids unnecessary treatment for many patients, and may prevent complications.

Treatment should be initiated as soon as the diagnosis and the indication for treatment have been established. The rationale for early treatment is based on studies by Leather et al.[14] and Redman et al.[16] showing a significant decrease in the number of midtrimester pregnancy losses in treated patients compared with untreated control patients. When the indication for treatment appears late in gestation, medications should be given without concern that blood pressure reduction may impair uteroplacental perfusion and affect fetal well-being. In fact, the study of Redman et al.[16] shows that treatment started late in gestation causes no harm to patients.

An ideal antihypertensive drug should maintain the cardiac, renal, cerebral, and uteroplacental perfusion. It should not increase the heart rate or the plasma volume when the blood pressure drops, it should have no side effects, and it should be given once daily. This optimal medication does not exist. However, several medications are adequate for the treatment of chronic hypertension during pregnancy (Box 12-4). Most experience has been with methyldopa. Recently, beta blockers have surfaced as a first-line drug.

BOX 12-4

Antihypertensive Drugs That May Be Used during Pregnancy

Diuretics
Thiazide

Drugs that decrease peripheral vascular resistance
Hydralazine
Labetalol
Calcium channel blockers
Prazosin

Drugs that decrease cardiac output
Beta blockers

Centrally acting drugs
Methyldopa

Diuretics. Diuretics, particularly thiazides, have been used for more than 30 years, and their efficacy and safety in nonpregnant patients with mild hypertension have been clearly demonstrated. In pregnant patients the situation is different, and both the efficacy and the safety of diuretics have been questioned. There are two old controlled studies[17,18] showing no improvement in perinatal mortality or in the incidence of preeclampsia with the use of thiazides, whereas another large study[19] shows a significant decrease in perinatal mortality. Also, diuretics may cause neonatal thrombocytopenia and maternal hyperuricemia and may decrease placental perfusion.[20] However, in a review of the literature Collins et al.[21] did not find evidence that diuretics were dangerous when given to pregnant women. The reason for these conflicting reports is probably the heterogeneity of the patients being studied, with respect to the expansion of their intravascular volume. Diuretics are useful in patients with intravascular volume expansion and may be detrimental in patients with decreased plasma volume, and their use in unselected populations will give mixed results.

Initially, diuretics decrease blood pressure by increasing urinary sodium excretion, decreasing the plasma volume and the extracellular fluid, and decreasing the CO. After 6 to 8 weeks of therapy, the CO returns to the prior level, the reduction in plasma volume and extracellular fluid is maintained, and the blood pressure remains low because of an effect on PVR.

The diuretic most commonly used during pregnancy is chlorothiazide. The usual dose is 25 mg every morning and may be increased to 50 mg daily, but larger doses usually have no greater antihypertensive effect.

Side effects of thiazides are mild and have little clinical significance. The most frequent biochemical changes are hypokalemia, hyperuricemia, and hyperglycemia, but rarely are these changes severe enough to cause symptoms or require therapy.

Drugs that affect peripheral vascular resistance

Hydralazine. Hydralazine has been used for almost 40 years and is the prototype of peripherally acting antihypertensive drugs. It is a vasodilator that acts directly on the smooth muscle fibers of the arterial circulation. It has no effect on postcapillary capacitance vessels. The main obstetric use of hydralazine is to rapidly lower blood pressure, via intravenous injection, in patients with severe preeclampsia. The medication is unsuitable as a first choice antihypertensive for long-term use during pregnancy.

Hydralazine increases cardiac output and plasma volume by vasodilation and reflex stimulation of the renin angiotensin system, respectively. Consequently, resistance to treatment or treatment failures is common when the drug is used for prolonged periods. However, hydralazine may be useful when combined with diuretics and beta blockers in patients not responding to single-drug therapy.

The exact mechanism of action of hydralazine is unknown. It requires an intact endothelium and is probably mediated by prostaglandins. The onset of action occurs rapidly after intravenous injection. The drug is usually given in 5- to 10-mg intravenous doses that are repeated at 10- to 20-minute intervals until the desired level of blood pressure is achieved. Orally, its action peaks in 3 to 4 hours and has a total duration of action of 6 to 12 hours. It is usually given twice daily in doses of 40 to 200 mg. Hydralazine is acetylated in the liver at a rate that is genetically determined. Patients with slow acetylation respond to relatively small doses of medication with significant decreases in blood pressure, whereas those with fast acetylation are relatively resistant to the hypotensive effect of the drug.

Hydralazine can cause headaches, anxiety, nausea, vomiting, facial flushing, and epigastric pain. Most importantly, it causes decreased uteroplacental blood flow when the hypotensive effect is rapid or severe. In approximately 10% of patients, hydralazine causes a reversible lupuslike syndrome. This lupus syndrome is limited to patients with slow acetylation and usually responds to discontinuation of the medication. The appearance of positive ANA titers in pregnant patients treated with hydralazine is rare.

Labetalol. Different than other beta blockers, labetalol acts by decreasing PVR with little or no decrease in CO. The drug has $beta_1$, $beta_2$, and $alpha_1$ blocking properties. The alpha-to-beta blockade ratio is 3:1 when given orally and 1:7 when given intravenously.

The main obstetric use of labetalol is for hypertensive emergencies in patients with severe preeclampsia. Labetalol is replacing hydralazine for rapid reduction of blood pressure in preeclampsia because it does not cause severe hypotension, headaches, and tachycardia and has no effect on uteroplacental blood flow. The drug is given intravenously, 20-mg initial dose, followed by 40 to 80 mg every 10 minutes, until the therapeutic response is achieved. It can also be given in IV drip, dissolving a 40-ml vial in 160 ml of normal saline and giving 2 ml/min (120 mg/hr) and adjusting the rate to the patient's response.

Labetalol can be used orally for long-term treatment of chronic hypertension. Approximately 75% of the drug is inactivated in the first liver pass. The initial dose is 100 mg twice daily. This dose may be increased according to the patient's response. The maintenance dose is usually 200 to 400 mg twice daily.

Calcium channel blockers. Calcium channel blockers act as antihypertensive agents by impeding the influx of calcium through slow calcium channels into vascular smooth muscle cells, causing vascular relaxation and decreasing the PVR. They also relax the uterus and are used as tocolytic agents. The calcium channel blockers most commonly used in obstetric patients are nifedipine and verapamil.

Nifedipine can be used as a single agent or in combination with other antihypertensives in the treatment of chronic hypertension during pregnancy. The usual dosage is 10 mg orally every 6 hours. It can be increased up to 20 mg every 4 hours. The medication is absorbed immediately and reaches a peak level serum concentration in

30 minutes. Biting the capsule before swallowing accelerates the absorption of the drug. Approximately 80% of nifedipine is eliminated by the kidney. The medication has no deleterious effects on uteroplacental blood flow.[22]

The most common nifedipine side effects are facial flushing and headaches. In some patients it may cause constipation or exaggerated hypotension.

Verapamil is another calcium channel blocker that may be used in the treatment of chronic hypertension during pregnancy. The usual starting dosage is 80 mg 4 times daily. One of the main uses of this drug is treatment of preeclamptic patients who remain hypertensive after delivery. It is also useful in the treatment of patients who had low renin hypertension before pregnancy.

Prazosin. Prazosin is a peripheral vasodilator that works by blocking postsynaptic alpha receptors. The medication does not cause changes in cardiac output but has a significant effect on capacitance vessels. Abrupt loss of venous tone with peripheral blood pooling has been invocated as the mechanism for the occasional occurrence of severe hypotension with the first dose of medication. On the positive side, the effect on the capacitance vessels combined with the effect on PVR are important advantages of the drug when used in chronic hypertensive patients who fail to adequately expand plasma volume during pregnancy. Prazosin in combination with a diuretic is highly effective for the treatment of severe hypertension refractory to other medications.

Prazosin reaches a peak plasma concentration approximately 3 hours after ingestion, is metabolized in the liver, and is excreted in the bile and feces. Prazosin is a safe drug for pregnant patients.[23,24] The initial dose should be 1 mg at bedtime to avoid first-dose hypotension. The dose may be increased according to the patient's response, but usually 2 to 4 mg twice daily is all that is necessary to achieve adequate blood pressure control.

The main side effect of prazosin is postural hypotension effect that affects approximately 1% of the patients. Dizziness and light-headedness are also frequent complaints.

Medications that decrease cardiac output

Beta adrenergic blockers. Beta blockers are perhaps the drugs of choice for initial treatment of pregnant women with chronic hypertension. The present understanding of the hemodynamics of mild chronic hypertension in pregnancy indicates that the majority of these patients have increased cardiac output and hyperkinetic circulation.[25] Propranolol reduces cardiac output between 15% and 30% and suppresses renin production by 60%. After a few weeks of treatment, there is also a drop in peripheral vascular resistance. The effect on PVR is indirect and most likely is an autoregulatory response using vasodilation to maintain adequate blood flow despite the drop in CO. These hemodynamic characteristics make therapy with beta blockers ideal for the majority of patients with chronic hypertension during pregnancy. Also, beta blockers are safe in pregnancy, and there is abundant literature[26-28] documenting the excellent outcome of pregnant patients treated with these compounds.

Beta blockers act on blood pressure by competing with endogenous catecholamines for beta adrenergic receptors. They leave alpha-mediated vasoconstriction unopposed. Different compounds have different affinity for beta receptors and are classified as cardioselective when they predominantly bind to beta-1 receptors or noncardioselective when they bind to both beta-1 and beta-2 receptors. Atenolol is predominantly a beta-1 or cardioselective type of beta blocker, whereas propranolol is noncardioselective.

Propranolol is an effective drug for the treatment of chronic hypertension during pregnancy and has virtually no side effects. Several prospective studies have demonstrated the safety of its administration during pregnancy. Propranolol is metabolized by the liver, and approximately 70% of the drug is removed in the first pass. It has a half-life of 3 to 6 hours, but its effects are longer, and it can be given once or twice daily without problems. The medication lowers the blood pressure within hours, and the antihypertensive effect is not modified by changes in posture or activity. Treatment usually is initiated at a dosage of 40 to 60 mg twice daily. The initial dosage is adjusted according to the response and the side effects. The maximum dose is usually 480 to 640 mg per day, although higher doses rarely cause side effects.

Most of the side effects and contraindications for the use of propranolol are caused by the nonspecific beta-1 and beta-2 blockade produced by the drug. Minor problems include fatigue, insomnia, and bad dreams. More serious side effects are bronchospasm and a blunted response to hypoglycemia, therefore preventing its use in patients with asthma and in patients with brittle diabetes, respectively. Prolonged administration of propranolol may cause fluid retention.

Atenolol is a selective beta₁ adrenergic blocking agent that has significant advantages over propranolol and is being used with increasing frequency in the treatment of pregnant patients. About 50% of a given oral dose is absorbed from the gastrointestinal tract. The medication has minimal or no hepatic metabolism and is eliminated by the kidneys.

The effect of atenolol is noticeable within 1 hour and is at maximum effect 2 to 4 hours after a dose is given. The effect of the drug on the blood pressure is relatively long, and therefore it can be given in a single daily dose. The side effects are minimal. Most patients with mild or moderate hypertension require only 50 mg daily. Doses above 100 mg daily are not useful.

The advantage of atenolol is its selectivity for beta-1 receptors. Therefore it does not cause bronchospasm and may be given with caution to patients with history of asthma. Also, because of its prolonged duration of action, it can be given in one or two daily doses.

Centrally acting drugs

Methyldopa. Methyldopa has been the most widely used antihypertensive drug during pregnancy, but lately it is being replaced by beta blockers as the first-choice drug. The site of action of the medication is the central nervous system. Methyldopa induces the synthesis of alpha-methylnorepinephrine that stimulates alpha receptors and decreases the sympathetic outflow from the central nervous system.

The effect of methyldopa is mainly on peripheral vascular resistance with little effect on cardiac output. The medication causes dilation of both the arterial circulation and the capacitance vessels, thereby allowing increases in intravascular volume to occur. Also, renal blood flow is maintained during treatment with methyldopa, and this property makes it the drug of choice in patients with actual or potential limitations in kidney function. Methyldopa reaches a maximum effectiveness in 4 to 6 hours, with a total duration of action of about 8 hours. A single bedtime dose is usually effective for blood pressure control, but to obtain maximum therapeutic efficiency, administration 2 or 3 times daily is necessary. The drug is primarily excreted in the urine and may accumulate in patients with severe impairment of renal function.

Methyldopa is the only antihypertensive medication that has been submitted to controlled trials during pregnancy[13,15] and has been shown to have beneficial effects. The usual starting dose is 250 mg of methyldopa 3 times a day. This amount may be increased up to a total of 2 g per day according to the patient's response.

The most common side effect of methyldopa is postural hypotension, which subsides rather quickly with a decrease in the amount of medication. Excessive sedation and depression are occasionally seen. Positive Coombs' and abnormal liver tests occur in approximately 10% of all patients. Hemolytic anemia is an uncommon complication.

In some patients, long-term administration of methyldopa causes salt and water retention. It seems that the kidneys of patients with chronic hypertension react to decreases in blood pressure caused by medications other than diuretics as though the pressure were too low, and fluid and sodium retention occur. This is manifested clinically by an increase in body weight beyond that expected for pregnancy alone, edema, and hemodilution. This situation may progress to a point at which *rebound* hypertension caused by the large intravascular volume expansion is observed. In these cases hydrochlorothiazide should be added to the treatment using an initial dosage of 25 mg/day, which may be increased to 50 mg/day if necessary. The result will be diuresis, decreased edema, lowering of the blood pressure, and decrease in body weight.

Selection of antihypertensive medications

Treatment individualization is an important determinant of therapeutic success in pregnant patients with chronic hypertension. The patients should be classified into one of the three categories shown in Box 12-5. Most patients with mild chronic hypertension belong to the increased cardiac output and hyperdynamic circulation groups, whereas the majority of those with severe forms of the disease belong to the group with increased PVR.

The prototype of patients with increased cardiac output and increased plasma volume is the obese patient with gestational diabetes. The first-choice drug in these patients is a thiazide diuretic. Diuretics will have an immediate blood pressure–lowering effect by decreasing the plasma volume. Continued administration will cause decreased PVR, and that will allow the intravascular volume to expand again, this time as a consequence of pregnancy, without causing elevation of the blood pressure. Sibai et al.[29] have

---

BOX 12-5

Hemodynamic Subtypes of Pregnant Patients with Chronic Hypertension

Increased cardiac output

White or black, obese, diabetes, renal disease, normal heart rate, increased plasma volume, increased uric acid, abnormally "normal" PVR

Hyperdynamic circulation

White, lean, young, migraine, cardiac awareness, increased CO, increased plasma volume, predominantly systolic hypertension, decreased PVR, Korotkoff V sound at zero

Increased vascular resistance

Black, lean, older, slower heart rate, no decrease in diastolic blood pressure or drop in hematocrit in the second trimester, no increase or minimal increase in plasma volume, absence of physiologic systolic murmur in pregnancy, minimally increased or normal CO

---

demonstrated that pregnant patients treated with diuretics can have a normal expansion of intravascular volume. The administration of thiazides should be monitored with serial hematocrit determinations to evaluate their effect on plasma volume. If the expected physiologic increase in plasma volume does not occur, it may be necessary to add a vasodilator with an effect on capacitance vessels, such as prazosin or methyldopa, or adjust the dose of diuretic to decrease urinary sodium losses.

The prototype of patients with hyperdynamic circulation is the young, lean, white woman with tachycardia and a blood pressure with Korotkoff V sound at zero. The first-choice drug in these patients is atenolol. The effect of atenolol in these patients will be immediate, and most of them will do well for a long time with a 50-mg daily dose.

Patients with increased PVR are typically older, predominantly black, have had chronic hypertension for many years, and characteristically show minimal or no decrease in blood pressure and no expansion of plasma volume in the second trimester of pregnancy. The drug of choice in these patients is a peripheral vasodilator, such

as a calcium channel blocker, labetalol, methyldopa, or prazosin. Prazosin or methyldopa is preferred because of the effect on the capacitance vessels.

The different steps of the decision-making process concerning antihypertensive treatment during pregnancy are summarized in Figure 12-1.

Management during pregnancy

There is no substitute for frequent clinical observations in the follow-up of pregnant patients with chronic hypertension. They should have prenatal office visits every 2 weeks until 32 or 34 weeks of gestation and then every week until the end of pregnancy. The critical variables to monitor during the prenatal visits are:

1. Blood pressure
2. Uterine growth
3. Preterm contractions
4. Fetal movements
5. Maternal weight

Blood pressure monitoring is of critical importance. The patient should measure her blood pressure at home twice daily and bring the written results at each office visit. Patients should be asked to call the doctor if the diastolic blood pressure is consistently above 100 mm Hg or the systolic blood pressure is above 160 mm Hg. If the diastolic blood pressure starts to decrease at the beginning of the second trimester, this is an indication of decreased PVR, expanded intravascular volume, and possibly a good outcome. Increased intravascular volume during pregnancy is necessary to ensure adequate placental blood flow. Further evidence of intravascular volume expansion is the finding of a grade II systolic ejection murmur at about 12 to 14 weeks of gestation. If the diastolic pressure remains above 80 mm Hg well into the second trimester and there is no systolic murmur, this is an indication of increased PVR and lack of intravascular volume expansion. Thus there is an indication for initiation of therapy. The blood pressure measurements taken at home are also the best index for measuring the patient's response to therapy. The goal is to keep diastolic blood pressure below 85 mm Hg[30] and systolic blood pressure below 140 mm Hg.

Monitoring maternal weight is also important in the prenatal follow-up of patients with chronic hypertension. Too much or too little weight gain is a concern, but preoccupation with the latter

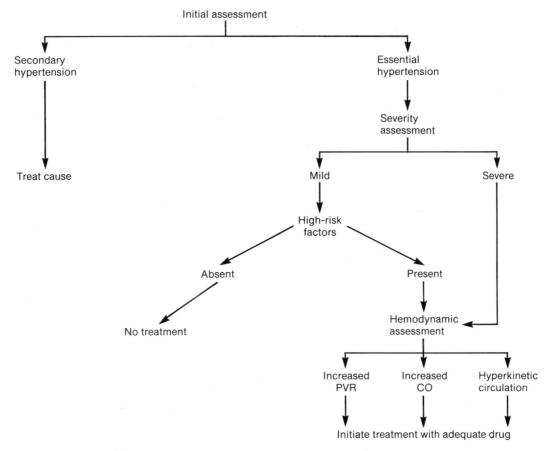

FIGURE 12-1 ◪ Sequence of steps in deciding treatment for pregnant patients with chronic hypertension.

should be greater. In fact, the pregnant patient with chronic hypertension who does not gain weight during pregnancy is at high risk for fetal malnutrition and other fetal problems. In contrast, too much weight gain may be normal and predictive of the birth of a large baby. Excessive weight gain may also be the consequence of unopposed methyldopa action or the first sign of superimposed preeclampsia.

Adequate fetal growth and activity are important clinical indicators of fetal well-being. Clinical evaluation of the fetal growth is imprecise, and ultrasound measurements should be obtained every 3 or 4 weeks. This evaluation is necessary even in patients with mild or well-controlled chronic hypertension.

It would be unusual to find monitoring signs of fetal hypoxia and acidosis in patients with

mild or well-controlled chronic hypertension who show normal fetal growth in serial ultrasound examinations. However, if there is any alteration in fetal growth or if the hypertension is inadequately controlled, it is necessary to institute other measures to evaluate fetal well-being. The simpler and more accurate tests for this purpose are the nonstress test with vibroacoustic stimulation and ultrasonic determination of fluid volume. These tests should be performed weekly after 32 weeks of gestation or earlier if there are clinical or ultrasound suggestions of impaired fetal growth, sudden deterioration of the maternal status, or decreased fetal movements.

Doppler waveform analysis of the umbilical artery may be useful for evaluating fetuses with inadequate growth. Umbilical Doppler analysis reflects downstream vascular impedance and is affected by conditions that compromise the placental vascular tree at the level of the tertiary villi. This type of placental compromise occurs frequently in patients with chronic hypertension and fetal growth retardation. There is evidence in the literature indicating that fetal growth retardation in the presence of normal umbilical Doppler analysis is a benign condition and the fetal prognosis is good. In contrast, an abnormal umbilical Doppler analysis suggests that there is placental compromise and the potential for fetal hypoxia is significant. However, an abnormal umbilical Doppler analysis should not be used as an indication for delivery except when exhibiting reversed diastolic flow. An abnormal Doppler analysis has only prognostic value and indicates the need for closer fetal surveillance.

Laboratory evaluation of pregnant patients with chronic hypertension is simple. An important test is the hematocrit/hemoglobin, used to determine whether plasma volume expansion occurs. Measurement of serum creatinine once early in pregnancy, then every 2 to 3 months, and biweekly dipstick measurements of protein in the first voided morning urine should be employed to monitor renal function. There is no need for monthly or periodic creatinine clearance tests and quantitative urinary protein determinations unless the serum creatinine level is more than 0.8 mg/dl or there is 2+ or more protein in qualitative examination of a random urine specimen.

Assessment of fetal pulmonary maturity is occasionally necessary in patients with chronic hypertension. However, in the majority of cases, early delivery is a consequence of either fetal or maternal deterioration, and determination of fetal lung maturity adds little to the plan of management.

Delivery

The large majority of patients who remain stable during the prenatal period will develop spontaneous labor and deliver at term or near term. In these patients cesarean section is usually necessary only for obstetric indications or for fetal heart rate monitoring suggestive of fetal hypoxia. Patients with moderate or severe hypertension and those with mild hypertension and high-risk factors may require preterm delivery because of maternal or fetal compromise.

◪   IMPORTANT POINTS   ◪

1. Chronic hypertension complicates approximately 1% to 3% of all pregnancies. To establish this diagnosis, it is necessary to document the presence of hypertension—140/90 mm Hg or above in repeated measurements—before pregnancy or before 20 weeks of gestation.

2. The overwhelming majority of pregnant women with chronic hypertension have essential hypertension. Rarely, the hypertension is secondary to renal artery stenosis, chronic renal disease, pheochromocytoma, or other causes.

3. Chronic hypertension usually starts with a phase of increased cardiac output (CO) and normal peripheral vascular resistance (PVR). In the next several years there is a gradual increase in PVR and a decrease in CO. The elevated blood pressure causes accelerated arteriosclerosis and results in damage to the heart, brain, kidney, and other organs. This process takes several years. Most pregnant women with chronic hypertension are in the earlier phases of this disease and have no evidence of end-organ damage.

4. The technique used for measuring blood pressure during pregnancy is important. Blood pressure should be taken with the patient in the sitting position with her arm supported in horizontal position at the level of the heart. A large cuff should be used for obese patients. Korotkoff IV should be used as end point for the diastolic pressure.

5. The most common maternal risks for patients with chronic hypertension during pregnancy are the development of superimposed preeclampsia and abruptio placentae. The most common fetal risks are fetal growth retardation, preterm delivery, and hypoxia and acidosis.

6. Severity classification is based on the magnitude of blood pressure elevation. Patients with persistent diastolic blood pressure greater than 110 mm Hg or systolic blood pressure greater than 160 mm Hg have severe hypertension. Most pregnant patients have mild hypertension.

7. In pregnant patients with mild chronic hypertension, factors other than the elevation

of blood pressure should be taken into consideration to determine whether they are at risk for complications and to determine the need for antihypertensive therapy.

8. The hemodynamic characteristics of patients with chronic hypertension during pregnancy are different. The majority have increased CO and normal PVR. Others have hyperkinetic circulation. Those at higher risk have elevated PVR and normal CO.

9. Self-monitoring of blood pressure is of fundamental importance in the management of patients with chronic hypertension and pregnancy. The dynamics of the blood pressure and the frequent occurrence of *white coat hypertension* make occasional measurements in the office unreliable for monitoring these patients.

10. Antihypertensive drugs should be a part of the treatment of patients with severe hypertension and patients with mild hypertension and high-risk factors.

11. Diuretics lower blood pressure initially by decreasing the plasma volume and after a few weeks by decreasing PVR. They are the first-choice drugs for hypertensive patients with expanded intravascular volume and increased CO.

12. Contrary to other beta blockers, labetalol acts by decreasing PVR with little change in CO. The main indication for the use of labetalol is the need to rapidly reduce blood presssure in patients with severe preeclampsia.

13. Prazosin is a peripheral vasodilator with a significant effect on capacitance vessels. The combination of prazosin and a diuretic is extremely effective for hypertension resistant to other drugs.

14. The cardioselective beta-1 blocker atenolol is the drug of choice in patients with hyperkinetic circulation.

15. Fetal growth should be assessed by periodic ultrasound measurements in all patients with chronic hypertension. There is no need for repeated creatinine clearance and quantitative protein determinations unless the serum creatinine is more than 0.8 mg/dl or more than 2+ protein is found in qualitative examination of a randomly obtained urine specimen.

REFERENCES

1. Lindheimer MD, Katz AI: Hypertension in pregnancy. *New Engl J Med* 1985;313:675-680.
2. Taufield PA, Ales KL, Resnick LM, et al: Hypocalciuria in preeclampsia. *N Engl J Med* 1987;316:715-718.
3. Huikeshoven FJM, Zuijderhoudt FMJ: Hypocalciuria in hypertensive disorder in pregnancy and how to measure it. *Eur J Obstet Gynecol Reprod Biol* 1990;36:81-85.
4. Arias F: Expansion of intravascular volume and fetal outcome in patients with chronic hypertension and pregnancy. *Am J Obstet Gynecol* 1975;123:610.
5. Arias F, Zamora J: Antihypertensive treatment and pregnancy outcome in patients with mild chronic hypertension. *Obstet Gynecol* 1979;53:489.
6. Dunlop JCH: Chronic hypertension and perinatal mortality. *Proc R Soc Med* 1966;59:838.
7. Rayburn WF, Zuspan FP, Piehl EJ: Self-monitoring of blood pressure during pregnancy. *Am J Obstet Gynecol* 1984;148:159-162.
8. Zuspan FP, Rayburn WF: Blood pressure self-monitoring during pregnancy: Practical considerations. *Am J Obstet Gynecol* 1991;164:2-6.
9. Curet LB, Olson RW: Evaluation of a program of bed rest in the treatment of chronic hypertension in pregnancy. *Obstet Gynecol* 1979;53:336-340.
10. Sibai BM, Anderson GD: Pregnancy outcome of intensive therapy in severe hypertension in first trimester. *Obstet Gynecol* 1986;67:517-522.
11. Sibai BM, Villar MA, Mabie BC: Acute renal failure in hypertensive disorders of pregnancy: Pregnancy outcome and remote prognosis in thirty-one consecutive cases. *Am J Obstet Gynecol* 1990;162:777-783.
12. Kincaid-Smith P, Bullen H, Mills J: Prolonged use of methyldopa in severe hypertension in pregnancy. *Br Med J* 1966;1:274-278.
13. Gallery EDM, Saunders DM, Hynyou SN, et al: Randomized comparison of methyldopa and oxprenolol for treatment of hypertension in pregnancy. *Br Med J* 1979;1:591-594.
14. Leather HM, Humpreys DM, Baker PB, et al: A controlled trial of hypotensive agents in hypertension in pregnancy. *Lancet* 1968;1:488-489.
15. Sibai BM, Mabie WC, Shamsa F, et al: A comparison of no medication versus methyldopa or labetalol in chronic hypertension during pregnancy. *Am J Obstet Gynecol* 1990;162:960-967.
16. Redman CWG, Beilin LJ, Bonnar J, et al: Fetal outcome in a trial of antihypertensive treatment in pregnancy. *Lancet* 1976;2:753.
17. Weseley AC, Douglas GW: Continuous use of chlorothiazide for prevention of toxemia of pregnancy. *Obstet Gynecol* 1962;19:355-358.
18. Flowers CE, Grizzle JE, Easterling WE, et al: Chlorothiazide as prophylaxis against a toxemia of pregnancy: A double-blind study. *Am J Obstet Gynecol* 1962;84:919-929.
19. Finnerty FA, Bepko FJ: Lowering the perinatal mortality and the prematurity rate. *JAMA* 1966;195:429-432.
20. Gant NF, Madden JD, Siiteri PK, et al: The metabolic clearance rate of dehydroisoandrosterone: III. The effect of thiazide diuretics in normal and future pre-eclamptic pregnancies. *Am J Obstet Gynecol* 1975;123:159-163.
21. Collins R, Yusuf F, Peto R: An overview of randomized trials of diuretics in pregnancy. *Br Med J* 1985;290:17.

22. Lindow SW, Davies N, Davey DA, et al: The effect of sublingual nifedipine on uteroplacental blood flow in hypertensive pregnancy. *Br J Obstet Gynaecol* 1988;95:1276.

23. Lubbe WF, Hodge JF: Combined alpha- and beta-adrenoceptor antagonism with prazosin and oxprenolol in control of severe hypertension in pregnancy. *N Z Med J* 1981;691:169-172.

24. Davey DA, Dommisse J: The management of hypertension in pregnancy. *S Afr Med J* 1980;14:551-556.

25. Lim YL, Walters WAW: Hemodynamics of mild hypertension in pregnancy. *Br J Obstet Gynaecol* 1978:86:198.

26. Eliahou HE, Silverberg DS, Reisin E, et al: Propranolol for the treatment of hypertension in pregnancy. *Br J Obstet Gynaecol* 1978;85:431.

27. Pruyn SC, Phelan JP, Buchanan GC: Long-term propranolol therapy in pregnancy: Maternal and fetal outcome. *Am J Obstet Gynecol* 1979;135:485.

28. Rubin RC: Beta blockers in pregnancy. *N Engl J Med* 1981;305:1323.

29. Sibai BM, Abdella TN, Anderson GD, et al: Plasma volume findings in pregnant women with mild hypertension: Therapeutic considerations. *Am J Obstet Gynecol* 1983;145:539.

30. Desforges JF: How far should blood pressure be lowered. *N Engl J Med* 1992;326:251-254.

13

HEMATOLOGIC PROBLEMS DURING PREGNANCY

The hematologic abnormalities that occur most frequently during pregnancy are those affecting the red cells and the hemostatic system. Other problems, such as those affecting the white cells, are rarely seen in pregnant women and are not covered in this chapter.

☑ PHYSIOLOGIC CHANGES OF THE RED CELL COUNT DURING PREGNANCY

Hemoglobin concentrations less than 12 g/dl and hematocrits below 36%, which define anemia in the general population, are not indicative of anemia in pregnant patients because of a physiologic change called *hemodilution of pregnancy*. This phenomenon was described by Scott and Pritchard,[1] who measured the hemoglobin/hematocrit (H/H) concentrations of a large group of healthy young women with proven normal iron and folate stores. They found an average drop in hematocrit of five units for a singleton and seven units for a twin pregnancy during the second trimester. This is a consequence of the intravascular volume expansion that starts at 8 to 10 weeks of gestation and reaches its maximum during the second trimester. Initially the increase in plasma volume is larger than the rise in red cell volume, and the net result is a drop in the H/H. This is misleading because the total number of red cells in the circulation is, in fact, increasing.

There are limits to the physiologic drop in H/H that occurs during pregnancy. Most authors consider anemia to be present if the hemoglobin concentration drops below 10 g/dl or the hematocrit falls below 30%. Anemia is the most common hematologic abnormality diagnosed during pregnancy. It is most often caused by iron deficiency and occasionally by more complex situations involving deficient production or accelerated destruction of erythrocytes.

☑ EFFECTS OF ANEMIA ON MOTHER AND FETUS

There is evidence indicating that preeclampsia and eclampsia occur more frequently in patients with iron-deficiency[2] or megaloblastic anemias[3] than in nonanemic gravidas. However, the relationship between anemia and preeclampsia-eclampsia has not been clarified. It is possible that preeclampsia interferes with the gastrointestinal absorption of blood-forming elements or causes hepatorenal dysfunction, thereby affecting the metabolism of folic acid or the production of erythropoietin.

Another maternal complication seemingly associated with maternal anemia is abruptio placentae. Studies in this area are contradictory. Some authors[4] have found a high correlation between folic acid deficiency and abruption, but others[5] have not.

Studies have shown that anemia during pregnancy is associated with stillbirths and neonatal deaths. The incidence of stillbirths and preterm births decreases significantly when iron is given to anemic mothers before they reach 30 weeks of gestation. What constitutes the mechanism behind the association of fetal problems and maternal anemia is purely speculative. The association between anemia and preterm delivery is poor.[6]

◼ EFFECTS OF PREGNANCY ON ANEMIC PATIENTS

The expansion of plasma volume and the utilization by the fetus of substrates necessary for the building of hemoglobin molecules will aggravate any preexisting anemia. Patients who are mildly anemic before pregnancy will become markedly anemic, and patients with severe anemia will become symptomatic by the end of the second trimester.

◼ IRON-DEFICIENCY ANEMIA

Aproximately 80% of all anemias in pregnancy result from iron deficiency. The reasons for the predominance of this etiologic factor are (1) the suboptimal iron content of the average American diet and (2) the insufficient iron stores in the majority of women during their reproductive years.

Iron requirements during pregnancy

The daily iron requirement for an adult is about 2 mg. Although the average diet in the United States provides between 5 and 15 mg of elemental iron per day, only about one tenth (0.5 to 1.5 mg) is absorbed. This amount of dietary iron is probably enough to compensate for the daily losses plus the monthly menstrual loss of an average female, but it is not adequate for the formation of large iron stores. Consequently, more than 20% of all women in the United States have no stored iron, and probably twice

that number have small stores that quickly become exhausted under the increased demands of pregnancy. The iron requirements of a normal pregnancy have been quantified by the Council on Foods and Nutrition as follows:

To compensate for external iron losses	170 mg
To allow expansion of maternal red cell mass	450 mg
Fetal iron	270 mg
Iron in placenta and cord	90 mg
TOTAL	980 mg

The gastrointestinal absorption of iron increases during the last two trimesters of pregnancy to about 1.0 to 3.0 mg per day. Even if this increased absorption is taken into consideration, the iron content of an unsupplemented diet cannot provide more than one to two thirds of the normal requirements of pregnancy. A pregnant woman must have at least 500 mg of stored iron at the beginning of pregnancy to fulfill the requirements of gestation without the need for iron supplementation. Even if this deposit is present, it will be completely exhausted at the end of gestation. It is also important to note that demands on maternal iron stores begin early in pregnancy, whereas increased gastrointestinal absorption of iron is apparent only after midgestation.

Pathophysiology and diagnosis

Iron in the human body is complexed to transferrin (transport form), ferritin (storage form), or heme (such as in hemoglobin, myoglobin, or iron-containing enzymes). The iron necessary for the synthesis of hemoglobin is carried as transferrin. In patients with nutritional iron deficiency, the iron stores become depleted to maintain the production of erythrocytes and satisfy the needs of the pregnancy. Once the iron stores become depleted, the molecules of transferrin become less than 15% saturated with iron, and erythropoiesis is impaired, resulting in microcytosis and hypochromia. Finally, the production of red cells by the bone marrow will decrease. Thus iron-deficiency anemia can be divided into three stages: (1) depletion of iron stores, (2) deficient erythropoiesis, and (3) frank iron-deficiency anemia. Ideally, iron-deficiency anemia should be detected and treated in its first stage.

Depletion of iron stores without overt signs of iron-deficiency anemia usually occurs during the first trimester of pregnancy. Iron is stored in the form of ferritin, a spheric protein that holds approximately 4500 iron atoms. The status of iron stores can be assessed by measuring stainable iron in bone marrow biopsy or by measuring the concentration of plasma ferritin that is in equilibrium with the iron stored in the tissues. One ng/ml of serum ferritin is equivalent to 8 mg of iron stores.

Since bone marrow aspiration is impractical for routine use, determination of serum ferritin is the best available method for evaluating the status of the iron stores during pregnancy.[7] Serum ferritin is measured by radioimmunoassay, and the values reported by different laboratories vary because ferritin from different sources is used to prepare the antibodies used in the assays. The normal range of serum ferritin is 50 to 155 ng/ml, and any value under 20 ng/ml is indicative of deficient iron stores.

The value of routine evaluation of the iron stores in pregnant women using serum ferritin determinations is controversial. Some investigators[8] believe that the diagnosis of iron deficiency is more accurate using ferritin than other tests. Others believe that iron supplementation for all pregnant women on the assumption that they have decreased iron stores probably costs less than screening all of them with serum ferritin determinations. Serum ferritin is not valuable for distinguishing between anemia caused by chronic disorders and iron-deficiency anemia.

Iron-deficient hematopoiesis without overt signs of iron-deficiency anemia can be diagnosed by measuring the serum transferrin (normal value 200 to 360 mg/dl), which increases with the severity of the iron-deficiency state. Transferrin concentration is usually greater than 360 μg/dl in patients with iron-deficient hematopoiesis. In contrast, the serum iron concentration (normal value 60 to 175 μg/dl) decreases and is usually below 60 μg/dl. The result of these changes is a decrease in transferrin saturation (normally 25% to 60%) to under 25%. Simultaneously, since there is not enough iron to convert protoporphyrin to hemoglobin, the concentration of protoporphyrin (30 to 70 μg/100 ml of red cells) increases to 2 to 3 times its normal concentration. Another change that occurs before generalized microcytosis and hypochromia is an abnormal (>15%) red cell distribution width (RDW).[9] The RDW is an index of the

BOX 13-1
Normal Red Cell Values in Women

Red blood cells	3.9 to 5.0×10^6 cells/μl
Hemoglobin level	12.1 to 15.1 g/dl
Hematocrit value	36.1% to 44.3%
MCV	80 to 97.6 μm^3
MCH	26.7 to 33.7 pg/cell
MCHC	32.7 to 35.5 g/dl
Reticulocyte count	0.5% to 1.5%

presence of a heterogenous red cell population with different diameters.

Alterations of the erythrocyte count and morphology mark the final stage in the evolution of iron-deficiency anemia. At this point, the most important tests for diagnosis are the blood smear and the red cell indices: mean corpuscular volume (MCV), mean corpuscular hemoglobin (MCH), and mean corpuscular hemoglobin concentration (MCHC). The normal red cell values are shown in Box 13-1.

Iron-deficiency anemia is characteristically microcytic and hypochromic. The blood smear shows abundant, small, well-rounded erythrocytes with pale centers. The MCV, MCH, and MCHC are low. Also, the serum transferrin iron-binding capacity, the serum iron concentration, the transferrin saturation, and the red cell protoporphyrin concentration show changes as described earlier. However, these tests are unnecessary for the diagnosis of frank iron-deficiency anemia. Anemia is a late manifestation in the spectrum of iron deficiency, and when it is present, the situation can be diagnosed easily without the need for complex and expensive laboratory determinations.

Prevention

Every pregnant woman needs iron supplementation during pregnancy, and it should be started as early as possible, usually when the patient is seen for her first prenatal visit. If the patient suffers from nausea and vomiting in early pregnancy, the administration of iron should be postponed until the gastrointestinal disturbances disappear in the second trimester. Multiple forms of iron are available, and they vary in their content of elemental iron (Box 13-2).

BOX 13-2

Different Types of Iron Supplements

	Molecular iron content (mg)	Elemental iron content (mg)
Ferrous sulfate	300	60
Ferrous gluconate	320	36
Ferrous fumarate	200	67

A pregnant woman needs only one tablet of iron per day for prophylaxis of iron-deficiency anemia. In fact, one tablet per day of any form of iron supplies enough iron to fulfill the needs of pregnancy provided that it is taken for at least the last two trimesters and that there is no pre-existing anemia. More than one tablet of iron per day for prophylaxis is unnecessary, since the excess iron is not absorbed, resulting in gastrointestinal side effects.

Treatment

Oral iron therapy. Oral administration of one 300-mg tablet of iron sulfate 3 times daily after meals is adequate treatment for most patients with iron-deficiency anemia. This dosage provides 180 mg per day of elemental iron, of which 15 to 25 mg per day are absorbed. The patient's response to this dosage is fast, and a significant increase in reticulocyte count is observable 5 to 10 days after initiation of oral therapy. Hemoglobin rises from 0.3 to 1.0 g per week, and this is reflected in a significant elevation in H/H values 2 to 3 weeks after initiation of treatment.

A prevalent problem associated with oral iron therapy is gastrointestinal intolerance, which is experienced by about 10% of patients undergoing treatment. The most common symptoms are nausea, vomiting, constipation, abdominal cramping, and diarrhea. Since the gastrointestinal side effects are dose-related, the treatment of choice is to reduce the dose to a tolerable level. Another useful maneuver is to give the iron pill with meals rather than after meals. Although this decreases the amount of iron that is absorbed and prolongs the time necessary to achieve normalization of the hematologic indices, it is frequently the only way to continue the treatment. Gastrointestinal toxicity depends on the amount of ionic iron, the absorbable form of iron, that contacts the gastrointestinal mucosa. Thus preparations containing less absorbable iron produce fewer side effects. It is cheaper to reduce the dosage of the preparation that is causing adverse effects than to change to a preparation with less absorbable iron.

Parenteral iron therapy. Parenteral iron therapy is rarely indicated and should be used only in patients who (1) have severe iron-deficiency anemia (hemoglobin less than 8 g/dl) a few weeks before their expected date of delivery and thus require rapid normalization of their hematologic indices that cannot be achieved with oral therapy; (2) cannot absorb iron (malabsorption syndromes); or (3) develop incapacitating side effects with oral iron. Parenteral iron therapy is hazardous and expensive when compared with oral administration. Up to 2% of patients receiving parenteral iron may develop acute severe systemic reactions such as hemolysis, hypotension, circulatory collapse, vomiting, muscle pain, and anaphylactic shock. Other patients suffer delayed reactions characterized by pyrexia, myalgias, and arthralgias.[10] Parenteral iron may also cause dark staining of the skin and inflammation at the site of application. The frequency of side effects with parenteral iron therapy is such that the manufacturer has recently recommended that the dosage not exceed 2 ml in a 24-hour period.

Before giving parenteral iron it is necessary to calculate the patient's iron deficit using one of the following formulas:

$$[(\text{Normal Hb} - \text{Patient's Hb}) \times \text{weight (kg)} \times 2.21] + 1000 = \text{Milligrams of iron needed}$$

For example, the iron required by a pregnant woman with a hemoglobin concentration of 7.1 g/dl and a weight of 140 pounds (63 kg) is:

$$[(14 - 7.1) \times 63 \times 2.21] + 1000 = \text{approx 1950 mg}$$

Another formula, simpler and easier to remember, is to give 250 mg of elemental iron for each gram of hemoglobin below normal. In the hypothetical case just mentioned the calculation is:

$$250 \text{ mg} \times 6.9 \text{ g} = 1725 \text{ mg}$$

The iron dextran preparation (Imferon) for intravenous or intramuscular administration is a solution containing 50 mg of elemental iron per milliliter. Since the maximal recommended dosage of intramuscular iron is 2 ml per day, several injections may be necessary to correct the calculated deficiency.

Some authors suggest diluting the iron dextran in normal saline solution (1.5 g/1000 ml), administering it initially at a rate of 1 ml/30 min, and if no side effects are apparent, continuing at a rate of 150 ml/hr. A syringe with epinephrine must be at hand, as well as an ampule of a suitable glucocorticoid for intravenous administration. The incidence of phlebitis at the site of administration increases with the use of diluted iron solutions.

◪ MEGALOBLASTIC ANEMIA
Incidence and pathophysiology

Only 3% to 4% of women with anemia during pregnancy have the megaloblastic variety. In the vast majority of cases, megaloblastic anemia is the result of a folic acid deficiency. Only 1 of every 8500 pregnant women with anemia has vitamin B_{12} deficiency.[11] The reason for the low incidence of megaloblastic anemia during pregnancy is the abundance of both folic acid and vitamin B_{12} in the American diet. Folate is present in fruits, green vegetables, and meats; vitamin B_{12} is found in meat, fish, poultry, and dairy products.

Folic acid deficiency may result from inadequate intake, poor absorption, or increased utilization, and all three mechanisms may occur during pregnancy. Folic acid deficiency usually results from inadequate ingestion, not because of unavailability but because prolonged cooking destroys the vitamin. Thus poor cooking habits combined with a lack of raw food in the diet eventually lead to the production of megaloblastic anemia.

Poor absorption of folate despite adequate ingestion occurs usually because ingested folic acid polyglutamates cannot be degraded to absorbable monoglutamates. The presence in the diet of an inhibitor of the enzyme responsible for this degradation or an acid intestinal pH leads to malabsorption. Decreased utilization of folate is seen in about 60% of patients with vitamin B_{12} deficiency.

Theoretically, inadequate ingestion, poor absorption, or increased use may also cause vitamin B_{12} deficiency. In practice, however, vitamin B_{12} deficiency only results from poor absorption, and perhaps the only situation in which inadequate ingestion should be suspected as a cause is in those who are strict vegetarians.

Poor vitamin B_{12} absorption may occur because of inadequate secretion of intrinsic factor (pernicious anemia), poor ileal absorption despite adequate amounts of intrinsic factor, or a pancreatic defect causing inadequate alkalinization of the intestinal content and poor removal of intrinsic factor binders. Until recently, almost all cases of megaloblastic anemia in pregnancy were caused by pernicious anemia. In the last few years, however, defects in ileal absorption have risen in frequency, mainly as a result of the popularization of gastrointestinal surgical procedures in the treatment of patients with morbid obesity.

Both folic acid and vitamin B_{12} deficiencies cause megaloblastic anemia by affecting DNA replication. Folic acid is an essential cofactor for one-carbon metabolism, and its deficiency affects particularly the synthesis of thymidine. In vitamin B_{12} deficiency, DNA replication is affected at the same step but by a mechanism that involves a defect in the conversion of circulating forms of folate to those involved in thymidine synthesis. As a consequence, more cells are in a nonresting state, trying to slowly complete the doubling of their DNA. When examined microscopically, these cells show more than the normal amount of DNA despite poor synthesis. Furthermore, since protein synthesis is not affected, these cells exhibit large, mature cytoplasms. These nuclear and cytoplasmic changes are the basic elements of megaloblastosis, and they affect not only the erythroid line but also the myeloid line, producing the hypersegmented neutrophils that are characteristic of megaloblastic degeneration.

The similarities in morphologic effects on red and white blood cells caused by folate and vitamin B_{12} deficiencies, as well as the fact that the anemia caused by the deficiency of one of them can be corrected by administering the other, cannot obscure the fundamental difference between the two processes. Vitamin B_{12} deficiency causes progressive demyelinization, but folate deficiency does not, and treatment of a vitamin B_{12} anemia with folate does not arrest the progression of neurologic damage. Therefore differential diagnosis between these two major causes of megaloblastic anemia is important and necessary.

Both folate and vitamin B_{12} deficiencies may mask an iron deficiency. Red cell synthesis is inhibited during the vitamin deficiency, available iron is underused, and increased saturation of transferrin occurs. As soon as therapy with folate or B_{12} is initiated, red cell synthesis starts again, use of iron is maximal, and iron deficiency becomes apparent.

Diagnosis

The first indication of megaloblastic anemia in pregnancy is usually an elevated MCV found on routine prenatal evaluation. In a few cases, the elevated MCV may be the result of hypothyroidism, but the presence of hypersegmented neutrophils obviates this diagnosis. As mentioned, folate deficiency is most commonly the cause of the megaloblastic changes. The clinician, however, should obtain serum levels of both folate and vitamin B_{12} to avoid missing the rare case of vitamin B_{12} deficiency. Other tests that may be useful in the differential diagnosis are the reticulocyte count, which usually is normal in vitamin B_{12} and elevated in folate deficiencies, and the urine formiminoglutamic acid (FIGLU), which is high in cases of folate deficiency.

The serum vitamin B_{12} level may be low in cases of folic acid deficiency, and the serum folate may be low in cases of vitamin B_{12} deficiency, reflecting the intimate biochemical relation that exists between these two nutrients. A serum level less than 100 pg/ml is diagnostic of vitamin B_{12} deficiency. A combination of a serum folate less than 3 ng/ml and a red cell folate less than 150 ng/ml is diagnostic of folate deficiency. Red cell folate is the best reflection of the amount of folate in tissue, it has fewer fluctuations in value, and it is the test of choice for the diagnosis of deficiency.

Therapy

Treatment of folic acid deficiency requires 1 mg per day of folic acid. No more than this is necessary, since the daily requirement probably does not exceed 100 to 200 µg even in the presence of anemia.

Treatment of vitamin B_{12} deficiency requires about 250 µg of parenteral cyanocobalamin every month. The oral preparations of vitamin B_{12} have unreliable absorption properties and are inadequate for long-term therapy.

In severely anemic patients, especially if they are near delivery, exchange transfusions of packed red cells followed by parenteral therapy with folic acid (1 mg/day for 1 week) or cyanocobalamin (100 µg/day for 1 week) may be necessary.

The reticulocyte count should show an appropriate response to therapy in 3 to 8 days. An underlying iron deficiency may be detected a few days after initiation of therapy for megaloblastic anemia if appropriate follow-up is carried out.

◢ HEMOLYTIC ANEMIAS

A normal red cell lives for about 120 days. This life span is shortened in the case of hemolytic anemias because of premature destruction of red cells, which may occur extravascularly (i.e., acquired immune hemolytic anemia) or intravascularly (i.e., microangiopathic hemolytic anemia of preeclampsia). When hemoglobin is liberated intravascularly, the alpha chains bind to haptoglobin—an alpha-2 globulin—and the hemoglobin-haptoglobin complex is rapidly cleared in the liver. Thus a decrease in plasma haptoglobin is a reliable sign of hemolysis. After the haptoglobin becomes saturated, free hemoglobin appears in the plasma. Hemoglobinuria occurs when the amount of hemoglobin in the plasma exceeds the reabsorptive capacity of the tubular cells of the kidney. The free plasma hemoglobin becomes oxidized to methemoglobin. Methemalbumin forms when heme groups of methemoglobin bind albumin molecules. To compensate for hemolysis, bone marrow erythropoiesis increases markedly, resulting in an increase in reticulocyte count. Thus the diagnostic hallmarks of intravascular hemolytic anemia include a decreased or absent haptoglobin and the presence of free hemoglobin, methemoglobin, methemalbumin, and reticulocytosis. Also, abnormalities in red cell morphology are frequently seen in the blood smear.

Extravascular hemolysis in the reticuloendothelial system liberates hemoglobin, which is converted to bilirubin. An increase in indirect bilirubin is apparent in the patient's serum. The products of bilirubin metabolism, fecal and urinary urobilinogen, also increase. Erythropoiesis markedly increases, and reticulocytosis occurs. Thus elevated unconjugated bilirubin, increased urinary urobilinogen, and reticulocytosis are the laboratory hallmarks of extravascular hemolysis. Although classification of these anemias according to the site of hemolysis is important for an adequate interpretation of the laboratory tests and for differential diagnosis, in many hemolytic processes, destruction occurs in both compartments, and laboratory tests are ambiguous.

Intravascular and extravascular hemolysis both cause a bone marrow response characterized by marked erythroid hyperplasia and reticulocytosis. In some cases the erythropoiesis is so active that there is passage of immature cell lines into the bloodstream. Also, in all cases of accelerated red cell destruction, plasma lactic dehydrogenase (LDH) increases as a consequence of the liberation of the erythrocyte isoenzyme.

Microangiopathic hemolytic anemia

Microangiopathic hemolytic anemia occurs during pregnancy in some patients with severe forms of preeclampsia-eclampsia or in the rare cases of thrombotic thrombocytopenic purpura, hemolytic uremic syndrome, and herpetic hepatitis. Characteristically, the blood smear shows fragmented red cells, schistocytes, and helmet cells. Thrombocytopenia is always present. Immunofluorescent studies show marked and generalized fibrinogen deposition in the microvasculature, especially in the kidney, liver, and brain. This condition usually disappears with prompt termination of pregnancy. Delivery is followed by progressive improvement in the indicators of hemolysis. This subject is further discussed in Chapter 10.

Acquired immune hemolytic anemia

In cases of acquired immune hemolytic anemia, the patient makes antibodies of the IgG type, or "warm antibodies," against red cell antigens, causing premature destruction of these cells. This abnormality may occur in association with several diseases (leukemia, lymphomas, viral infections) or as a consequence of an immune reaction to certain drugs (penicillin, sulfas, quinidine). However, the most frequent cause of this abnormality in pregnant women is collagen vascular disease. On a few occasions, no cause can be discovered; thus the disorder is termed *idiopathic acquired immune hemolytic anemia*.

In immune hemolytic anemia, IgG antibodies and complement coat the red cell surface, and reticuloendothelial cells, which contain receptors for both IgG and complement, bind them. When the red cells detach, some membrane fragments remain on the reticuloendothelial cells. As a consequence of this loss of membrane fragments, the erythrocytes are transformed into spherocytes and are easily destroyed in the spleen.

The diagnosis of immune hemolytic anemia is made with the direct Coombs' test. In this test, red cells of the patient are mixed with antihuman globulin antiserum, and since they are coated with IgG and complement, agglutination occurs immediately.

Diagnosis of a connective tissue disorder, usually lupus erythematosus, causing the synthesis of antibodies against red cell antigens is made with laboratory tests to determine antinuclear antibody (ANA) titers and anti-DNA antibodies. These tests are negative in idiopathic immune hemolytic anemia.

Treatment of immune hemolytic anemia consists of the administration of immunosuppressive drugs. Glucocorticoids, used in doses equivalent to between 60 and 100 mg of prednisone per day, are first choice. These steroids act preferentially by interfering with the reticuloendothelial cell recognition of the IgG and complement covering the erythrocyte surface and, to a smaller extent, by interfering with the process of antibody synthesis.

In cases not responsive to glucocorticoids, the drug of choice is azathioprine. Splenectomy may be necessary to arrest the hemolytic process. However, not all patients respond to surgery. The degree of splenic entrapment of radioactively tagged red cells, determined before a surgical procedure is carried out, may identify those patients who would benefit from splenectomy.

Some patients with lupus-induced hemolytic anemia during pregnancy may exhibit hemoglobin concentrations under 5 g/dl. Transfusions seem to be clearly indicated in these cases, but most patients quickly hemolyze the transfused red cells. The only hope of finding some compatible blood in these desperate situations is by in vivo crossmatching. For this purpose, a small amount of red cells from the potential donor is tagged with 51Cr and given to the patient. If the red cells are hemolyzed, radioactive chromium will be released from the cells and found in the plasma. If no hemolysis occurs, the radioactivity will remain contained in the red cells. In the majority of cases, the best management is to wait for the patient's response to glucocorticoids rather than to transfuse. In some critical patients, however, cells that are quickly destroyed must be given anyway to keep the patient alive until the effect of the immunosuppressant drugs is apparent.

Hemolytic anemias associated with hemoglobinopathies

The abnormalities in hemoglobin synthesis most commonly found in pregnant patients in the United States are (1) sickle cell trait, (2) beta thalassemia minor, and (3) sickle cell disease (SCD).

Sickle cell trait. Sickle cell trait is present in about 10% of the black population of the United States. There is evidence[12] that these patients are not at greater risk for abnormal reproductive performance than are individuals without the trait. The only problem for these patients is the possibility of transmission of the abnormal gene to their descendants. Patients with sickle cell trait should have preconceptional counseling, and the man should be examined to determine whether or not he also carries the trait. If the man is a carrier, there is a 25% chance that an infant with homozygous SCD will result. As opposed to patients with SCD, patients with sickle cell trait require iron supplementation during pregnancy.

Beta thalassemia minor. Beta thalassemia minor is second in frequency to sickle cell trait among pregnant women with hemoglobinopathies. This disease is characterized by diminished synthesis of hemoglobin beta chains. These patients have a microcytic, hypochromic anemia with hemoglobin levels that range from 8 to 10 g/dl.[13] The diagnosis is frequently missed, and the patients are repeatedly treated with large doses of oral, and in some instances parenteral, iron without therapeutic response. This is dangerous because they may develop hepatic and cardiac hemosiderosis from iron overload. To avoid this problem, hemoglobin A_2 and serum iron determinations should be ordered for every pregnant patient with mycrocytic, hypochromic anemia who does not respond to oral iron by developing an elevation of her reticulocyte count or hemoglobin concentration. Patients with beta thalassemia minor characteristically show hemoglobin A_2 concentrations greater than 3.5% and normal or increased serum iron concentrations.

Patients with beta thalassemia minor have reproductive performance similar to patients with normal hemoglobin. They do not require iron supplementation during pregnancy unless there is laboratory evidence of iron deficiency. If it is necessary to raise their red cell concentrations, the only way to do it is through transfusions.

Sickle cell disease. Although sickle cell trait and beta thalassemia minor are seen more often during pregnancy than SCD, the latter is the most important hemoglobinopathy encountered during pregnancy because of the severity of the complications associated with this disease. Pregnant patients with SCD are affected by the following problems:

1. *A significant maternal mortality.* Approximately 2% to 7% of women with SCD die during pregnancy. The causes of maternal deaths are multiple, but pulmonary infection, pulmonary infarcts, and pulmonary embolization are predominant.
2. *A high incidence of severe maternal morbidity.* Morbidity is frequent, severe, and prolonged in pregnant patients with SCD. Painful vasoocclusive episodes (sickle cell crisis), infections, cerebrovascular accidents, and preeclampsia-eclampsia are common in these patients.
3. *A high incidence of spontaneous abortion.* Early reproductive failure affects close to 20% of all pregnant patients with SCD.
4. *A high incidence of stillbirths and neonatal deaths.* Approximately 14.2% of all pregnancies in patients with SCD end with the delivery of stillborn infants. Neonatal mortality is also high, approximately 84.5 per 1000 live births.
5. *A high incidence of low birth weight infants.* The incidence of infants with birth weights under 2500 g in patients with SCD is 37.5%. A large number of these infants are born at term but are growth retarded. Intrauterine growth retardation is also present in a large number of the stillborn babies delivered by patients with SCD.

The problems associated with SCD during pregnancy have decreased in frequency and severity with advances in perinatal medicine. A study from the University of Southern California[14] has shown a decrease in maternal mortality from 4.1% before 1972 to 1.7% after 1972 and a decrease in perinatal mortality from 52.7% to 22.7% in the same period.

Blood transfusions are used to decrease the incidence and severity of pregnancy-related problems in patients with SCD. Transfusions can be given prophylactically or used only when specific indications, such as sickle cell crisis, infection, or arrest of erythropoiesis, appear.

The purpose of prophylactic administration of red cells containing hemoglobin A_1 is to prevent fetal and maternal problems. Two methods have been used for prophylactic transfusions. In the first,[15] the patient has one partial exchange transfusion at 28 weeks of gestation to achieve a hematocrit value of 35% and a concentration of hemoglobin A_1 of at least 40%. The procedure is repeated if a crisis occurs, if the hematocrit value drops under 25%, if the hemoglobin A_1 drops under 20%, or when the patient reaches 36 to 38 weeks of gestation. In the second method,[16] packed red cells are given by partial exchange transfusion or, more commonly, by simple infusion, starting as soon as the diagnosis of pregnancy is established and then intermittently throughout the rest of the pregnancy. The objective of the transfusions is to keep the hematocrit value above 25% and the concentration of hemoglobin S under 50%.

Proponents of the first method believe that most of the serious complications in patients with SCD appear in the last trimester of pregnancy, that these complications are prevented by this method, and that fewer transfusions are given than with the other method. Those who use the protocol with intermittent transfusions beginning early in pregnancy believe that it is better to correct the maternal oxygen-carrying capacity as early as possible to avoid problems both in middle and in late pregnancy.

There is no agreement on the value of prophylactic transfusion for pregnant patients with SCD. In April of 1979, the National Institutes of Health had a Consensus Development Conference on transfusion therapy in pregnant patients with SCD and concluded that the risks and benefits have not been established and this treatment is not ready for routine clinical use. Of the dangers associated with prophylactic transfusion protocols, the most important are (1) the development of hemosiderosis, (2) the development of alloantibodies, making it difficult to carry out future transfusions, and (3) the possibility of transmitting infective agents.

One recent investigation compared the benefits and risks of prophylactic transfusions initiated at the start of the observation period with transfusions given only in emergency situations.[17] The authors found that prophylactic transfusion patients had significant pain relief and lower rates of SCD-associated complications. However, no difference between the groups was found in other respects such as obstetric complications, alloimmunization, and perinatal outcome. It seems, therefore, that transfusion only when

there is a specific indication is, at present, the best method for managing SCD in pregnancy. With this approach, the hazards associated with prophylactic transfusions are decreased.

Partial exchange transfusions may be carried out manually using phlebotomy followed by infusion or using automated erythrocytopheresis with a cell separator. This technique allows a fast and rigorously controlled exchange that is valuable for the patient in crisis or congestive heart failure.

Patients with SCD do not require iron supplementation during pregnancy unless laboratory evidence of iron deficiency is obtained. In contrast, they need adequate folic acid supplementation to compensate for the increased consumption of folate caused by the active process of cell replication that takes place in their bone marrow.

Patients with sickle cell–hemoglobin C disease and sickle cell–beta thalassemia disease may have problems during pregnancy similar to those of patients with SCD, but the frequency and severity of these problems are substantially less. A similar relatively benign situation occurs in patients with SCD who have elevated (greater than 10%) concentrations of fetal hemoglobin. In these two groups of patients, the need for prophylactic transfusions is less than in patients with SCD.

◼ APLASTIC ANEMIAS

Aplastic anemias occur rarely during pregnancy, and fewer than 50 cases have been reported in the literature. In most of these cases, no association has been found between the anemia and exposure to chemicals, medications, or infections that may have affected the bone marrow. The disease has a serious prognosis, and the maternal mortality is about 30%.[18] However, recent advances in the treatment of aplastic anemias using bone marrow transplantation, antithymocyte globulin (ATG), high-dose corticosteroids, and cyclosporine may improve the maternal outcome.

◼ ALTERATIONS OF THE HEMOSTATIC SYSTEM

The hemostatic system seals vascular leaks and prevents bleeding. Alterations in this system causing lack of clot formation or thrombosis are of interest to the obstetrician because they are serious and relatively common problems during pregnancy.

Adequate hemostasis is maintained through a

precise interaction between the vessel wall, the platelets, the coagulation system, and the fibrinolytic system. The vessel wall participates actively in the hemostatic process by vasoconstriction and by production of substances necessary to inhibit platelet aggregation. Platelets are necessary for the formation of the primary hemostatic plug and for the production, storage, and release of substances required for the enlargement of the temporary clot. The coagulation system participates in the hemostatic process through a series of reactions that culminate in the transformation of fibrinogen into fibrin. The fibrinolytic system prevents the continuous enlargement of the hemostatic plug by breaking down fibrin into fibrin degradation products. The harmonious interaction of these four components is necessary to maintain the integrity of the vascular system.

Pregnancy brings about physiologic changes in the hemostatic system that result in a hypercoagulable state. This is the result of an increase in several of the factors involved in the coagulation cascade and also of a depressed activity of the fibrinolytic system. Teleologically, these alterations represent the preparation of the mother to tolerate the hemostatic challenge that occurs at the time of parturition.

An adequate evaluation of the hemostatic system requires testing for abnormal blood vessel wall/platelet interaction (bleeding time), platelet count, prothrombin time (PT), partial thromboplastin time (PTT), and testing for abnormal fibrinolysis (D dimer). Most laboratories also include in this evaluation a quantitative measurement of fibrinogen.

The abnormalities of the hemostatic system most frequently seen by the obstetrician are caused by a disruption of the integrity of the vessel walls. In the majority of cases, this problem requires a surgical solution and measures to maintain the intravascular volume. This subject is treated extensively in Chapter 9 (Third-Trimester Bleeding) and Chapter 21 (Postpartum Complications).

Immune thrombocytopenic purpura

The majority of patients with thrombocytopenia (platelet count $<150/mm^3$) during pregnancy are healthy women.[19] Only 21% of these patients had preeclampsia or immune thrombocytopenia and are at risk of having babies with low platelet counts ($<50,000/mm^3$).

Immune thrombocytopenic purpura (ITP) is a disorder occasionally seen during pregnancy and is characterized by an antibody-mediated destruction of maternal platelets. The patients are usually asymptomatic, but may complain of easy bruising or bleeding, and frequently have petechiae. Laboratory evaluation reveals thrombocytopenia and enlarged platelets, but normal erythrocyte and leukocyte counts. The diagnosis of ITP is made by exclusion after finding no evidence of collagen vascular disease, drug mediation, or isoantibodies.

When ITP appears during pregnancy, both the mother and the fetus are affected. Maternal problems result not only from the disease but also from therapy. Maternal platelet counts may reach levels lower than $20,000/mm^3$, leading to gastrointestinal, urinary, or intracranial bleeding. Also, splenectomy, corticosteroid therapy, and immunosuppressant therapy have side effects that may be serious in the pregnant woman with ITP. The greatest concern in these cases, however, is with the fetal effects of ITP. Perinatal mortality is close to 20%, and the majority of infant deaths are caused by intracranial bleeding resulting from fetal or neonatal thrombocytopenia. The fetal and neonatal thrombocytopenia is the result of transplacental passage of maternal antiplatelet antibodies that bind to antigenic sites on the surface of the infant's platelets and facilitate their destruction in the spleen. Since the antigenic composition of the infant's platelets is unknown, it is impossible to predict without measuring the baby's platelet count whether or not fetal thrombocytopenia is present.

To diagnose ITP, it is necessary to demonstrate the presence of antiplatelet antibodies in the maternal serum. One method, similar to the direct Coombs' test, measures the antibodies attached to the platelet surface (platelet-associated [PA]–IgG). A second test, similar to the indirect Coombs' test, investigates the presence of antiplatelet antibodies circulating in the patient's plasma (circulating PA-IgG). The direct test has an inverse relationship to the maternal platelet count and to the patient's clinical picture, but its correlation with the fetal and neonatal platelet count is controversial.[20,21] The circulating IgG may have a better correlation with the existence and the severity of fetal thrombocytopenia. In general, however, measurements of maternal circulating or platelet-bound antibodies are unreliable for predicting fetal or neonatal platelet counts. The antigenic composition of the surface of the fetal platelets is different from that of the mother, and the concentration of maternal antibodies is irrelevant if those antibodies do not react with the infant's platelets. The important concept is that if any of these antibodies (direct or indirect) is present in the maternal blood, fetal thrombocytopenia may occur, and measurement of the baby's platelet count is necessary to determine the route of delivery.

The maternal platelet count cannot predict the fetal platelet count. It has been suggested that if the maternal platelet count in nonsplenectomized mothers is greater than 150,000/mm^3, the probability of neonatal thrombocytopenia is almost nil.[22] However, 27% of the babies born to mothers with platelet counts greater than 100,000/mm^3 are thrombocytopenic.

In view of the unreliability of maternal tests in assessing the presence or absence of fetal thrombocytopenia, it is necessary to measure the fetal platelet count before labor to determine the presence and extent of fetal compromise. Thus patients with ITP who have direct or indirect PA-IgG antibodies present in their bloodstreams should have percutaneous umbilical blood sampling at 37 to 38 weeks of gestation. The cordocentesis should be performed in Labor and Delivery, close to the operating room in case the baby needs expeditious delivery because of complications that may be caused by the procedure. Cesarean section delivery would be the best route of delivery if cordocentesis shows that the fetal platelet count is under 50,000/mm^3. Cordocentesis should be avoided in patients in whom access to the umbilical cord is difficult (posterior placentas), and the fetal platelet count should be measured in a scalp sample obtained in the early stages of labor when the cervix reaches 2 to 3 cm of dilation.

Measurement of the fetal platelet count by using a scalp sample requires the collection of blood using a procedure similar to that for measuring fetal pH. The blood must be collected in a special pipette (Unopette Test System 5855 from Becton-Dickinson). The test must be performed early in labor to avoid the error introduced when a caput has formed and to minimize fetal trauma during labor if the fetus has thrombocytopenia. If the fetal platelet count is greater than 50,000/mm^3, the probability of neonatal thrombocytopenia or intracranial bleeding is very small, and vaginal delivery would be safe. If

the fetal platelet count is less than 50,000/mm^3, cesarean section delivery is indicated.

The patient with ITP who has had a splenectomy may have a high concentration of PA-IgG despite a normal platelet count because splenectomy does not change the ability of the mother to make antiplatelet antibodies. Therefore a splenectomized pregnant woman with a normal platelet count may have abundant antibodies that cross the placenta, causing fetal thrombocytopenia. Splenectomized patients with antiplatelet antibodies require measuring of the fetal platelet count by cordocentesis or by scalp sample early in labor before vaginal delivery is allowed.

When the thrombocytopenic patient with ITP is seen early in gestation, the therapy of choice is glucocorticoid treatment. Prednisone, 60 to 100 mg/day, must be given until the platelet count is above 150,000/mm^3. The dosage should be tapered to reach the minimum required to keep the count at the 150,000/mm^3 level. However, a positive maternal response to corticosteroid therapy does not necessarily mean that a similar response has occurred in the fetus, and it is necessary to measure the fetal platelet count.

Corticosteroids have been used shortly before delivery to improve the maternal and the fetal platelet counts and to facilitate vaginal delivery. In the only controlled study of this approach to the problem,[23] fetuses from women treated with glucocorticoids had adequate responses that allowed labor without adverse effects. In seven pregnancies in which glucocorticoid therapy was not given, four infants had purpura at the time of delivery, and one of the four had periumbilical hemorrhage. Also, the neonatal platelet counts were significantly lower in untreated cases. However, there were only 19 cases in this study, and 6 of the 12 treated pregnancies resulted in babies with platelet counts under 50,000/mm^3. It seems, therefore, that corticosteroid treatment before delivery is not beneficial to all fetuses of mothers with ITP and that more studies are necessary before this mode of therapy should be accepted.

High doses of immunoglobulin (400 mg/g/day for 5 days) have been successfully used for the treatment of pregnant patients with ITP.[24] The mechanism of action of the immunoglobulin has not been elucidated, but interference with antibody attachment to platelets and inhibition of antiplatelet antibody production are possibilities.

The response to immunoglobulin is fast and lasts for several days, but is expensive.

◪ COAGULATION DISORDERS

Congenital disorders of the coagulation system are rare during pregnancy. On a rare occasion, an obstetrician has the opportunity to care for a patient with von Willebrand's disease, the main inherited coagulation defect seen in women of reproductive age.

Von Willebrand's disease

Von Willebrand's disease is a disorder resulting from a quantitative or qualitative deficiency in von Willebrand's factor, which is necessary for platelet adhesion. This coagulopathy is rarely found during pregnancy, and only a few well-studied cases have been reported in the literature.[25] This disorder is usually inherited in an autosomal dominant pattern, but there are rare autosomal recessive cases. Characteristically, these patients have prolonged bleeding times and moderate-to-marked decreases in von Willebrand's factor activity. The von Willebrand factor (VIII:Ag or VWF:Ag), the major component of the factor VIII complex, is a high–molecular weight glycoprotein produced by endothelial cells. In some cases, the factor VIII coagulant (VIII:C), the other component of the factor VIII complex, is also decreased.

The most sensitive test for detecting von Willebrand's disease involves observing the ability of the patient's plasma to agglutinate forma-linized-washed platelets in the presence of ristocetin. This test is named ristocetin cofactor assay or von Willebrand's factor activity. Also, factor VIII:Ag can be measured directly by means of radioimmunoassay. However, this test may be negative in as many as 20% of patients.

The diagnosis of von Willebrand's disease must be suspected in any pregnant patient with an abnormal bleeding tendency, particularly with recurrent postpartum bleeding. Such a patient should be screened with bleeding time, PTT, PT, and platelet count. If the platelet count is normal and the bleeding time and PTT are abnormal, the probability of von Willebrand's disease is high, and a definite diagnosis should be obtained by means of the ristocetin cofactor assay. The diagnosis is more difficult when the PTT and the bleeding time are normal. In such a case, an aspirin challenge may be necessary to establish the diagnosis.

The course of pregnancy in the majority of patients with von Willebrand's disease is benign. The most frequent complication is bleeding during labor, delivery, or the postpartum period.[26] Pregnancy causes an increase in von Willebrand's factor, and the probability of bleeding is inversely related to the magnitude of such an increase. In general, if von Willebrand's factor rises to about 50% of the normal concentration, the probability of intrapartum or postpartum bleeding is almost nil. If the concentration of von Willebrand's factor by the end of pregnancy is less than 25% of normal and the bleeding time is prolonged by more than 20 minutes, the patient must be treated with cryoprecipitate to prevent abnormal bleeding.

Each bag of cryoprecipitate contains approximately 100 U of von Willebrand's factor. In general, 15 to 25 bags of cryoprecipitate should be given as the initial dose, and 7 to 12 bags should be given every 12 hours to keep the level of the factor at around 30% or normal.

Desmopressin (Stimate) is a vasopressin analogue that has been used successfully in patients with von Willebrand's disease to promote the release of the von Willebrand factor from endothelial cells. There is limited experience with the use of this medication during pregnancy.

Disseminated intravascular coagulation

Disseminated intravascular coagulation (DIC) is a syndrome that can be associated with many different conditions. It is characterized by increased turnover of coagulation factors, platelet destruction, activation of the fibrinolytic system, formation of thrombi in the microcirculation, and uncontrolled thrombin activity. For a discussion of this subject, the reader should turn to Chapter 9 (Third-Trimester Bleeding).

◪ THROMBOEMBOLIC DISEASES

If the series of reactions leading to clot formation were not adequately counterbalanced, each interruption of a vessel wall would result in the formation of a clot that would enlarge continuously, causing generalized coagulation. This does not occur because of mechanisms that inhibit coagulation. The most important of these is the activity of the inhibitors antithrombin III and protein C. Antithrombin III antagonizes the action of activated factors XII, XI, IX, X, and II, whereas protein C destroys factors V and VIII. The anticoagulant heparin binds to antithromb

III and enhances its ability to inactivate thrombin and factor X. Full activation of protein C requires the intervention of another enzyme, protein S. Any reduction in the activity of antithrombin III, protein C, or protein S will lead to a state of hypercoagulability.

Deficiencies in the activity of all three of the natural anticoagulants have been described during pregnancy.[27-29] Individuals with these deficiencies tend to have extensive thrombosis of maternal and fetal placental vessels. All women who have had episodes of thromboembolism should be tested for possible deficiencies in the activities of these anticoagulants.

The thromboembolic diseases occurring most frequently during pregnancy are (1) the intravascular deposition of fibrinogen-like material that occurs in the course of severe preeclampsia and eclampsia, (2) deep vein thrombosis (DVT) of the lower extremities, and (3) pulmonary embolism. The first of these problems is reviewed in Chapter 10. In this chapter the discussion is limited to the last two problems.

Deep vein thrombosis

The incidence of thrombophlebitis of the legs in the antepartum period is approximately 2.0 per 1000 pregnancies (about the same as for nonpregnant women). The large majority of cases of antepartum thrombophlebitis are superficial (1.7 per 1000 pregnancies), and DVT is a rare event (3.6 of each 10,000 pregnancies).

The incidence of superficial thrombophlebitis increases 7 times (12 per 1000 pregnancies), and the incidence of DVT increases 4 to 5 times (15 per 10,000 pregnancies) during the postpartum period compared to the antepartum period.[30] It is paradoxical that the postpartum period is the time of significant risk for thromboembolic complications, since this is the time during which a rapid rise in plasma and whole blood fibrinolytic activity occurs.[31]

The majority of patients who develop thrombophlebitis during pregnancy belong to a population characterized by the presence of one or more of the following risk factors: (1) cesarean-section delivery, (2) obesity, (3) use of estrogen to suppress lactation, (4) obstetric complications involving prolonged bed rest (e.g., prolonged labor, multiple labor inductions, difficult deliveries), (5) age greater than 30 years and high parity, and (6) deficiency of a natural anticoagulant activity (antithrombin III, protein C, protein S).

The clinical diagnosis of lower extremity DVT is in error 50% of the time. Therefore, when this diagnosis is being considered, the clinical impression must be confirmed with laboratory tests. The most commonly used are continuous Doppler ultrasound, duplex Doppler ultrasound, impedance plethysmography, fibrinogen ^{125}I scanning, and contrast venography.

The gold standard for the diagnosis of DVT is contrast venography. Unfortunately, venography has side effects (e.g., pain, local chemical phlebitis, accidents caused by the contrast dye) in one of every four patients and, therefore, is not the procedure of choice. Its use is limited to those instances in which noninvasive tests give uncertain results. Venography is the most accurate method for the diagnosis of thrombosis in the calf. In 80% of pregnant patients, however, the thrombosis starts in the iliac and femoral veins and can be diagnosed by noninvasive methods.

Continuous Doppler ultrasound is the test of choice for the diagnosis of popliteal, femoral, or iliac thrombosis but is less accurate for calf thrombosis. Also, patients in the third trimester of pregnancy have impaired venous return and may have false-positive results. In the last few years, the combination of real-time ultrasound and gated Doppler ultrasound (duplex Doppler) is used increasingly to diagnose DVT. Duplex Doppler has a 92% to 95% sensitivity and a 97% to 100% specificity when compared with venography in nonpregnant patients for the diagnosis of DVT.[32] The recent advent of color Doppler imaging most likely will increase the accuracy of the method.

Another test is impedance plethysmography (IPG) using the occlusive cuff technique. This method measures the changes in electrical impedance that occur when there are changes in the blood volume of the leg. When the venous return is impaired with a cuff applied to the thigh, there is a local increase in blood volume followed by a rapid decrease when the cuff pressure is released. These changes in volume are reflected by changes in electrical impedance, which is altered when DVT is present. The test is highly specific (less than 5% false positives) and very sensitive (less than 5% false negatives) for the diagnosis of popliteal and suprapopliteal DVT, and there is at least one report of its use in pregnant patients as a screening test for DVT.[33]

Fibrinogen ^{125}I scanning is an excellent technique for the diagnosis of DVT in the calf and lower thigh, but unfortunately it has very limited use during pregnancy because the radioactive iodine will cross the placenta and accumulate in the fetal thyroid gland. The use of fibrinogen ^{125}I scanning in the postpartum period is limited to women who are not breastfeeding, because the radioactive isotope will contaminate the breast milk and will reach the thyroid gland of the newborn.

Once the diagnosis of DVT has been established, treatment with intravenous heparin is mandatory. Of those patients who have episodes of DVT during pregnancy and who receive no treatment, 20% to 35% experience a recurrence.[34] If untreated, 19% of pregnant patients with DVT develop pulmonary embolism, and 29% of those with pulmonary embolism die. The amount of heparin necessary to obtain full anticoagulation—1.5 to 2.0 times PTT control values—may be calculated using the following formula:

$$\text{Heparin infusion rate} = \text{Css} \times \text{K} \times \text{V}$$

where:

Css = steady state concentration of heparin in serum (usually 0.2 to 0.3 U/ml, which is the therapeutic level)

K   = elimination constant (0.832 U/hr)

V   = volume of distribution (varies from 60 ml/kg in the first trimester to 90 ml/kg in the third trimester)

A patient in the second trimester of pregnancy weighing 140 lb (63 kg) will require:

$$\text{Heparin infusion rate} = 0.25 \times 0.832 \times 63 \times 70 = 917 \text{ U/hr}$$

The treatment is monitored by daily measurements of the PTT, and the goal is to maintain the PTT between 1.5 and 2.0 times the normal control PTT value (60 to 80 seconds).

Treatment with intravenous heparin is continued for a minimum of 7 days or until the pain has subsided completely. If the patient has already delivered at the end of the heparin treatment, she is switched to oral anticoagulants, and full anticoagulation is continued until the Doppler ultrasound or the venogram is negative. Some authors recommend a minimum of 3 months of anticoagulation with warfarin (Coumadin) after delivery.

If the patient has not delivered at the end of the 7 days of intravenous heparin treatment,

subcutaneous administration of therapeutic doses of heparin should be started and continued until delivery. After delivery the patient should be switched to warfarin or maintained on prophylactic heparinization (5000 U subcutaneously every 12 hours).

Heparin is the drug of choice for keeping the patient with DVT fully anticoagulated during pregnancy. Heparin therapy has a low rate of maternal and fetal complications and is an effective drug for the prophylaxis and treatment of DVT.[35] Warfarin has been used for this purpose, but the associated occurrence of fetal congenital abnormalities[36] and spontaneous intracranial bleeding with fetal death in utero are reasons to avoid this drug during pregnancy.

Once the patient is discharged from the hospital, full anticoagulation with heparin is difficult because of the need for parenteral administration of the drug. The following three modes of treatment are available:

1. Repeated subcutaneous injections of heparin by the patient herself every 6 to 8 hours in amounts that vary from 6000 to 12000 U, with the treatment monitored by PTT measurements carried out 1 hour before injection. This method causes wide fluctuations in blood clotting, with increased risk of bleeding complications, and produces multiple small, painful, darkly stained hematomas at the injection sites. These local problems decrease with the use of the calcium salt of heparin (Calciparine).

2. Repeated intravenous injections of heparin administered by the patient herself via a heparin lock placed and secured in a peripheral vein of the arm. This method also causes wide swings in blood coagulation and requires a knowledgeable patient capable of adequately handling the heparin lock.

3. Continuous subcutaneous or intravenous injection of heparin using a micropump. With the development of sophisticated, small, programmable pumps for continuous intravenous or subcutaneous infusion, it is possible to inject continuously small volumes of highly concentrated solutions of heparin and secure a steady level of hypocoagulation. However, these pumps are expensive and may fail, producing bleeding or inadequate coagulation levels.

Pulmonary embolism

Pulmonary embolism (PE) occurs rarely during pregnancy. Friend and Kakkar[37] reported an incidence of 2.7 per 1000, but almost certainly this is a high estimate resulting from overdiagnosis. In about 95% of the cases, PE is the result of DVT of the ileo-femoral veins, and in the majority of cases, it occurs in the immediate postpartum period.

All the clinical signs and symptoms of PE are inconsistent and unreliable, and only a pulmonary angiogram provides absolute evidence. Typically, these patients have arterial PO_2 below 80 mm Hg and pCO_2 below 40 mm Hg. The test most often used for PE diagnosis is the ventilation-perfusion (V/Q) scan. The Prospective Investigation of Pulmonary Embolism Diagnosis (PIOPED) found that PE was present in 88%, 33%, and 12% of patients with V/Q scans indicating high, intermediate, and low probability of embolization, respectively.[38] Thus to compensate for the low specificity of V/Q scanning, it is necessary to obtain a pulmonary angiogram in patients with clinical assessment suggestive of PE and a V/Q scan indicating intermediate probability of embolization. Figure 13-1 shows the sequence of steps that we follow in the evaluation of patients suspected of PE. If the clinical presentation is strongly suggestive of PE, the diagnostic studies must be initiated after giving the patient an intravenous injection of 10,000 U of heparin, and the treatment with heparin must be discontinued later depending on the results of the diagnostic workup. It is also important to look for proximal DVT of the lower extremities in all cases in which PE is suspected, since DVT is present in about 95% of all cases of PE.

With respect to the diagnostic protocol (Figure 13-1), the following are the most important points to remember:

1. Most patients with PE have clear chest x-ray films.
2. A positive perfusion scan is sine qua non evidence of PE. If the perfusion scan is *negative*, the patient does not have PE, and no further testing is necessary.

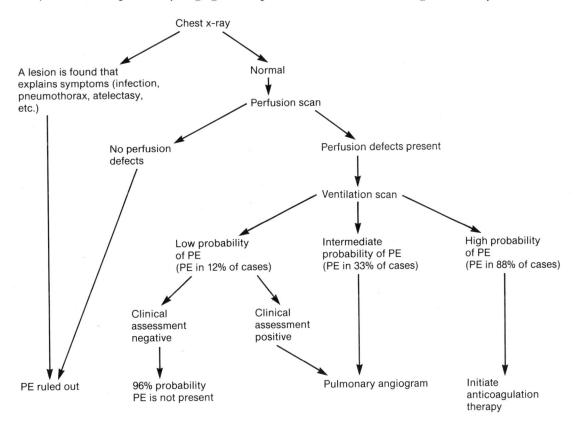

FIGURE 13-1 ◪ Diagnostic steps to take for patients suspected of pulmonary embolization.

3. A ventilation-perfusion mismatch is not diagnostic of PE, since there are other causes of pulmonary vascular obstruction (i.e., inflammation). However, the probability of PE is high.

4. Pulmonary angiography is the only procedure that will establish definitely the diagnosis of PE.

The duration of anticoagulation therapy for patients with PE is controversial. Traditionally, patients have been managed with continuous heparin infusion for 10 days, with oral anticoagulation started on day five and continued for several months. Other investigators have proposed giving continuous intravenous heparin for 5 days, with oral anticoagulation started on day one and continued for several months.[39] The duration of full anticoagulation with warfarin is variable, but most authors recommend a period of 3 months.

◼ IMPORTANT POINTS ◼

1. Anemia is present during pregnancy if the hemoglobin concentration is less than 10 g/dl or the hematocrit is less than 30%. These values are lower than in the nonpregnant state because of the physiologic hemodilution that occurs during pregnancy.

2. Iron deficiency is responsible for approximately 80% of all anemias during pregnancy. The main reasons for this are inadequate dietary iron and insufficient iron stores to meet the demands of pregnancy.

3. Ideally, iron deficiency should be diagnosed when iron stores are depleted but abnormal erythropoiesis is not yet present. The best test to assess the status of the iron stores is serum ferritin.

4. In patients with iron-deficiency anemia, an abnormal red cell distribution width (RDW) occurs before generalized microcytosis and hypochromia.

5. A pregnant woman needs only one 300-mg ferrous sulfate tablet daily to prevent iron-deficiency anemia. Treatment of overt disease requires higher doses.

6. Although most cases are the result of folic acid deficiency, laboratory investigation of patients with megaloblastic anemia during pregnancy should include a serum vitamin B_{12} level. This avoids missing the rare patient who has vitamin B_{12} deficiency and may suffer progressive demyelinization.

7. The most common hemolytic anemia observed during pregnancy occurs in patients with severe preeclampsia and HELLP syndrome. The blood smear in these patients shows schistiocytes, burr cells, helmet cells, and fragmented cells.

8. A microcytic, hypochromic anemia and a hemoglobin A_2 level greater than 3.5% are characteristic features of patients with beta thalassemia minor.

9. In the management of pregnant patients with sickle cell disease a controversy exists between proponents of prophylactic transfusion and proponents of transfusion for specific indications. Prophylactic transfusions decrease the frequency of painful crises and disease-associated complications but have no effect on obstetric complications, alloimmunization, or perinatal outcome.

10. Platelet counts under 150,000/mm^3 are relatively common in pregnancy, but only 21% of those patients have preeclampsia or immune thrombocytopenia.

11. To diagnose idiopathic thrombocytopenic purpura (ITP), it is necessary to demonstrate the presence of antiplatelet antibodies in the maternal serum.

12. The maternal platelet count cannot be used to predict the fetal platelet count. Patients with ITP should have percutaneous umbilical blood sampling to measure the fetal platelets. If the platelet count is less than 50,000/mm^3, cesarean section is indicated.

13. Every woman of reproductive age with deep vein thrombosis or pulmonary embolization should be tested for possible deficiency of the natural anticoagulants antithrombin III, protein C, and protein S.

14. The gold standard for the diagnosis of DVT is contrast venography, but it has side effects in 25% of the patients. Duplex Doppler ultrasound is the test of choice for the diagnosis of popliteal, femoral, or iliac thrombosis but is less accurate for calf thrombosis.

15. The amount of heparin necessary to obtain full anticoagulation with a continuous intravenous infusion may be calculated using an equation that involves the volume of distribution of the drug, the steady state concentration to be achieved, and the rate of elimination of the medication.

16. A ventilation-perfusion mismatch is not diagnostic but indicates a high probability of pulmonary embolization. Angiography is the gold standard for the diagnosis of pulmonary embolization.

REFERENCES

1. Scott DE, Pritchard JA: Iron deficiency in healthy young college women. *JAMA* 1967;199:897-900.
2. Roszkowski I, Wojcick J, Zaleska K: Serum iron deficiency during the third trimester of pregnancy: Maternal complications and fate of the neonate. *Obstet Gynecol* 1966;28:820-825.
3. Gatenby PPB, Lillie EW: Clinical analysis of 100 cases of severe megaloblastic anemia of pregnancy. *Br Med J* 1960;2:1111-1114.
4. Hibbard BM: The role of folic acid in pregnancy with particular reference to anemia, abruption, and abortion. *Br J Obstet Gynaecol* 1964;27:155.
5. Whalley PJ, Scott DE, Pritchard JA: Maternal folate deficiency and pregnancy wastage: I. Placental abruption. *Am J Obstet Gynecol* 1969;105:670-677.
6. Klebanoff MA, Shiono PH, Berendes WH, et al: Facts and artifacts about anemia and preterm delivery. *JAMA* 1989;262:511-515.
7. Thompson WB: Comparison of tests for diagnosis of iron depletion in pregnancy. *Am J Obstet Gynecol* 1988;159:1132-1134.
8. Goepel E, Ulmer HU, Neth RD: Premature labor contractions and the value of serum ferritin during pregnancy. *Gynecol Obstet Invest* 1988;26:265-273.
9. Osborne PT, Burkett LL, Ryan GM, et al: An evaluation of red cell heterogeneity (increased red blood cell distribution width) in iron deficiency of pregnancy. *Am J Obstet Gynecol* 1989;160:336-339.
10. Stein ML, Gunston KD, May RM: Iron dextran in the treatment of iron-deficiency anemia of pregnancy: Haematological response and incidence of side-effects. *S Afr Med J* 1991;79:195-196.
11. Bitran JD, Miller JB, Golomb HM: Megaloblastic anemia during pregnancy. *J Reprod Med* 1977;19:186-192.
12. Pritchard JA, Scott DE, Whalley PJ, et al: The effect of maternal sickle cell hemoglobinpathies and sickle cell trait on reproductive performance. *Am J Obstet Gynecol* 1973;117:662-673.
13. White JM, Richards R, Byrne M, et al: Thalassaemia trait and pregnancy. *J Clin Pathol* 1985;38:810-817.
14. Powers DR, Sandhu M, Niland-Weiss J, et al: Pregnancy in sickle cell disease. *Obstet Gynecol* 1973;41:865-872.
15. Morrison JC, Schneider JM, Whybrew WD, et al: Prophylactic transfusions in pregnant patients with sickle cell hemoglobinopathies: Benefit versus risk. *Obstet Gynecol* 1980;56:274-280.
16. Cunningham FG, Pritchard JA, Mason R, et al: Prophylactic transfusions of normal red blood cells during pregnancies complicated by sickle cell hemoglobinopathies. *Am J Obstet Gynecol* 1979;135:994-1001.
17. Koshy M, Burd L, Wallace D, et al: Prophylactic red-cell transfusions in pregnant patients with sickle cell disease: A randomized comparative study. *N Engl J Med* 1988;319:1447-1452.
18. Aitchison RG, Marsh JC, Hows JM, et al: Pregnancy-associated aplastic anemia: A report of five cases and review of current management. *Br J Haematol* 1989;73:541-545.
19. Burrows RF, Kelton JG: Thrombocytopenia at delivery: A prospective survey of 6715 deliveries. *Am J Obstet Gynecol* 1990;162:731-734.
20. Clines DB, Dusak B, Tomaski A, et al: Immune thrombocytopenic purpura and pregnancy. *N Engl J Med* 1982;206:826-831.
21. Kellton JG, Inwood JM, Barre RM, et al: The prenatal prediction of thrombocytopenia in infants of mothers with clinically diagnosed immune thrombocytopenia. *Am J Obstet Gynecol* 1982;144:449-454.
22. Carloss HW, McMillan R, Crosby WH: Management of pregnancy in women with immune thrombocytopenic purpura. *JAMA* 1980;244:2756-2758.
23. Karpatkin M, Porges RF, Karpatkin S: Platelet counts in infants of women with immune thrombocytopenic purpura. *JAMA* 1980;244:2756-2758.
24. Mizunuma H, Takahaski Y, Taguchi H, et al: A new approach to idiopathic thrombocytopenic purpura during pregnancy by high dose immunoglobulin G infusion. *Am J Obstet Gynecol* 1984;148:218-219.
25. Noller KL, Bowie EJW, Kempers RD, et al: Von Willebrand's disease in pregnancy. *Obstet Gynecol* 1973;41:865-872.
26. Chediak JR, Alban GM, Maxey B: Von Willebrand's disease and pregnancy: Management during delivery and outcome of offspring. *Am J Obstet Gynecol* 1986;155:618-624.
27. Brenner B, Shapira A, Bahari C, et al: Hereditary protein C deficiency during pregnancy. *Am J Obstet* 1987;157:1160-1161.
28. Hellgren M, Tengborn L, Abildgaard U: Pregnancy in women with congenital antithrombin III deficiency: Experience of treatment with heparin and antithrombin. *Gynecol Obstet Invest* 1982;14:127-141.
29. Rose PG, Essig GF, Vaccaro PS, et al: Protein S deficiency in pregnancy. *Am J Obstet Gynecol* 1986;155:140-141.
30. Kierkegaard A: Incidence and diagnosis of deep vein thrombosis associated with pregnancy. *Acta Obstet Gynecol Scand* 1983;62:239-243.
31. Arias F, Andrinopoulos G, Zamora J: Whole-blood fibrinolytic activity in normal and hypertensive pregnancies and its relation to the placental concentration of urokinase inhibitor. *Am J Obstet Gynecol* 1979;133:624-629.
32. White RH, McGaham JP, Daschbach MM, et al: Diagnosis of deep vein thrombosis using duplex ultrasound. *Ann Intern Med* 1989;111:297-304.
33. Clarke-Pearson DL, Creasman WT: Diagnosis of deep venous thrombosis in obstetrics and gynecology by impedance phlebography. *Obstet Gynecol* 1981;58:52-57.
34. Villasanta U: Thromboembolic disease in pregnancy. *Am J Obstet Gynecol* 1965;93:142-160.
35. Ginsberg JS, Kowalchuk G, Hirsch J, et al: Heparin therapy during pregnancy: Risks to the fetus and mother. *Arch Intern Med* 1989;149:2233-2236.
36. Tawes RL, Kennedy PA, Harris EJ, et al: Management of deep vein thrombosis and pulmonary embolism during pregnancy. *Am J Surg* 1982;144:141-145.

37. Friend JR, Kakkar VV: Deep vein thrombosis in obstetrics and gynecological patients, in Kakkar VV, Jouhar AJ (eds): *Thromboembolism: Diagnosis and treatment.* London. Churchill Livingstone, 1972, pp 131-138.

38. The PIOPED investigations: Value of ventilation/perfusion scan in acute pulmonary embolism: Results of the prospective investigation of pulmonary embolism diagnosis (PIOPED). *JAMA* 1990;263:2753.

39. Hull RD, Raskob GE, Rosenbloom D, et al: Heparin for 5 days as compared with 10 days in the initial treatment of proximal venous thrombosis. *N Engl J Med* 1990;322:1260-1264.

14

RENAL DISEASE DURING PREGNANCY

To better understand the effect of pregnancy complications on renal function, as well as the effect of pregnancy on preexistent kidney disease, the obstetrician should have an adequate understanding of the anatomic and functional changes that occur in the kidneys and the urinary system during gestation. The first part of this chapter is dedicated to the analysis of those changes.

◪ CHANGES IN THE KIDNEYS AND THE URINARY TRACT DURING NORMAL PREGNANCY

The most important anatomic change in the urinary tract during pregnancy is the dilation of the collecting system. The renal calices, the renal pelvis, and the ureters start to dilate in the second trimester and remain enlarged for several weeks after delivery. The cause of this dilation is unknown, although many people believe that it is mediated by placental progesterone. After 18 weeks of gestation, compression of the ureters by the uterus at the level of the pelvic brim is another factor contributing to dilation and stasis of urine in the upper part of the collecting system.[1]

Because of these changes, the frequency and severity of urinary tract infections increases.

Also, these anatomic changes make 24-hour urine collections imprecise because a significant amount of urine may remain unmeasured.

The principal physiologic changes that occur in the kidney during pregnancy are:
1. Increase in renal plasma flow (RPF)
2. Increase in glomerular filtration rate (GFR)
3. Changes in tubular reabsorption of glucose, sodium, amino acids, and uric acid

The increase in RPF begins in the second trimester and probably is caused by the combined effect of an increased cardiac output and a decrease in renal vascular resistance resulting from increased production of renal prostaglandins. It has been calculated that approximately 25% of the cardiac output during pregnancy is destined to flow through the kidneys.

The most important consequence of the increased RPF is a 50% increase in the GFR, to an average of 137 ml/min. Knowing this, one can properly interpret laboratory data during pregnancy. A 24-hour creatinine clearance of 110 ml/min, perfectly normal outside of pregnancy, is inadequate during gestation and implies the presence of some factor affecting renal hemodynamics. Also, the serum creatinine and urea nitrogen concentrations will be lower than in the nonpregnant situation. The average serum creatinine concentration during pregnancy is 0.6 mg/dl, and a value above 0.8 mg/dl is suspicious. Similarly, the average blood urea nitrogen (BUN) value during pregnancy is 9 mg/dl, and any value greater than 13 mg/dl is abnormal.

The renal handling of glucose is markedly altered during pregnancy, and glucosuria in the presence of normal blood sugar occurs frequently. This happens because of the increased GFR combined with an impaired tubular reabsorption of glucose. The presence of sugar in the urine is a factor that promotes urinary tract infections during pregnancy.

The average plasma sodium concentration during pregnancy is 136 mEq/L. This slight decrease in plasma sodium concentration during pregnancy is a result of the increased amount of filtered sodium caused by the increased GFR. In fact, during pregnancy the amount of sodium presented to the tubules for reabsorption is approximately 30,240 mEq/day, whereas the nonpregnant woman filters only about 20,160 mEq.[2] Although the efficiency of tubular sodium reabsorption during pregnancy is remarkable, the serum sodium equilibrates at a slightly lower level than it does in the nonpregnant status.

As a result of the increased GFR, serum uric acid concentration decreases slightly during the second trimester, but it returns to normal nonpregnant levels (4 to 6 mg/dl) during the third trimester. Some investigators believe that preeclampsia selectively affects the tubular reabsorption and causes a characteristic elevation of uric acid.

Maternal position has a profound influence on renal function. RPF, GFR, sodium excretion, and urinary production all decrease when the patient is recumbent. All these indices return to normal when the patient assumes the lateral decubitus position. Also, the dorsal decubitus position worsens the compression of the ureters by the pregnant uterus.

◪ RENAL DISEASE AND PREGNANCY

The two presentations of kidney abnormalities that obstetricians encounter most commonly are:
1. The acute onset of signs and symptoms of renal disease in patients with no history of kidney problems before pregnancy
2. The occurrence of pregnancy in a patient with known renal disease

The problems posed by each of these situations are different and require separate analysis.

◪ NEW ONSET OF RENAL DISEASE DURING PREGNANCY
Acute pyelonephritis

Infections of the urinary tract occur frequently during gestation. Approximately 4% to 10% of all pregnant women have asymptomatic bacteriuria, and if untreated, 25% of them will develop acute pyelonephritis.

Usually, a single bacterial species is the cause of acute pyelonephritis. Also, the overwhelming majority of cases of pyelonephritis are ascending infections caused by perineal bacteria. The most common offenders are gram-negative bacilli (*Escherichia coli, Klebsiella pneumoniae, Proteus mirabilis*) or enterococci.

E. coli is responsible for more than 80% of all acute upper urinary tract infections. There is evidence indicating that some strains of *E. coli* have fimbriae (P-fimbriae) that bind to specific glycoprotein receptors on the surface of the epithelial cells, a property that increases their virulence and their selectivity for the urinary tract.[3] Bacterial virulence is not the only important factor implicated in the severity of urinary tract infections. Another factor is individual susceptibility. It has been demonstrated that women with nonsecretor Lewis blood group phenotypes are highly susceptible to urinary tract infections. Another important factor is the presence of anatomic or functional abnormalities in the urinary tract, such as occur in women with vesicoureteral reflux that allows a direct route for ascending infection.

Since in the large majority of pregnant patients, acute pyelonephritis is preceded by asymptomatic bacteriuria, detecting patients with bacteriuria and treating them should decrease the incidence of pyelonephritis. However, the screening of pregnant women in search for those with asymptomatic bacteriuria has not been universally accepted. It is argued that screening only once early in gestation will not detect more than one third of those women that develop pyelonephritis, and to increase the rate of detection, a second screening would be necessary later in pregnancy. Thus, in populations with a low prevalence of asymptomatic bacteriuria, universal screening is not justified.[4]

The criteria commonly used to make the diagnosis of asymptomatic bacteriuria is the growth in solid culture of 100,000 or more colonies of a single bacterial species per milliliter of freshly voided urine collected by the midstream catch technique. However, some investigators believe that urine counts of 20,000 to 50,000 also represent active infection.[5] Depending on the population under study, 4% to 10% of all pregnant women will fulfill this criterion.

Several antibiotic regimens can be successfully used for the treatment of asymptomatic bacteriuria. One of the most commonly used is nitrofurantoin, 400 mg daily for 7 days. Ampicillin, cephalexin, and trimethoprim-sulfamethoxazole can be used instead with similar success. The results of treatment should be confirmed by repeated urine cultures, and the treatment should be repeated until bacteriuria is eradicated. If bacteriuria persists after two courses of treatment, it is necessary to give one dose of antibiotic (500 mg cephalexin or 100 mg nitrofurantoin) every night for the duration of the pregnancy. Continuous daily treatment is also necessary for patients who have relapses after successful treatments or who are reinfected by a different bacterial species.

Histologically, acute pyelonephritis is characterized by infiltration of the renal interstitium and the tubules by polymorphonuclear leukocytes, with formation of white cell casts. Healing of the acute lesion will lead to cortical scarring and calyceal dilation.

Acute pyelonephritis usually occurs in the second and third trimesters of pregnancy. It is manifested by the onset of malaise, fatigue, chills, and back pain that is usually located in the upper lumbar area. In some patients, changes in the characteristics of the urine and symptoms of low urinary tract infection occur. Also, patients frequently complain of nausea, vomiting, and uterine contractions. On physical examination the patients have fever, are dehydrated, and have costovertebral angle (CVA) tenderness. Frequently it is possible to see changes in the urine, which may look turbid or bloody. Urinalysis will demonstrate red cells, leukocytes, and white cell casts, and in the majority of patients, microscopic examination of unspun urine will show bacteria. Most patients show some signs of renal dysfunction, such as slightly elevated serum BUN and creatinine and creatinine clearance that is abnormally low for pregnancy.[6]

Acute pyelonephritis during pregnancy may have serious consequences. Some of them are effects of endotoxin, which can cause septic shock or pulmonary injury. There is evidence in the literature indicating that pregnant women are more susceptible to the effects of endotoxin than are nonpregnant individuals. Some other consequences of acute pyelonephritis, such as chronic renal infection, are the result of incomplete or delayed treatment or of coexistent obstruction.

Treatment of pregnant patients with acute pyelonephritis should be aggressive to avoid progression of the disease and the occurrence of serious complications. Patients should be admitted to the hospital, hydrated, treated with antibiotics, and carefully monitored. Laboratory evaluation should include assessment of their renal function and electrolytes, and also a hemogram. A specimen of urine obtained by catheterization should be sent to the laboratory for culture and for sensitivity testing. Blood cultures should be obtained when the patients have chills or temperature elevation.

Patients with acute pyelonephritis during pregnancy need assessment of their vital signs at least every 4 hours. Tachycardia and hypotension may indicate early endotoxic shock. These patients also require continuous monitoring with pulse oximetry.[7] Desaturation should be followed by chest x-ray examination to rule out the possibility of acute respiratory distress syndrome (ARDS). They also require continuous fetal monitoring. Preterm labor is a frequent problem, and patients require continuous observation for uterine contractions.

The two fundamental aspects of the treatment of patients with acute pyelonephritis are the administration of intravenous fluids and intravenous antibiotic therapy. These patients are frequently dehydrated and oliguric and require rapid expansion of intravascular volume with crystalloid solutions. The antibiotic of choice for acute pyelonephritis used to be ampicillin, 2 g IV every 4 to 6 hours. Unfortunately, the microbial resistance of gram-negative bacteria to ampicillin is increasing.[8] For that reason, pending the results of laboratory identification of the infectious species and its sensitivity to antibiotics, the best therapeutic option is to give a combination of ampicillin/sulbactam and aztreonam. Both antibiotics should be administered intravenously. A cephalosporin is a good alternative treatment for patients allergic to ampicillin. However, it should be remembered that up to 10% of patients with significant allergic reactions to ampicillin are also allergic to cephalosporins.

Most patients respond quickly to hydration and antibiotic therapy. Once they have been afebrile for 24 to 48 hours, they may be switched to oral antibiotics. Follow-up with urine cultures is necessary. Recurrence of bacteriuria demands antibiotic treatment for the duration of pregnancy.

Patients who do not respond quickly to therapy require additional testing to rule out the possibility of obstruction. A renal sonogram is indicated initially, and if necessary, a *modified intravenous pyelogram (IVP)*, only one or two x-ray exposures following the administration of contrast medium, should be obtained. Ureteral stents and percutaneous nephrostomy may be necessary in patients with demonstrated urinary obstruction.

Acute nephrolithiasis

Acute nephrolithiasis is a rather unusual complication of pregnancy that occurs once in every 1500 deliveries,[9] usually during the second and third trimesters. The main symptoms are severe flank and lower-quadrant pain with microscopic hematuria. Pregnant patients with renal stones should be managed as if they were not pregnant, with two exceptions:

1. The use of x-ray examinations should be kept to a minimum.
2. In cases requiring surgical intervention, palliative measures are the first choice, and definitive procedures should wait until the postpartum period.

If a pregnant patient develops symptoms suggestive of ureteral calculi, the following should be done:

1. All urines should be strained for the passage of gravel or stones.
2. The urine should be cultured. The finding of a *Proteus mirabilis* infection in a patient with a history of chronic recurrent urinary tract infections is strongly suggestive of the presence of magnesium ammonium phosphate (struvite) stones.
3. A 24-hour urine collection for quantitative determination of calcium and uric acid should be obtained. Hypercalciuria (greater than 250 mg/day) suggests the presence of calcium oxalate stones, whereas hyperuricemia (greater than 800 mg/day) suggests uric acid stones. However, a diagnostic error can easily be made during pregnancy because hypercalciuria may be found in normal patients who are taking large amounts of calcium.

4. A careful family history should be elicited. If the disease exists in several members of the family, cystinuria or hyperoxaluria may be present. In patients with a family history of calculi, a 24-hour urine collection should be sent to the laboratory for cystine and oxalic acid determination.
5. The urine pH should be determined several times a day for several days. A pH that is persistently acidic suggests uric acid stones; a persistently alkaline urine suggests magnesium ammonium phosphate stones.
6. Serum calcium, uric acid, and electrolytes should be measured. If hypercalcemia is present, it will be necessary to rule out the possibility of hyperparathyroidism, a situation frequently associated with calcium oxalate stones. Hyperchloremia suggests renal tubular acidosis and calcium phosphate calculi. Hyperuricemia suggests uric acid stones (Table 14-1).
7. A renal ultrasound must be ordered. It is useful for the detection of stones in the upper urinary tract and for the diagnosis of upper urinary tract obstruction.

If the diagnosis of nephrolithiasis or ureterolithiasis cannot be established with certainty by the mentioned laboratory tests and the patient's symptoms warrant further diagnostic procedures, a flat plate of the abdomen and a limited IVP should be done. Approximately 80% of calculi can be seen by x-ray examination. A limited IVP is useful only if a positive diagnosis is reached, and a negative IVP does not necessarily prove the absence of stones. The technique results in a fetal exposure to 0.1 to 1.0 rad.

Treatment of patients with acute nephrolithiasis during pregnancy depends on the severity and duration of their symptoms and the presence of obstruction. When acute hydronephrosis develops as a consequence of obstruction, cystoscopic passage of a ureteral stent and stone manipulation using retrograde ureteral catheterization may be attempted.[10] If this fails, a percutaneous nephrostomy should be performed. Operative removal of ureteral stones in the late second and third trimesters is difficult because of the increased vascularization and problems generated by the pregnant uterus. Such surgery is a last resource and, ideally, should be postponed until after delivery.[11]

More than 50% of patients admitted to the hospital with symptoms of renal lithiasis pass the

TABLE 14-1 ◪ Laboratory studies in patients with renal stones

Test	Finding	Diagnostic possibility
Urine culture	*Proteus mirabilis*	Struvite stones
24-hour urine collection for calcium	Hypercalciuria (>250 mg/day)	Calcium oxalate stones
24-hour urine collection for uric acid	Hyperuricosuria (>800 mg/day)	Uric acid stones
Urine pH (several days)	Acid	Uric acid stones
	Alkaline	Struvite stones
Serum calcium	Hypercalcemia	Hyperparathyroidism
Serum uric acid	Hyperuricemia	Uric acid stones
Plasma chloride	Hyperchloremia	Renal tubular acidosis

stones spontaneously.[12] For most of these patients, analgesics and intravenous fluids maintaining urinary output at 2 L/day is all that is necessary. With no evidence of obstruction, spontaneous passage of the stones should be expected and intervention deferred. If the situation fails to improve after a reasonable period, attempting cystoscopic extraction is justified.

Once the acute crisis is over, further treatment depends on the cause of the nephrolithiasis. For example, a low calcium diet and thiazide diuretics are beneficial for patients with idiopathic hypercalciuria. Patients with uricosuria and uric acid stones benefit from a low purine diet. Those affected by hyperparathyroidism stop producing stones once the underlying problems are corrected. Magnesium ammonium phosphate stones require intensive treatment for chronic urinary tract infections.

Acute renal failure

The incidence of acute obstetric renal failure is 1 in 10,000 in industrialized countries, but is a serious problem in developing countries where the incidence varies from 1 of every 2000 to 1 of every 5000 pregnancies.[13] This is due in part to the availability of voluntary pregnancy termination that has made acute renal failure caused by septic abortion a rare event.[14] For practical purposes, acute obstetric renal failure occurs mainly as a complication of severe preeclampsia or following hemorrhagic shock caused by placenta previa or abruptio placentae.

Definition. The term *acute renal failure* describes an abrupt decline in renal function characterized by a urine output of less than 400 ml/24 hr or less than 20 ml/hr.

Etiology. Acute renal failure in pregnancy usually results from a severe deficit in blood flow to the renal cortical region. In 60% of the cases, hypoperfusion is caused by preeclampsia. In 30% the underlying problem is severe bleeding resulting from placenta previa or abruptio placentae. In 5% severe nephrotic syndrome, malignant hypertension, or hemolytic uremic syndrome are the causes of inadequate perfusion. In a small number of cases, obstetric renal failure is the consequence of ureteral obstruction by an overdistended uterus or results from an acute inflammatory process such as lupus nephritis.

Pathophysiology. Renal hypoperfusion in preeclamptic patients results from decreased intravascular volume, spasm of afferent arterioles, and subendothelial deposits of fibrinogen occluding the glomerular capillaries. In patients with placenta previa and abruptio placentae, acute intravascular volume depletion and severe reactive vasospasm are responsible for the decreased renal perfusion. In patients with abruptio placentae, acute disseminated intravascular coagulation with formation of microvascular thrombi in the renal vasculature is a contributory factor to the decreased renal blood flow.

Studies using radioactive tracers have shown that after severe hypovolemia, blood flow to the renal cortex decreases, whereas the perfusion to the medullar area is preserved.[15] Cortical ischemia results in a marked decrease in the glomerular filtration rate, concentrating ability, and urinary volume. This stage of severe impairment in renal function used to be named *prerenal azotemia*, but more recently the term *prerenal disease* is more commonly used. If cortical hypoperfusion persists, the functional changes will be followed by acute tubular necrosis (ATN) or cortical necrosis. Renal hypoperfusion may occur in patients with adequate intravascular volume if there is low perfusion pressure caused by heart failure or decreased plasma colloid osmotic pressure caused by nephrotic syndrome.

TABLE 14-2 ▨ Laboratory studies in the differential diagnosis of acute renal failure

	Prerenal failure	Acute tubular necrosis or bilateral cortical necrosis
U/P osmolality ratio	>1.2	<1.2
Urinary sodium	<20	>40
U/P creatinine ratio	>40	<20
FE_{Na}	<1	>3

The initial renal response to hypoperfusion is to preserve intravascular volume and maintain body sodium. This results in the production of concentrated urine with a low sodium concentration, usually less than 20 mEq/L. If the situation remains uncorrected, the kidney will lose its ability to concentrate the urine and save sodium, and this will be reflected in a urine/plasma (U/P) osmolality ratio close to 1.0 and a urinary sodium concentration greater than 20 mEq/L, frequently in the 50-to-70 mEq/L range (Table 14-2).

Diagnosis. Obstetric patients with acute renal failure may be seen in a variety of clinical situations. Some patients are diagnosed with renal failure after the onset of an obstetric emergency such as eclampsia, abruptio placentae, or placenta previa. Others develop oliguria or anuria in the course of a hospital stay. Irrespective of the clinical presentation, there are some measures to be carried out immediately. These are discussed below.

Hemodynamic monitoring. Insertion of a central venous pressure (CVP) line or Swan-Ganz catheter is important for diagnosis and monitoring of therapy. An elevated CVP or pulmonary wedge pressure (PWP) suggests ATN or cortical necrosis, and intravenous fluids should be restricted. In contrast, if the CVP or PWP are low, intravascular volume depletion is present, and intravenous fluids should be administered.

Urine examination. Complete anuria is rare and indicates obstructive uropathy or profound kidney damage. In most cases of acute renal failure, it is possible to obtain a sample of urine, which should be sent for sodium and osmolality evaluation. A urine osmolality above 500 mosm/kg indicates good tubular function and prerenal disease. Urine osmolality below 400 mosm/kg

suggests ATN. A U/P osmolality ratio larger than 1.2 indicates that the oliguria or anuria is prerenal. In cases of ATN, the U/P osmolality ratio is 1.0 or close to 1.0, indicating the kidney's lack of capacity to concentrate the urine. The urinary sodium is high in ATN, reflecting the inability of the kidneys to reabsorb sodium, and is usually below 20 mEq/L in prerenal disease.

Perhaps the more effective test for differentiating prerenal disease from ATN is the fractional excretion of sodium, or FE_{Na} test.[16] This test depends on the different handling of sodium in prerenal failure, when the tubes avidly reabsorb sodium, compared with ATN, when sodium reabsorption is impaired because of tubular damage. The FE_{Na} is calculated using the following equation:

$$FE_{Na} = \text{U/P sodium/U/P creatinine} \times 100$$

A FE_{Na} less than 1.0 indicates prerenal azotemia, and a value larger than 3.0 indicates ATN.

Smelling the urine is a simple clinical test that may be valuable in making the differential diagnosis between prerenal failure and ATN. The urine of patients in ATN smells like water, whereas in patients with prerenal azotemia, the urine has a distinguishable odor. Examination of the urine sediment is also valuable in making the differential diagnosis. The urine sediment of patients in ATN characteristically contains numerous renal tubular cells, renal tubular cell casts, and muddy-brown pigment casts. Many nephrologists accept pigment casts as a pathognomonic sign of ATN.

Blood chemistry. It is important to obtain laboratory information to monitor the evolution of the renal situation and the effects of therapy. Serum BUN, uric acid, and creatinine are useful for evaluating the renal ability to excrete nitrogen products. Of particular importance is the plasma BUN/creatinine ratio. In prerenal disease there is significant urea reabsorption, increasing the BUN/creatinine ratio to 20:1 or more. Potassium should be measured frequently because elevations of this ion are common in the course of acute renal failure and may reach a point at which hemodialysis becomes mandatory. The serum sodium concentration should be measured, especially in patients who have received diuretics and crystalloid solutions.

Management. The initial treatment of prerenal disease and ATN is similar. The majority of pregnant patients in acute renal failure have prerenal disease, and their oliguria will reverse with adequate management. There are certain steps that should be taken to reestablish the urine flow. These are discussed below.

Intravascular volume expansion. Packed red cells, fresh frozen plasma, salt-poor albumin, low–molecular-weight dextran, cryoprecipitate, and crystalloid solutions may be used to treat intravascular volume deficits depending on the nature of the primary problem and the presence of complications. For example, in cases of abruptio placentae it is necessary to expand volume and improve oxygen-carrying capacity, and the agent of choice is packed red cells. Cryoprecipitate and fresh frozen plasma are used if there is a deficit in coagulation factors. In patients with preeclampsia and low serum albumin concentration, the agents of choice for volume expansion are crystalloid solutions and salt-poor albumin. The administration of hypertonic solutions (7.5% NaCl) may be lifesaving for patients in profound shock.[17]

Intravascular volume expansion should be monitored by frequent CVP measurements. The CVP reflects right atrial filling pressure and indicates the capacity of the right heart to accept a fluid load. The CVP should remain between 10 and 15 cm H_2O during treatment, and any elevation above 15 cm H_2O should be followed by a decrease in the rate of fluid administration.

In most patients intravascular volume expansion may be achieved by administering 500 to 1000 ml of normal saline solution over 30 to 60 minutes. This should cause a modest elevation of the CVP and result in increased urine production. Some people prefer to use a *synthetic extracellular fluid solution* (750 ml of 0.9% NaCl, 225 ml of 5% dextrose in water, and 25 ml of a solution of sodium bicarbonate containing 3.75 g/50 ml) for the fluid challenge. After the fluid challenge, administration of isotonic NaCl should be continued at 125 to 200 ml/hr. The treatment goals are to maintain a normal CVP and a urinary output above 30 ml/hr. Unfortunately, the response to a fluid challenge usually is transient and is necessary to increase the administration of intravenous fluids. In patients with severe preeclampsia, this may result in pulmonary edema. These patients have increased capillary permeability and low colloid osmotic pressure, and the intravenous fluids move rapidly from the intravascular into the interstitial

space. When the difference between the plasma colloid osmotic pressure (usually 21 to 25 mm Hg) and the pulmonary wedge pressure (usually 6 to 10 mm Hg) is reduced to less than 3 mm Hg, pulmonary edema may occur.

Delivery. The development of oliguria-anuria in an obstetric patient is, in the majority of cases, an indication for delivery. Delivery is beneficial for the infant, who is removed from a progressively hostile environment, and also has advantages for the mother. Patients who have had oliguria or anuria for several hours before delivery often begin to produce copious amounts of urine after delivery. This raises the possibility that compression of the ureters was present. However, in the majority of cases the diuresis that follows delivery is a consequence of better renal perfusion resulting from redistribution of the cardiac output. Approximately 25% of the cardiac output in pregnant patients is destined to fulfill the needs of the placental circulation. This need disappears abruptly after delivery, which is followed by a redistribution of the cardiac output and increased blood flow to the kidneys. Another advantage of delivery is that it is possible to use large doses of diuretics and perform diagnostic procedures using x-ray and radioactive isotopes without fear of causing harm to the fetus.

It is important to caution against the systematic use of delivery in the treatment of mild or moderate preeclamptic patients with oliguria. These patients are frequently delivered because of a "drop in urine output." However, in many cases the diagnosis of oliguria is questionable, and the condition is not adequately evaluated and treated. Delivery is indicated when the urine output is less than 20 ml/hr for 2 or more hours despite adequate volume expansion, after treatment with furosemide, and when vaginal delivery is not expected within 2 to 4 hours. To proceed to cesarean section because of a low urinary output without attempting to understand and treat the cause of the problem is not advisable.

Diuretics. Two groups of pregnant patients in acute renal failure should be given diuretics: (1) patients in prerenal failure who fail to respond to an intravenous fluid challenge because of *third spacing* formation and (2) patients in early stages of ATN.

Third space formation caused by increased capillary permeability and decreased plasma colloid oncotic pressure occurs frequently in patients with preeclampsia and in those who have sustained a large blood loss without adequate replacement. In these patients the renal tubules respond inadequately to volume expansion, and it is necessary to force diuresis with small doses of furosemide. Diuresis, in turn, will promote fluid mobilization from the interstitial into the intravascular space.

Whether ATN can be prevented or ameliorated with high doses of furosemide is a controversial issue.[18,19] Some argue that patients who respond to this treatment have mild forms of ATN and may have done well without furosemide. Some believe that obstetric patients with oliguria unresponsive to volume expansion should receive furosemide because this drug has relatively few severe side effects and may help to reestablish normal renal function or produce a milder type of ATN. Starting with 40 mg IV is preferred. If there is no response in 30 minutes, the dose is increased to 100 mg. If there is no diuresis, 300 mg is administered 30 minutes later. If the 300-mg dose does not induce diuresis, the patient is considered to be in ATN and managed accordingly.

Dialysis. After the diagnosis of ATN is established (0.5 mg/dl or greater elevation of plasma creatinine, U/P osmolality ratio near 1.0, urinary sodium more than 40 mEq/L, elevated CVP, lack of response to furosemide), the role of the obstetrician is to expedite delivery, to restrict the fluid intake to an amount equal to the urine output plus the insensible losses, and to refer the patient to a place with adequate facilities for hemodialysis. Dialysis is indicated in patients who develop cardiovascular overload during the oliguric phase of ATN, hyperkalemia that could not be controlled with the use of potassium exchange resins, pericarditis, uremic encephalopathy, electrolyte imbalances, or metabolic acidosis. However, in recent years obstetric patients with ATN are being dialyzed before the development of these complications.

The most common indication for dialysis in patients with obstetric renal failure is fluid overload. For this reason fluid restriction is mandatory as soon as the diagnosis of ATN is established. It is difficult to maintain an adequate caloric intake with severe fluid restriction. One of the advantages of prophylactic dialysis is that it allows a more liberal fluid intake and makes it easier to adjust the diet to an optimal caloric and protein intake.

Prognosis. The majority of obstetric patients with ATN recover without sequelae. Most exhibit normal creatinine clearances and blood chemistries 6 to 12 months later.

Renal cortical necrosis. This severe form of acute renal failure is usually associated with catastrophic obstetric complications such as severe hypovolemia caused by abruptio placentae or placenta previa or vascular collapse in patients with severe preeclampsia. Histologically, this condition is characterized by necrosis of all the elements of the renal cortex including extensive necrosis and thrombosis of the renal vessels.

Clinically, renal cortical necrosis is characterized by the sudden onset of severe oliguria or anuria in a patient with life-threatening complications of pregnancy. The urine is frankly hematuric, and the urinary red cells are dysmorphic and hypochromic, with the appearance of collapsed empty sacs. Hematologic abnormalities characteristic of disseminated intravascular coagulation may be present. The BUN and plasma creatinine increase rapidly.

On many occasions it is difficult to differentiate renal cortical necrosis from ATN. However, the evolution of these conditions is different, and prolonged oliguria and anuria with little or no improvement of renal function characterize renal cortical necrosis.

The prognosis for patients with renal cortical necrosis is poor. The majority do not recover or have only partial recovery of renal function and require chronic dialysis.

Acute renal failure caused by obstructive uropathy. There are a few reported cases of severe oliguria caused by obstructive uropathy during pregnancy. Obstructive uropathy usually results from ureteral compression at the level of the pelvic brim by an overdistended uterus.[20,21] This is more likely to occur in twin pregnancies and in patients with severe polyhydramnios.

In obstructive uropathy, complete anuria is a frequent finding, whereas in prerenal and renal oliguria, urine production rarely ceases completely. Therefore the possibility of obstructive uropathy should be considered when complete anuria develops in a patient with an overdistended uterus. In these cases termination of pregnancy is followed by profuse diuresis.

Nephrotic syndrome

A nephrotic syndrome is characterized by the presence of proteinuria greater than 3 g/day, serum albumin less than 3 g/dl, edema, and hypercholesterolemia. This complication occurs approximately once every 1500 pregnancies.[22]

Etiology and diagnosis. The etiology of nephrotic syndrome during pregnancy is varied. The most common causes are:

1. Preeclampsia and eclampsia
2. Lupus nephritis
3. Diabetic nephropathy
4. Chronic and acute renal diseases

The most important sign in the differential diagnosis among these conditions is hypertension. Although all of them may produce elevation of blood pressure, the presence of hypertension strongly suggests preeclampsia. If the patient is not hypertensive, preeclampsia may be ruled out, and a search for other diseases should be initiated.

The second most valuable element in the differential diagnosis of nephrotic syndrome during pregnancy is examination of the urine sediment. The presence of red cells and red cell casts is diagnostic of acute glomerulonephritis. A benign sediment with large, coarse granular casts is the usual finding in preeclampsia. The presence of lipid droplets, cellular casts, and birefringent lipids points to chronic renal disease.

Other laboratory tests useful in the differential diagnosis of nephrotic syndrome are the ANA titer, the complement panel, and the urinary protein electrophoresis. A positive ANA titer suggests systemic lupus erythematosus, and this may be confirmed by an elevated titer of anti-DNA antibodies.

The finding of alterations in the complement panel (C3, C4, and CH50) is also useful.[23] There are several renal conditions that cause a decrease in complement levels. The most common are poststreptococcal glomerulonephritis (PSGN), membranous-proliferative glomerulonephritis (MPGN), the nephritis of patients with chronic bacteremia, and lupus nephritis. PSGN is rare during pregnancy. Normal antistreptolysin (ASO) and antihyaluronidase titers are useful for ruling out this disease. MPGN, especially the variety called *dense deposit disease* or MPGN type II, characteristically depresses C3, whereas C4 remains normal. This is a disease of children and is extremely rare during pregnancy. Patients with chronic infectious processes who develop nephrotic syndrome are unusual in obstetrics. Thus

for all practical purposes, a decrease in complement levels in a pregnant patient with nephrotic syndrome indicates the presence of lupus nephritis.[24]

The diagnosis of lupus nephritis during pregnancy is difficult to make, and it is frequently confused with preeclampsia. In lupus nephritis the ANA titer is positive; the CH50, C3, and C4 values are below normal limits; and frequently there are signs of extrarenal disease such as hemolytic anemia, thrombocytopenia, or cutaneous alterations. There are five different histologic types of lupus nephritis, but most cases of severe nephrotic syndrome correspond to the membranous variety.

Urinary protein electrophoresis is another test of value in the analysis of pregnant patients with nephrotic syndrome.[25] With this method it is possible to determine the predominant molecular size of the urine proteins, which in turn is an index of glomerular permeability. This is done by comparing the clearance of IgG, with a molecular weight of 160,000, to the clearance of transferrin, with a molecular weight of 88,000. The ratio of gamma globulin, formed mainly by immunoglobulins with molecular weights greater than 150,000, to albumin, with a molecular weight of 69,000 serves the same purpose. A gamma globulin/albumin ratio of 0.1 or less indicates a selective proteinuria. If the proteinuria is not selective and a large amount of gamma globulin is lost in the urine, the ratio will be greater than 0.1. High selectivity suggests that the patient will benefit from glucocorticoid therapy.

The preferential excretion of small-molecular-weight proteins is characteristic of minimal change disease, although it also occurs in a few cases of membranous glomerulonephritis, focal glomerulosclerosis, and MPGN. The proteinuria that occurs in cases of multiple myeloma and acute leukemia or when there is a defect in tubular reabsorption of amino acids (Fanconi's syndrome) is also selective but rarely is large enough to fulfill the definition of nephrotic syndrome. Thus for practical purposes, the finding of a selective proteinuria in a pregnant patient with nephrotic syndrome is strongly suggestive of the presence of minimal change disease. Minimal change disease is the most common cause (95%) of nephrotic syndrome in children, but its prevalence decreases during adulthood, being the cause of only 10% of the cases observed af-

---

BOX 14-1

Differential Diagnoses of Nephrotic Syndrome during Pregnancy

1. *Preeclampsia:* Elevated blood pressure, negative ANA titer, normal complement, nonselective proteinuria, benign urinary sediment
2. *Lupus nephritis:* Positive ANA titer, positive DNA antibodies, low complement, nephritic sediment
3. *Diabetic nephropathy:* History of insulin-dependent diabetes of long duration
4. *Acute glomerulonephritis* (usually IgA nephropathy, minimal change disease, or focal glomerulonephritis): Negative ANA titer, inflammatory urinary sediment with red cell casts

---

ter age 40. In contrast, membranous glomerulonephritis is unusual in children but is the underlying problem in about 50% of the cases of nephrotic syndrome occurring after 30 years of age.

Renal biopsy is occasionally necessary for diagnosis of patients with nephrotic syndrome.[26] Although the complications of this procedure are few in experienced hands,[26] it is more difficult to perform during pregnancy, and when it is absolutely necessary, it is better to postpone it until the postpartum period.

Figure 14-1 is a summary of the diagnostic steps to be followed in the study of patients with nephrotic syndrome during pregnancy. Box 14-1 is a summary of the differential diagnoses among the four most common causes.

Management. In the majority of pregnant patients, the cause of nephrotic syndrome is preeclampsia, and the most important part of their treatment is delivery. Patients with lupus nephritis or minimal change disease should be treated with prednisone, 60 to 100 mg/day, and delivered if there is no rapid improvement. When the cause of the nephrotic syndrome is unknown, treatment should be symptomatic.

Diet. These patients need a diet rich in high-quality protein and poor in cholesterol and saturated fats. Sodium intake should be restricted before the development of edema.

Anticoagulation. Patients with nephrotic syndrome have a tendency to develop renal vein thrombosis. This tendency is aggravated by pregnancy and by hypoalbuminemia. Heparin, 5000 U subcutaneously every 12 hours, should be used and continued during the postpartum period.

Diuretics. These patients usually become edematous early in the course of their disease, but they should not be treated with diuretics unless they are uncomfortable and do not respond to dietary salt restriction, decreased physical activity, and periods of rest in the lateral supine position. If a diuretic is required, furosemide is the agent of choice.

Albumin. The administration of albumin to patients with nephrotic syndrome is controversial. However, if edema progresses to a state of anasarca and plasma albumin concentration is 2 g or below, salt-poor albumin may be indicated.

Glucocorticoids. Glucocorticoids are indicated when lupus erythematosus or minimal change disease is the cause of the nephrotic syndrome.

Prophylactic antibiotics. Pregnant patients with nephrotic syndrome are at high risk for the development of urinary tract infections. For this reason they should receive prophylactic antibiotic treatment. Preferred treatments are 500 mg ampicillin, 500 mg cephalosporin, or 200 mg nitrofurantoin taken at bedtime.

Follow-up. Pregnant patients with nephrotic syndrome frequently develop superimposed preeclampsia. They should check their blood pressure at home. If hypertension develops, they should be admitted to the hospital, and the majority will require delivery.

These patients should be weighed daily. Their renal function should be monitored periodically by measuring their BUN, creatinine, and uric acid. They often develop anemia unresponsive to iron therapy because of urinary losses of transferrin. They should be transfused if their hematocrit drops below 25%.

Fetal monitoring. The fetuses of these patients are at risk for growth retardation, preterm delivery, and antepartum fetal distress. These complications usually occur when the maternal condition worsens. The complication having the largest impact on the fetal outcome is maternal hypertension. If this occurs, the patient's management will depend on the severity of the hypertension. As a general rule, if the mother remains stable, the risk of fetal complications is small. The best methods for assessing the fetal status are serial ultrasound examinations to fol-

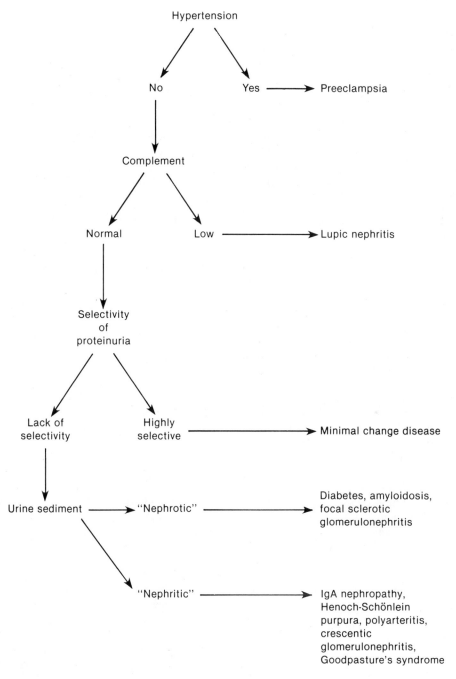

FIGURE 14-1 ▨ Differential diagnosis of the cause of nephrotic syndrome during pregnancy.

low fetal growth and weekly nonstress tests (NSTs) and fluid volume evaluation.

Acute glomerulonephritis

Acute glomerulonephritis (AGN) occurs rarely during pregnancy and is frequently confused with preeclampsia or with idiopathic nephrotic syndrome. The diagnosis of AGN should be considered in patients who develop proteinuria without hypertension and have inflammatory urinary sediment containing red cell casts. Patients with AGN during pregnancy, especially those with highly selective proteinuria, should be treated with prednisone, 60 to 100 mg daily.

Hemolytic-uremic syndrome

Hemolytic-uremic syndrome (HUS) is a condition characterized by the sudden onset and rapid progression of hemolytic anemia, thrombocytopenia, and renal failure, usually occurring in the postpartum period.[27] In a majority of cases hypertension is present. The onset of symptoms is usually preceded by a flulike syndrome. The disease may occur at any time from 1 day to 10 weeks after delivery. The predominant opinion is that HUS is a disease of unknown origin, independent of pregnancy, and closely related to thrombotic thrombocytopenic purpura.

The essential anatomic feature in HUS is damage to the glomerular capillaries by subendothelial deposits of fibrin. These deposits reduce the vascular lumen and cause parenchymal changes. Formation of microthrombi, especially in the afferent arterioles, is another feature contributing to tissue ischemia. Erythrocytes and platelets are fragmented during their passage through the affected vessels causing microangiopathic hemolytic anemia and thrombocytopenia.

The most important differential diagnosis in patients with HUS is preeclampsia with HELLP (Hemolytic anemia, Elevated Liver enzymes, Low Platelet count) syndrome. The best criteria to use to avoid confusing the two conditions are:

1. Patients with HUS should not have signs or symptoms of preeclampsia before delivery, at the time of delivery, or in the immediate postpartum period.
2. The diagnosis of HUS is more likely if there is a symptom-free period of several days after delivery.

The differentiation between preeclampsia and HUS is important from a prognostic viewpoint,

since recovery is the rule in preeclampsia and death or chronic renal insufficiency are the usual courses for postpartum HUS. The differential diagnosis is also important for management because plasmapheresis and heparin are indicated in HUS and may not be needed in the HELLP syndrome.

There is evidence indicating that plasmapheresis improves the outcome of patients with HUS.[28] Also, most survivors reported in the literature have been treated with heparin. Antihypertensive drugs, anticonvulsants, antiplatelet medications, and dietary management are also important in the management of this almost uniformly fatal disease.

■ PREGNANCY IN PATIENTS WITH KNOWN RENAL DISEASE

When a pregnant patient known to have renal disease arrives in the obstetrician's office, three main questions arise:

1. What are the fetal and maternal prognoses?
2. What are the possible complications and risks?
3. What are the basic principles of the patient's management?

The correct answers to these questions depend on the nature and severity of the underlying renal disease, but some general answers are valid. For instance, the general concept that maternal and fetal prognoses are directly related to the presence of hypertension and the severity of the renal condition applies irrespective of the type of renal disease affecting the individual patient. It is also generally accepted that the most common maternal and fetal complications in these patients are superimposed preeclampsia, deterioration of renal function, fetal growth retardation, and preterm birth.

Maternal and fetal prognoses

One important concern for the pregnant woman with renal disease is whether pregnancy will accelerate the progression of her condition. Most reports on this subject involve patients with moderate or mild renal insufficiency because when renal function is severely impaired pregnancy rarely occurs. Katz et al.[29] analyzed 121 pregnancies in 89 patients with renal disease, 26 with chronic diffuse glomerulonephritis, 12 with focal glomerulonephritis, 7 with membranous glomerulonephritis, and 21 with interstitial nephritis. Renal function declined in 16% of these pregnancies, most often in patients with chronic diffuse glomerulonephritis. Increased proteinuria occurred in 47% of these patients and in 39 pregnancies was greater than 3 g/24 hr. They concluded that in patients with normal or only mildly impaired renal function, pregnancy does not accelerate renal damage. This conclusion has been supported by two recent studies. One retrospective study of 72 patients with chronic renal disease found that approximately 15% of them had worsening of renal function during pregnancy and less than one third recovered renal function to levels similar to those existing before pregnancy.[30] A similar proportion of pregnant patients with renal disease had deterioration of renal function in another study in Dallas.[31]

Hou et al.[32] gathered data from 25 pregnancies in 23 patients with moderate renal insufficiency as defined by a serum creatinine of 1.4 mg/dl or greater before pregnancy. In 14 women renal function was stable or declined at a degree consistent with the natural history of their disease, but in 7 women they found a decrease in renal function greater than expected from the natural history of their disease. This indicates that when renal insufficiency is moderate, a significant number of patients will have a decline in renal function.

The fetal prognosis for women with chronic renal disease is favorable as long as they do not develop superimposed preeclampsia early in pregnancy and their renal function is not severely affected. In the Katz et al. series,[29] fetal survival was 94%. However, 24% were growth retarded and 20% were preterm. Patients with advanced degrees of renal insufficiency have a more obscure prognosis, and their fetal survival rate is only about 50%.

The most reliable prognostic indicator of the outcome of pregnancy is the presence of hypertension. It is exceptional for patients with diastolic blood pressure of 100 mm Hg or more, despite treatment, to undergo pregnancy without having serious complications.[33] Patients who are normotensive have better prognoses. Even patients with creatinine clearance between 20 and 30 ml/min and serum creatinine between 2.5 and 3.5 mg/dl may have a good outcome as long as hypertension is not a part of their disease.

Second to hypertension, the most valuable prognostic index for patients with chronic renal disease during pregnancy is the degree of renal functional impairment. Patients with creatinine clearances under 30 ml/min, and especially under 20 ml/min, have poor prognoses. The prognosis for such a patient is better if the creatinine clearance is between 50 and 70 ml/min. Patients usually have good prognoses if their serum creatinine concentrations are 1.4 mg/dl or less, but the prognoses become guarded for patients with values above that level.[32]

Another important prognostic sign is the presence or absence of proteinuria. As a general rule, if the patient has 2+ or more in qualitative tests or 3 g or more in 24-hour urine collections at the beginning of pregnancy, the tendency will be toward increased protein losses and development of nephrotic syndrome. Patients without proteinuria at the beginning of pregnancy have better prognoses.

The histologic characteristics of the renal lesion also have prognostic value. Patients with diffuse glomerulonephritis,[29] membranoproliferative glomerulonephritis,[34] and focal glomerulosclerosis[35] frequently have poor outcomes. Patients with IgA nephropathy usually have a good prognosis, but some investigators have reported frequent and serious complications such as 30% incidence of fetal death, 22% incidence of prematurity, and 26% incidence of declining renal function during pregnancy.[36,37] Patients with diffuse mesenchymal changes and superimposed focal proliferation have much worse prognoses than patients with other histologic features.[38]

Complications

Hypertension. The development of severe hypertension is the most common and serious complication for patients with renal disease during pregnancy. The prognosis is worse when hypertension occurs before 28 weeks of gestation and is resistant to conventional treatment. Hypertension is the most important reason for the perinatal mortality and the preterm delivery associated with renal disease during pregnancy.[39] Maternal mortality may occur because of intracranial bleeding, abruptio placentae, or renal shutdown. Fetal mortality may occur because of decreased placental blood flow, abruptio placentae, or intrapartum hypoxia.

Fetal growth retardation. Infants born to patients with renal disease often show weight, length, and head circumference that are well below average for their gestational ages. This inadequate development occurs more often and is more severe in patients with high blood pressure. However, intrauterine growth retardation also occurs in normotensive patients.

Fetal growth retardation occurs in approximately 10% of normotensive and 35% of hypertensive patients with chronic renal disease. The diagnosis is almost certain when, in addition to a fetal weight less than expected, the ultrasound examination shows abnormal head/abdomen and femur/abdomen ratios (see Chapter 16).

Preterm birth. There are two main reasons for the high incidence of preterm birth in patients with renal disease. In about half of the cases, it results from necessary medical intervention because of maternal or fetal problems. In the other half of the cases, preterm birth is the consequence of preterm labor, usually resulting from placental vascular insufficiency.

Fetal distress. Antepartum and intrapartum fetal distress occur frequently in pregnancies complicated by intrauterine growth retardation. All patients with renal disease should have weekly NST and fluid volume estimations starting as early as 26 weeks if their renal function is severely impaired. These fetuses may not tolerate the stress of labor.

Management

General measures. Interruption of work is necessary for patients when complications develop and also necessary for patients who are symptomatic from the beginning of pregnancy. In all cases, physical activity should be moderate, and periods of bed rest in the lateral supine position are beneficial. The diet should be rich in high-quality protein. Sodium intake may require adjustments if the patient is hypertensive and does not respond adequately to therapy or if there is excessive accumulation of sodium and water.

Antihypertensive treatment. If the patient is hypertensive at the beginning of pregnancy, a serious effort should be made to reduce her blood pressure to a normal range with medications. Methyldopa, hydralazine, labetalol, and calcium channel blockers should be used, and diuretics should be added if necessary. If the blood pressure cannot be maintained within a normal range with these drugs, the prognosis is poor, and the possibility of complications is high.

Monitoring renal function. The functional status of the kidneys should be monitored by making determinations of serum creatinine every 4 to 6 weeks and by making daily qualitative determinations of urinary protein. At the beginning of the prenatal care, a creatinine clearance determination is of value, but for subsequent checkups, measurements of serum creatinine are adequate. Any elevation of serum creatinine of 0.2 mg/dl or greater requires evaluation with a creatinine clearance. The patient should be instructed to check for albuminuria in the first urine voided every morning and to call the obstetrician if significant changes are apparent. It is unnecessary to order periodic 24-hour urine collections for quantitative protein determinations unless there is significant proteinuria demonstrated with Albustix strips.

Excessive retention of sodium and water with marked peripheral edema is a frequent problem in the pregnant patient with renal disease. If this occurs, the patient should be certain that she is taking a low-sodium diet, decreasing work time, avoiding prolonged periods of standing up or sitting, and increasing her daily rest time in the lateral supine position. If these measures are not successful and the patient becomes uncomfortable with her edema, diuretics may be used. The degree of intravascular volume constriction caused by the diuretic should be monitored with serial hematocrit values.

If the patient has nephrotic syndrome, she should be managed as described earlier. These patients may need intravenous albumin to partially compensate for urinary losses, to mobilize fluid out of the interstitial space, and to maintain the integrity of the intravascular volume.

Fetal evaluation. Fetal growth should be monitored with serial ultrasound examinations. The first ultrasound should be performed at 16 to 18 weeks, with follow-up examinations every 4 weeks thereafter. Any deviation from normal is significant and requires initiation of additional fetal surveillance.

Delivery. The renal patient who remains stable during pregnancy may go to term and develop spontaneous labor. If the patient is unstable or symptomatic, delivery should be performed as soon as fetal pulmonary maturity is reached. If the mother becomes severely ill, immediate delivery is indicated without fetal lung maturity evaluation.

Chronic pyelonephritis

Chronic pyelonephritis, also called reflux nephropathy, is a condition characterized by severe scarring of the kidneys resulting from persistent or recurrent infections that occur most commonly in patients with vesicoureteral reflux. These patients may have flare-ups of renal infection during pregnancy. They should have antibiotic prophylaxis with ampicillin 500 mg, nitrofurantoin 200 mg, or cephalosporin 500 mg every night for the duration of pregnancy.

Hyponatremia may occur in pregnant patients with chronic pyelonephritis when they receive diuretics because these agents may intensify their sodium-losing tendency. They also frequently exhibit glycosuria in the presence of normal blood sugar levels.

Pregnant patients with renal transplants

Most patients with renal transplants tolerate pregnancy well if their kidney function is adequate and if hypertension is not present.[40] Most of these patients are taking azathioprine and prednisone when they become pregnant, and they should continue taking these agents during gestation. So far, no congenital malformations have been reported as a consequence of the use of these medications. Recently cyclosporin has become the most commonly used immunosuppressive agent in renal transplantation. The effects of this agent on the fetus are unknown at this time. Patients taking cyclosporin may be switched to azathioprine during pregnancy.

The most common problems for these patients are preterm labor, preeclampsia, and preterm delivery. Rejection episodes during pregnancy are rare and difficult to diagnose. Delivery should be accomplished without delay if the patient develops preterm rupture of the membranes because of the risk of infection. Vaginal delivery is the route of choice.

Pregnant patients in chronic dialysis

Patients in chronic dialysis occasionally become pregnant. Also, renal failure may occur during gestation requiring the use of dialysis. Both hemodialysis and peritoneal dialysis have been used successfully in these cases.[41] The majority of patients can continue their pregnancies until the baby reaches a gestational age with adequate chances of survival outside the uterus. Complications, mainly preterm labor, hypertension, hypotension, hypoglycemia, vaginal bleeding, fetal growth retardation, and placental separation, are common.

◪ IMPORTANT POINTS ◪

1. The most important changes that occur in the kidneys during pregnancy are dilation of the collecting system, increase in renal plasma flow and glomerular filtration rate, and changes in the tubular reabsorption of glucose, sodium, amino acids, and uric acid.

2. The average serum creatinine concentration during pregnancy is 0.6 mg/dl. The average BUN is 9 mg/dl. The average creatinine clearance is 137 ml/min.

3. *E. coli* is responsible for more than 80% of all acute upper urinary tract infections. The selectivity and virulence of *E. coli* for the urinary tract may be explained by the presence, in some strains, of fimbriae that bind to specific glycoproteins on the surface of epithelial cells.

4. Universal screening for symptomatic bacteriuria during pregnancy is not universally accepted.

5. Acute pyelonephritis during pregnancy is a serious complication. Some patients develop septic shock and pulmonary and hematologic problems.

6. Approximately 80% of all urinary stones have calcium and can be seen by x-ray examination in a flat plate of the abdomen.

7. Obstruction of the urinary tract by a stone requires cystoscopic ureteral catheterization, dislodgment of the stone, and passage of a ureteral stent. If this is not possible, percutaneous nephrostomy should be performed.

8. In the majority of cases, acute renal failure in pregnancy is the result of severe hypoperfusion caused by preeclampsia or by hypovolemia caused by abruptio placenta or placenta previa.

9. Inadequate renal perfusion results in redistribution of the blood flow with production of cortical ischemia. This causes a marked decrease in the glomerular filtration rate, concentrating ability, and urinary volume. These functional changes (prerenal disease) may progress to parenchymal damage (acute tubular necrosis).

10. Complete anuria after an ischemic insult to the kidneys suggests renal cortical necrosis.

11. The BUN/creatinine ratio and the fractional excretion of sodium are two useful tests in making the differentiation between prerenal disease and ATN.

12. The initial treatment of prerenal disease and ATN is the same and involves hemodynamic monitoring, intravascular volume expansion, furosemide, and delivery.

13. Whether ATN can be prevented or ameliorated with high doses of furosemide is a controversial issue. It is believed by some that furosemide should be given to patients with severe oliguria unresponsive to volume expansion because the potential benefit is large and the drug has relatively few severe side effects.

14. Although many of the conditions causing nephrotic syndrome during pregnancy may cause elevation of blood pressure, the presence of this sign is strongly suggestive of the possibility of preeclampsia.

15. The finding of a decrease in complement levels in patients with nephrotic syndrome during pregnancy is strongly suggestive of the possibility of lupus nephropathy.

16. Most studies indicate that pregnancy does not accelerate renal damage in patients with renal disease and normal or only mildly impaired kidney function. However, complications will frequently occur if the patient has preeclampsia, proteinuria, or elevated serum creatinine.

17. The fetal prognosis for women with chronic renal disease is favorable if they do not develop superimposed preeclampsia before 28 weeks of gestation and if their renal function is not severely affected. Patients with advanced renal insufficiency have a more guarded fetal prognosis.

REFERENCES

1. Rasmussen E, Nielsen FR: Hydronephrosis during pregnancy: A literature survey. *Eur J Obstet Gynecol Reprod Biol* 1988;27:249-259.
2. Davison JM, Dunlop W: Renal hemodynamics and tubular function in normal human pregnancy. *Kidney Int* 1980;18:152.
3. Latham RH, Stamm WE: Role of fimbriated *Escherichia coli* in urinary tract infections in adult women: Correlation with localization studies. *J Infect Dis* 1984;149:835.
4. Campbell-Brown M, McFadyen IR, Seal DV, et al: Is screening for bacteriuria in pregnancy worth while? *Br Med J* 1987;294:1579-1582.
5. Stamm WE, Counts GW, Running KR, et al: Diagnosis of coliform infection in acutely dysuric women. *N Engl J Med* 1982;307:463.
6. Gilstrap LC, Cunningham FG, Whalley PJ: Acute pyelonephritis in pregnancy: An anterospective study. *Obstet Gynecol* 1981;57:409.
7. Pearl ML, Dattel BJ: The pulse oxymeter for respiratory distress associated with pyelonephritis in pregnancy. *J Rep Med* 1990;35:724-726.
8. Dunlow S, Duff P: Prevalence of antibiotic-resistant uropathogensin obstetric patients with acute pyelonephritis. *Obstet Gynecol* 1990;76:241-244.
9. Lattanzi DR, Cook WA: Urinary calculi in pregnancy. *Obstet Gynecol* 1980;56:462-466.
10. Loughlin KR, Bailey RB: Internal ureteral stents for conservative management of ureteral calculi during pregnancy. *N Engl J Med* 1986;315:1647-1649.
11. Rodriguez PN, Klein AS: Management of urolithiasis during pregnancy. *Surg Gynecol Obstet* 1988;166:103.
12. Hendricks SK, Ross SO, Krieger J: An algorithm for diagnosis and therapy of management and complications of urolithiasis during pregnancy. *Surg Gynecol Obstet* 1991;172:49-54.
13. Grunfeld JP, Pertuiset N: Acute renal failure in pregnancy: 1987. *Am J Kidney Dis* 1987;9:359-362.
14. Pertuiset N, Grunfeld JP: Acute renal failure in pregnancy. *Baillieres Clin Obstet Gynecol* 1987;1:873-890.
15. Hollenberger NK, Epstein M, Rosen SM, et al: Acute oliguric renal failure in man: Evidence for preferential renal cortical ischemia. *Medicine* 1968;47:455-470.
16. Espinel CH: The FE_{Na} test. *JAMA* 1976;236:579-581.
17. DeFelippe J, Timoner J, Valasco IT, et al: Treatment of refractory hypovolemic shock by 7.5% sodium chloride injections. *Lancet* 1980;2:1002-1004.
18. Epstein M, Schneider NS, Befeler B: Effect of intrarenal furosemide on renal function and intrarenal hemodynamics in acute renal failure. *Am J Med* 1975;58:510-516.
19. Fries D, Pozet D, Dubois N, et al: The use of large doses of furosemide in acute renal failure. *Postgrad Med J* 1971;47(suppl):18.
20. O'Shaughnessy R, Weprin SA, Zuspan FP: Obstructive renal failure by an overdistended pregnant uterus. *Obstet Gynecol* 1980;55:247-249.
21. Homans DC, Blake GD, Harrington JT, et al: Acute renal failure caused by ureteral obstruction by a gravid uterus. *JAMA* 1981;246:1230-1231.
22. Weisman SA, Simon NM, Herdson PB, et al: Nephrotic syndrome in pregnancy. *Am J Obstet Gynecol* 1973;117:867-883.
23. West CD, McAdams AJ, McConville JM, et al: Hypocomplementemic and normo-complementemic persistent (chronic) glomerulonephritis; Clinical and pathologic characteristics. *J Pediatr* 1965;67:1089.
24. Buyon JP, Cronstein BN, Morris M, et al: Serum complement values (C3 and C4) to differentiate between systemic lupus activity and preeclampsia. *Am J Med* 1986;81:194-200.
25. Boyer M: Selectivity of proteinuria. *Major Probl Clin Pediatr* 1974;11:432.
26. Packham D, Fairley KF: Renal biopsy: Indications and complications in pregnancy. *Br J Obstet Gynaecol* 1987;94:935-939.
27. Robson JS, Martin AM, Ruckley VA, et al: Irreversible postpartum renal failure. *Q J Med* 1968;37:423.

28. Bell WR, Braine HG, Ness PM, et al: Improved survival in thrombotic thrombocytopenic purpura-hemolytic uremic syndrome. *N Engl J Med* 1991;325:398-403.
29. Katz AI, Davison JN, Hayslett JP, et al: Pregnancy in women with renal disease. *Kidney Int* 1980;18:192-206.
30. Abe S, Amagasaki Y, Konishi K, et al: The influence of antecedent renal disease on pregnancy. *Am J Obstet Gynecol* 1985;153:508-514.
31. Cunningham FG, Cox SM, Hartstad TW, et al: Chronic renal disease and pregnancy outcome. *Am J Obstet Gynecol* 1990;163:453-459.
32. Hou SH, Grossman SD, Madias NE: Pregnancy in women with renal disease and moderate renal insufficiency. *Am J Med* 1985;78:185-194.
33. Felding CP: Obstetric aspects in women with histories of renal disease. *Acta Obstet Gynecol Scand* 1969;48:1-43.
34. Leichter HE, Jordan SC, Cohen AH, et al: Postpartum renal failure in patients with membranoproliferative glomerulonephritis type II. *Am J Nephrol* 1986;6:382-385.
35. Barcelo P, Lopez-Lillo J, Cabero L, et al: Successful pregnancy in primary glomerular disease. *Kidney Int* 1986; 30:914-919.
36. Packham D, Whitworth JA, Fairley KF, et al: Histologic features of IgA glomerulonephritis as predictors of pregnancy outcome. *Clin Nephrol* 1988;30:22-26.
37. Kincaid-Smith PS, Whitworth JA, Fairley KF: Mesangial IgA nephropathy in pregnancy. *Clin Exp Hypertens* 1980;821-838.
38. Packham DK, North RA, Fairley KF, et al: IgA glomerulonephritis and pregnancy. *Clin Nephrol* 1988;30:15-21.
39. Felding CF: The obstetric prognosis in chronic renal disease. *Acta Obstet Gynecol Scand* 1968;47:166-172.
40. Hous S: Pregnancy in organ transplant recipients. *Med Clin North Am* 1989;73:667-683.
41. Yasin SY, Beydun SN: Hemodialysis in pregnancy. *Obstet Gynecol Surv* 1988;43:655-667.

15

DIABETES AND PREGNANCY

Abnormalities of carbohydrate metabolism occur frequently during pregnancy, and between 1% and 3% of all pregnant patients will show glucose intolerance. The largest number of these patients is comprised of individuals with genetic or metabolic predisposition toward diabetes and who are incapable of compensating adequately for the diabetogenic effects of pregnancy, that is, patients with gestational diabetes. A smaller group is formed by women who had diabetes diagnosed before they became pregnant.

◪ CARBOHYDRATE METABOLISM DURING PREGNANCY

The most important reason that pregnancy uncovers the diabetic tendencies of asymptomatic women is the progressive increase in insulin resistance that occurs during gestation. Other reasons for the diabetogenic tendency of pregnancy are the increased lipolysis and the alterations in gluconeogenesis that normally occur (Box 15-1).

During pregnancy a given dose of insulin has a greater hypoglycemic effect when administered in the first trimester than in the last. This diminished effectiveness stems mainly from the antagonistic effect of placental human chorionic somatomammotropin. Insulin destruction by the kidney and placental insulinases, as well as the

antiinsulin effects of other hormones (cortisol, estriol, progesterone) produced in large amounts during pregnancy, contribute to insulin resistance.

As a result of the physiologic changes of pregnancy, the normal fasting blood sugar is 65 ± 9 mg/dl. The mean nonfasting blood sugar level is 80 ± 10 mg/dl. Postprandial elevations normally never exceed 140 mg/dl.[1]

BOX 15-1

Diabetogenic Effects of Pregnancy

Insulin resistance

Production of placental somatomammotropin
Increased production of cortisol, estriol, and progesterone
Increased insulin destruction by kidney and placenta

Increased lipolysis

The mother uses fat for her caloric needs and saves glucose for fetal needs

Changes in gluconeogenesis

The fetus uses preferentially alanine and other amino acids and deprives the mother of a major gluconeogenic source

---

◪ EFFECTS OF DIABETES ON PREGNANCY

The great majority of women with carbohydrate intolerance during pregnancy do not have signs or symptoms. Unfortunately, carbohydrate intolerance during pregnancy causes significant increases in fetal and maternal morbidity.

The maternal consequences of abnormal carbohydrate metabolism during pregnancy are important (Box 15-2). These women have a greater incidence of preeclampsia, infection, postpartum bleeding, and cesarean deliveries.[2] The incidence of preeclampsia is approximately 15%, and it is associated with poor glycemic control and end-organ damage.[3]

The consequences to the fetus are more serious than those to the mother (Box 15-3). Among these effects, fetal macrosomia is of great interest to the obstetrician because of the difficulty in diagnosing it and the controversies surrounding its management. Fetal macrosomia is discussed extensively later in this chapter.

◪ EFFECTS OF PREGNANCY ON DIABETES

Pregnancy imposes a heavy burden on the patient who is diabetic (Box 15-4). These patients have a tendency toward metabolic instability and will need frequent monitoring, strict therapy, and a highly regulated life-style. For diabetic patients who already have organ damage, pregnancy may accelerate it and necessitate intensive testing and therapeutic procedures.

The complex interaction between abnormal carbohydrate metabolism and pregnancy should be explained to each patient immediately after the diagnosis is made, and when the patient has overt diabetes, the explanation should ideally occur before pregnancy.

◪ PRECONCEPTION COUNSELING OF THE DIABETIC PATIENT

Counseling of the diabetic patient planning pregnancy should emphasize the following points.

1. *Importance of blood glucose control.* The patient should be informed that inadequate blood sugar control often results in a higher incidence of first-trimester abortion, fetal congenital abnormalities, fetal macrosomia, polyhydramnios, and stillbirths. She should understand that the frequency of these abnormal outcomes approaches that

---

BOX 15-2

Effects of Diabetes on the Mother

Preeclampsia
Affects 10% to 25% of all pregnant diabetic patients

Infection
High incidence of chorioamnionitis and postpartum endometritis

Postpartum bleeding
High incidence caused by exaggerated uterine distention

Cesarean section
High incidence in pregnant diabetic patients

BOX 15-3

Effects of Diabetes on the Fetus

Congenital abnormalities	Hyaline membrane disease
Hypoglycemia	Hypocalcemia
Hyperviscosity syndrome	Apnea and bradycardia
Macrosomia	Traumatic delivery

BOX 15-4

Effects of Pregnancy on Diabetes

More insulin is necessary to achieve metabolic control
Progression of diabetic retinopathy
Worsening of diabetic nephropathy
Increased risk of death for patients with diabetic cardiomyopathy

---

of the nondiabetic population if the blood sugar is strictly controlled before conception and during the pregnancy. It is important to emphasize that the time of highest risk of fetal malformations is during the periconception period and the period of organogenesis and that the risk can be greatly reduced by adequate glycemic control before pregnancy and during early pregnancy.[4] The fear of anatomic deformities in the offspring is a powerful motivation for controlling blood glucose levels before conception.

2. *Importance of self-monitoring.* The next step is to emphasize that strict control is best achieved through self-monitoring of blood glucose levels. The patient should be informed that frequent measurements are critical because they allow early detection and immediate correction of abnormalities. The patient should be told that pregnancy will produce various gastrointestinal symptoms that will cause fluctuations in the ingestion of food and, therefore, cause changes in blood sugar levels. She should also understand that during pregnancy the fetus continuously obtains nutrients from the mother's bloodstream and this, combined with the other factors mentioned, produces significant changes in blood sugar levels that need to be recognized promptly to institute appropriate therapy. It should also be emphasized that frequent monitoring will decrease the probability of serious complications, such as ketoacidosis, because alterations in blood glucose levels will be detected and treated before metabolic derangement occurs.

3. *Importance of fetal surveillance during the diabetic pregnancy.* The different problems affecting the fetus and the methods of detecting them should be explained during preconception counseling. Emphasis should be placed on the problem of diabetic embryopathy and the need for determination of glycohemoglobin early in pregnancy, measurement of maternal serum alpha-fetoprotein at approximately 16 weeks of gestation, fetal anatomic survey at about 20 weeks, and fetal echocardiogram at about 24 weeks to rule out the most common fetal malformations. Fetal growth should be monitored with serial ultrasound examinations to detect macrosomia or growth retardation. Fetal well-being should be assessed during the last several weeks by using tests such as the contraction stress test (CST), the nonstress test (NST), or the modified biophysical profile (MBPP). The reasons for these tests should be carefully explained to the mother to increase her motivation and compliance.

4. *Financial cost of the diabetic pregnancy.* The prospective pregnant patient with diabetes frequently does not realize the amount of time that she will have to spend providing adequate care for her pregnancy. In many cases the patient has a demanding job that is incompatible with frequent office visits and intense perinatal testing. She may need to leave her job, adding a financial strain to those already present. Also, medical disability plans and insurance programs frequently do not cover the time loss and the expenses associated with the care of a complicated pregnancy. Patients should check with their employer and insurance companies to assure that they may take the necessary medical leave and that their expenses will be covered.

Education of the pregnant patient with newly diagnosed diabetes

Patients who develop diabetes during pregnancy usually know little about diet and blood glucose monitoring and therefore require education about these subjects. Those patients who do not respond to dietary measures and so require insulin need additional instruction about self-administration of insulin.

The pregnant patient with newly diagnosed diabetes should be counseled by a nutritionist. The nutritionist will obtain a nutritional history, and the patient will be taught about the caloric requirements of pregnancy, the caloric value of different foods, the importance of meal timing, the need for a balanced diet, and other aspects of a caloric-restricted meal plan. This knowledge will be reinforced in follow-up visits to the nutritionist. The number and frequency of visits will depend on the results of the treatment and the patient's compliance with the diet.

The obstetrician, a nurse, or a diabetes educator should inform the patient of the advantages of home glucose monitoring. The patient should learn the approximate values above or below which she should call the physician for further instructions. Then she should learn the procedure for self-monitoring her blood sugars, with emphasis on the details so she will obtain consistent and reliable results. The patient should perform the procedure several times under observation so she can develop the proper technique.

The patient in need of insulin treatment should be taught about the different types of insulin available, emphasizing those that she is going to receive. The onset, the peak, and the duration of action of regular and slow-release insulin are concepts that the patient should firmly grasp. The concentration of insulin in units per milliliter and the measurement of a given number of units in insulin syringes are also important points of the instruction. The patient should then be taught to inject herself using an aseptic technique and to alternate the sites of injection. Using sterile distilled water, the patient should practice injecting an orange. The instructor should use this opportunity to correct mistakes and improve her technique. Ideally, the patient will be supervised the first few times to assure that she does not make any serious errors.

The patients must be able to recognize and treat hypoglycemic reactions. They should be instructed to carry sugar or candy with them to be ingested if hypoglycemia develops when other carbohydrates are not immediately available. Also, the patient and her husband should be instructed in the administration of glucagon in case of severe hypoglycemic reactions.

◤ DIAGNOSIS

The vast majority of pregnant women with diabetes have gestational diabetes defined as carbohydrate intolerance of varied severity with onset or first recognition during the present pregnancy. Unfortunately, this condition has no reliable signs or symptoms and can be diagnosed only through the use of laboratory tests.

Screening for diabetes during pregnancy

An area of controversy is whether screening for diabetes during pregnancy should be routine or whether it should be limited to patients at risk for diabetes during pregnancy (Box 15-5). There is substantial evidence in the medical literature indicating that screening should be universal. One study found that if only high-risk patients are screened, approximately 35% of gestational diabetes patients will not be discovered.[5]

The best screening test for gestational diabetes is the measurement of plasma glucose 1 hour after ingesting 50 g of glucose.[6] It is not necessary to follow any special diet before the test. If the plasma glucose 1 hour after the load is greater than 140 mg/dl (135 mg/dl if the patient has been fasting overnight), the patient may have gestational diabetes and requires further testing. If the plasma glucose is below 140 mg/dl, the patient is not at risk. The 50-g oral glucose screening test has excellent sensitivity and specificity.

BOX 15-5

Risk Factors Requiring Diabetic Screening

1. Obesity (>200 pounds or >15% of nonpregnant ideal body weight)
2. Positive family history of diabetes (sibling or parent)
3. History of stillbirth
4. History of delivery or a large infant (>4000 g)
5. Glycosuria
6. History of unexplained neonatal death
7. History of congenital anomaly
8. History of prematurity
9. History of preeclampsia as a multipara
10. Polyhydramnios
11. History of traumatic delivery with associated neurologic disorder in the infant
12. Poor reproductive history (>3 spontaneous abortions in the first or second trimester)
13. Chronic hypertension
14. Recurrent severe moniliasis
15. Recurrent urinary tract infections
16. Age >30 years
17. History of diabetes in a previous pregnancy

Plasma glucose values should not be substituted with capillary reflectance meter glucose values.[7]

The best time to screen is between 24 and 30 weeks of gestation. Patients at high risk may have the test earlier (18 to 22 weeks), but if it is negative, they should have the test repeated between 26 and 30 weeks.

Patients with an abnormal screening test should be given a 3-hour glucose tolerance test (GTT). Patients whose 1-hour screening test produced plasma glucose values larger than 200 mg/dl should have a fasting glucose measurement. Any patient whose fasting glucose is frankly abnormal, 120 mg/dl or greater, is diabetic and does not need a 3-hour GTT.

Glucose tolerance test (3 hours)

To prepare for the 3-hour GTT, patients should be instructed to consume daily diets containing approximately 200 g of carbohydrate for at least 3 days before the test. This will minimize false-positive results.

Normal values for the 3-hour GTT are shown in Box 15-6. If two or more of these values are abnormal, the patient has gestational diabetes. If

---

BOX 15-6

Upper Limits of Normal for the 3-Hour Glucose Tolerance Test during Pregnancy*

Fasting	96 mg/dl	(5.3 nmol/L)
One hour	172 mg/dl	(9.6 nmol/L)
Two hours	156 mg/dl	(8.49 nmol/L)
Three hours	131 mg/dl	(7.31 nmol/L)

*Venous plasma glucose (capillary blood measurements are approximately 15% lower).

---

only one value is abnormal, the patient cannot be diagnosed as having gestational diabetes, although she is at risk for complications,[8] such as macrosomia (18.0%) and preeclampsia-eclampsia (7.9%). Patients with no abnormal values in their 3-hour GTT have a risk for these complications of 6.6% and 3.3% respectively. Even those patients with a normal 3-hour GTT after an abnormal screening test are at risk for macrosomia when compared with patients who have a normal screening value.[9-11] These findings suggest that minimal alterations in maternal carbohydrate metabolism may have a significant impact on the fetus and that patients with minimal alterations also require strict glycemic control to decrease the frequency of abnormal outcomes.[12]

Renal glycosuria

Some patients have a normal GTT but show significant glycosuria during the test. The presence of glucose in the urine when the blood glucose level is within normal limits is called *renal glycosuria* and is thought to be the result of a low threshold for the elimination of glucose by the kidneys. Renal glycosuria occurs frequently during pregnancy. In fact, the average renal threshold for glucose is 155 ± 17 mg/dl during pregnancy, compared with 197 ± 6.5 mg/dl in the nonpregnant patient. During pregnancy, glycosuria can occur at blood sugar levels as low as 70 to 100 mg/dl. Women with renal glycosuria during pregnancy are at high risk for preterm delivery and for fetal macrosomia.[13]

Most pregnant patients with renal glycosuria have normal kidneys, and the abnormality disappears after delivery. In some cases, however, renal glycosuria during pregnancy is a manifestation of renal tubular damage caused by chronic

pyelonephritis. Such patients frequently develop recurrent urinary tract infections and have asymptomatic bacteriuria.

Management of renal glycosuria consists of (1) performing frequent urine testing to detect asymptomatic bacteriuria, (2) instructing the patient to have several small meals per day, rather than three large meals, to avoid postprandial elevations in the blood sugar and glycosuria, and (3) staying alert for early signs and symptoms of preterm labor.

Patients with renal glycosuria may lose as much as 100 g/day of glucose in the urine. Such large losses leave less glucose for their caloric needs, and their lipolysis is activated to a maximum. Unfortunately, this causes production of ketones and a tendency towards ketoacidosis (starvation ketosis). Therefore it is not surprising that these patients gain little weight during pregnancy and require dietary counseling to compensate for their abnormal metabolic situation.

◪ CLASSIFICATION

After diagnosis diabetic patients should be classified to indicate the severity of their condition and the prognosis of the pregnancy. One system is that proposed by the National Diabetes Data Group (Box 15-7). Type I corresponds to the old juvenile-onset diabetes (JOD) and type II, or non-insulin-dependent diabetes, corresponds to the old adult-onset diabetes (AOD). This system is inadequate during pregnancy because it lacks further categorization according to the stability of the disease and to the presence or absence of target organ damage. These criteria are important in determining a prognosis for the pregnancy.

The classification system most commonly used is that of Priscilla White (Box 15-8). This system[14] separates patients into groups according to the age of onset and the years of duration of the disease and the presence or absence of micro- and macrovascular changes. White's classification has been valuable because it has established a basis of comparison among different institutions for the management of pregnant diabetic patients. Unfortunately, White's classification system is not ideal. The number of groups is large, and patients in the same group may have completely different prognoses. For example, some patients in class C may be metabolically stable and have predictable insulin needs during pregnancy and excellent outcomes, whereas other patients in

---

BOX 15-7

National Diabetes Data Group Classification of Diabetes

New name	*Old name*
Type I (IDDM): Insulin-dependent diabetes mellitus	Juvenile diabetes Juvenile-onset diabetes Ketosis-prone diabetes Brittle diabetes
Type II (NIDM): Non-insulin-dependent diabetes mellitus	Adult-onset diabetes Maturity-onset diabetes Ketosis-resistant diabetes Stable diabetes Maturity-onset diabetes of youth
Type III (GCI): Gestational carbohydrate intolerance Nonobese Obese	Gestational diabetes

From National Diabetes Data Group: Classification and diagnosis of diabetes mellitus and other categories of glucose intolerance. *Diabetes* 1979;28:1039.

BOX 15-8

White's Classification of Diabetes during Pregnancy

Gestational diabetes: Discovered during pregnancy; glycemia may or may not be maintained by diet alone and insulin may be required

Class A: Discovered before pregnancy; controlled with diet alone; any duration or age of onset

Class B: Onset 20 yr or older or duration less than 10 yr

Class C: Onset age 10-19 yr or duration 10-19 yr

Class D: Onset age under 10 yr; duration over 20 yr; background retinopathy

Class R: Proliferative retinopathy or vitreous hemorrhage

Class F: Nephropathy with over 500 mg/day proteinuria

Class RF: Criteria for both classes R and F coexist

Class H: Arteriosclerotic heart disease clinically evident

Class T: Prior renal transplantation

From Hare JW, White P: Gestational diabetes and the White classification. *Diabetes Care* 1980;3:394.

BOX 15-9

Classification of Pregnant Patients with Diabetes

1. Gestational diabetes, non-insulin-dependent
   a. Low-risk
   b. High-risk
2. Insulin-dependent diabetes without end-organ damage
   a. Stable
   b. Unstable
3. Insulin-dependent diabetes with end-organ damage

---

the same group may be unstable, prone to ketosis, and have a high probability for a poor outcome. Thus the most serious defect of White's classification system is the failure to recognize that metabolic instability is the principal prognostic factor in the insulin-dependent diabetic pregnant patient. Because of its poor predictive value, White's classification is being replaced by other systems.

Another system used to classify pregnant patients with diabetes is shown in Box 15-9. The first group has gestational diabetes. These women can obtain adequate metabolic control with diet alone. Patients with gestational diabetes who require insulin for adequate control are reclassified and managed as are those who have insulin-dependent diabetes. The largest number of pregnant women with diabetes that the obstetrician sees have gestational diabetes. This is not a homogeneous group but can be subdivided depending on the presence of certain high-risk factors.

The second group in this classification is patients with insulin-dependent diabetes and no end-organ damage. This group includes patients in White's classes B and C, and some in class D. Also included in this group are patients with gestational diabetes who require insulin. These patients are subdivided into two subgroups according to the stability of their diabetes. Patients having had several episodes of ketoacidosis in the 2 years preceding pregnancy, wide variations in blood sugar values, frequent severe hypoglycemic reactions, the need for more than two injections of insulin per day, or problems with noncompliance form the unstable group. They are difficult to manage, require frequent admissions to the hospital, and are at high risk for fetal complications. Most of these unstable patients are type I, or have JOD. Patients who have metabolically stable insulin-dependent diabetes without end-organ damage are usually obese, and many are type II or have AOD. In these patients the fundamental disorder is insulin resistance, but in type I patients the problem is insufficient insulin. Stable patients tend not to develop diabetic ketoacidosis or severe hypoglycemic reactions. They follow a predictable course of increasing insulin requirements with the progression of pregnancy. The prognosis for these patients is usually good, and their main complication is fetal macrosomia.

The third group of pregnant diabetic patients is formed by those who are insulin-dependent and have end-organ damage. They correspond to classes F, R, RF, H, and T and some class D patients in White's classification. In these patients the severity and the duration of their disease has caused alterations in the microvasculature leading to organ damage. For the majority of these patients, the prognosis of the pregnancy is guarded. In addition to multiple fetal problems, these mothers may suffer further organ deterioration resulting from the effects of pregnancy and delivery.

■ GESTATIONAL DIABETES

Patients with gestational diabetes are a heterogeneous group of patients whose disease onset or first recognition occurs during the present pregnancy. Some of these patients may have type II diabetes that was asymptomatic before pregnancy, some others may have preclinical type I or type II diabetes that became apparent under the metabolic demands of pregnancy, and a few may have type I or type II diabetes and had the onset of their disease coincident with pregnancy. Gestational diabetes affects 1% to 2% of all pregnancies. In most of these patients, it is mild and can be adequately controlled with diet alone, but a minority of these patients will require insulin.

The effect of gestational diabetes on the mother is small. The most common problems are an increased incidence of preeclampsia, about twice that found in the control population, pyelonephritis, and polyhydramnios.[15] Also, the incidence of cesarean section in this group of patients is higher than in a nondiabetic population.

The effects on the fetus are more frequent and of more concern. The most common complication is macrosomia, which may affect up to 40% of the babies whose mothers have gestational diabetes. Fetal macrosomia, defined as a birth weight greater than or equal to 4000 g is associated with a high incidence of fetal trauma during delivery,[16,17] and there are indications that fetal macrosomia may be a precursor of obesity during extrauterine life. Also, infants of mothers with gestational diabetes frequently develop problems in the neonatal period. The most common of these are hyperbilirubinemia, hypoglycemia, hypocalcemia, and hyperviscosity syndrome. Finally, the incidence of fetal death and stillbirths is higher in gestational diabetic mothers than in nondiabetic populations.

As mentioned before, some gestational diabetic patients are at higher risk for complications (Box 15-10). These patients should be identified soon after the diagnosis is made because they need antepartum fetal surveillance testing and they may require delivery before their estimated date of delivery (EDD).

Nutritional management of the gestational diabetic patient

The initial management of the gestational diabetic patient consists of dietary regulation. To determine the number of calories that the pa-

---

BOX 15-10

Indicators of High-Risk Gestational Diabetes

History of stillbirth
History of neonatal death
History of fetal macrosomia
Concomitant obesity and/or hypertension
Development of oligohydramnios, polyhydramnios preeclampsia, or fetal macrosomia
Inadequate metabolic control with diet alone

TABLE 15-1 ▨ Ideal body weight and recommended caloric intake during pregnancy

Height (without shoes)	Nonpregnant ideal body weight (kilograms)	Recommended caloric intake (35 kcal/kg)
4'10"	48.6	1701
4'11"	50.0	1750
5'0"	51.4	1799
5'1"	52.7	1845
5'2"	54.1	1894
5'3"	55.9	1957
5'4"	58.2	2037
5'5"	60.0	2100
5'6"	61.8	2163
5'7"	63.6	2226
5'8"	65.7	2300
5'9"	67.3	2356
5'10"	69.1	2419

Data from Metropolitan Life Insurance tables.

tient should have in her diet, it is necessary to know her ideal body weight in kilograms (Table 15-1). The number of calories required to maintain 1 kg of body weight (usually 35 calories) is multiplied by the ideal body weight in kilograms to obtain the total calories that the patient should consume during a 24-hour period. Some individuals add 300 calories to cover the additional needs of the pregnancy. This is not absolutely necessary, and it should be limited to the third trimester, when the caloric needs are increased.

The daily caloric allowance should be distributed among the different food groups in such a way that 50% to 60% of the calories come from complex carbohydrates. Also, to avoid wide variations in blood sugar levels, the total caloric intake is split into three meals and three snacks or into three meals and a bedtime snack. The patient should then be referred to the nutritionist for a more detailed explanation of the dietary plan.

Some patients find that the amount of food provided by their new diet exceeds what they were ingesting before its institution. Usually these are obese patients who had been on restricted diets before pregnancy. In these cases, the caloric intake can be reduced to between 25 and 30 kcal/kg of ideal weight until the patient feels comfortable with the diet. When this restriction is made, the patient should have daily checks for acetone in the urine. If she starts to consistently show marked acetonuria (>3+ in qualitative examinations), she should increase her caloric intake. If the ketonuria disappears only when the caloric intake is increased to a point that precipitates postprandial hyperglycemia, the patient will need insulin therapy.

There is controversy about how much weight should be gained during a gestational diabetes pregnancy. The classic teaching is that the patient should gain approximately 25 lb and should not persistently spill large amounts of acetone in the urine. More recent information[18,19] indicates that obese diabetic patients may not gain weight and may even lose some weight during pregnancy without adverse consequences. In fact, gestational diabetic patients who are truly compliant with their diets should gain less than 15 lb or have no weight gain during their pregnancies. Continuous weight gain in these patients means that they are eating more than their allowance or that they are retaining large amounts of water. Also, elimination of small or moderate amounts of acetone in the urine is not necessarily a poor prognostic sign. Usually, it suggests that they are using their own fat rather than dietary carbohydrates for their caloric needs. Dietary intervention is more effective in preventing fetal macrosomia if the mother is maintained just above the ketonuric threshold.[20]

The patient with gestational diabetes should be instructed in blood sugar self-determination using a Glucometer. She should measure her fasting blood sugar and 2-hour postprandials. The objective of the dietary treatment is to maintain the fasting value under 105 mg/dl and the 2-hour postprandials under 120 mg/dl. Others use as the goal of treatment a 1-hour postprandial under 140 mg/dl. If these objectives are not met within 2 weeks of the institution of dietary regulation, the patient needs insulin therapy.

Insulin therapy

The dose and administration of insulin depends on the severity and characteristics of the metabolic problems. If there is persistent elevation in fasting blood sugar levels, treatment should start with a small amount (5 to 10 U) of intermediate-acting NPH (isophane suspension) insulin at bedtime, and this should be modified according to the patient's response to therapy. If the problem is persistent elevation of postprandial values, treatment may be started with a relatively small dose (10 to 15 U) of NPH insulin before breakfast, or a mixture of NPH and regular insulin (15 U NPH + 5 U regular) before breakfast or a small dose of regular insulin (10 U) before the meal causing the postprandial elevation. Control of postprandial blood sugars seems to be fundamental in the prevention of fetal macrosomia.[21] The amount and type of insulin, the number of doses, and the timing of administration will vary according to the patient's response to the treatment. The majority of patients with insulin-dependent gestational diabetes have predictable responses to insulin therapy, and the dosage adjustments are easy to perform. These patients do not have tendencies toward ketoacidosis or hypoglycemic crises, and side effects of the medication are rare. Human insulin is the drug of choice for initial treatment.

Oral hypoglycemic agents should not be used in pregnant patients. These agents may induce severe, prolonged fetal hyperinsulinemia and neonatal hypoglycemia. Also, they may aggravate neonatal hyperbilirubinemia by competing for albumin binding sites.

Management of the low-risk gestational diabetic patient

Low-risk gestational diabetic patients who achieve adequate control with diet and do not develop macrosomia, polyhydramnios, or preeclampsia do not require antepartum fetal surveillance testing before 40 weeks of gestation. In fact, the risk of fetal distress in these patients is as low as in nondiabetic patients, and they can

be monitored with kick counts and with vibroacoustic stimulation at each office visit.

There is no reason to deliver low-risk gestational diabetic patients before term. They may be allowed to develop spontaneous labor and to deliver at term. Once the uncomplicated gestational diabetic patient reaches 40 weeks, one must evaluate cervical ripeness, the amount of amniotic fluid, fetal size, and fetal well-being. If these are normal, the pregnancy may continue for 1 more week. However, these patients should be delivered once they reach 41 weeks of gestation.

Management of the high-risk gestational diabetic patient

High-risk gestational diabetic patients, as well as low-risk patients who develop problems during pregnancy, should have antepartum fetal surveillance testing starting at approximately 34 weeks of gestation. There is controversy over which test is the best for monitoring these patients. Weekly or twice per week nonstress test (NST) is most popular. However, the biophysical profile (BPP), the modified biophysical profile (MBPP), and the contraction stress test (CST) are also used. Some prefer to use weekly CSTs because it is believed that late decelerations (the end point of the CST) appear in the hypoxic fetus before changes in reactivity (the end point of the NST,) or decreased fetal movements (the end point of the BPP). Thus the CST should provide earlier warning of the presence of fetal distress. Patients with contraindications to the CST are managed with weekly MBPP.

The high-risk gestational diabetic patient should be delivered at term (38 to 40 weeks). One exception is the patient with a macrosomic fetus. When this is apparent clinically and by ultrasound examination, labor should be induced as soon as the cervix is ripe and fetal lung maturity is attained. Unfortunately, the cervix of these patients is often unripe, and induction of labor is unsuccessful. Therefore if the cervix is unripe, it is best to wait because vaginal delivery will be more likely when spontaneous labor develops, even if the baby has gained additional weight.

Insulin-dependent gestational diabetic patients do not need their daily dose of insulin if they develop spontaneous labor, are being induced, or are being delivered by cesarean section. The blood sugar should be measured every

4 hours during labor, and deviations from normal should be corrected as needed.

Long-term prognosis

Gestational diabetes may recur in a future pregnancy. In fact, approximately 55% of patients, usually obese patients and those with prior macrosomic infants, will show glucose intolerance in a subsequent pregnancy.[22]

It is important to repeat the glucose tolerance test after delivery in gestational diabetic women who had elevated fasting serum glucose levels during pregnancy or who were diagnosed with gestational diabetes before 24 weeks of gestation. In these patients the incidence of diabetes mellitus is between 9% and 44%.[23] Other gestational diabetic patients should occasionally measure their fasting and postprandial blood sugars during the first 6 weeks postpartum to be certain that the abnormality has disappeared. In the majority of cases, the need for a restricted diet or for insulin disappears after delivery.

Gestational diabetic patients should be informed that they are at high risk for developing type II diabetes later in their lives. Roughly 40% to 60% will develop overt diabetes when they are in their fifth decade. Obviously, weight loss, dietary control, and exercise will help prevent overt diabetes later in life.[24]

◾ MANAGEMENT ASPECTS COMMON TO ALL INSULIN-DEPENDENT DIABETIC PATIENTS

The incidence of insulin-dependent diabetes in a given obstetric population is 1 in 200 to 1 in 1000. Most of these patients have their diabetes diagnosed preconceptionally and are able to self-administer insulin and to properly use a Glucometer. The majority are compliant, measure their blood sugars frequently, and follow their diets. However, a few of these diabetic patients do not take their condition seriously and are more difficult to manage. Repeated efforts are required to improve their education and their motivation so that they will meet the multiple demands of their pregnancies. The most common problems found with these patients are reluctance to follow restricted diets and failure to measure their blood sugars frequently.

The care of all insulin-dependent diabetic patients during pregnancy has the following objectives:

1. Detection of diabetic embryopathy
2. Strict control of blood sugar levels
3. Detection of fetal macrosomia
4. Detection of fetal distress and prevention of antepartum death
5. Decision about timing of delivery
6. Decision about cesarean section vs. vaginal delivery
7. Adequate intrapartum and postpartum management

Detection of diabetic embryopathy

With current care, perinatal mortality of the insulin-dependent diabetic patient has been drastically reduced. The main contributor to perinatal mortality and morbidity in these patients is congenital malformations of the fetus (Box 15-11). The most frequent abnormalities involve the heart and the central nervous system.[25] Most common are anencephaly, spina bifida, transposition of the great vessels, and ventricular septal defects. The lesion most associated with diabetic embryopathy, the *caudal regression syndrome*, is actually less common, with an incidence of 1.3 per 1000 diabetic pregnancies.

BOX 15-11

Most Common Anomalies in Infants of Diabetic Mothers

Central nervous system
Anencephaly
Holoprosencephaly
Encephalocele

Heart and great vessels
Transposition of the great vessels
Ventricular septal defect
Aortic coarctation
Atrial septal defect

Skeletal and spinal
Caudal regression syndrome

Genitourinary
Renal agenesis
Ureteral duplication

Gastrointestinal
Anal atresia

Efforts to detect diabetic embryopathy should start soon after conception by measuring the patient's glycosylated hemoglobin or hemoglobin A_{1c}.[26] This hemoglobin fraction is glycosylated in a nonenzymatic reaction that is directly dependent on the concentration of sugar in the bloodstream. If this test is performed 4 to 6 weeks after conception, it will reflect the levels of blood sugar that the patient had in the periconception period. There is good evidence indicating that levels of hemoglobin A_{1c} greater than 8.5% are associated with a 20% to 25% probability of fetal developmental abnormalities. When the concentration of glycosylated hemoglobin is normal, the probability of major malformations is less than 2%.

Women at high risk for congenital malformations of the fetus, as indicated by their hemoglobin A_{1c}, should have ultrasound examination with vaginal probe at 8 to 10 weeks. Some defects such as anencephaly and holoprosencephaly can be detected very early using this technique. Also, blighted ova will be easily detected at this time.

The search for diabetic embryopathy should also include measurements of maternal serum alpha-fetoprotein (MSAFP) at 16 weeks. Normally, MSAFP is lower in diabetic patients, and the necessary corrections should be made by the laboratory. An abnormal MSAFP often indicates the need for follow-up with genetic amniocentesis, as explained in Chapter 2.

At 18 to 20 weeks of gestation, a detailed anatomic survey of the fetus, level II examination using high-resolution ultrasound, should be performed. This will permit the detection of major malformations not seen on earlier ultrasound examinations.

The final step in the search for fetal abnormalities is performing a fetal echocardiogram at 24 to 26 weeks of gestation. Unfortunately, some of the most common cardiac abnormalities associated with diabetes (i.e., transposition of the great vessels and aortic coarctation) are difficult to detect and require considerable performer expertise.

Strict control of blood glucose levels

A fundamental objective of the care of every pregnant patient with insulin-dependent diabetes is strict control of the blood sugar. To monitor whether the patient is achieving this objective, the patient should measure fasting and 2-hour postprandial levels daily. The concentration of glucose in the blood is determined visually (Visidex strips) or by using a machine (e.g., Glucometer, Accu-Chek, Glucoscan, One-Touch). The values obtained should be recorded with the time at which each measurement is made and the time of food ingestion. The patient should bring this information to each prenatal visit so the obstetrician may change the patient's regimen as needed.

The most common cause of elevations in the blood sugar above the established limits (105 mg/dl fasting, 140 mg/dl 1 hour after meals, or 120 mg/dl 2 hours after meals) is dietary indiscretion. The first question for the obstetrician to ask when there are unexpected wide variations in blood sugar values is whether there have been changes in the amounts or in the quality of the food intake. Diabetic patients need to be questioned frequently about this and need reassurance about the importance of measuring the amount of food they eat and avoiding eating anything outside of their meal plan. Some patients with long-standing diabetes falsely believe that they can calculate the weight or size of a given portion of food without the use of a scale or a measuring tape. They need continuous reinforcement about the need to measure their food accurately. Other diabetic patients do not follow dietary instructions because they have grown up with the idea that they can eat anything they want to eat and that the resulting blood sugar variations can be corrected by adjustments in their insulin dose. These patients should be given frequent and detailed explanations concerning the need to follow a different, more restricted meal plan during pregnancy to avoid wide fluctuations in their blood sugars and thereby avoid the resulting effects such fluctuations would have on the fetus.

A frequent problem affecting blood sugar control is variable timing of meals and insulin injections. Some patients follow an erratic schedule and constantly change the intervals between meals and insulin injections, thus making adequate control extremely difficult. They should be instructed that during pregnancy they should follow a more organized schedule resulting in a more predictable response to treatment and facilitating tight glucose control.

The effect of subcutaneous injection of regular insulin starts after 15 minutes, peaks at 4 hours, and has a duration of 6 to 8 hours. The

TABLE 15-2 ◪ Pharmacokinetics of insulin preparations given subcutaneously

Type of insulin	Beginning of action (hours)	Peak of action (hours)	Duration of effect (hours)
Regular	¼	4 to 6	6 to 8
NPH	3	8 to 12	18 to 24
Semilente	½	4 to 6	12 to 16
Lente	3	8 to 12	18 to 28

effect of subcutaneous NPH insulin begins 3 hours after injection, peaks 8 to 12 hours later, and lasts a total of 18 to 24 hours (Table 15-2).

No regimen for insulin administration is applicable to all diabetic pregnant patients. Many of them can achieve control with two doses of a combination of short- and intermediate-acting insulin. Some patients require three or more daily doses.

In general, the morning dose of regular insulin is determined by the glucose level 2 hours after breakfast or immediately before lunch. The evening dose of regular insulin is determined by the glucose level following the evening meal and the blood sugar at bedtime. The morning dose of NPH is reflected in the blood sugar after lunch and before supper, and the evening NPH dose is reflected by the fasting blood sugar and the presence or absence of nocturnal hypoglycemia.

There is no place for the use of "sliding scales" based on blood sugar concentrations in pregnant women with diabetes. To allow these patients to change insulin dosages based solely on blood sugar values is potentially dangerous. Before an insulin dose is changed, it is necessary to take into consideration other factors such as size and time of the last meal, direction of the plasma glucose change, time of the last dose of insulin, type of insulin used in the last dose, time of the day or night the blood value was obtained, and patient's prior experience under similar conditions.

Detection of fetal macrosomia

Since fetal macrosomia is the most frequent fetal complication of pregnant diabetic patients, a particular effort should be directed toward its diagnosis and management. Thus, unless the pa-

tient is not obese and periodic fundal measurements are normal, all pregnant diabetic patients should have ultrasound examinations of the fetus every 4 weeks, starting at 20 weeks of gestation, to monitor the fetal growth. The macrosomic fetus at some time will be above the 95th percentile for one or more variables, most frequently the abdominal circumference. By the end of the pregnancy, clinical estimation and sonographic evaluation usually concur in the diagnosis of large fetal size.

The positive predictive value for the detection of macrosomia exceeds 90% when the abdominal circumference or the estimated fetal weight is above the 95th percentile.[27] However, there is a significant margin of error, and the baby's birth weight may differ from the ultrasonic estimation of fetal weight by as much as 25%.[28] This translates into a maximum error of as much as 1000 g if the estimated fetal weight is 4000 g.

The management of macrosomia is controversial. Most authorities agree that primary cesarean section is justified if the estimated fetal weight at the end of the pregnancy is 4500 g or more. The controversy arises when the estimated fetal weight is between 4000 and 4500 g. Some investigators argue that in the macrosomic fetus, the shoulder and trunk fat pads are relatively larger than the head. This would favor shoulder dystocia at the time of birth. For this reason, these authorities advise cesarean delivery for infants of diabetic mothers if the infant's estimated weight is greater than 4000 g.[29] Others believe that the margin of error of sonographic weight estimates in patients at term and the relatively small number of fetal injuries, approximately 1 in 500 deliveries, when the fetus is between 4000 and 4500 g do not justify cesarean delivery.

If the baby is between 4000 and 4500 g, with good arguments in favor of both vaginal delivery and cesarean section, flexibility in the management of these patients is best. Ideally, they should develop spontaneous labor and deliver vaginally. However, any abnormality of labor such as protracted active phase or protracted descent, failure to descend, or secondary arrest of cervical dilation indicates the need for cesarean section delivery. No vacuum or forceps should be used in these patients. Persistent occiput posterior presentations that do not rotate spontaneously should be delivered by cesarean section. Finally, the obstetrician should be prepared for the possibility of shoulder dystocia and should be versed in the maneuvers necessary to relieve it. (For management of shoulder dystocia see Chapter 8.) Also, if the estimated fetal weight is closer to 4500 than to 4000 g, it is, perhaps, better to proceed to a primary cesarean delivery.

Another problem related to fetal macrosomia is the induction of labor 2 or 3 weeks before the EDD. The rationale of this management is to avoid cesarean section that may be necessary if the baby remains *in utero* and continues to grow for 2 or 3 more weeks. There are two conditions that are indispensable for this approach to be successful. First, it is necessary to have evidence of adequate fetal lung maturity if induction of labor is performed before 39 weeks of gestation. Second, the patient must have a ripe cervix with a Bishop's score of 6 or more because otherwise she will likely deliver by cesarean section. If the cervix is unfavorable, it is best to wait for it to ripen or for spontaneous labor to develop. The chance for vaginal delivery of a large baby after spontaneous labor is better than that after an induction if the cervix is unripe.

Prevention of fetal distress and antepartum death

There is universal agreement that insulin-dependent diabetic patients need some method of fetal surveillance during the last 6 to 10 weeks of pregnancy. However, the best test to use and when to start the testing are preferential points. Some investigators prefer weekly oxytocin challenge tests (OCTs); others prefer twice per week NSTs or weekly BPPs. Weekly OCTs are preferred because this test offers earlier indications of fetal compromise.

Initiation of antepartum surveillance depends on the severity and stability of the maternal diabetes. Mothers with brittle diabetes, those who require more than 100 U of insulin per day, or those with growth-retarded fetuses should have fetal surveillance as early as 28 weeks. Stable, type II insulin-dependent diabetic mothers may start fetal surveillance as late as 34 weeks.

Timing of pregnancy termination

There is no need to terminate the pregnancy before term in stable insulin-dependent diabetic patients. However, once these patients reach their EDD, they should be delivered. This will avoid adding the potential fetal complications resulting from prolongation of pregnancy to the potential fetal complications of diabetes.[30]

The unstable insulin-dependent diabetic patient should be managed differently. These patients are better served by delivering them as soon as fetal lung maturity, lecithin to sphingomyelin (L/S) ratio greater than 2.4 and phosphatidylglycerol (PG) positive, is attained. Fetal and maternal complications in the unstable patient are high, and there is no advantage of further pregnancy prolongation once the fetus's lungs are mature.

Mode of delivery

It is not necessary to deliver all insulin-dependent diabetic patients by cesarean section. Although there are multiple indications for operative delivery of these patients, more than 50% of them can be safely delivered vaginally.

Intrapartum and postpartum management

Insulin requirements of insulin-dependent diabetic patients during labor and delivery are low. They should be told to eat their usual evening meal and bedtime snack the evening before induction or cesarean delivery. They should also have their usual evening insulin dose. Their regular morning dose of insulin will not be given the day of induction or cesarean delivery. Instead, a continuous infusion of insulin, 50 U in 500 ml of lactated Ringer's solution is started at 6:00 AM at 0.5 U of insulin per hour. This dosage is adjusted according to the patient's blood sugar values, measured hourly. This insulin infusion is discontinued soon after delivery.

Postpartum there is a sudden loss of insulin resistance, and the majority of patients do not require insulin for 24 to 48 hours. Once a patient shows fasting or postprandial elevations of her blood sugar, insulin therapy should be restarted, using one half to two thirds of the dosage that the patient was receiving *before* pregnancy. Naturally, this is adjusted according to the patient's response.

◪ MANAGEMENT OF UNSTABLE INSULIN-DEPENDENT DIABETIC PATIENTS

The care of unstable insulin-dependent diabetic patients presents a significant challenge to the obstetrician because these patients are difficult to control, require frequent office visits and frequent telephone communication, and also require frequent hospital admissions for metabolic regulation. These patients should be under the care of a specialist in maternal-fetal medicine. "Split" management between a general obstetrician and an internist or diabetologist is an open invitation for a poor outcome. Some of the most common problems that these patients develop are:

1. Somogyi phenomenon
2. Dawn phenomenon
3. Hypoglycemic episodes
4. Changes in peak of action and duration of insulin action
5. Problems peculiar to patients on continuous infusion pumps

Somogyi phenomenon

Somogyi phenomenon[31] should be suspected in patients who have high fasting blood sugars and also complain of sleep disturbances such as nightmares or nocturnal sweating. Nocturnal hypoglycemia followed by an exaggerated counterregulatory response produces the elevated fasting blood sugar. Documenting hypoglycemia between 1:00 AM and 5:00 AM cinches the diagnosis. The treatment is to decrease, rather than increase, the amount of long-acting or intermediate-acting insulin that the patient takes before supper or at bedtime.

Dawn phenomenon

Some patients have high fasting blood sugars in the absence of nocturnal hypoglycemia. This is called the *Dawn phenomenon.*[32] The mechanism responsible for this has not yet been clarified. The solution is to increase the amount of intermediate-acting insulin given before supper or to administer it at bedtime rather than before supper. However, one must avoid large changes in insulin dosage because, for a given patient, the severity of the Dawn phenomenon may be variable, and its occurrence may be irregular.

Hypoglycemic episodes

Severe hypoglycemia requiring assistance is a common emergency in unstable, insulin-dependent diabetic patients. The majority of these patients are type I, requiring relatively large amounts of insulin. Most likely the root of their problem is some degree of impairment in their counterregulatory mechanisms. It seems that patients with long-standing diabetes have an obtunded response of their counterregulatory hormones, epinephrine, growth hormone, and cortisol, to hypoglycemia. Also, it seems that when large amounts of insulin are required for metabolic control, the blood glucose threshold for the release of counterregulatory hormones is lowered. Therefore these patients may have marked hypoglycemia without eliciting a compensatory response.

An integral part in the prevention and treatment of hypoglycemic reactions is educating those living with the patient because often in such situations, the patient will be unable to respond to her own needs. The husband and/or relatives should be able to recognize the behavioral changes that accompany hypoglycemia and should know the emergency treatment of the situation.

In mild-to-moderate reactions, treatment consists of giving the patient some liquid containing carbohydrate. A glass of milk, orange juice, sugar water, or even pancake syrup dissolved in water is an effective treatment for most episodes. For severe reactions administration of glucagon is necessary. Given intramuscularly or subcutaneously, 1 mg of glucagon is sufficient if the patient is unconscious. As soon as she awakens, oral carbohydrates should be given because the effect of glucagon is transient. If the patient remains unconscious after the glucagon injection, she should be transferred immediately to an emergency room for intravenous glucose administration. Usually, 20 ml of 50% glucose is adequate to awaken the patient, but in severe cases the injection may have to be repeated. Treatment with 5% or 10% dextrose may have to be continued for several hours until the blood sugar levels remain in the normoglycemic range.

Changes in insulin pharmacokinetics

Unstable pregnant insulin-dependent diabetic patients may have marked variations in the time of onset, time of peak of action, and total duration of action of the insulin preparation they are using. This happens more frequently in patients with long-standing diabetes and may have several explanations. Two of the most likely are the development of insulin antibodies and irregular absorption from the injection site. Irrespective of the mechanism, these alterations in the pharmacokinetics of insulin complicate the management of these patients and should be suspected in long-standing diabetic patients with large fluctuations in blood sugar levels that do not respond predictably to dosage changes. In these cases it is necessary to measure the blood sugar every hour for 24-hour periods and to graphically plot the values, the time of meals, and the time of insulin administration. These 24-hour profiles will reveal that the time of peak action and the total duration of action of insulin are prolonged.

If altered insulin pharmacokinetics is diagnosed or strongly suspected, the patient must switch to human insulin if she is not taking it already. Many of these long-standing diabetics are using beef or pork insulin, and the problem is the presence of antiinsulin antibodies. If that is the case, these patients will show predictable responses to human insulin. When switching to human insulin, it is best to start patients at doses one half to two thirds of what they were previously receiving because these patients may develop hypoglycemia with equivalent doses of human insulin.

The problem of irregular absorption from the injection site is also closely related to changes in the pharmacokinetics of insulin. It is well known that absorption is more rapid when insulin is injected in extremities, where activity increases regional blood flow. A more steady rate of absorption is obtained from subcutaneous injections in the abdomen. Absorption is also erratic when the same areas are used repeatedly, and patients should be encouraged to rotate the sites of injection frequently.

Insulin pumps

Patients on continuous subcutaneous insulin infusion micropumps constitute a special group. The majority of them are deeply motivated and closely monitor their blood sugars. Most have long-standing diabetes and have a fair knowledge of their disease and the relationship of glucose levels to diet, insulin, and exercise.

The most common problem found in these patients is hypoglycemia of varied severity. Because their diabetes is long-standing, the efficacy of their counterregulatory mechanisms is limited, and they can have prolonged, severe hypoglycemia. Such episodes mandate a reduction in the preprandial boluses or in the daytime nocturnal basal rate, depending on the timing of the hypoglycemic crises. A second common problem with these patients is infection at the injection site. Emphasis on aseptic technique and frequent changing of injection site may minimize this. An exaggeration of one of the objectives of their treatment, that of the patient's independence and self-management of her disease, may also be a problem. Frequently, these patients think that physician input in their treatment is unnecessary, and they find it difficult to follow recommendations.

◢ MANAGEMENT OF INSULIN-DEPENDENT DIABETIC PATIENTS WITH END-ORGAN DAMAGE

Patients with insulin-dependent diabetes and end-organ damage are at high risk for both maternal and fetal complications. As with the unstable insulin-dependent diabetic patient, these patients should be under the care of a specialist in maternal-fetal medicine.

Twenty years ago it was believed that pregnancy was contraindicated in these patients. Therapeutic abortion or surgical sterilization was frequently advised. Today most of these patients can have a successful pregnancy. However, vascular complications will not only generate significant fetal risks but also will shorten the maternal life span.

Diabetic nephropathy

The characteristic features of patients with diabetic nephropathy are proteinuria and hypertension in the first or second trimester. These signs are usually mild in early pregnancy, but by 20 to 24 weeks of gestation, most of these patients have increases in proteinuria, blood pressure, and serum creatinine.[33] Hypertension and edema are almost always present, and by the third trimester it is difficult to determine whether the symptoms are caused solely by the diabetic nephropathy or by superimposed preeclampsia.

The main fetal disorders occurring in patients with diabetic renal disease are prematurity and fetal growth retardation. Prematurity results from preterm labor and from intentional medical intervention because of aggravation of the disease in the third trimester. The incidence of preterm delivery in these patients is approximately 45%. Fetal growth retardation affects approximately 20% of these pregnancies, and it should be diagnosed early to institute adequate fetal surveillance and to prevent fetal death.

Another concern with these patients is the potential for proliferative retinopathy. Of patients with diabetic nephropathy, 90% have retinopathy, but only 20% of them have the proliferative type. A complete ophthalmologic examination is necessary in all patients with diabetic kidney disease. Another concern is the reduced longevity for these patients once diabetic nephropathy is diagnosed. Usually, end-stage renal disease will occur within 2 to 4 years, and the best hope for survival is through renal transplantation.

Diabetic retinopathy

Diabetic retinopathy affects approximately 40% of all insulin-dependent diabetic patients. Unfortunately, pregnancy seems to accelerate the progression of diabetic retinopathy.[34] In approximately 80% of the cases, the lesion is not severe and is called *background retinopathy*. The other 20% of these patients have neovascularization along the retinal surface, and this is named *proliferative retinopathy*. The important group to identify is the latter because the new vessels are fragile and may bleed profusely with the changes in intraocular pressure that occur during labor, thereby leading to sudden vision loss. Therefore labor is contraindicated in these patients because Valsalva efforts may increase intraocular pressure causing vitreal hemorrhage and retinal detachment.

Diabetic cardiomyopathy

The maternal and fetal prognosis for patients with diabetic cardiomyopathy is very poor. Maternal and fetal mortality occur frequently.[35] These patients need to be identified early in pregnancy and will require intensive care to increase the probability of a good outcome.

◪ DIABETIC KETOACIDOSIS

Fortunately, diabetic ketoacidosis (DKA) does not occur very often in pregnant diabetic patients. This low incidence is the result of strict compliance by most of these women. Occasionally, however, the pregnant diabetic patient does develop DKA. This is a serious emergency that requires adequate treatment to save maternal and fetal lives.

DKA results from a deficit in insulin and the response to that deficit by counterregulatory hormones. As a result of decreased cellular glucose consumption and increased neoglucogenesis, the blood sugar concentration reaches high levels. This severe hyperglycemia causes osmotic diuresis with depletion of the intravascular volume and electrolyte changes. Simultaneously, an increase in lipolysis produces excessive ketone bodies that titrate the body buffers, resulting in a high anion gap and metabolic acidosis. If uncorrected, this may lead to maternal and fetal death. This emergency requires early diagnosis and aggressive treatment with identification and elimination of the precipitating event.

The diagnosis of DKA requires (1) a blood sugar concentration > 250 mg/dl; (2) ketone bodies in urine and plasma; (3) arterial pH < 7.3; and (4) serum bicarbonate < 15 mEq/L. The initial laboratory evaluation of these patients requires measurements of blood glucose, serum and urine ketones, blood gases, electrolytes, complete blood count, electrocardiogram, and chest x-ray examination. Some of these examinations should be repeated frequently to monitor the evolution of the disease.

Upon admission to the hospital, an intravenous line should be placed and hydration started with 1000 ml of normal saline in the first hour. If the patient is in shock, plasma expansion with colloid solutions may be indicated. If the serum potassium is low, 40 mEq of potassium chloride should be given intravenously during the first hour after admission. If the arterial pH is below 6.9, 88 mg of sodium bicarbonate should be given every 2 hours until the pH rises above 7.0.

Insulin therapy should be started soon after the initial laboratory evaluation. Typically, an initial intravenous bolus of 0.2 U/kg is given and followed by a continuous infusion of insulin using 0.1 U/kg/hr. With this treatment, blood glucose should decrease by 70 to 100 mg/dl per hour. If blood glucose levels do not decline by at least 30% in the first 2 to 3 hours, insulin administration should be increased to twice the initial dosage. Once the blood sugar is between 150 and 200 mg/dl, the IV fluids should be changed from normal saline to 5% dextrose in half normal saline, and the insulin dosage should be adjusted to avoid hypoglycemia. Administration of phosphate solutions to patients with DKA is no longer recommended.

A fundamental part of the treatment of DKA is the identification of the precipitating events. Frequently it is a viral or bacterial infection. In the latter case, treatment with antibiotics is necessary to adequately control the ketoacidosis.

The prognosis of DKA during pregnancy is guarded. With modern, aggressive treatment, maternal mortality is approximately 2%. The prognosis is worse if the patient has symptoms of central nervous system dysfunction or is in shock on arrival. Fetal mortality is high in all cases.

◪ PRETERM LABOR IN THE PREGNANT DIABETIC PATIENT

The use of intravenous beta-adrenergic drugs to stop preterm labor in pregnant diabetic patients is to be discouraged. These agents increase glycogenolysis and lipolysis and, consequently, also increase the tendency toward metabolic acidosis. Most diabetic patients require continuous intravenous insulin to antagonize the diabetogenic effect of the labor-inhibiting medications. The potential morbidity from the intravenous administration of beta-adrenergic agents to diabetic pregnant patients contraindicates their use.

The drug of choice for initial tocolysis in the diabetic patient is IV magnesium sulfate. Once the contractions have subsided, the patient may be maintained on calcium channel blockers. Oral terbutaline, in doses no more than 2.5 mg every 4 to 6 hours, may be used in patients who do not tolerate nifedipine. Before 32 weeks of gestation, indomethacin may also be used.

A significant number, approximately 40%, of these patients are in preterm labor as a result of intrauterine infection. Amniocentesis with Gram stain and culture of fluid should be performed in every diabetic patient who requires treatment with intravenous magnesium sulfate.

◪ PREMATURE RUPTURE OF MEMBRANES IN THE PREGNANT DIABETIC PATIENT

Every time a pregnant diabetic patient has spontaneous rupture of the membranes there is a strong possibility that infection is present. Obstetric infections occur more easily in diabetic patients, and they may be more severe than in nondiabetic patients. Thus expectant management of diabetic patients with premature rupture of membranes should be the exception rather than the rule.

◪ THE INFANT OF THE DIABETIC MOTHER

Infants of diabetic mothers (IDMs) frequently have significant problems, which are often preventable by prepartum intervention. The obstetrician caring for pregnant diabetic women should explain these problems to them as part of the preconception counseling or the pregnancy counseling.

The most common problems affecting the infant of the diabetic mother are:

1. Congenital malformations
2. Neonatal hypoglycemia
3. Neonatal hyperbilirubinemia
4. Neonatal respiratory distress syndrome
5. Hyperviscosity syndrome
6. Feeding problems

Congenital abnormalities

Congenital abnormalities were reviewed earlier in this chapter (p. 289). In summary, congenital abnormalities are the most frequent cause of neonatal mortality and morbidity in the pregnant diabetic patient. This is a problem that is potentially preventable through strict control of maternal blood sugar levels in the periconception period.

Neonatal hypoglycemia

Neonatal hypoglycemia is the problem that most frequently affects infants of diabetic mothers. In the majority of cases, neonatal hypoglycemia is caused by excessive insulin production by the newborn's pancreatic beta cells, which are enlarged and hyperactive as a result of maternal hyperglycemia. Strict regulation of blood sugars in the days before delivery may prevent this problem.

Neonatal hyperbilirubinemia

Neonatal hyperbilirubinemia is a frequent problem in the IDM, usually caused by immaturity of the infant's liver function and, specifically, by the bilirubin catabolic system, glucuronosyl transferase. Administration to the mother of medications that induce the production of the necessary enzymes for bilirubin degradation may prevent hyperbilirubinemia. Phenobarbitol offers promise in this respect, but more research is necessary before it can be adopted for routine clinical use.

Neonatal respiratory distress syndrome

Neonatal respiratory distress syndrome (RDS) caused by hyaline membrane disease has decreased significantly during the past decade. Among the most important factors responsible for this decrease are the availability of better tests to determine fetal pulmonary maturity, the availability of surfactant treatment, and the decreased frequency of diabetic patients delivering preterm. However, cases of RDS caused by pulmonary hypertension or by diabetic myocardiopathy still occur sporadically.

Hyperviscosity syndrome

Hyperviscosity is diagnosed when the neonatal hematocrit is 65% or more. Many of these infants are asymptomatic, but others have RDS, necrotizing enterocolitis, renal vein thrombosis, or cerebral infarcts. The cause of this abnormality is not completely clear, but the evidence suggests that it is caused by excessive production of erythropoietin in response to chronic fetal hypoxia. If this hypothesis is proven, the hyperviscosity syndrome may also be preventable.

Feeding problems

Poor feeding is a common problem in infants of diabetic mothers and is often associated with other neonatal complications. It is also a common reason for prolonged stays in the nursery. Prevention of this problem requires more knowledge about its cause.

◢ IMPORTANT POINTS ◣

1. There is a progressive increase in insulin resistance during pregnancy. This results from several factors, the most important being the antiinsulin effect of the placental hormones human chorionic somatomammotropin, progesterone, and estriol and the accelerated destruction of insulin by kidney and placental insulinases.

2. Pregnant diabetic women have a greater than normal incidence of preeclampsia, infection, postpartum bleeding, and cesarean delivery.

3. The risk of fetal anomalies in the pregnant diabetic patient can be greatly reduced by adequate glycemic control during the periconception period.

4. There are no reliable signs or symptoms allowing clinical identification of patients with gestational diabetes. This condition can be diagnosed only through the systematic screening of all pregnant women with a 1-hour 50-g glucose tolerance test.

5. Gestational diabetic patients truly compliant with their diets gain little or no weight during pregnancy and may show small acetonuria. Dietary intervention in these patients is more effective in preventing fetal macrosomia if the mother is maintained just above the ketonuric threshold.

6. The patient with gestational diabetes should measure her fasting blood sugar and the 2-hour postprandials. The objective of treatment is to maintain the fasting blood sugar under 105 mg/dl and the 2-hour postprandials under 120 mg/dl. Control of postprandial blood sugars is fundamental in the prevention of fetal macrosomia.

7. The high-risk gestational diabetic patient should have antepartum surveillance starting at 34 weeks of gestation and should be delivered between 38 and 40 weeks.

8. The detection of diabetic embryopathy involves determination of glycosylated hemoglobin 4 to 6 weeks after conception, measurement of MSAFP at 16 weeks, detailed fetal anatomic survey with ultrasound at 20 weeks, and fetal echocardiography at 24 weeks.

9. There is no place for the use of "sliding scales" based on blood sugar concentrations in pregnant insulin-dependent diabetic patients. Before an insulin dose is given, it is necessary to take into consideration factors such as size and time of last meal, direction of the plasma glucose change, time of the last insulin dose, type of insulin used in the last dose, time of day the blood value is obtained, level of activity, and patient's prior experience under similar blood sugar conditions.

10. Most authorities agree that primary cesarean section is justified in pregnant diabetic patients if the estimated fetal weight at term is 4500 g or more. There is controversy over the need for cesarean delivery when the estimated fetal weight is between 4000 and 4500 g.

11. Postpartum there is a sudden loss of insulin resistance, and the majority of pregnant diabetic patients do not need insulin for 24 to 48 hours.

12. The diagnosis of diabetic ketoacidosis requires (1) a plasma glucose concentration greater than 250 mg/dl; (2) ketone bodies in urine and plasma; (3) arterial pH less than 7.3; and (4) serum bicarbonate less than 15 mg/dl.

13. The drug of choice for initial tocolysis in the pregnant diabetic patient is magnesium sulfate. Once the contractions have subsided, the patient may be maintained on oral nifedipine.

REFERENCES

1. Cousins L, Rigg L, Hollingsworth D, et al: The 24-hour excursion and diurnal rhythm of glucose, insulin, and C-peptide in normal pregnancy. *Am J Obstet Gynecol* 1980;136:483.
2. Cousins L: Pregnancy complications among diabetic women: Review 1965-1985. *Obstet Gynecol Surv* 1987;42:140-148.
3. Siddigi T, Rosenn B, Mimouri F, et al: Hypertension during pregnancy in insulin-dependent diabetic women. *Obstet Gynecol* 1991;77:514-519.
4. Kitzmiller JL, Gavin LA, Gin GD, et al: Preconception care of diabetes: Glycemic control prevents congenital anomalies. *JAMA* 1991;265:731-736.
5. Coustan DR, Nelson C, Carpenter MW, et al: Maternal age and screening for gestational diabetes: A population-based study. *Obstet Gynecol* 1989;73:557.
6. O'Sullivan JB, Mahan CM, Charles D, et al: Screening criteria for high-risk gestational diabetes patients. *Am J Obstet Gynecol* 1973;116:895.
7. Dacus JV, Schulz K, Sibai BM, et al: Comparison of capillary and plasma glucose values in screening and oral glucose tolerance testing in pregnancy. *J Reprod Med* 1990;35:1150-1152.
8. Langer O, Brustman L, Anyaegbunam A, et al: The significance of one abnormal glucose tolerance test value on adverse outcome in pregnancy. *Am J Obstet Gynecol* 1987;157:758-763.
9. Leikin EL, Jenkins JH, Pomerantz GA, et al: Abnormal glucose screening tests in pregnancy: A risk factor for fetal macrosomia. *Obstet Gynecol* 1987;69:570.
10. Lindsay MK, Graves W, Klein L: The relationship of one abnormal glucose tolerance value and pregnancy complications. *Obstet Gynecol* 1989;73:103.
11. Tallarigo L, Giampetro O, Pennmo G, et al: Relation of glucose tolerance to complications of pregnancy in nondiabetic women. *N Engl J Med* 1986;315:989-992.
12. Langer O, Anyaegbunam A, Brustman L, et al: Management of women with one abnormal oral glucose tolerance test value reduces adverse outcome in pregnancy. *Am J Obstet Gynecol* 1989;161:593-599.
13. Chen WW, Sese L, Tantakesen P, et al: Pregnancy associated with renal glycosuria. *Obstet Gynecol* 1976;47:37.
14. Hare JW, White P: Gestational diabetes and the White classification. *Diabetes Care* 1980;3:394.
15. Cousins L: Pregnancy complications among diabetic women: Review 1965-1985. *Obstet Gynecol* 1980;136:483.
16. Nathanson JN: The excessively large fetus as an obstetric problem. *Am J Obstet Gynecol* 1950;60:54-63.
17. Wikstrom I, Axelsson O, Bergstrom R, et al: Traumatic injury in large-for-dates infants. *Acta Obstet Gynecol Scand* 1988;67:2959.
18. Coetz EJ, Jackson WU, Berman PA: Ketonuria in pregnancy—with special reference to calorie-restricted food intake in obese diabetics. *Diabetes* 1980;29:177.
19. Maresh M, Gillmer MDG, Beard RW, et al: The effect of diet and insulin on metabolic profiles of women with gestational diabetes mellitus. *Diabetes* 1985;34(suppl 2):88.
20. Jovanovic-Peterson L, Peterson CM: Dietary manipulation as a primary treatment strategy for pregnancies complicated by diabetes. *J Am Coll Nutr* 1990;9:320-325.
21. Jovanovic-Peterson L, Peterson CM, Reed GF, et al: Maternal postprandial glucose levels and infant birth weight: The diabetes in early pregnancy study. *Am J Obstet Gynecol* 1991;164:103-111.
22. Philipson EH, Super DM: Gestational diabetes mellitus: Does it recur in subsequent pregnancy? *Am J Obstet Gynecol* 1989;160:1324-1331.
23. Kjos SL, Buchanan TA, Greenspoon JS, et al: Gestational diabetes mellitus: The prevalence of glucose intolerance and diabetes mellitus in the first two months postpartum. *Am J Obstet Gynecol* 1990;163:93-98.
24. Grant PT, Oats JN, Beischer N: The long-term follow-up of women with gestational diabetes. *Aust NZ J Obstet Gynecol* 1986;6:17.
25. Gabbe SG: Congenital malformations in infants of diabetic mothers. *Obstet Gynecol Surv* 1977;32:125-132.
26. Reece EA, Hobbins JC: Diabetic embryopathy: Pathogenesis, prenatal diagnosis, and prevention. *Obstet Gynecol Surv* 1986;41:325-335.
27. Timor-Tritsch IE, Itskovitz J, Brandes JM: Estimation of fetal weight by real-time sonography. *Obstet Gynecol* 1981;57:653-656.
28. Benson CB, Doubilet PM, Saltzman DH: Sonographic determination of fetal weights in diabetic pregnancies. *Am J Obstet Gynecol* 1987;156:441-444.
29. Benedetti TJ, Gabbe SG: Shoulder dystocia: A complication of fetal macrosomia and prolonged second stage of labor with midpelvic delivery. *Obstet Gynecol* 1978;52:526-529.
30. Eden RL, Seifert LS, Winegar A, et al: Maternal risk states and postdate pregnancy outcome. *J Reprod Med* 1988;33:53.
31. Somogyi M: Exacerbation of diabetes by excess insulin action. *Am J Med* 1959;26:169-191.
32. Bolli GB, Gerich JE: The "Dawn phenomenon"—A common occurrence in both non-insulin-dependent and insulin-dependent diabetes mellitus. *N Engl J Med* 1984;310:746-750.
33. Reece EA, Coustan DR, Hayslett JP, et al: Diabetic nephropathy: Pregnancy performance and fetomaternal outcome. *Am J Obstet Gynecol* 1988;159:56-66.
34. Klein BEK, Moss SE, Klein R: Effect of pregnancy on progression of diabetic retinopathy. *Diabetes Care* 1990;13:34-40.
35. Silfin SL, Wapner RJ, Gabbe SG: Maternal outcome in class H diabetes mellitus. *Obstet Gynecol* 1980;55:749-751.

PART FOUR
Fetal Disorders

16

FETAL GROWTH RETARDATION

The ability to reach an optimal birth weight results from the interaction between the fetal growth potential and the environment. The growth potential varies from race to race and from individual to individual. This is one reason for significant differences in birth weight among fetuses of the same gestational age. For example, the mean birth weight of the Cheyenne Indians in the United States is 3700 g, whereas it is only 2400 g for newborns of the Lummy tribe in New Guinea.

The fetus requires several substrates for normal growth. The most important are oxygen, glucose, and amino acids. Oxygen crosses the placenta by simple diffusion and is necessary for the formation of chemical energy in the form of adenosine triphosphate (ATP). Glucose crosses the placenta by facilitated diffusion, is used in the formation of energy, and provides the carbon building blocks for the synthesis of lipids, glycogen, nucleotides, and other molecules. Amino acids cross the placenta by active transport and are essential for the synthesis of protein. Any persistent decrease in the availability of any of these substrates will limit the ability of the fetus to reach his or her growth potential. Persistent and severe substrate deficiency may threaten the ability of the fetus to survive.

The availability of substrates necessary for fetal growth may be limited by pathologic condi-

tions affecting the mother, the placenta, and the fetus. A partial list of these conditions is shown in Box 16-1. The maternal conditions most frequently associated with poor fetal growth are chronic hypertension, preeclampsia, and chronic renal disease. The most common placental problem causing impaired fetal growth is abnormal placentation characterized by small size and inadequate changes in the spiral arteries. Suboptimal growth as a consequence of fetal disease occurs in chromosomal abnormalities, infections, and multifactorial malformations.

The problems in diagnosing and managing pregnancies with impaired fetal growth are substantial. This is because of the lack of a precise definition of fetal growth retardation, our ignorance about individual fetal growth potential, the occurrence of fetal growth retardation in patients without recognizable high-risk factors, the proliferation of measurements to assess fetal growth, the difficulties in estimating gestational age, and the differences of opinion between investigators about the ideal time to deliver these fetuses.

◼ DEFINITION

Fetal growth retardation used to be diagnosed at birth by the pediatricians. They invented the term *small for gestational age* to designate newborns with birth weight less than the 10th per-

---

BOX 16-1

Maternal, Placental, and Fetal Conditions Frequently Associated with Fetal Growth Retardation

Maternal

Preeclampsia
Chronic hypertension
Chronic renal disease
Connective tissue disorder
Diabetes with vascular lesions
Sickle cell anemia
Cardiac disease class III or IV
Severe malnutrition
Smoking
Alcohol ingestion

Placental

Abnormal placentation
Chronic villitis
Placental infarcts
Placental hemangiomas
Chorioangiosis
Hemorrhagic endovasculitis
Placenta previa

Fetal

Chromosomal abnormalities
Multifactorial defects
Infections
Multifetal pregnancies

---

centile for their gestational age and less than 2500 g (SGA babies) and to distinguish them from babies with low birth weights resulting from preterm delivery (preterm babies).[1] This distinction is important because the complications associated with each of these conditions are different. The preterm newborn exhibits complications predominantly related to the immaturity of several organs. In contrast, SGA babies are affected by metabolic and nutritional problems.

With the development of ultrasound scanning, obstetricians became capable of diagnosing growth retardation *in utero*, and the term *intrauterine growth retardation (IUGR)* was designed to indicate fetuses with birth weight below the 10th percentile for their gestational ages. The similarity between the definitions of IUGR and SGA is obvious. The two terms are frequently used in an interchangeable manner, and both attempt to identify fetuses or newborns that are small for reasons other than being preterm.

There are multiple problems with the definitions of SGA and IUGR babies. One problem is the variation in birth weight for gestational age standards.[2] For example, the 10th percentile at 40 weeks is 2980 g in an Australian study[3] and 2535 g in a study done in Denver, Colorado.[1] It is obvious that the incidence of SGA and IUGR babies will change depending on the birth weight curve used by the person evaluating the newborn or the fetus. The table designed by Brenner et al.[4] is useful for evaluating infants born in the United States at about sea level (Table 16-1). Brenner's fetal growth table may be inappropriate for other countries or for babies born at different altitudes.

Another problem is that the terms *SGA* and *IUGR* do not separate normal and healthy fetuses that have a weight below the 10th percentile from those who are small because of intrauterine malnutrition. This differentiation is important and ideally should be made during pregnancy, so that perinatal resources may be focused on the fetuses at risk instead of being used for the assessment of all small fetuses.

The confusion in defining these fetuses will lessen if SGA and IUGR are not used as equivalent terms. The term *IUGR* should be applied to fetuses affected by a pathologic restriction in their ability to grow.[5,6] This diagnosis should be confirmed in the neonatal period by findings such as low ponderal index, decreased subcutaneous fat, hypoglycemia, hyperbilirubinemia, necrotizing enterocolitis, hyperviscosity syndrome, or any other of the characteristic complications of these babies. The term *SGA* should be applied to all babies with birth weights below the 10th percentile for their gestational age without implying a pathologic restriction in their growth. The terms SGA and IUGR are used within that context in this chapter.

◼ INCIDENCE

The incidence of newborns with birth weight below the 10th percentile (SGA babies) should be, by definition, close to 10%. The incidence of newborns affected by intrauterine malnutrition (IUGR babies) is approximately 2% to 5% in the United States, but it varies in different geographic areas.

◼ ANTEPARTUM COMPLICATIONS
Stillbirth

There is a definite relationship between uterine malnutrition and the incidence of stillbirths.

TABLE 16-1 ◪ Fetal weight percentiles throughout pregnancy

Gestational age (Menstrual weeks)	Smoothed percentiles				
	10	25	50	75	90
8	—	—	6.1°	—	—
9	—	—	7.3°	—	—
10	—	—	8.1°	—	—
11	—	—	11.9°	—	—
12	—	11.1	21.1	34.1	—
13	—	22.5	35.3	55.4	—
14	—	34.5	51.4	76.8	—
15	—	51.0	76.7	108	—
16	—	79.8	117	151	—
17	—	125	166	212	—
18	—	172	220	298	—
19	—	217	283	394	—
20	—	255	325	460	—
21	280	330	410	570	860
22	320	410	480	630	920
23	370	460	550	690	990
24	420	530	640	780	1080
25	490	630	740	890	1180
26	570	730	860	1020	1320
27	660	840	990	1160	1470
28	770	980	1150	1350	1660
29	890	1100	1310	1530	1890
30	1030	1260	1460	1710	2100
31	1180	1410	1630	1880	2290
32	1310	1570	1810	2090	2500
33	1480	1720	2010	2280	2690
34	1670	1910	2220	2510	2880
35	1870	2130	2430	2730	3090
36	2190	2470	2650	2950	3290
37	2310	2580	2870	3160	3470
38	2510	2770	3030	3320	3610
39	2680	2910	3170	3470	3750
40	2750	3010	3280	3590	3870
41	2800	3070	3360	3680	3980
42	2830	3110	3410	3740	4060
43	2840	3110	3420	3780	4100
44	2790	3050	3390	3770	4110

From Brenner WE, Edelman DA, and Hendricks CH: A standard of fetal growth for the United States of America. *Am J Obstet Gynecol* 1976;126:555-564.

°Median fetal weights may be overestimated. Few fetuses are delivered at these gestational ages.

One study found that approximately 20% of all stillborn infants show signs of growth retardation.[7] Another study found that IUGR was associated with and probably responsible for 26% of stillbirths among infants with a birth weight less than 2500 g.[8] Fetal death in IUGR babies may occur at any time but is more frequent after 35 weeks of gestation.[9,10]

Oligohydramnios

Oligohydramnios is a common finding in severe IUGR.[11] The amniotic fluid volume is normal with mild IUGR. The relationship between fluid volume and fetal growth was studied by Chamberlain et al.[12] They found that the incidence of IUGR when the amniotic fluid volume was normal was 5%. When oligohydramnios was present, the incidence of IUGR was approximately 40%. These findings have been confirmed by other investigators.[13]

The most likely cause of oligohydramnios in IUGR babies is decreased fetal urinary output caused by redistribution of the blood flow with preferential shunting to the brain and decrease in renal perfusion.

Intrapartum fetal acidosis

Fetal monitoring signs of acidosis such as late decelerations, severe variable decelerations, decreased beat-to-beat variability, and episodes of bradycardia are more frequent in IUGR than in normal growth fetuses.[14] Acidosis occurs during labor in as many as 40% of IUGR fetuses.[15] As a result, the incidence of cesarean delivery of IUGR fetuses is high.[16]

◪ NEONATAL COMPLICATIONS

At birth the IUGR infant shows signs of soft tissue wasting. The skin is loose and thin, and there is little subcutaneous fat. The abdomen is scaphoid, the ribs are protuberant, and the muscle mass of the arms, buttocks, and thighs is reduced. The umbilical cord is limp, thin, and frequently meconium stained. Most of the time it is apparent that the head circumference is larger than the abdominal circumference. Also, in the majority of cases, the birth weight and the placental weight are below the 10th percentile. In contrast, the healthy SGA baby has symmetric development of the head and abdomen and a normal amount of subcutaneous fat.

The neonatal course of the IUGR infant is different from that of the baby that is small and healthy. The latter rarely has significant problems and in the majority of cases goes home after an uneventful stay in the nursery. In contrast, the IUGR infant frequently develops complications. The most important complications are:

1. Related to perinatal asphyxia and acidosis: persistent fetal circulation, meconium aspi-

ration syndrome, hypoxic-ischemic encephalopathy
2. Metabolic alterations: hypoglycemia, hypocalcemia, hyperviscosity syndrome, hyperglycemia, and hypothermia
3. Related to the specific cause of fetal
growth retardation: infections, congenital
malformations, chromosomal abnormalities

Meconium aspiration syndrome

Meconium aspiration was a major cause of
mortality and morbidity in the IUGR baby. The
use of amnioinfusion before birth and proper resuscitative techniques after birth has significantly
decreased the severity of this problem. These
techniques are described in Chapter 8.

Persistent fetal circulation

Persistent fetal circulation is a common sequela of perinatal hypoxia and acidosis. The
pathophysiology is characterized by severe pulmonary vasoconstriction with persistent blood
flow through the ductus arteriosus. The main
signs are hypoxia with moderate hypercarbia,
right-to-left shunting without evidence of intrinsic heart disease, and cardiomegaly. The treatment is adequate ventilation, minimal stimulation, and the use of pulmonary vasodilators.

Hypoxic-ischemic encephalopathy

Hypoxic-ischemic encephalopathy is a nonspecific diagnosis used to describe a variety of neurologic signs and symptoms occurring after episodes of severe perinatal asphyxia. The injury to
the brain may range from cerebral edema to diverse forms of intracranial bleeding to nonspecific asphyxial injuries. The symptoms include
seizures, irritability, twitching, and apnea. Treatment is symptomatic and supportive.

Hypoglycemia

Hypoglycemia occurs in approximately 25% of
term and in as many as 67% of preterm IUGR
infants.[17] The condition is caused by lack of adequate glycogen stores in liver and muscle and
decreased subcutaneous fat. Another important
component of neonatal hypoglycemia is a relative deficiency of hepatic gluconeogenic enzymes. The most common definition of hypoglycemia is a blood sugar below 30 mg/dl. The
symptoms are nonspecific: jitteriness, twitching,
apnea, tachypnea, and, occasionally, seizures.
Early feeding, orally or intravenously, can minimize or prevent hypoglycemia.

Hypocalcemia

Hypocalcemia, particularly during the first day
of life, is common in IUGR babies. Relative hy-
poparathyroidism, increased calcitonin level
caused by chronic asphyxia, and increased phos-
phorus level resulting from increased tissue ca-
tabolism seem to be responsible for this problem. Symptoms are nearly identical to those of
hypoglycemia.

Hyperviscosity syndrome

The hyperviscosity syndrome affects approximately 18% of all IUGR babies.[18] The main
manifestation is polycythemia, defined as a central hematocrit in excess of 65% or hemoglobin
concentration above 22 g/dl. Blood viscosity is
linearly related to the hematocrit at levels below
60%, but the relationship becomes exponential
once the hematocrit increases beyond 65%.[18]
Polycythemia is probably caused by a chronic hypoxic stimulation of the fetal hematopoietic system. Hyperviscosity slows the blood flow in the
microcirculation with production of pulmonary
infarcts and necrotizing enterocolitis. The destruction of a large number of red cells results in
hyperbilirubinemia. Also, volume overload may
lead to pulmonary edema and congestive heart
failure. Treatment of the hyperviscosity syndrome involves partial exchange transfusions
with plasma or albumin replacing blood.

Deficient temperature control

The IUGR fetus has poor temperature control
and a tendency toward hypothermia resulting
from deficient energy stores and the small size
of the subcutaneous fat layer. The treatment
consists of artificial warmth during the first few
days of life.

◼ ETIOLOGY

Many different conditions affecting the
mother, the placenta, or the fetus may impair
the ability of the fetus to grow.

Most frequent causes of IUGR

Placental insufficiency. In cases of IUGR
the placental weight is usually below the 10th
percentile, and there is a reduction in the number of stem and villous capillaries. The reduction
in villous capillaries results from a deficit in the
formation of tertiary villi.[19,20] This, in turn, is responsible for the decrease in parenchyma and
the increase in stroma seen in these placentas.
Also, there are clumps of syncytial villi forming

knots into the intervillous space, and the latter frequently contains fibrin deposits and clots. The spiral arteries preserve their muscular layer because of incomplete penetration by trophoblastic cells.

These placental changes are unspecific and also found in maternal conditions associated with IUGR such as chronic hypertension, preeclampsia, chronic renal disease, systemic lupus, sickle cell anemia, and insulin-dependent diabetes. They are also seen in a significant number of patients with idiopathic preterm labor. It seems that different conditions associated with impaired fetal growth produce similar histologic changes in the placenta. The extent of the placental changes is related to the severity of the maternal disease.

Maternal vascular disease. Maternal vascular disease (e.g., chronic hypertension, preeclampsia, renal disease) is a frequent cause of IUGR. These patients have small placentas with histologic changes similar to those described for placental insufficiency.

The group of Khong et al.[21] has investigated the relationship between maternal disease and abnormal placentation. These authors have demonstrated the presence of trophoblastic invasion of the spiral arteries during normal pregnancy and its absence or deficiency in cases of fetal growth retardation. They postulated that a deficient trophoblastic invasion is common to preeclampsia and to idiopathic fetal growth retardation. The extent of this abnormality and the efficiency of the maternal compensatory mechanisms will determine whether the abnormality will manifest clinically as fetal growth retardation, preeclampsia, or a combination of both.

Genetic syndromes. There is an increased prevalence of genetic syndromes among IUGR babies. The frequency of congenitally abnormal babies among severely affected IUGR fetuses is approximately 10% but may be as high as 33%. The majority of genetically affected babies have symmetric measurements.

IUGR is common in chromosomal disorders, especially in somatic trisomies. IUGR also occurs in patients with familial disautonomy, osteogenesis imperfecta, and other multifactorial disorders. Single gene mutations do not affect fetal growth as much as chromosomal defects. The possibility of a fetal congenital disorder should always be considered in patients with "idiopathic" or "unexplained" IUGR.

The mechanism of fetal growth impairment caused by genetic syndromes is unknown. The placenta of a baby affected with autosomal trisomies sometimes exhibits histologic features that suggest to the experienced pathologist the presence of a genetic problem. Chromosomal defects may cause alterations in placental function resulting in fetal malnutrition. Also, they may affect the growth potential.

Maternal habits. *Smoking* is a well-recognized cause of impaired fetal growth. The reduction in fetal growth is between 150 to 400 g at term. Tobacco chewing gravidas and passive smokers also have reduced fetal weight. The mechanism behind the decrease in fetal growth has not been completely elucidated, but it probably results from the combination of factors such as reduced intervillous blood flow, the effect of carbon monoxide and thiocyanate on the fetus, and reduced prostacyclin production.

Maternal alcohol ingestion is another well-recognized cause of fetal growth retardation. The alcohol effect is synergistic with that from smoking. In one series of 76 babies with fetal alcohol syndrome, IUGR occurred in 91%.[22] The fetal effect of alcohol is more severe in heavy drinkers.

The chronic ingestion of *heroin, morphine, cocaine,* and other addictive substances is frequently associated with fetal growth retardation. The mechanism is not clear but most likely involves a direct drug effect on the fetus and maternal malnutrition, a condition that is prevalent in these individuals.

Multifetal gestation. Multiple gestations are associated with impaired fetal growth of one or more of the fetuses in approximately 21% of the cases.[23] The most common reasons for impaired growth in twins are abnormal placentation, decreased placental size, or abnormal placental vascular anastomosis. The problem occurs more frequently in twins with monochorionic placentation.

Less frequent causes of IUGR

Cord and placental abnormalities. Abnormal insertion of the umbilical cord, torsion of the cord, hemangiomas of the placenta, and placenta previa are situations frequently associated with the presence of IUGR fetuses. The overall prevalence of these abnormalities is low.

Fetal infection. Intrauterine infections are not a common cause of IUGR. The majority of bacterial infections have relatively acute courses and end in preterm labor, preterm rupture of membranes, or fetal death. Viral infections may be chronic and may affect fetal growth; however, the only viral infection clearly associated with impaired fetal growth is congenital rubella.

Chronic villitis. Occasionally, the pathologist describes lymphocytic and histiocytic infiltration of the villi indicating the presence of *chronic villitis*.[24] Chronic villitis is probably viral in origin, but there is no rigorous evidence that this is the case. IUGR is present in approximately 30% of patients with chronic villitis.

Maternal malnutrition. There is evidence that severe maternal malnutrition can cause fetal growth retardation. Studies of women pregnant during the siege of Leningrad in World War II[25] and the Dutch famine in the winter of 1944[26] demonstrated that severe protein caloric malnutrition, especially during the second half of the pregnancy, causes decreased fetal weight; in the case of the siege of Leningrad, fetal weight loss was on the average 530 g. Fortunately, this is a problem that for practical purposes is nonexistent in the United States. The average caloric intake of women in the low socioeconomic sectors of the United States population is adequate for normal fetal growth. The opposite is true for other countries in which protein caloric malnutrition is endemic. In these countries, maternal malnutrition is a major cause of IUGR.

Another example of IUGR resulting from maternal malnutrition is found in women who have had gastric bypass operations for the treatment of morbid obesity. They have an incidence of IUGR babies of 20% to 40%.[27]

Maternal medications. The use of certain medications during pregnancy is associated with IUGR babies. Cancer chemotherapeutic agents, warfarin (Coumadin) and phenytoin (Dilantin), are drugs that have the potential to cause IUGR. Fortunately, these medications are used rarely during pregnancy.

◪ CLASSIFICATION

The method commonly used to classify patients with small fetuses is based on the presence or absence of symmetry among different anatomic structures. Type I IUGR corresponds to fetuses that are symmetrically small and have normal head-to-abdomen and femur-to-abdomen ratios. Type II IUGR corresponds to fetuses that have an abdominal circumference that is smaller than the head circumference and the femur length. Type III, or intermediate IUGR, corresponds to fetuses that are symmetric initially but become asymmetric later in the pregnancies. The principal characteristics of type I and type II IUGR are shown in Box 16-2.

The main problems with the morphologic classification of IUGR into types I, II, and III are the heterogeneity and the diverse outcome of the fetuses in each of these groups. Some investigators prefer an etiologic classification of small fetuses and subdivide them into the following groups:

1. *Intrinsic IUGR.* These fetuses are small because of fetal conditions, such as intrauterine infection or chromosomal abnormality.

BOX 16-2
Comparison of IUGR Babies and Small, Healthy Babies

IUGR	*Small and healthy*
Birth weight usually < 10% but may be < 25%	Birth weight < 10%
Birth weight usually < 2500 g but may be larger	Birth weight < 2500 g
Low ponderal index	Normal ponderal index
Decreased subcutaneous fat	Normal subcutaneous fat
Frequently develops complications in the neonatal period such as hypoglycemia, hyperbilirubinemia, hypocalcemia, hyperviscosity, necrotizing enterocolitis	Usually have an uneventful neonatal course

2. *Extrinsic IUGR.* The growth failure is caused by an element outside of the fetus, such as a placental condition or a maternal disease.
3. *Combined IUGR.* In these patients there are both extrinsic and intrinsic factors acting in conjunction to bring about the growth failure.
4. *Idiopathic IUGR.* The cause of the fetal growth failure is unknown.

The etiologic classification has little prognostic value, and all four groups may contain severely affected babies. Also, the morphologic and the etiologic classifications do not include babies that are small and healthy.

Another simple classification (Box 16-3) can be used that designates as "small fetuses" all those suspected of being SGA or IUGR by clinical evaluation and ultrasound examination. The small fetuses are divided into two groups:

1. Fetuses that are small and healthy
2. Fetuses affected by a pathologic restriction in their ability to grow, or true IUGR

BOX 16-3

Classification of Impaired Fetal Growth (Small Fetuses)

1. Small and healthy
2. True IUGR
   a. Symmetric
   b. Asymmetric

IUGR fetuses are subdivided into symmetric and asymmetric categories depending on the relative size of their head, abdomen, and femur (Box 16-4).

◪ DIAGNOSIS
Clinical diagnosis

Medical and obstetric history. The patient's medical history contains important elements (see Box 16-1) needed to identify patients at high risk for IUGR. Mothers with significant medical or obstetric problems such as chronic hypertension, severe toxemia of pregnancy, chronic renal disease, twin pregnancies, and advanced insulin-dependent diabetes are at high risk for having IUGR fetuses. The obstetric history is also of importance, and a patient with prior delivery of an IUGR baby is at high risk of having a similar problem in the present pregnancy.

Weight gain. Decreased maternal weight gain during pregnancy is a relatively insensitive sign of inadequate fetal growth. The association between poor maternal weight gain and small babies was demonstrated in the Perinatal Collaborative Study.[28] Other studies[29] have found that this association has questionable clinical value and that the weight gain is normal in a significant number of mothers who deliver small babies. Maternal weight gain is an insensitive index to use in differentiating IUGR babies from babies who are small and healthy.

Uterine fundal height. Measurement of the uterine fundal height is the most common method used to clinically estimate fetal growth. This method does not discriminate IUGR babies

---

BOX 16-4

Comparison of Symmetric and Asymmetric IUGR Fetuses

Symmetric	*Asymmetric*
Symmetrically small	Head larger than abdomen
Normal ponderal index	Low ponderal index
Normal head/abdomen and femur/abdomen ratios	Elevated head/abdomen and femur/abdomen ratios
Genetic disease, infection	Placental vascular insufficiency
Complicated neonatal course; poor prognosis	Usually have unexpectedly benign neonatal course and do well if complications are prevented or adequately treated

from small and healthy babies. Fundal height measurements should be measured in centimeters from the upper border of the pubic symphysis to the top of the fundus of the uterus. In many cases the uterine fundus is deviated toward one side of the abdomen, and measurements taken in the middle will be inaccurate. Also, it is a good idea to place the numbered side of the tape against the patient's skin so that the numbers cannot be seen during the measurement. Fundal height measurements are open to error in patients too obese or too thin, in nulliparas with a strong anterior abdominal wall, in multiparas with flaccid anterior abdominal muscles, and in patients with breech presentations or transverse lies.

The fundal height values should be plotted against a standard curve derived from a normal obstetric population. A useful curve was constructed by Belizan and coworkers.[30] These investigators were able to successfully identify 38 of 44 (86%) SGA fetuses with this curve. They had only 10% false-positive results. This curve has been compared with others and found to have the best predictive value.[31] Another study[32] found that 44% of pregnancies with abnormal uterine fundal height growth resulted in small babies, and 75% of small babies were adequately identified using this method.

Diagnosis by ultrasound examination

Biparietal diameter. The first attempts to diagnose IUGR fetuses by ultrasound examination used serial measurements of the fetal biparietal diameter (BPD). This method demonstrated two distinct patterns of impaired fetal growth.[32] Some fetuses exhibit continuous BPD growth during the entire pregnancy, but the measurements remain at all times below the 10th percentile for the gestational age. This type of abnormal growth was named *slow growth profile*. Other fetuses exhibit normal BPD growth during the first two trimesters of pregnancy followed by arrest of growth during the last trimester. This pattern was called *late flattening profile*. Fetuses demonstrating late flattening profile are more likely to be true IUGR babies and to develop antepartum and neonatal problems than fetuses with slow growth profile.

Unfortunately, the sensitivity and specificity of serial BPD measurements are too low to be used as the primary method for evaluating the suspected small fetus.[33,34] This is not surprising,

since the head is one of the last organs affected by fetal malnutrition. Also, late in pregnancy, the fetal head begins to undergo a molding process as it dips into the pelvis, making it difficult to obtain adequate measurements.

Abdominal circumference. The accuracy of routine fetal measurements in the diagnosis of small babies is shown in Table 16-2. The best single measurement is the abdominal circumference (AC), which has a negative predictive value of 99%. This means that finding a normal AC practically rules out the possibility that the baby is small. Unfortunately, the positive predictive value of AC measurements is not adequate, but when used together with the BPD, head circumference, femur length (FL), and estimated fetal weight (EFW), it reaches a satisfactory accuracy.

Estimated gestational age. Modern obstetric ultrasound equipment has computer programs that estimate the gestational age of the fetus by averaging routine fetal measurements. The difference between the ultrasound-derived and the clinically estimated gestational age gives the obstetrician a quantitative idea of the severity of the fetal growth impairment. This method is useful only if the gestational age is reliable.

Estimated fetal weight. Several investigators have developed mathematical equations to estimate the fetal weight. A formulation commonly used is that of Hadlock et al.[35] Fetal weight estimates are usually within 5% to 10% of the true fetal weight. This margin of error is unimportant when the birth weight is less than 2000 g. However, with larger fetal sizes, the error of the method may be as large as 1 pound for a term fetus. Also, the method requires precise knowledge of the gestational age.

Fetal weight estimates are valuable in the diagnosis of small fetuses but do not differentiate between IUGR babies and babies who are small and healthy. The method has a sensitivity of 87% and a specificity of 87% when the estimated fetal weight is below the 10th percentile for the gestational age.[36] Chervenak et al.[37] found that when the estimated fetal weight is below the 0.5% confidence limit, the probability that the fetus is small is 82%. If the estimated fetal weight is between the 0.5% and 20% confidence limits, the probability that the fetus is small is 24%.

Head-to-abdomen ratio. A useful measurement in the evaluation of small babies is the head-to-abdomen circumference ratio (H/A ra-

TABLE 16-2 ◪ Expected accuracy of ultrasound measurements in the diagnosis of small babies in a general population assuming a 10% prevalence of SGA

Parameter	Ultrasound variables°					
	BPD	FL	AC	FL/AC	PI	EFW
Sensitivity (%)	75	45	95	55	55	65
Specificity (%)	70	97	60	75	71	96
Predictive value (%)						
Positive	21	64	21	20	18	65
Negative	96	94	99	94	92	96

From Brown HL, Miller Jr JM, Gabert HA, et al: Ultrasonic recognition of the small-for-gestational-age fetus. *Obstet Gynecol* 1987;69:631-635.

°BPD = biparietal diameter; FL = femur length; AC = abdominal circumference; FL/AC = femur length/abdominal circumference; PI = ponderal index; EFW = estimated fetal weight.

tio). This ratio compares the most preserved organ in the malnourished fetus, the brain, with the most compromised, the liver, and is of significant value in identifying asymmetric IUGR babies. When a baby is small and symmetric, the liver will be preserved and the H/A ratio will be normal. The H/A ratio decreases with gestational age, and precise knowledge of the patient's dates are required for adequate interpretation.

The AC should be measured at the level of the bifurcation of the hepatic vein in the center of the fetal liver. Measurements taken at the entrance of the umbilical vein in the abdomen are in an oblique cross section and produce erroneously large values. The fetal head circumference should be measured at the level of the thalami. An advantage of using the head circumference instead of the BPD is that the effect of head molding is minimized.

Campbell and Thomas[38] examined 568 normal pregnancies with good clinical dating and developed a normal curve for the H/A ratio in relation to gestational age. Then they measured the H/A ratio in 31 fetuses who were later classified as SGA at birth. The patients carrying these fetuses had been referred because of poor uterine fundal growth, medical complications affecting pregnancy, or abnormal BPD growth. Of these 31 fetuses, 22 had H/A ratios above the 95th percentile. Clinically, the fetuses were wasted, suffered intrapartum fetal distress, and had other stigmata of intrauterine malnutrition. The other nine SGA babies were symmetrically small. Fetal malnutrition should be suspected when the H/A

ratio is abnormally high. A small fetus with normal H/A ratio may be a symmetric IUGR or may be small and healthy.

Femur-to-abdomen ratio. Another popular measurement in the evaluation of patients suspected of carrying small fetuses is the femur-to-abdomen ratio (F/A ratio). This method compares the femur length (FL), which is minimally affected by fetal growth impairment, with the abdominal circumference (AC), which is the most affected measurement. The FL is easy to obtain and is not affected by molding or abnormal fetal presentations or positions. The F/A ratio remains constant after 20 weeks. The normal value for this index is 22 ± 2. An upper limit of 23.5 (90th percentile) has a sensitivity of 63.3% and a specificity of 90% for the diagnosis of IUGR in a general population.[39]

When the F/A ratio is abnormally high, fetal malnutrition should be strongly suspected. When the F/A ratio is normal, the baby may be small and healthy or may have symmetric IUGR, but it is unlikely that the baby is suffering from severe malnutrition.

Fetal ponderal index. Another ultrasound measurement useful for the diagnosis of fetal malnutrition is the fetal ponderal index (PI). The PI is gestational age–independent and has a constant value throughout the second part of the pregnancy. The normal value for the fetal PI is 8.325 ± 2.5 (2SD). The fetal PI is obtained by dividing the estimated fetal weight by the third power of the femur length.[40] The use of the third power of the femur length magnifies considerably any error in femur measurements. Despite this possibility of error, the fetal PI is useful in the evaluation of the small baby.[41] The fetal PI has a negative predictive value of 96.4%. Unfortunately, the positive predictive value is only 35.7%.[41] A fetal PI of 7.0 or less should be considered abnormal and strongly suggestive of fetal malnutrition.

Abdominal circumference growth rate. Another gestational age–independent index useful in the evaluation of the potential IUGR fetus is the rate of growth of the abdominal circumference, which is linear from 15 weeks' gestation onward. A growth rate less than 1 cm in 2 weeks correctly identifies most IUGR babies.[42]

Oligohydramnios. Oligohydramnios is a late sign of fetal malnutrition. Amniotic fluid volume is measured with the four-quadrant technique,[43] which consists of measuring the largest pool of fluid found in each of the four quadrants of the uterus. The measurements are added, and the result is the amniotic fluid index (AFI). The fluid is decreased if the AFI is less than 10 cm and markedly decreased if less than 5 cm.

Doppler waveform analysis. The development of Doppler ultrasound has provided the obstetrician with a new tool for the assessment of IUGR fetuses. There is experimental evidence suggesting that Doppler waveforms may be used to assess resistance to blood flow.[44,45] Vessels with low resistance will produce waveforms with significant flow during diastole, whereas vessels with high resistance will show decreased diastolic flow. The measurement most commonly used to indicate the varied degrees of vascular resistance is the systolic/diastolic ratio (S/D ratio). During pregnancy, the umbilical (Figure 16-1) and the uterine (Figure 16-2) arteries have low resistance and low S/D ratios.

In one of the first studies on this subject, Fleischer et al.[46] studied 189 women at risk for having small babies. The neonates of these women were divided into four groups based on their quartile birth weights per sex and gestational age. The researchers found that the negative predictive value of a normal S/D ratio was 95%. The positive predictive value of an S/D ratio greater than 3.0 was 49%. However, other investigators[47] have found that ultrasound estimation of fetal weight is a better predictor of IUGR than umbilical Doppler assessment. In another study 2097 patients had umbilical Doppler assessment at 28, 34, and 38 weeks' gestation, and no abnormal features or indices of neonatal outcome were predicted.[48]

The average of nine umbilical velocimetry studies resulted in 46% sensitivity, 87.5% specificity, 47.5% positive predictive value, and 86.5% negative predictive value for the diagnosis of IUGR.[49] The average of three studies on uteroplacental velocimetry and IUGR are 53%, 74%, 50.6%, and 72.3% respectively.[49] It is clear from these numbers that umbilical velocimetry is better than uteroplacental velocimetry for the diagnosis of IUGR. It is also clear that Doppler assessment is not the perfect answer for the diagnosis of IUGR. This is logical since the cause of IUGR is varied, and Doppler waveform should only be used to identify IUGR caused by placental vascular disorders.

An exciting possibility of Doppler examination is that it may be useful in making the critical distinction between the fetus that is small and healthy and the one who is truly growth retarded. Rochelson et al.[50] studied 54 SGA newborns, 42 with high and 12 with normal S/D ratios. Only one of the babies with normal S/D ratios showed signs of fetal distress during labor, whereas 25 of the 42 babies with abnormal S/D ratios exhibited electronic monitoring signs of distress before or during labor. Two of the mothers in the normal S/D ratio group had hypertension as compared with 50% of the mothers in the abnormal S/D ratio group. Fourteen women in the abnormal S/D ratio group had decreased amniotic fluid. There were four stillbirths and two neonatal deaths in the abnormal S/D ratio group and none in the normal S/D group. This study strongly suggests that measurement of the umbilical artery S/D ratio can distinguish between the malnourished fetus that is at high risk and the SGA fetus that is at little or no risk. Similar findings have been reported by Trudinger et al.[51] These authors reported that small babies with normal umbilical and uterine waveforms are not at increased risk of fetal or neonatal morbidity. In another study[52] 124 of 179 babies had normal S/D ratios, and there was only one abnormal outcome and one delivery before 34 weeks. The incidence of cesarean section for fetal distress was 3.8%. These data suggest that small fetal size in the presence of normal umbilical velocimetry is a benign condition. Other authors[53,54] have also found normal Doppler studies in babies that are small but healthy and markedly abnormal findings in compromised, malnourished babies.

As mentioned before, there are multiple observations indicating that in cases of fetal malnu-

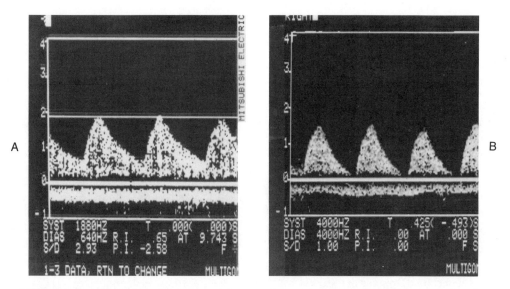

FIGURE 16-1 ◪ Umbilical artery Doppler waveforms. **A,** Waveforms with normal diastolic flow. **B,** Absent diastolic flow in a growth-retarded fetus.

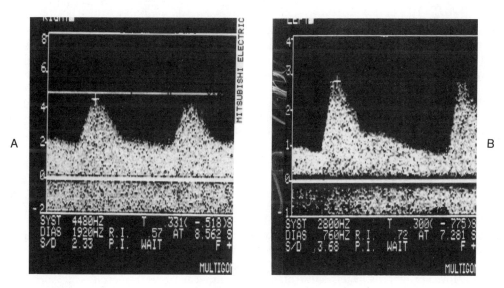

FIGURE 16-2 ◪ Uterine artery Doppler waveforms. **A,** Uterine waveforms with normal diastolic flow. **B,** Decreased end-diastolic flow and early diastolic notching.

trition there is at least partial preservation of the fetal head growth. Theoretically, this "sparing" effect protects the integrity of the fetal brain in the face of diminished availability of nutrients. Arduini et al.[55] studied 75 patients at risk for having truly growth-retarded babies. Of these 75 patients, 53% had hypertension, 24% were heavy smokers, 14.7% had a history of malnourished fetuses, and 8% had renal disease. The study was done at 26 to 28 weeks of gestation and before any of the fetuses exhibited ultrasonic signs of growth impairment. At birth, 52 neonates (69.3%) had normal birth weights, and 23 (30.7%) were small and had signs of malnutrition. According to these investigators, the ratio between the pulsatility index of the fetal umbilical and carotid arteries predicted the occurrence of fetal malnutrition with a specificity of 92.3%, a sensitivity of 78.2%, and positive and negative predictive values of 81.8% and 91.5%, respectively. The authors believe that increased flow to the brain precedes evidence of fetal growth retardation by ultrasound measurements. Similar observations have been made by Wladimiroff et al.[56,57] Other investigators[58] have found different results.

Another potential use of Doppler ultrasound is in antepartum surveillance in situations in which electronic fetal monitoring is unreliable, such as in pregnancies less than 30 weeks' gestation. McGowan et al.[59] used Doppler waveform to evaluate 15 preterm, severely growth-retarded infants and found that Doppler assessment was a more sensitive predictor of the severity of fetal compromise than a nonreactive nonstress test or decreased variability of the fetal heart rate.

◼ MANAGEMENT

The first step in managing suboptimal fetal growth is to identify patients at high risk for small infants. The second step is to differentiate the truly malnourished or IUGR fetus from those that are small but healthy. The third step is to establish adequate methods of fetal surveillance for patients with IUGR fetuses and deliver them under optimal conditions.

Identification of patients carrying small fetuses

The identification of patients at high risk for carrying small fetuses is relatively simple. A careful history and physical examination allow the physician to recognize high-risk factors (see Box 16-1) such as chronic hypertension, maternal renal disease, and history of a small baby in a prior pregnancy. However, approximately 40% of all small newborns are born to mothers who have no high-risk factors. To identify these patients it is necessary:

1. To determine the reliability of the dates in all obstetric patients and to consider at high risk all patients with unreliable dates
2. To perform serial measurements of the uterine fundal height in all obstetric patients and to consider at high risk all patients with inadequate fundal growth

With the help of these methods it is possible to separate from the overall obstetric population patients at high risk for having small fetuses. They are:

1. Patients with high-risk factors
2. Patients with unreliable dates
3. Patients with abnormal uterine growth

To identify patients with small fetuses among patients at risk, it is necessary to use ultrasound assessment. The first examination should be used to confirm the clinical estimation of gestational age. When the patient is being evaluated because of unreliable dates or inadequate fundal growth, the finding of fetal measurements in agreement with the clinical dating is reassuring. In that situation, there is no reason for concern, and no further evaluation is necessary unless a new indication appears. If the ultrasound measurements are smaller than expected for the clinical dating, the baby is small or the dates are in error, and further evaluation is necessary.

The finding of ultrasound measurements in agreement with the clinical dating is also reassuring in the case of patients with high-risk factors such as chronic hypertension and renal disease. However, these patients should have serial evaluations of the fetal growth until the time of delivery. Normal fetal growth, and particularly normal measurements of the abdominal circumference, indicate that the fetus is growing normally and will have a normal weight at birth. Suboptimal fetal growth indicates that the patient has an IUGR fetus.

Differentiation of the small and healthy fetus from the true IUGR fetus

The differentiation between asymmetric IUGR fetuses and other small fetuses is made by ultrasound measurements and by Doppler assessment. The most important measurements are the F/A ratio, the H/A ratio, the fetal PI, and the umbilical S/D ratio. When all of these tests were applied to a population of small fetuses, a sensitivity of 90%, specificity of 88%, positive predictive value of 90%, and negative predictive value of 88% were found for the diagnosis of asymmetric IUGR.

The umbilical artery S/D ratio is simple to obtain and, when elevated, indicates a high probability that the fetus is truly IUGR. Reversed flow or the absence of flow during diastole (see Figure 16-1, *B*) are signs of serious fetal compromise. The large majority of fetuses with normal S/D ratios are small and healthy, and a few are IUGR for reasons other than placental vascular insufficiency. In these cases antepartum surveillance may be limited to fetal movement count and vibroacoustic stimulation at each office visit.

Uterine artery Doppler assessment does not have the specificity or sensitivity of umbilical artery Doppler assessment in the prediction of IUGR. However, Ducey et al.[60] found that the 3% incidence of IUGR found in hypertensive patients with normal umbilical and uterine waveforms increased to 51% when the umbilical and uterine Doppler waveforms were both abnormal.

Antepartum surveillance of the IUGR fetus

Once the asymmetric IUGR fetus is identified by a combination of ultrasound measurements and Doppler studies, the perinatal resources should be used for fetal surveillance and for determination of the optimal time for delivery. Electronic monitoring of the fetal heart, amniotic fluid assessment, amniocentesis for determination of fetal lung maturity, and percutaneous fetal blood sampling are some of the methods that may be used for the evaluation of the IUGR fetus.

Nonstress test. The most important test in the follow-up of the IUGR fetus is the nonstress test (NST). As long as the NST shows adequate variability and accelerations and no decelerations, the fetal situation is not deteriorating, and expectant management is possible. Decrease in beat-to-beat variability, loss of reactivity, lack of accelerations, and occurrence of variable decelerations are signs indicating exhaustion of the fetal reserves and the need for prompt delivery.

Depending on the clinical circumstances, the frequency of NST testing varies from once every week to every day. Daily NSTs are indicated for patients with severe IUGR and with S/D ratios above 6. Less severe cases can be adequately monitored with twice per week or weekly NSTs. However, it is important to remember that IUGR fetuses that have reactive NSTs until the time of delivery have a high incidence of intrapartum fetal distress and an increased rate of cesarean section.

The contraction stress test (CST) or the biophysical profile (BPP) may be used to follow abnormal NSTs. Delivery of the baby is the best management when the backup test suggests fetal compromise. However, on many occasions the alterations in the NST are severe enough to justify delivery in the absence of a backup test. Preterm IUGR babies should be delivered in hospitals with intensive care neonatal nurseries.

Fluid volume. Amniotic fluid volume assessment is important in the follow-up of the IUGR fetus. This evaluation should be performed every week, and the frequency of NST testing should be increased if the amount of fluid decreases. Delivery may be indicated if oligohydramnios develops.

The most important ultrasound criteria indicating a severely compromised IUGR fetus is the presence of oligohydramnios. To find oligohydramnios in a patient carrying a small fetus requires prompt evaluation with an NST and with Doppler assessment. If the Doppler evaluation shows reversed diastolic blood flow, the fetal prognosis is poor, and delivery is the best management. If the diastolic flow is absent but not reversed and the pregnancy is under 32 weeks' gestation, the fetus should be monitored with daily NSTs and movement count and steroids used to accelerate lung maturity. Delivery will be determined by the results of the NST. Loss of long-term and short-term beat-to-beat variability and the presence of spontaneous decelerations will be indications for termination of pregnancy.

Amnioinfusion is a useful technique for improving ultrasound visualization and ruling out gross fetal congenital malformations in patients with severe oligohydramnios. Many cases of severe IUGR with oligohydramnios are caused by bilateral renal agenesis, and amnioinfusion is a great help in the diagnosis of this lethal condition.

Amniocentesis. There are few advantages in keeping an IUGR baby inside the uterus once fetal lung maturity has been reached. In IUGR babies, amniocentesis should be performed every week starting at 36 weeks, and the pregnancy should be delivered when the fetal lungs are mature or if meconium is present.

Cordocentesis. Umbilical cord blood sampling is rarely indicated in the management of the IUGR fetus. Perhaps the most common indication for umbilical cord blood sampling is the need to make a rapid determination of the fetal karyotype when a chromosomal defect is suspected. Some investigators have suggested using umbilical cord blood sampling to assess the degree of fetal hypoxia and acidosis. There are few occasions when this evaluation is necessary or useful. Nicolini et al.[61] found similar umbilical blood gases measurements in IUGR fetuses that survived and in those who died in the perinatal period. This study indicates that fetal blood sampling has a limited role in the evaluation of IUGR fetuses. Also, umbilical cord sampling is dangerous in the IUGR fetus, and these babies frequently develop prolonged, severe bradycardia during this procedure, requiring emergency cesarean delivery.

Delivery of the IUGR fetus

The management of labor and delivery is an important part of the care of the IUGR fetus. The reason for this is that, excluding congenital defects, intrapartum asphyxia is the major cause of perinatal morbidity and mortality for the IUGR fetus.

The full-term fetus has a large capacity for tolerating the stress of labor. This is substantially reduced in the IUGR baby because of the marked depletion of energy stores in the liver and subcutaneous tissues. With hypoxia, the energy reserves are rapidly consumed, and the fetus must switch to anaerobic metabolism for the generation of energy. Unfortunately, anaerobic metabolism produces a large number of hydrogen ions, and metabolic acidosis then appears.

Low et al.[62] found moderate-to-severe acidosis in 48% of IUGR babies during labor. Other authors[63,64] have found fetal heart rate monitoring tracings suggesting fetal distress in 30% to 35% of IUGR pregnancies. All studies have found an increased number of low 5-minute Apgar scores in IUGR fetuses when compared with babies of normal growth. Because of the high incidence of intrapartum asphyxia, labor and delivery in IUGR babies should be managed aggressively.

Direct fetal monitoring using scalp electrode and uterine pressure catheter should be initiated as early as possible. Amnioinfusion should be performed early in labor if the amniotic fluid volume is decreased. Even mild signs of distress should be followed with scalp stimulation or fetal scalp pH sampling. The second stage of labor, with its well-known tendency toward low pH values, should be kept to a minimum. To shorten the duration of the second stage, it is useful to instruct the patient in an adequate technique for bearing down and to use forceps when the vertex is well below plus 2 station.

The best choice for pain relief during labor in patients with IUGR fetuses is epidural anesthesia. However, these patients may develop hypotension even after proper intravascular volume loading with lactated Ringer's solution. Also, epidural anesthesia is associated with prolongation of the second stage of labor. These inconveniences are not unsurmountable, and epidural anesthesia in the hands of a competent obstetric anesthesiologist is the procedure of choice for these patients. Paracervical block anesthesia is not recommended in these patients, nor is the use of meperidine or diazepam for pain relief or sedation.

The placenta of an IUGR baby needs careful examination by a competent placental pathologist.[65] In many cases placental pathology provides evidence about the cause of the growth retardation. Stem artery thrombosis causing infarcts, fibrin deposition, insufficient invasion of spiral arteries, anomalies in the cord insertion, and the presence of arteriovenous malformations are some of the possible findings in the placenta of an IUGR baby.

Ideally, a neonatologist should be present at the time of delivery of an IUGR baby. The neonatal course of the infant will be better if sophisticated neonatal treatment begins shortly after childbirth rather than later when complications occur.

A summary of the plan of management is shown in Figure 16-3.

■ LONG-TERM PROGNOSIS

Today a large proportion of IUGR babies survive the neonatal period. Therefore more and more attention is focused on their long-term growth and development. The main question is whether these babies will recover completely from the intrauterine malnutrition or whether they will permanently suffer the consequences of the fetal insult.

The first follow-up studies of IUGR babies born between 1950 and 1960 found a significant incidence of poor growth and neurologic and developmental sequelae. However, more recent studies have demonstrated better outcomes.

A nearly universal finding is that IUGR babies as a group remain smaller than their appropriate-for-gestational-age cohorts in follow-up examinations. This occurs despite the occurrence, in some cases, of "catch-up growth" during the first 6 months of life. Several years after birth, 30%

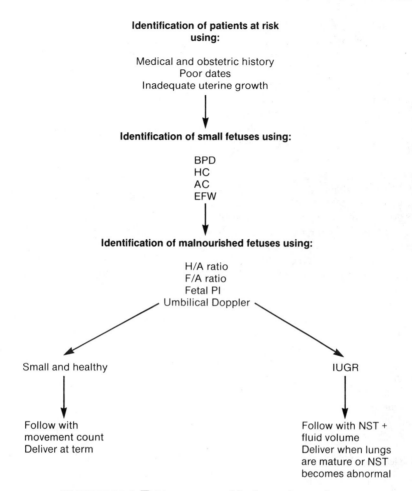

Identification of patients at risk using:

Medical and obstetric history
Poor dates
Inadequate uterine growth

Identification of small fetuses using:

BPD
HC
AC
EFW

Identification of malnourished fetuses using:

H/A ratio
F/A ratio
Fetal PI
Umbilical Doppler

Small and healthy

IUGR

Follow with
movement count
Deliver at term

Follow with NST +
fluid volume
Deliver when lungs
are mature or NST
becomes abnormal

FIGURE 16-3 ◪ Management of fetal growth retardation.

of IUGR babies will remain below the 30th percentile for weight of children of their age, and only 10% to 20% will be above the 50th percentile.[29,66,67]

Several studies have looked for characteristics that may help differentiate those IUGR babies who will remain growth stunted and those who will move into more normal growth patterns. Fitzhardinge and Stevens[68] found that if growth is to catch up, acceleration of growth has to occur during the first 6 months of life. They also found that the degree of initial growth failure does not have predictive value and that babies that are severely affected at birth have as good a chance as less affected infants of growing to normal percentiles. In another study,[69] it was found that infants whose growth retardation starts be-

fore 34 weeks of gestation are more likely to be below the 10th percentile at 4 years of age than are babies whose growth impairment is diagnosed after 34 weeks.

A major concern extrapolated from animal studies is that chronic intrauterine malnutrition may lead to a permanent decrease in brain cell number. Koops[70] reviewed the literature on neurologic sequelae of IUGR. It was found that babies with congenital anomalies and infections had a significant incidence of major neurologic problems later in life. Babies who did not have these problems had only a 1% incidence of motor deficits and a 6% incidence of seizures later in life. However, minimal brain dysfunction (hyperactivity, decreased attention span, learning difficulties, poor coordination) was diagnosed in

25%. Speech defects were also present in 33% of boys and 26% of girls tested. Other investigators[69] found a mean developmental quotient depressed by nearly 10 points in infants whose growth failure had a very early onset as compared with either late-onset or normal control subjects. Other studies[71,72] have found equal or improved outcomes in IUGR babies delivered before 36 weeks when compared with AGA preterm infants.

In summary:

1. The length of the insult seems to be more important than its severity in terms of both somatic growth and neurologic development: the earlier in pregnancy that IUGR is detected, the greater the probability of developmental problems later in life.

2. The probability of developmental problems is lower when there is catch-up growth during the first 6 months of life.

3. The worst prognosis is for babies with IUGR caused by congenital infections or abnormalities or chromosomal defects.

4. IUGR babies experiencing asphyxia at birth have a higher chance than AGA babies also suffering from intrapartum asphyxia of developing neurologic problems in their childhood.

◪ IMPORTANT POINTS ◪

1. The fetus requires several substrates for normal growth. The most important are oxygen, glucose, and amino acids. The availability of substrates may be limited by pathologic conditions affecting the mother, the placenta, or the fetus.

2. The term *small for gestational age,* or SGA, designates newborns with birth weight less than the 10th percentile for their gestational age and less than 2500 g. The term *intrauterine growth retardation,* or IUGR, should be used to designate fetuses or newborns of any birth weight affected by intrauterine malnutrition.

3. The prenatal diagnosis of IUGR should be confirmed in the neonatal period by findings of decreased subcutaneous fat, abnormal ponderal index, hypoglycemia, hyperviscosity, necrotizing enterocolitis, or any of the complications of intrauterine malnutrition.

4. To classify a newborn as SGA, it is necessary to use an adequate table of birth weight for gestational age. The Brenner's table is useful for infants born in the United States at sea level.

5. The main antepartum complications of true IUGR fetuses are an increased incidence of stillbirth, oligohydramnios, and antepartum fetal distress.

6. The main intrapartum complications of the true IUGR baby are fetal hypoxia, acidosis, and high rate of cesarean delivery.

7. The neonatal complications of the true IUGR baby are multiple and include hypoglycemia, hyperbilirubinemia, meconium aspiration, persistent fetal circulation, hypoxic-ischemic encephalopathy, hypocalcemia, hyperviscosity syndrome, and necrotizing enterocolitis.

8. The most common causes of IUGR are placental vascular insufficiency, maternal vascular disease, and genetic syndromes.

9. In the majority of cases, clinical findings and ultrasound measurements allow only the diagnosis of "small fetus." The majority of small fetuses are healthy. Only a modest proportion of small fetuses are truly undernourished or IUGR.

10. To distinguish between fetuses who are small and healthy and those who are true IUGR, the best indicators are the H/A ratio, F/A ratio, fetal ponderal index, abdominal circumference growth, and umbilical artery Doppler assessment.

11. Umbilical artery Doppler assessment does not identify all small fetuses. However, it helps to identify asymmetric IUGR fetuses at high risk for antepartum and intrapartum hypoxia. Small fetal size in the presence of normal umbilical Doppler measurements almost always is a benign condition.

12. Patients with high-risk factors, unreliable dates, and abnormal uterine growth are at risk for carrying small fetuses.

13. The most important tests for monitoring an IUGR fetus are the NST and the amniotic fluid volume. As long as these tests remain normal, expectant management is adequate.

14. Amnioinfusion with saline solution should be one of the initial steps in the intrapartum

management of the IUGR fetus with decreased amniotic fluid volume.

15. The placenta of all IUGR babies should be examined by a competent placental pathologist. In many cases the placenta will provide evidence about the cause of the problem.

16. The earlier in gestation IUGR is detected, the greater the possibility of developmental problems later in life. The worse prognosis is for IUGR caused by congenital infections, congenital abnormalities, and chromosomal defects.

REFERENCES

1. Lubchenco LO, Hansman G, Dressler M, et al: Intrauterine growth as estimated from liveborn birth-weight data at 24 to 42 weeks gestation. *Pediatrics* 1963;32:793-800.
2. Goldenberg RL, Cutter GR, Hoffman HJ, et al: Intrauterine growth retardation: Standards for diagnosis. *Am J Obstet Gynecol* 1989;161:271-277.
3. Kitchen WH, Robinson HP, Dickinson AJ: Revised intrauterine growth curves for an Australian hospital population. *Aust Paediatr J* 1983;19:157-161.
4. Brenner WE, Edelman DA, Hendricks CG: A standard of fetal growth for the United States of America. *Am J Obstet Gynecol* 1976;126:555.
5. Seeds JW: Impaired fetal growth: Definition and clinical diagnosis. *Obstet Gynecol* 1984;64:303-310.
6. Altman DG, Hytten FE: Intrauterine growth retardation: Let's be clear about it. *Br J Obstet Gynaecol* 1989;96:1127-1128.
7. Manara LR: Intrapartum fetal morbidity and mortality in intrauterine growth-retarded infants. *J Am Osteopath Assoc* 1980;80:101.
8. Morrison I, Olsen J: Weight-specific stillbirths and associated causes of death: An analysis of 765 stillbirths. *Am J Obstet Gynecol* 1985;152:975.
9. Usher RH: Clinical and therapeutic aspects of fetal malnutrition. *Pediatr Clin North Am* 1970;17:169.
10. Tejani N, Mann LI, Weiss RR: Antenatal diagnosis and management of the small-for-gestational age fetus. *Obstet Gynecol* 1976;47:31.
11. Manning FA, Hall LM, Platt LD: Qualitative amniotic fluid volume determination by ultrasound: Antepartum detection of intrauterine growth retardation. *Am J Obstet Gynecol* 1981;139:254.
12. Chamberlain PF, Manning FA, Morrison I, et al: Ultrasound evaluation of amniotic fluid volume: I. The relationship of marginal and decreased amniotic fluid volumes to perinatal outcome. *Am J Obstet Gynecol* 1984;150:245.
13. Philipson EH, Sokol RJ, Williams T: Oligohydramnios: Clinical associations and predictive value for intrauterine growth retardation. *Am J Obstet Gynecol* 1983;146:271.
14. Low JA, Pancham SR, Worthington D: Fetal heart rate deceleration patterns in relation to asphyxia and weight-gestational age percentile of the fetus. *Obstet Gynecol* 1976;47:14.
15. Lin CC, Moawad AH, Rosenow P, et al: Acid-base characteristics of fetuses with intrauterine growth retardation during labor and delivery. *Am J Obstet Gynecol* 1980;137:553.
16. Mann LI, Tejani NA, Wiss RR: Antenatal diagnosis and management of the small-for-gestational age fetus. *Am J Obstet Gynecol* 1974;120:995.
17. Oh W: Considerations in neonates with intrauterine growth retardation. *Clin Obstet Gyncol* 1977;20:99.
18. Tudehope DI: Neonatal aspects of intrauterine growth retardation. *Fetal Medicine Review* 1991;3:73-85.
19. Lee MML, Yeh M: Fetal microcirculation of abnormal human placenta: I. Scanning electron microscopy of placental vascular casts from small-for-gestational-age fetuses. *Am J Obstet Gynecol* 1986;154:1133.
20. Althabe O, Labarrere C, Teleuta M: Maternal vascular lesions in placentas of small-for-gestational-age infants. *Placenta* 1985;6:265.
21. Khong TY, DeWolf F, Robertson WB, et al: Inadequate maternal control to placentation in pregnancies complicated by preeclampsia and small-for-gestational-age infants. *Br J Obstet Gynaecol* 1986;93:1049.
22. Jones KL, Smith DW: Recognition of the fetal alcohol syndrome in early infancy. *Lancet* 1973;2:999.
23. Galbraith RS, Karchmar EJ, Piercy WN, et al: The clinical prediction of intrauterine growth retardation. *Am J Obstet Gynecol* 1979;133:281.
24. Althabe O, Labarrere C: Chronic villitis of unknown etiology and intrauterine growth-retarded infants of normal and low ponderal indexes. *Placenta* 1985;6:369.
25. Anatov AN: Children born during the siege of Leningrad in 1942. *J Pediatr* 1947;30:250.
26. Stein ZA, Susser MW: The Dutch famine 1944-45 and the reproductive process: Effects on six indexes at birth. *Pediatr Res* 1975;9:70.
27. Ingardia CJ, Fisher JR: Pregnancy after jejunoileal bypass and the SGA infant. *Obstet Gynecol* 1978;52:215.
28. Niswander KR (ed): *The Women and Their Pregnancies: The Collaborative Perinatal study of the National Institute of Neurological Diseases and Stroke.* Philadelphia, WB Saunders Co, 1972.
29. Low JA, Galbraigh RS: Pregnancy characteristics of intrauterine growth retardation. *Obstet Gynecol* 1974;44:12.
30. Belizan JM, Villar J, Nardin JC, et al: Diagnosis of intrauterine growth retardation by a simple clinical method: Measurement of uterine height. *Am J Obstet Gynecol* 1978;131:643.
31. Pattison RC, Antenatal detection of small-for-gestational-age babies. *South Afr Med J* 1988;74:282-283.
32. Campbell S, Dewhurst CJ: Diagnosis of the small-for-dates fetus by serial ultrasound cephalometry. *Lancet* 1971;2:1002.
33. Arias, F: The diagnosis and management of intrauterine growth retardation. *Obstet Gynecol* 1977;49:293.
34. Queenan JT, Kubarish SF, Cook LN, et al: Diagnostic ultrasound for detection of intrauterine growth retardation. *Am J Obstet Gynecol* 1976;124:865.
35. Hadlock FP, Harrist RB, Sharman RS, et al: Estimation of fetal weight with the use of head, body, and femur measurements. A prospective study. *Am J Obstet Gynecol* 1985;151:333.
36. Divon MY, Guidetti DA, Braverman JJ, et al: Intrauterine growth retardation—A prospective study of the diag-

nostic value of real-time sonography combined with umbilical artery flow velocimetry. *Obstet Gynecol* 1988; 72:611.

37. Chervenack FA, Romero B, Berkowitz RL, et al: The use of sonographic estimated fetal weight in the prediction of intrauterine growth retardation. *Am J Perinatol* 1984;1:298.

38. Campbell S, Thomas A: Ultrasonic measurement of the fetal head-to-abdominal circumference ratio in the assessment of growth retardation. *Br J Obstet Gynaecol* 1977;84:165.

39. Hadlock FP, Deter RL, Harrist RB, et al: A date-independent predictor of intrauterine growth retardation: Femur length/abdominal circumference ratio. *Am J Radiol* 1983;141:979.

40. Yagel S, Zacut D, Igelstein S, et al: In utero ponderal index as a prognostic factor in the evaluation of intrauterine growth retardation. *Am J Obstet Gynecol* 1987;157: 415-419.

41. Vinzileos AM, Lodeiro JG, Feinstein SJ, et al: Value of fetal ponderal index in predicting growth retardation. *Obstet Gynecol* 1986;67:584.

42. Divon MY, Chamberlain PF, Sipos L, et al: Identification of the small for gestational age fetus with the use of gestational age-independent indexes of fetal growth. *Am J Obstet Gynecol* 1986;155:1197.

43. Phelan JP, Smith CV, Broussard P, et al: Fluid volume assessment with the four-quadrant technique at 36-42 weeks' gestation. *J Reprod Med* 1987;32:540-542.

44. Clapp JF, Szeto HH, Larrow R, et al: Umbilical blood flow response to embolization of the uterine circulation. *Am J Obstet Gynecol* 1980;138:60.

45. Giles WB, Trudinger BJ, Baird PJ: Fetal umbilical artery flow velocity waveforms and placental resistance: Pathological correlation. *Br J Obstet Gynaecol* 1985;92:31.

46. Fleischer A, Schulman H, Farmakides G, et al: Umbilical artery velocity waveforms and intrauterine growth retardation. *Am J Obstet Gynecol* 1985;151:502.

47. Divon MY, Guidetti DA, Barverman JJ, et al: Intrauterine growth retardation—a prospective study of the diagnostic value of real-time sonography combined with umbilical artery flow velocimetry. *Obstet Gynecol* 1988; 72:611-614.

48. Beattie RB, Dornam JC: Antenatal screening for intrauterine growth retardation with umbilical Doppler ultrasonography. *Br Med J* 1989;298:631-635.

49. Low JA: The current status of maternal and fetal blood flow velocimetry. *Am J Obstet Gynecol* 1991;164:1049-1063.

50. Rochelson BL, Schulman H, Fleischer A, et al: The clinical significance of Doppler umbilical artery velocimetry in the small for gestational age fetus. *Am J Obstet Gynecol* 1987;156:1273.

51. Trudinger BJ, Giles WB, Cook CM: Velocity waveforms in the maternal uteroplacental and fetal umbilical placental circulations. *Am J Obstet Gynecol* 1985;152:155.

52. Burke G, Stuart B, Crowley P, et al: Is intrauterine growth retardation with normal umbilical artery blood flow a benign condition? *Br Med J* 1990;300:1044.

53. Rewer PJ, Simmons EA, Reitman GW, et al: Intrauterine growth retardation: Prediction of perinatal distress by Doppler ultrasound. *Lancet* 1987;2:415.

54. Dempster J, Mires GJ, Patel N, et al: Umbilical artery velocity waveforms: Poor association with small-for-gestational- age babies. *Br J Obstet Gynaecol* 1989;96:692-696.

55. Arduini D, Rizzo G, Romanini C, et al: Fetal blood flow velocity waveforms as predictors of growth retardation. *Obstet Gynecol* 1987;70:7.

56. Wladimiroff JW, Tonge HM, Stewart PA: Doppler ultrasound assessment of cerebral blood flow in the human fetus. *Br J Obstet Gynaecol* 1986;93:471-475.

57. Wladimiroff JW, VanBel F: Fetal and neonatal cerebral blood flow. *Semin Perinatol* 1987;11:335-346.

58. Veille J-C, Cohen I: Middle cerebral artery blood flow in normal and growth-retarded fetuses. *Am J Obstet Gynecol* 1990;162:391-396.

59. McGowan LM, Erskine LA, Ritchie K: Umbilical artery Doppler blood flow studies in the preterm small-for-gestational-age fetus. *Am J Obstet Gynecol* 1987;156:655.

60. Ducey J, Schulman H, Farmakides G, et al: A classification of hypertension in pregnancy based on Doppler velocimetry. *Am J Obstet Gynecol* 1978;157:680.

61. Nicolini U, Nicolaidis P, Fisk NM, et al: Limited role of fetal blood sampling in prediction of outcome in intrauterine growth retardation. *Lancet* 1990;336:768-772.

62. Low JA, Pancham SR, Piercy WN, et al: Intrapartum fetal asphyxia: Clinical characteristics, diagnosis, and significance in relation to pattern of development. *Am J Obstet Gynecol* 1977;129:857.

63. Cetrulo CL, Freeman R: Bioelectric evaluation in intrauterine growth retardation. *Clin Obstet Gynecol* 1977; 20:1979.

64. Pdendall H: Fetal heart rate patterns in patients with intrauterine growth retardation. *Obstet Gynecol* 1976;48: 187.

65. Rayburn W, Sander C, Compton A: Histologic examination of the placenta in the growth-retarded fetus. *Am J Perinatol* 1989;6:58-61.

66. Hill DE: Physical growth and development after intrauterine growth retardation. *J Reprod Med* 1978;21:335.

67. Low JA, Galbraith RS, Muir D, et al: Intrauterine growth retardation: A preliminary report of long-term morbidity. *Am J Obstet Gynecol* 1978;130:534.

68. Fitzhardinge PM, Stevens EM: The small-for-date infant: I. Later growth patterns. *Pediatrics* 1972;49:671.

69. Fancourt R, Campbell S, Harvey D, et al: Follow-up study of small-for-date babies. *Br Med J* 1976;1:1435.

70. Koops BL: Neurologic sequelae in infants with intrauterine growth retardation. *J Reprod Med* 1978;21:352.

71. Churchill JA, Masland RL, Maylov AA, et al: The etiology of cerebral palsy in preterm infants. *Dev Med Child Neurol* 1974;16:143.

72. Vohr BR, Oh W, Rosenfeld AG, et al: The preterm small-for-gestational-age infant: A two years' follow up study. *Am J Obstet Gynecol* 1979;133:425.

17

FETAL DISMORPHOLOGY

Andres Sarmiento*
Fernando Arias

Before the generalized use of obstetric ultrasound, the majority of fetal malformations were recognized at the time of delivery, and it was the responsibility of the pediatrician to answer questions from the parents about the unfortunate outcome of the pregnancy. At the present time, ultrasound technology has made it possible to recognize a large number of fetal abnormalities and changes in the amniotic fluid and placenta during the antenatal period. This situation has created a need for the practicing obstetrician to become familiar with the diagnosis, prognosis, and treatment of these abnormalities. This chapter is dedicated to the description of the most common problems found with the use of ultrasound equipment in the physician's office.

◪ POLYHYDRAMNIOS

One of the anomalies most commonly found during routine office ultrasound examination in the office is polyhydramnios. It affects approximately 0.4% to 1.5% of all pregnancies.[1] Traditionally, any volume of amniotic fluid greater than 2000 ml has been considered polyhydramnios. Since quantitative evaluation of the fluid volume is impractical, the most commonly used definition is by ultrasound assessment. Clinically, the diagnosis may be suspected by finding a uterine size larger than expected for the gestational age, easy ballottement of the fetus, difficulty in defining fetal parts, and faded heart tones. The clinical diagnosis of polyhydramnios should always be confirmed by ultrasound. One definition is the finding of a pocket of fluid measuring 8 cm or more in vertical diameter.[2] Another definition is an amniotic fluid index (AFI) greater than 25 cm.[3] Traditionally, polyhydramnios has been classified as acute when it occurs before 24 weeks of gestation and chronic when the diagnosis is made in the third trimester.

The amount of amniotic fluid in the amniotic cavity is a variable dependent on fetal and maternal factors. The alteration of any factor that regulates the fetomaternal equilibrium may induce an abnormal increase in fluid volume. The factors involved in this regulation are fetal swal-

*Andres Sarmiento, M.D., Department of Obstetrics and Gynecology, Universidad Militar Nueva Granada, Hospital Militar Central, Bogotá, Colombia, South America.

BOX 17-1

Causes of Polyhydramnios

Maternal (15%)
Rh isoimmunization
Diabetes

Placental (<1%)
Placental chorioangioma
Circumvallate placenta syndrome

Fetal (18%)
Multiple pregnancy
Fetal anomalies
  CNS abnormalities
  GI abnormalities
  GU abnormalities
  Skeletal malformations
  Fetal tumors
  Cardiac anomalies
  Chromosomal abnormalities
  Genetic syndromes
  Hematologic disorders
  Intrauterine infections
  Miscellaneous

Idiopathic (65%)

---

lowing, micturition, respiratory movements, and uteroplacental blood flow.

The conditions associated with polyhydramnios can be divided into maternal, fetal, placental, and idiopathic (Box 17-1).

Maternal causes

Rh isoimmunization. The use of prophylactic Rh(D) immune globin has made isoimmunization an uncommon cause of polyhydramnios. This is clearly shown by comparing the study of Queenan and Gadow,[1] performed 20 years ago when Rh isoimmunization was the cause of 11.5% of all cases of polyhydramnios, with recent reports in which the incidence is as low as 1%.[4]

Diabetes mellitus. Polyhydramnios is present in 1.5% to 66% of all diabetic pregnancies. Diabetes mellitus may be responsible for approximately 14% of all cases of polyhydramnios.[3] The etiology of polyhydramnios in diabetic patients is unknown. Fetal hyperglycemia with polyuria and increased osmolarity of the amniotic fluid caused by high glucose concentration have been proposed.

Placental causes

The most common placental causes of polyhydramnios are placental chorioangioma and the circumvallate placenta syndrome.

Fetal causes

Multiple pregnancy. Polyhydramnios has been reported in 25% of monozygotic twins with twin-to-twin transfusion syndrome. The recipient twin may develop polyuria, congestive heart failure, hydrops, and polyhydramnios. Usually the donor sac becomes oligohydramniotic. These events may be seen as early as the middle part of the second trimester. Multiple pregnancy accounts for 4.9% of all cases of polyhydramnios.[3]

Fetal anomalies. Fetal anomalies are responsible for approximately 12.7% of all the cases of polyhydramnios.[3] The most common lesions are:

Abnormalities of the central nervous system (CNS). Including anencephaly, hydrocephaly, encephalocele, spina bifida, microcephaly, holoprosencephaly, and hydranencephaly

Gastrointestinal (GI) abnormalities. Include esophageal atresia, annular pancreas, jejunal atresia, diaphragmatic hernia, duodenal atresia, omphalocele, gastroschisis, and midgut volvulus

Genitourinary (GU) abnormalities. Partial or complete renal obstruction, most commonly ureteropelvic obstruction

Skeletal malformations. Including multiple arthrogryposis, osteogenesis imperfecta, achondroplasia, and thanatophoric dwarfism

Fetal tumors. Including cystic congenital adenomatoid malformation of the lung, sacrococcygeal teratoma, and malignant cervical teratoma

Cardiac abnormalities. Severe congenital heart disease and persistent cardiac arrhythmias account for cardiac-related polyhydramnios

Chromosomal abnormalities. Several chromosomal abnormalities are associated with polyhydramnios; the most frequent are Down syndrome and trisomies 13 and 18

Genetic syndromes. Including hydrolethalus syndrome, multiple congenital anomalies, myotonia dystrophica, and Pena Shokeir syndrome

Hematologic disorders. Homozygous alpha thalassemia and fetomaternal hemorrhage

Intrauterine infections. Rubella, syphilis, or toxoplasmosis

Miscellaneous. Fetal retroperitoneal fibrosis and nonimmune hydrops fetalis

Idiophatic causes

Idiopathic polyhydramnios was the most frequent finding in several studies. Most mild cases of polyhydramnios are idiopathic. In a study of 102 cases of polyhydramnios, only 16% of the mild cases, defined as a vertical amniotic fluid pocket greater than 8 cm but less than 12 cm, had a cause. In severe cases, defined as a vertical pocket greater than 16 cm, an etiologic factor was identifiable in 91%.[3] In approximately 65% of the cases, polyhydramnios is idiopathic.

Complications

There is an increased fetal and maternal morbidity and mortality associated with polyhydramnios. Maternal complications include pregnancy-induced hypertension, preterm labor, premature rupture of membranes (PROM), and respiratory discomfort. Intrapartum complications include placental abruptio, cord prolapse, placental insufficiency, and an increased incidence of cesarean section. Postpartum hemorrhage is also more frequent in these patients.

Fetal morbidity and mortality is significant in cases of polyhydramnios, and several studies report an incidence of complications between 16% and 69%. The major causes of mortality are congenital abnormalities incompatible with life. Morbidity is usually associated with minor abnormalities and with prematurity and its complications.[4]

Management

A level II ultrasound examination should be performed on every patient in whom the physician finds polyhydramnios to detect congenital and placental abnormalities and to confirm gestational age. Fetal karyotype must be obtained using amniocentesis, cordocentesis, or placental biopsy. Fetal swallowing studies are also indicated. Basic laboratory studies include maternal antibody screen, diabetic screening, and TORCH (toxoplasmosis, other viruses, rubella, cytomegalovirus, herpes) serology. If these evaluations are negative, the case should be considered as idiopathic polyhydramnios.[5]

Serial amniotic fluid decompression is the treatment of choice for severe polyhydramnios when a conservative management is intended. This method not only relieves maternal discomfort, but also reduces excessive intrauterine pressure that can induce preterm labor. An alternative treatment is the use of prostaglandin synthetase inhibitors. Indomethacin has been proven effective in reducing the amount of amniotic fluid.[6] It probably acts by decreasing the fetal urinary output or by increasing the reabsorption of fluid via the lungs. A recommended dosage is 2.2 mg/kg/day administered orally every 6 hours. This treatment should be suspended at 32 weeks of gestation to avoid neonatal hemodynamic complications. Periodic ultrasonographic surveillance during treatment in search for signs of ductal constriction, such as tricuspid regurgitation, is warranted.[7]

◪ OLIGOHYDRAMNIOS

Oligohydramnios affects approximately 3.9% of all pregnancies. It has been defined as the absence of an amniotic fluid pocket, or one measuring less than 1 cm in vertical diameter. This definition encompasses only severe cases, and it is becoming more popular to use an AFI of less than 5 cm to define this condition.

Causes

In the majority of cases, oligohydramnios occurs in the setting of postterm pregnancy or is an expected event following PROM. This chapter deals with oligohydramnios that is an unexpected finding in the course of a routine ultrasound examination. The most likely causes for this occurrence are undetected PROM, severe intrauterine growth retardation (IUGR), fetal congenital abnormalities, especially those involving the urinary tract, and leaking fluid following amniocentesis or chorionic villi sampling (CVS) (Box 17-2).

Undetected PROM. Occasionally patients confuse leaking amniotic fluid with an increase in vaginal discharge caused by pregnancy, and this poses a diagnostic problem for the obstetrician who then finds decreased fluid in a routine ultrasound examination. To compound the situation, verification of the presence of PROM by fern testing is equivocal during the second trimester.

The prognosis for patients with PROM in the second trimester is guarded. The interested reader can find more information on this subject in Chapter 5.

Severe fetal growth retardation. One of the signs of severe fetal malnutrition is decreased amniotic fluid volume. This usually happens within the context of maternal diseases

---

BOX 17-2

Causes of Oligohydramnios

Postterm pregnancy
PROM
Fetal renal anomalies
Renal agenesis
Urethral obstruction
Prune belly syndrome
Bilateral multicystic dysplastic kidneys

Nonrenal fetal abnormalities
Triploidy
Thanatophoric dwarfism
Thyroid gland agenesis
Skeletal dysplasias
Congenital heart block
Multiple anomalies

Chronic abruptio
Leaking fluid following amniocentesis or CVS

---

such as chronic hypertension, connective tissue disorders, severe preeclampsia, and chronic renal disease. The interested reader can find more about this subject in Chapter 16.

Fetal congenital abnormalities. Severe fetal congenital abnormalities may be associated with oligohydramnios. Predominant among them are those affecting the urinary system, especially renal agenesis. Other conditions associated with decreased amniotic fluid are obstructive uropathy, prune belly syndrome, multicystic dysplastic kidneys, thanatophoric dwarfism, agenesis of the thyroid gland, skeletal dysplasias, congenital heart block, and multiple anomalies.[8,9]

Leaking fluid following amniocentesis or CVS. Leaking fluid is a low-frequency complication affecting less than 1% of patients undergoing amniocentesis or CVS. In the majority of cases, the patient is aware that she is leaking fluid, and oligohydramnios can be documented on ultrasound examination. In almost all of these patients, the leaking will stop, and the fluid will return to normal following a period of bed rest.

Diagnosis

The history and physical examination will provide valuable information for the differential diagnosis. In most cases it will be necessary to perform amnioinfusion to improve ultrasound visu-

alization and to confirm or rule out the possibility of PROM.

Amnioinfusion in patients with oligohydramnios is not a simple procedure. The needle should be advanced slowly with continuous ultrasound visualization, and when its tip has reached the interface between the fetus and the membranes, warmed saline solution should be infused. In the majority of cases, 250 to 350 ml of saline solution will be necessary to achieve optimal ultrasound transmission and perform a careful level II examination. A normal fetus will swallow the infused fluid, and its bladder will be easily seen with ultrasound after approximately 20 minutes. The bladder will not be seen in fetuses with renal agenesis.

Before ending the amnioinfusion, 1 ml of indigo carmin is injected inside the amniotic sac. The patient is instructed to wear a tampon for a few hours following the procedure and observe it for evidence of blue discoloration. This finding will confirm the presence of PROM.

Prognosis and management

The prognosis for patients with oligohydramnios in the second trimester is poor because the two most common causes, PROM and fetal congenital anomalies, are not amenable to successful treatments. Also, pulmonary hypoplasia occurs frequently in fetuses deprived of amniotic fluid for several weeks. The best outcomes are obtained in fetuses with severe IUGR that occasionally can be saved by early delivery and intensive neonatal care.

Pulmonary hypoplasia is an almost uniformly lethal neonatal condition characterized by small, anatomically immature lungs, pulmonary hypertension, and surfactant deficiency. Pulmonary hypoplasia affects approximately 60% of fetuses with prolonged oligohydramnios before 28 weeks. The amniotic fluid pressure is abnormally low in patients with oligohydramnios, and this causes a reversal of the normal amniotic-tracheal pressure gradient with the loss of pulmonary fluid and alveolar collapse.

Several techniques have been described for the antenatal diagnosis of pulmonary hypoplasia with ultrasound. All of them are unreliable. The most commonly used methods are the thoracic-to-abdominal circumference ratio and the lung length.

The option of termination of pregnancy should be offered to patients with lethal fetal abnormalities or with PROM before 20 weeks. One exception is those patients with PROM following amniocentesis or CVS in whom recovery is the rule. For patients with PROM after fetal viability, the management will be dictated by their gestational age as explained in Chapter 5. For patients with severe IUGR, the best option probably is delivery. However, expectant management with intensive fetal monitoring may be an option depending on the gestational age.

◢ NONIMMUNOLOGIC FETAL HYDROPS

Nonimmune hydrops fetalis (NIFH) is defined as the extracellular accumulation of fluid in tissues and serous cavities, without evidence of circulating antibodies against red blood cell antigens. Sonographic examination must demonstrate fluid accumulation in at least two sites.

The incidence of NIHF has been estimated to be around 1 in 1500 to 1 in 3500 live births. Before the introduction of anti-D gamma globulin prophylaxis in 1960, 80% of cases of hydrops fetalis were caused by Rh isoimmunization. Now that Rh disease can be successfully prevented, NIFH constitutes 75% of all cases of hydrops seen in developed countries.[10]

Causes

NIFH is the result of a heterogeneous group of conditions. Approximately 120 separate diseases have been reported in association with NIFH. With the introduction of new antenatal diagnostic techniques, the constant improvement of ultrasound imaging, and detailed postnatal histopathologic examination, new causes are described frequently.

The numerous causes of NIFH have been categorized into different groups (Box 17-3) for the purpose of diagnosis and management.

Cardiovascular. Cardiovascular malformations, arrhythmias, and neoplasms are responsible for approximately 20% of all cases of NIFH. The common mechanism that leads to fetal hydrops is congestive heart failure. Fetal arrhythmias are susceptible to treatment and have a reasonably good outcome, whereas cardiac malformations and neoplasms are associated with an extremely poor prognosis.[11]

Idiophatic. Despite thorough investigation, as many as 15% to 30% of cases of NIFH have to be classified as idiopathic.

Chromosomal abnormalities. Chromosomal abnormalities are found in 10% to 16% of all

BOX 17-3
Causes of Nonimmunologic Fetal Hydrops

Cardiovascular	19.3%
Idiopathic	15.7%
Chromosomal abnormalities	13.0%
Cystic hygroma	10.7%
Hematologic disorders	10.0%
Pulmonary malformations	6.0%
Miscellaneous	4.7%
Malformation syndrome	4.3%
Hydrothorax/chylothorax	3.7%
Infections	2.7%
Genitourinary anomalies	2.3%
Gastrointestinal anomalies	2.3%

From Hansman M, Gembruch U, Bald R: Management of the fetus with nonimmune hydrops, in Harrison MR, Golbus MS, Filly RA (eds): *The Unborn Patient.* Philadelphia, WB Saunders Co, 1991, p 248.

cases of NIFH. The most frequent chromosomal anomalies are trisomy 21 and Turner's syndrome. Other less common abnormalities are trisomies 13, 16, and 18, triploidy, mosaicism, and unbalanced translocation.[12] The underlying mechanisms responsible for the development of hydrops in these fetuses are cardiovascular anomalies, hypoalbuminemia, and lymphatic malformations.

Cystic hygroma. This malformation is described on p. 334.

Hematologic disorders. Alpha-thalassemia major with severe fetal anemia and high-output cardiac failure has been reported in approximately 7% to 10% of cases of NIFH.[8,13] Thalassemia is transmitted as an autosomal recessive trait and is more frequent in Southeast Asia, Mediterranean countries, and Central Africa. However, with increasing migration tendencies, this disease has become a worldwide health problem. The prenatal evaluation of patients from this geographic origin should include testing for red blood cell corpuscular volume and hemoglobin electrophoresis if this test is abnormal. If the thalassemia trait is present in the mother, the father should be tested, since the disease can be present only if both parents are carriers.

Pulmonary malformations. The pulmonary malformations most commonly associated with

NIFH are the cystic adenomatoid malformation of the lung, the chest wall hamartoma, and the extralobar intrathoracic lobe sequestration. Congenital diaphragmatic hernia is another anomaly frequently associated with NIFH.

Infections. Approximately 1.6% to 5% of all cases of NIFH are caused by infection. Several microorganisms can cause NIFH. Of all the PRATSCHEC agents (parvovirus, rubella, AIDS, toxoplasma, syphilis, cytomegalovirus, herpes, echovirus, and coxsackievirus), only rubella and AIDS have not been reported in association with NIFH. *Parvovirus B-19* is the most common viral infection associated with NIFH. The fetal hydrops is caused by severe fetal anemia. Unlike other agents, parvovirus does not produce fetal malformations. *Cytomegalovirus* (CMV) is also a common infectious cause of NIFH. The major diagnostic criteria include IUGR, microcephaly, cerebral echogenic densities, a positive maternal IgM-specific titer for CMV and, ideally, a positive viral culture from fetal blood or amniotic fluid.[14]

Other causes. Other less frequent causes of NIFH are:

Skeletal dysplasia
Multiple gestation
Gastrointestinal anomalies
Mendelian syndromes
Umbilical cord anomalies
Maternal disease
Fetomaternal hemorrhage
Genitourinary anomalies
Placental tumors
Lysosomal storage disorders
Fetal hepatic neoplasms

Diagnosis

The ultrasound diagnosis of NIFH is simple (Figure 17-1). Common sonographic findings include polyhydramnios, skin edema greater than 5 mm in thickness, ascites, placental enlargement, pericardial or pleural effusions, and cardiomegaly. It is recommended that NIFH not be diagnosed when fluid accumulation is limited to one body cavity. However, since a unique fluid accumulation may be the first sign of developing NIFH, follow-up sonographic examination is warranted.

Once the diagnosis has been made, a complete workup should be performed. This should include:

1. Complete maternal health history including determination of pedigree and investigation of teratogenic or infectious exposures
2. Complete maternal blood workup including blood group and typing, antinuclear antibody, glucose screen, hemoglobin electrophoresis, viral antibody titers, Kleihauer test, and glucose-6-phosphate dehydrogenase activity
3. Ultrasound level II examination
4. Cordocentesis for fetal karyotype, viral titers, blood count, blood gases, cultures, liver function, and metabolic testing
5. Fetal echocardiography

Prognosis

The prognosis for the fetus with NIFH is poor. The perinatal death rate is between 40% and 98%. The prognosis depends on the underlying cause of the hydrops. Anatomic malformations, found in approximately 40% of the cases, have the worst prognosis and indicate a lethal condition in virtually all cases. The karyotype, severity of anemia, and amount and location of fluid collections are also important prognostic features. Only cases of CMV infection and cardiac arrhythmias without structural malformations have spontaneous resolution of the hydrops.[15] The risk of recurrence is low unless the cause is genetic.

Preeclampsia, preterm labor, PROM, postpartum hemorrhage, and difficulty in removing the placenta are other factors associated with NIFH and contributing to the poor prognosis.

Management

The management of NIFH must be individualized, and decisions should be made in conjunction with the parents. Termination of pregnancy is an option before fetal viability. In viable fetuses the management varies widely depending on the cause and prognosis. In cases with severe anatomic malformations or chromosomal anomalies, the management should be expectant. In contrast, fetuses with no anatomic anomalies and treatable problems such as tachyarrhythmia or parvovirus anemia should be aggressively managed.

Amniocentesis has been used to remove excessive amniotic fluid, relieve maternal discomfort, and diminish the risk of premature labor. Fetal paracentesis and thoracentesis have also been used in selected cases to decrease the pos-

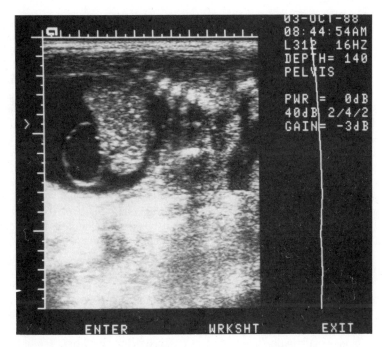

FIGURE 17-1 ◪ Nonimmunologic fetal hydrops. There are fluid collections in the abdomen and the thorax. The bladder is distended, and there is no amniotic fluid. This fetus had obstructive uropathy caused by posterior urethral valves.

sibility of dystocia and facilitate neonatal resuscitation.[9,11] Other therapies that have been used with promising results are intraperitoneal injection of red blood cells or albumin, intrauterine transfusion to treat parvovirus-induced fetal anemia, and thoracoamniotic shunting in cases of pleural effusions.

◪ FETAL ARRHYTHMIAS

Fetal arrhythmia (FA) is any irregularity of the cardiac rhythm not associated with uterine activity. Fetal arrhythmias are diagnosed in approximately 1% to 2% of all pregnancies. Fortunately, only 10% of these arrhythmias are considered potential sources of fetal morbidity.[16]

The heart begins to beat in a synchronized fashion at about 21 to 22 days of intrauterine life. At this early gestational age, the heart contracts without any identifiable conducting system, and the initial pacemaker is in the sinus venosus. Later, after day 24, when interatrial and interventricular septa are formed, the cardiac rate increases, and it is primarily directed by the sinus node through the newly formed conductive system. The sinus node is identifiable by the

sixth week, and the atrioventricular node is formed by the tenth week. By the sixteenth week of gestational age, the conductive system of the heart is functionally mature.

Classification

Several classifications have been proposed for fetal arrhythmias. One that classifies them according to regularity and rate is preferable.[14]

Irregular rhythms. Irregular rhythms are atrial or ventricular ectopic beats occurring more than 1 in every 10 beats. They account for over 85% of all FAs.[17] Usually the diagnosis is made incidentally during electronic monitoring or sonography. The cause may be atrial, ventricular, or nodal. However, most of them are atrial premature beats. In 1% to 2% of cases, an anatomic anomaly can be identified, and only 1% to 2% of them evolve into a sustained tachyarrhythmia. In the majority of cases, this type of arrhythmia resolves spontaneously during pregnancy or disappears during labor or immediately after delivery.

Tachyarrhythmias. Rapid rhythms are recurrent episodes of tachycardia greater than 180 bpm, lasting more than 10 seconds, and detected at least on two occasions, one day apart.[18] They affect 0.4% to 0.6% of all pregnancies and correspond to approximately 10% of all fetal arrhythmias. Most of them are supraventricular in origin and include sinus tachycardia, paroxysmal supraventricular tachycardia, and, rarely, Wolff-Parkinson-White syndrome, atrial fibrillation, and atrial flutter. Ventricular tachycardia occurs occasionally. Anatomic abnormalities, including cardiac tumors and Ebstein's malformation, are present in approximately 5% to 10% of the cases.

Paroxysmal supraventricular tachycardia (PST) is by far the most common fetal rapid arrhythmia and the one that has more clinical importance.[16,19] Persistent PST can lead to heart failure that may be diagnosed by the presence of various degrees of hydrops. The presence or absence of hydrops is the most important prognostic factor in the management of these fetuses.

Bradycardia. Fetal bradycardia is a rhythm of less than 100 bpm sustained during at least 10 seconds. Bradycardia, especially when associated with cardiac malformations, has an obscure prognosis. Fortunately, this type of arrhythmia is present in only 1 of 20,000 live births, and only 5% of fetal arrhythmias are classified as bradycardia. Fetal bradycardia may be caused by blocked premature contractions, complete heart block, sinus arrhythmia, congenital cardiac malformations, maternal medication, viral infections, maternal collagen vascular disease, umbilical cord or head compression, or profound fetal hypoxia.

Unfortunately, 40% of fetuses with complete heart block have anatomic malformations, the most common being atrioventricular canal defects and outflow vessel abnormalities. These fetuses usually develop hydrops and die in utero or shortly after birth. The prognosis is better for fetuses without anatomic abnormalities of the heart and with a heart rate of 50 bpm or above. The finding of a fetus with complete heart block and no associated congenital anomalies suggests that the arrhythmia originates from a maternal connective tissue disorder. In these cases maternal antibodies destroy the fetal cardiac conductive system.

Diagnosis

Fetal arrhythmias usually are an incidental finding during routine fetal assessment. They should be investigated by two-dimensional fetal echocardiography. One of the components of this examination, the M-mode ultrasound, can establish the type of arrhythmia, identify pericardial effusions, and measure wall thickness, chamber size, and fractional shortening. Doppler is another part of the fetal echocardiogram that is useful for assessing the adequacy of flow across the chambers and outflow tracts and for determining the degree of heart block. Through the use of this technique, it has been suggested that the heart flow is maintained within normal range until the heart rate drops below 50 beats/min or exceeds 230 beats/min.[17] Color flow mapping is another component of the fetal echocardiogram that is useful for identifying aberrant blood flow and congenital malformations.

There are maternal conditions that have to be considered when fetal arrhythmia is present. They are tachycardia, fever, intake of caffeine, and abnormal thyroid function.

Management

Irregular rhythms. Irregular rhythms should be managed expectantly. They are benign, and the possibilities of developing a rapid rhythm are only 1% to 2%.

Tachyarrythmias. The most common presentation is PST. Several management alternatives may be chosen, depending on the characteristics of each case.

In the absence of hydrops
1. Deliver the fetus at term
2. Use expectant management of the immature fetus
3. Administer antiarrhythmic agents

Administration of antiarrhythmic agents to the mother for nonhydropic fetuses is controversial. Most investigators recommend that the fetus be treated immediately after diagnosis, instead of waiting for hydrops to develop.

In the presence of hydrops. If PST is associated with hydrops, the condition must be considered a serious threat to the fetus and should be managed as a medical emergency by giving antiarrhythmic drugs to the mother. Therapy should start with high doses of digoxin, trying to maintain the maternal serum level between 1.5 and 2.0 ng/ml. Since digoxin absorption during pregnancy is erratic and the placental transfer is only about 40%, the maternal serum level should be tested periodically. Also, checking the maternal electrocardiogram for evidence of toxicity is warranted. It is necessary to continue the treatment for at least 3 weeks before considering it unsuccessful.

The second drug that can be used by itself, or in association with digoxin, is verapamil. Although the placental transfer is only 10% to 20%, its usefulness has been reported in several studies. Other drugs useful in the treatment of PST include procainamide, propranolol, furosemide, and quinidine. The presence of ventricular tachycardia contraindicates the use of digoxin or verapamil. If the arrhythmia persists and hydrops worsens despite a well-controlled medical treatment, the patient should be delivered.

Fetal administration of medications through cordocentesis has been reported. However, the risk involved in repeated procedures makes this approach less than ideal.

Bradycardia. When bradycardia is caused by blocked premature contractions, the heart rate frequency is above 50 beats/min, and there are no anatomic cardiac abnormalities. In cases of complete heart block, close examination should be made to detect anatomic abnormalities, ventricular hypertrophy, and development of hydrops. In cases with abnormal cardiac anatomy, the prognosis is poor, and the usual outcome is death in utero or shortly after birth. Experiences with in-utero treatment have been disappointing. Expectancy is the treatment of choice, and a good outcome is the most common result.

◢ ANENCEPHALY

Anencephaly is the absence of the cranial vault and cerebral hemispheres. It is the most common type of neural tube defect. Its incidence is approximately 1:1000 births in the United States, but in Ireland and Wales reaches 5:1000. The incidence has been estimated to be 5 times greater in abortion material than at birth. Females are affected more frequently than males, with a ratio of 4:1. The risk of recurrence is 5% after one affected child and 13% after 2 affected children. Because of this high risk of recurrence, every patient who has had a previous anencephalic child should be screened with ultrasound early in the second trimester.

The exact etiology of anencephaly is unknown. The defect is caused by a failure in the closure of the rostral neuropore at an early embryonic stage.

Pathologically, anencephaly is characterized by the absence of the structures derived from the forebrain and skull. The forebrain and midbrain are absent or replaced by rudimentary fibrovascular tissue and scattered islands of neural elements covering the crown of the head, or cerebrovasculosa. The cerebellum and midbrain are less involved or completely spared. The base of the skull and the facial bones are not affected, but the supraorbital region of the frontal bone and the parietal occipital squama of the temporal bone are absent. Other features that characterize these fetuses are bulging eyes, short neck, and a large tongue.

Diagnosis

Anencephaly was the first fetal anomaly detected in utero by sonography. The diagnosis is usually made by demonstration of an absence of the bony skull vault and of the brain cephalad to the orbits (Figure 17-2). The diagnosis may be suspected in the first trimester during examination with endovaginal probe, but usually it is not certain until after 14 weeks of gestation.[20] The accuracy of the sonographic diagnosis is 100% in experienced hands. Differential diagnosis must be made with severe forms of microcephaly, encephalocele, acrania, exencephaly, and with the cranial defects associated with an amniotic band syndrome.[21]

Screening for neural tube defects is usually done during the second trimester by estimation of maternal serum alpha-fetoprotein (MSAFP). Although this screening procedure is reliable, it does not differentiate anencephaly from other causes of elevated MSAFP. As explained in Chapter 2, an elevated MSAFP should be followed with ultrasound examination to rule out the possibility of anencephaly.

Polyhydramnios is present in approximately 35% of anencephaly cases. Its cause is not completely understood; diminished fetal swallowing, secretion of cerebrospinal fluid directly into the amniotic cavity, and excessive micturition have been implicated as possible etiologic factors.

Associated anomalies

The incidence of associated anomalies in anencephaly is approximately 30%, and half of them are spinal defects. The most frequent is spina bifida, which may be found in 27% of anencephalic babies. Other less common anomalies are hydronephrosis in 16%, cleft lip in 10%, omphalocele in 6%, and cardiac anomalies in 4% of the cases.

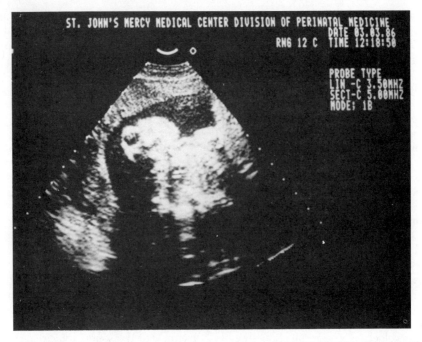

FIGURE 17-2 ▧ Anencephaly. Prominent eyes and absence of the cranial vault are apparent.

Prognosis and management

Anencephaly is uniformly fatal. Most fetuses deliver prematurely, although 15% of cases deliver postterm. Approximately 30% of these fetuses are born alive and die within the first hours of life. However, rare cases of survival for several months have been reported.

Since anencephaly has a lethal prognosis and its sonographic diagnosis is highly reliable, it is one of the few universally accepted indications for termination of pregnancy during the third trimester.[22] The use of anencephalic fetuses for organ transplantation is surrounded by ethical questions and is not accepted in many institutions.

▧ SPINA BIFIDA

Spina bifida, anencephaly, and encephalocele constitute a group of congenital anomalies known as neural tube defects (NTDs). Spina bifida is a midline defect of the spine resulting in exposure of the contents of the neural channel. The incidence of spina bifida in the United States is approximately 1 to 2 per 1000 births. The incidence is higher in England, approximately 4.5 per 1000 births. Caucasians apparently are at higher risk. The recurrence rate in England is 50 per 1000 after one affected child and 90 per 1000 after two affected children. In the United States the recurrence risk is 15 to 30 per 1000 after the first affected child and 57 per 1000 after two affected children.

Recent British studies[23] report a decline in the prevalence of NTDs during the past decade. The reasons for this trend are unknown, and only a part of this tendency may be attributed to antenatal testing. Other explanations include environmental factors, vitamin deficiency, and malnutrition, but they are inconclusive. The implications of this epidemiologic change are unknown and require further investigation.

NTDs are multifactorial in origin. Approximately 90% of fetuses with NTD are born to women who have no predisposing factors. However, malformations that follow a Mendelian pattern of inheritance, trisomies 18 and 13 or triploidy; exposure to valproic acid, thalidomide, or aminopterin; and maternal diabetes are etiologically related factors.

Classification

The term *spina bifida* encompasses several types of spinal abnormalities. Classically, spina bifida has been divided into *aperta* (open) or *oc-*

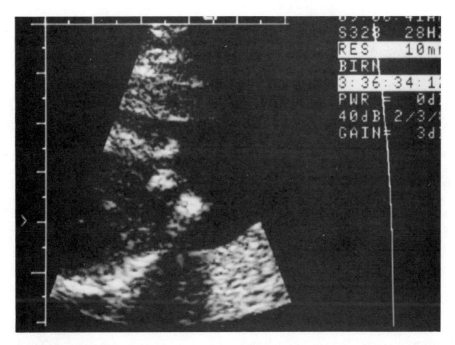

FIGURE 17-3 ◪ Spina bifida. There is an open space between the abnormally separated posterior ossification centers in this transverse scan of a 20-week fetus with open spina bifida.

culta (closed). The latter represents approximately 20% of the cases of spina bifida. Spina bifida occulta usually is a small, clinically asymptomatic defect, covered by skin, that can only be diagnosed through radiographic examination. In rare cases the lesion may be apparent by the presence of a subcutaneous lipoma. In open spina bifida, the defect is usually covered by a thin meningeal membrane, giving the appearance of a cystic tumor. If the mass contains spinal fluid and meningeal tissue, it is known as meningocele. If it contains spinal fluid and neural tissue, it is referred to as myelomeningocele. Spina bifida affects the lumbosacral region of the spine in more than 63% of the cases. Ventral defects of the spine are extremely rare.

Associated anomalies

One typical central nervous system lesion associated with spina bifida is hydrocephalus caused by the presence of an Arnold-Chiari malformation type II. In this type of anomaly, the cerebellar vermis is herniated through the foramen magnum, displacing the fourth ventricle inside the neural canal and causing obstructive hydrocephalus. Other associated central nervous system malformations include holoprosenceph-

aly, agenesis of the corpus callosum, and polymicrogyria. Limb deformities include clubfoot and dislocation of the hip. The pathogenesis of these defects is related to the unopposed action of muscle groups caused by a defect in the peripheral nerve corresponding to the involved myotomes.[24] Other less frequently seen abnormalities affect the gastrointestinal and renal systems. Chromosomal anomalies have also been reported.

Diagnosis

Spina bifida is the NTD most difficult to diagnose by sonography. To diagnosis the condition, the sonographer must be completely familiar with the normal appearance of the fetal spine.

The spine can be visualized in any of three main planes of examination: coronal, transverse, or sagittal. For the diagnosis of spina bifida, the ideal visualization is in the transverse plane. In this plane the three bony structures of the spinal axis are clearly seen. They are the two lateral processes of the vertebra and the midline vertebral body. In cases of spina bifida, typically there is absence of the posterior laminae, and the lateral vertebral processes are set apart. The soft tissue covering the defect is also absent (Figure 17-3).

There are central nervous system sonographic signs useful in the diagnosis of spina bifida.[25] They are the "lemon" sign and the "banana" sign. The former is a scalloping deformity of the frontal calvarium, best seen when scanning in the ventricular plane. It is so called because the cranium resembles the form of a lemon (Figure 17-4). In a study of 130 cases of spina bifida,[26] the lemon sign was found in 98% of fetuses with a gestational age of 24 weeks or less. However, as many as 1% of normal patients may have the lemon sign. The sign disappears spontaneously before 34 weeks.

The banana sign describes the curved shape of the cerebellar hemispheres wrapped around the posterior midbrain that is compressed into the posterior fossa because of an Arnold-Chiari malformation. The demonstration of an obliterated cisterna magna complements the diagnosis. In one study[25] the predominant cerebellum abnormality found in fetuses at 24 weeks or less was the banana sign (72%), whereas after this gestational age, a sonographic "absence" of cerebellum was found in 81% of the patients. In another study[27] visualization of the banana sign had a sensitivity of 96% and a negative predictive value of 100% for the diagnosis of spina bifida.

Other useful sonographic signs include the identification of a clubfoot and associated hydrocephalus. The latter has been reported in as many as 90% of cases of spina bifida, but only in 75% of cases before 24 weeks.

The accuracy of ultrasound to diagnose spina bifida depends on the experience of the ultrasonographer, the type of population studied (low or high risk) and the resolution of the equipment used. Several recent studies have demonstrated a diagnostic sensitivity of over 83% and a specificity of near 99%.

A method extensively used to improve the diagnosis of spina bifida is screening with MSAFP. This topic is treated extensively in Chapter 2.

Prognosis

The prognosis of spina bifida depends on the localization of the lesion, its extent, and its association with hydrocephalus or other abnormalities. Lesions localized high in the spine have the worst prognosis. In general, treated patients have a 40% rate of survival at 7 years of age. Of the survivors, only 25% have no major sequelae. The rest have several degrees of physical disability or neurologic impairment. At the present time, it is impossible to predict antenatally the outcome of patients with spina bifida.

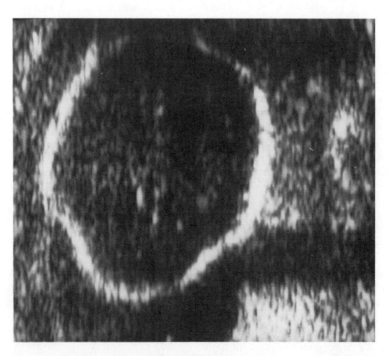

FIGURE 17-4 ▰ Lemon sign.

Management

Termination of the pregnancy is an option when the diagnosis is made early in gestation. Management of viable fetuses concerns mainly the timing and the mode of delivery. These fetuses should be delivered at term, with the exception of those developing a rapidly progressive hydrocephalus. However, even in these fetuses lung maturity should be assured before delivery. The mode of delivery is controversial. Some report a 14% incidence of cerebral brain injury with neurologic deficit after vaginal delivery in patients with myelomeningocele. On the other hand, a recent study of 72 infants with spina bifida,[28] followed for 1 year after delivery, failed to demonstrate any benefit of abdominal over vaginal delivery. Delivery should take place in a tertiary center, where a team of neurosurgeons, pediatricians, and rehabilitation therapists is available for immediate evaluation.

◪ HYDROCEPHALUS

Congenital hydrocephalus is an etiologically heterogeneous condition resulting in an abnormal increase in cerebrospinal fluid within the ventricular and subarachnoid spaces of the brain. Hydrocephalus is one of the most common congenital abnormalities. Its overall incidence ranges from 0.12 to 2.5 per 1000 births in the United States, and it is as high as 6 per 1000 births in the United Kingdom. It seems to have predilection for males. The incidence of isolated hydrocephalus is lower, ranging between 0.39 and 0.87 per 1000 births.[29]

The risk of recurrence of hydrocephaly after a first affected child is approximately 2%. A more precise risk can be calculated if the underlying cause is known. For example, the risk in X-linked aqueductal stenosis is approximately 25%.

Physiopathology

The cerebrospinal fluid is formed in the choroid plexus and cerebral capillaries of the ventricular system and flows in a unidirectional fashion from the lateral ventricles into the third ventricle across the foramen of Monro and to the fourth ventricle through the aqueduct of Sylvius. From the fourth ventricle it moves through the foramen of Luschka into the basal cisterns and reaches the subarachnoid space by moving across the foramen of Magendie. The fluid is then reabsorbed by the pacchionian granulations, which are distributed along the superior sagittal sinus.

In most patients with hydrocephalus, there is an alteration in cerebrospinal fluid dynamics, usually the result of an obstructive process, causing an increase in intraventricular pressure. There are other causes of an increase in cerebrospinal fluid, such as destructive brain processes or developmental anomalies in which the affected tissue areas are replaced by fluid, but in those cases the intraventricular pressure usually remains normal.

The cause and the site of the obstruction are the most important features in the pathogenesis of hydrocephalus. The amount of fluid produced and its rate of flow and absorption are also determining factors of the severity of ventricular dilation.

Diagnosis

The prenatal diagnosis of hydrocephalus is usually made by the demonstration of a dilated ventricular system in an ultrasound examination (Figure 17-5). The most widely used measurement has been the lateral ventricular-to-hemisphere width (LVW/HW) ratio in the biparietal and coronal planes. This ratio is approximately 0.71 at 15 weeks and decreases to 0.37 at 25 weeks. These figures reflect the normal decrease in the ventricular-to-brain ratio that occurs as the fetus develops. The LVW/HW ratio is useful after 24 weeks, and any value over 0.5 can be considered abnormal.[28] However, its reliability in the detection of hydrocephalus before 24 weeks is controversial. Other morphologic criteria, such as the asymmetric appearance of the choroid plexus, the size and configuration of the horns, and the diameter of the atria of the lateral ventricles, have been useful in the early diagnosis of the condition.[30-32]

Unlike the LVW/HW, the diameter of the atria remains constant during the second and third trimesters,[30] and its enlargement is the earliest sonographic sign of hydrocephalus. The mean value for the diameter of the atria from 15 to 35 weeks is 7.6 ± 0.6 mm and should not exceed 10 mm. The transverse atrial diameter is the most accurate measurement for the detection of hydrocephalus during the second and third trimesters (Figure 17-6).

An accurate diagnosis and classification of fetal hydrocephalus requires a systematic sonographic evaluation of the posterior fossa, the third and fourth ventricles, the subarachnoid space, and the bony calvaria and a careful examination of the fetal spine. The latter has special

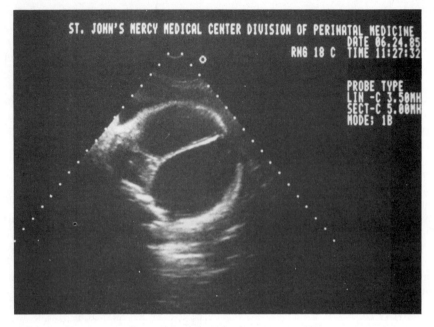

FIGURE 17-5 ◪ Hydrocephalus. Marked dilation of both lateral ventricles in this fetus with aqueductal stenosis.

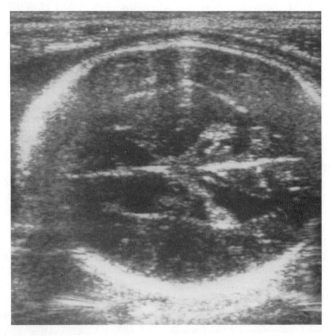

FIGURE 17-6 ◪ Hydrocephalus. Fetus with mildly dilated ventricles and atrial diameter larger than 10 mm. The choroid plexus is shrunk within the atrium.

importance since as many as 30% of hydrocephalic fetuses have associated spina bifida, most commonly in the lumbar area.

Associated anomalies

Hydrocephalus is associated with other anomalies in over 50% of the cases. This association may be as high as 84%. Intracranial anomalies are present in 37% of the cases, the most common being cephalocele, arachnoid cyst, agenesis of corpus callosum, and arteriovenous malformations. Extracranial anomalies exist in approximately 63% of the patients. These include myelomeningocele, scoliosis, spinal dysraphism, and vertebral body anomalies. In the renal system the most common anomalies are hydronephrosis and dysplastic kidneys. Ventricular septal defects, Fallot tetralogy, and hypoplastic left heart syndrome are the most common cardiac abnormalities. Gastrointestinal malformations are less common and include omphalocele, gastroschisis, tracheoesophagic fistula, and malrotation of the bowel. Finally, chromosomal abnormalities are seen in 11% of the patients. These include Down syndrome, trisomies 13 and 18, balanced translocations, and mosaicisms.

Classification

There are several classifications for hydrocephalus. The most useful divides hydrocephalus into three major groups, which differ in etiology, sonographic manifestations, and prognosis.

Aqueductal stenosis. Aqueductal stenosis is the most common cause of hydrocephalus, accounting for approximately 38% to 43% of the cases. It has predilection for females. The condition results from the narrowing of the aqueduct of Sylvius, which leads to a characteristic dilation of the lateral and third ventricles. Aqueductal stenosis may be produced by diverse agents. Several studies have demonstrated that it may be inherited as an X-linked recessive trait. Infectious processes related to the disease include syphilis, toxoplasmosis, CMV, and influenza virus. The real role of teratogenic factors is unknown, and the incidence of associated neoplastic processes is extremely low.

Aqueductal stenosis must be suspected when the sonogram shows dilated third and lateral ventricles and a normal fourth ventricle. These sonographic features are infrequent, and the differential diagnosis with other forms of hydrocephaly is sometimes impossible to make in utero. Careful examination of the fetal spine is warranted in search for associated spina bifida.

Communicating hydrocephalus. Communicating hydrocephalus is a form of ventricular dilation caused by an obstruction in the flow of cerebrospinal fluid outside the ventricular system. It accounts for 38% of all cases of hydrocephalus. It has been associated with hemorrhage, obliteration of the superior sagittal sinus, and absence of pacchionian granulations, but in most cases the etiology is unknown.

Communicating hydrocephalus should be suspected after finding sonographic dilation of the ventricular system, including the fourth ventricle and the subarachnoid cistern. However, dilation of the latter is not always present, and the differential diagnosis with aqueductal stenosis may be difficult if not impossible to make. Serial sonographic studies are advisable to evaluate progression and to attempt to define a cause.

Dandy-Walker malformation. The Dandy-Walker syndrome includes three classic features: hydrocephalus, posterior fossa cyst, and a defect in the cerebellar vermis. It accounts for approximately 5% to 10% of cases of hydrocephalus. Its cause is unknown, although it has been associated with Mendelian disorders, chromosomal abnormalities, infectious processes such as CMV, toxoplasmosis, and rubella, and exposure to coumadin and alcohol. Approximately 80% of patients with Dandy-Walker malformation have hydrocephalus.[33] However, the degree of hydrocephalus varies; some cases with open foramina of Luschka and Magendie may never develop hydrocephalus in utero. The incidence of associated cerebral defects is as high as 68%.

Dandy-Walker malformation should be suspected in the presence of a cyst in the posterior fossa and associated hydrocephalus. The differential diagnosis must include arachnoid cyst and dilation of the cisterna magna.

Prognosis

The incidence of early neonatal death and poor neurologic outcome and life expectancy are directly related to the presence and severity of the associated anomalies.[34] The mortality for hydrocephalus is 67% overall, but it drops to 37% for fetuses without anomalies outside of the central nervous system. In the past some studies[35] suggested that cortical mantle thickness was a prognostic factor, but long-term follow-up has failed to demonstrate any correlation with neurologic outcome.

Management

Once the diagnosis of hydrocephalus has been made, amniocentesis for determination of fetal karyotype and viral cultures should be performed. A level II ultrasound should be performed for the diagnosis of associated anomalies. The delivery should be delayed until fetal lung maturity is assured. Since only about 37% of hydrocephalic fetuses have some degree of macrocephaly,[34] cesarean section should not be routinely practiced, and a trial of labor should be offered in a vertex presentation. Cephalocentesis should be reserved for macrocephalic fetuses with severe associated anomalies that assure a dismal prognosis. Cesarean section should be performed for the macrocephalic fetus without associated malformations or for obstetric indications.[35]

In-utero shunting procedures have had disappointing results, even in fetuses who have early and progressive hydrocephalus and are too immature for delivery. In a study of 44 cases, the intraoperative mortality was 10%, and the overall procedure-related mortality was 17%. Only 35% of the treated fetuses were normal on serial postoperative testing, whereas 65% had varying degrees of neurologic and systemic defects. The incidence of false-negative sonographic examination for associated malformations was a discouraging 22%.[36]

◪ CYSTIC HYGROMA

Cystic hygroma is a malformation of the lymphatic system characterized by the presence of single or multiloculated fluid-filled cavities in the fetal posterior cervical region. The incidence of cystic hygroma is poorly defined and probably ranges between 5 and 15 per 1000 live births. The risk of recurrence, if associated with chromosomal abnormalities, is around 1%. However, if the cause is related to an autosomal-related condition, the risk may be as high as 25%.[37]

Cystic hygromas result from a drainage defect in the fetal lymphatic system. In the normal fetus the lympathic vessels drain into two sacs lateral to the jugular veins. At approximately 40 days of gestation, these sacs develop communications into the venous system and become the terminal portions of the right lymphatic duct and

the thoracic duct. Failure to develop these communications leads to an accumulation of lymph in cystic structures localized in the posterior triangles of the neck and in other tissues. This series of events and their resulting phenotypic features comprises the so-called jugular lymphatic-obstruction sequence. Theoretically, this sequence can be reversed by the formation of alternative routes of lymph drainage, and there are reported cases of in-utero regression of the disease.[38] Webbing of the neck and puffiness of the extremities are characteristic postnatal features in these cases.

The most commonly associated chromosomal abnormality in patients with cystic hygroma is Turner's syndrome. Other conditions are trisomy 21, trisomy 18, and several forms of mosaicism. Malformation syndromes, such as Noonan's syndrome, Robert's syndrome, fetal-alcohol syndrome, and familial pterygium colli are also related. In-utero exposure to aminopterin and trimethadione has also been reported in relation with cystic hygroma.

Diagnosis

The diagnosis of cystic hygroma can be made with high reliability through sonographic examination. A large cystic mass occupying the posterolateral aspect of the fetal neck is characteristic (Figure 17-7). Sometimes the cystic contents are interrupted by septae that occasionally can be incomplete. Large septated, multilocular hygromas seem to a have a worse prognosis than nonseptated ones.

A differential diagnosis must be made with encephalocele, meningocele, cystic teratoma, twin sac of a blighted ovum, a subcorial placental cyst, a nuchal bleb, and with an amniotic band syndrome.

Prognosis

Two types of cystic hygromas have been described, each with a different prognosis. In one type the diagnosis is usually made after 30 weeks of gestation. It consists of a localized lymphatic defect without associated fetal hydrops or other abnormalities. This condition has a fairly good prognosis, and surgical repair may be performed at any time during the neonatal period. This type forms the group of cystic hygromas familiar to the pediatricians.[39]

The second type of cystic hygroma is that of cases diagnosed early in pregnancy. In the first

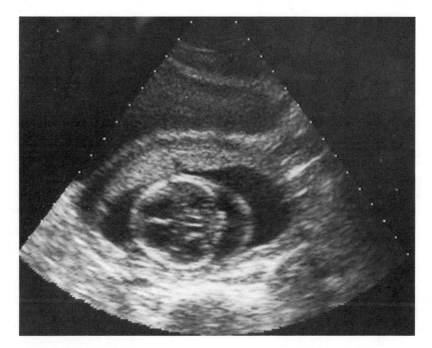

FIGURE 17-7 ◢ Cystic hygroma. A cystic formation is apparent in the posterior aspect of the fetal head. Karyotype revealed trisomy 21.

trimester the lesion has the sonographic appearance of a nuchal membrane and is associated with chromosome abnormalities in approximately 60% of the cases. The majority of fetuses with normal chromosomes have spontaneous resolution of the lesion before 20 weeks. In the second trimester the lesion has the sonographic characteristics of a cystic hygroma and may be associated with nonimmunologic hydrops. The cystic lesion may be multiloculated, and the frequency of chromosome abnormalities is greater than 80%. Fetal death usually occurs shortly after diagnosis. The cause of death has been related to chronic fetal hypoxemia caused by compression of the thoracic structures by the generalized edema. The association with hydrops fetalis is the most important prognostic factor.[40] When hydrops is present, the fetal mortality rate is near 100%.

Management

A detailed sonographic evaluation for cardiac anomalies, pleural or pericardial effusions, and skin edema should be performed after the diagnosis of cystic hygroma. The fetal karyotype should be obtained, and expectancy for spontaneous resolution should follow a normal result.

There is no available in-utero treatment for cystic hygroma. Because of its extremely poor prognosis, termination of pregnancy should be an option when the diagnosis is made before viability and the chromosomes are abnormal. In cases of late diagnosis without associated hydrops, expectant management is indicated. Intrapartum management should be conservative. Cesarean section should be reserved for patients with isolated cystic lesions and no associated hydrops. Gigantic cystic masses may cause dystocia, and if present in a nonhydropic fetus, a cesarean section should be performed.

◢ HYPOPLASTIC LEFT HEART SYNDROME

Hypoplastic left heart syndrome (HLHS) is a condition characterized by underdevelopment of the left side of the heart. It encompasses several degrees of hypoplasia of the aorta, aortic valve, mitral valve, left atrium, and left ventricle.

The incidence of this anomaly is estimated to be 10% to 15% of all congenital cardiac anomalies. The cause is unknown. Its risk of recurrence is only 0.5%. However, some investigators[41] have suggested the possibility of an autosomal recessive inheritance in some cases with a recurrence risk of approximately 25%.

In fetuses with HLHS the ascending aorta is usually hypoplastic, and in as many as 80% of the cases, aortic coarctation is present. An important physiopathologic role is played by the aortic atresia, which causes a diminished right-to-left shunt at the level of the atria. The left heart is nonfunctional, and the right heart maintains both the pulmonary and the systemic circulations. This hemodynamic alteration makes the fetal systemic perfusion ductus–arteriosus dependent. Hence the onset of cardiac decompensation in HLHS fetuses is delayed until several hours after birth.

Diagnosis

The prenatal diagnosis of HLHS relies on ultrasound, Doppler, color flow mapping, and M-mode echocardiography. HLHS alters the normal appearance of the four-chamber view of the heart (Figure 17-8). This view is of great importance in the evaluation of the fetus in routine obstetric ultrasound examinations. It has 92% sensitivity, 99.7% specificity, and 95.8% positive predictive and 99.4% negative predictive values in the detection of congenital heart disease.[42]

The demonstration of a dilated and hypertrophic right ventricle, atrium, and tricuspid valve, associated with hypoplasia of left heart structures and the aortic arch, makes the diagnosis. Most of the time, the left heart structures and the ascending aorta are hard to identify.

The precise diagnosis of HLHS is not always feasible. Adequate visualization of the cardiac structures is sometimes difficult after 30 weeks, when increased amounts of bone calcium produce rib and vertebral shadowing. Hydrops is not a constant feature in fetuses with HLHS. However, its presence should raise the suspicion of an additional obstructive or regurgitant lesion in the right heart.

Prognosis

The prognosis of fetuses with HLHS is extremely poor. Approximately 95% of all affected infants die within the first months of life. HLHS is responsible for 25% of all cardiac deaths in the first week of life. The presence of accompanying hydrops makes the prognosis more obscure.

Management

A careful sonographic examination should be performed in search for associated anomalies. A karyotype should be obtained. Sonographic eval-

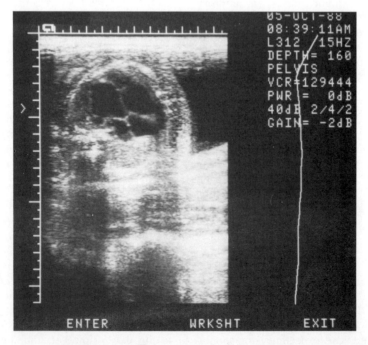

FIGURE 17-8 ◪ Four-chamber view of the heart.

uation must be done periodically to detect signs of heart failure. The presence of signs of heart failure indicates an extremely poor prognosis. If the diagnosis is made before the fetus is viable, termination of pregnancy should be offered. In the intrapartum management of these fetuses, the option of not performing a cesarean section in case of fetal distress should be considered. If an aggressive management is decided on, the delivery should occur in a tertiary center where a cardiovascular team should be available to undertake surgical care of the neonate. If the fetus is delivered in a hospital without adequate resources for neonatal cardiac surgery, prostaglandin E_1 should be used to prevent closure of the ductus until the infant is transferred to another facility. Palliative procedures include atrial septectomy and banding of the pulmonary artery with the creation of an aortopulmonary shunt. Surgical postnatal treatment of these neonates with the Norwood procedure or with cardiac transplantation has elevated mortality.[43]

◢ DIAPHRAGMATIC HERNIA

Congenital diaphragmatic hernia (CDH) is a herniation of the abdominal contents into the fetal thorax through a diaphragmatic defect. CDH occurs in approximately 1 of every 2000 to 5000 births. It is a sporadic malformation with a risk of recurrence of 2%. A familial recurrence has also been reported. These familial cases have a higher male-to-female ratio, a high incidence of bilateral defects, and a lower incidence of associated life-threatening malformations than sporadic cases.[44]

The cause of CDH is unknown. Maternal ingestion of thalidomide, quinine, and antiepileptic drugs has been associated with sporadic cases.

The development of the diaphragm begins at approximately 3 weeks of intrauterine life and is mostly complete by the ninth week, when a well-defined septum dividing the thorax and abdomen can be identified. The formation of the diaphragm is achieved by the fusion of four developmental compartments: the ventral or septum transversus, the lateral aspects formed from muscular components of the body wall, the dorsal esophageal mesentery, and the pleuroperitoneal membrane. Diaphragmatic defects may result from a delayed fusion of the four compartments or from a primary diaphragmatic malformation. In either case, the diaphragmatic defect permits the migration of the abdominal contents into the thoracic cavity. The negative pressure created by fetal breathing movements will contribute to this process.

From a pathologic point of view, CDH includes five different types of defects: hernia of Bochdalek, hernia of the foramen of Morgagni, diaphragmatic eventration, agenesis of the diaphragm, and esophageal hiatal hernia. The prenatal diagnosis of CDH only includes the first three categories. Diaphragmatic agenesis and esophageal hiatal hernia are rare entities with little relevance in prenatal diagnosis.

Bochdaleck's hernias account for as many as 90% of the fetal diaphragmatic anomalies. They are caused by a defect in the closure of the pleuroperitoneal membranes. They usually appear as a posterolateral defect, affecting the left hemithorax in 80% of the cases. The small bowel is involved in 90% of the cases, the stomach in 60%, the colon in 56%, and the spleen in 54%. The pancreas, liver, and kidneys may also be involved, but to a lesser extent.[44-46]

Approximately 5% of CDHs are eventrations of the diaphragm. They are characterized by a sac of herniated viscera covered by abdominal peritoneum, which elevates a weak aponeurotic diaphragm. Usually they involve the whole hemidiaphragm and are more common in the right side than in the left, although bilateral cases have also been reported.

Hernias of the foramen of Morgagni account for approximately 2% of all diaphragmatic defects. They appear in the anteromedial retrosternal portion of the diaphragm, most commonly in the right hemithorax, and often lack a peritoneal covering. They are usually caused by a maldevelopment of the septum transversus. The most commonly herniated organ is the liver, followed by the colon, the stomach, and the small bowel. Herniation into the pericardial sac also has been reported.

The displacement of intrabdominal content into the thoracic compartment alters the normal development of the lungs. Fetal lung development is an active process that begins around 5 to 6 weeks and continues throughout gestation and after birth. In the normal fetus, the bronchial tree is completely developed, and a full number of airways are established by 16 weeks. The alveoli develop through a canalicular phase that ends at approximately 24 weeks and then goes through a terminal sac period until the fetus reaches term. The alveolar development continues in the postnatal period until approximately 8 years of age. Normal expansion of the pulmonary tissue and fetal breathing movements are necessary to assure normal lung growth.

The severity of pulmonary developmental abnormalities depends on when and to what extent viscera herniate into the chest. If the herniation occurs before the sixteenth week of intrauterine life, the number of bronchial divisions will be reduced. If the compression is persistent, the airway size will be diminished, and the number and size of saccule, alveoli, and preacinar and intraacinar vessels will be decreased. The potential for further growth and development after surgical decompression will depend on the time at which the insult was initiated.

Associated anomalies

Excluding lung hypoplasia and gut malrotation, which are part of the pathophysiologic sequence of the disease, CDH is related to other anomalies in 16% to 57% of the cases. Classically, CDH has been associated with neural tube defects, omphalocele, and oral cleft. Other anomalies include the cardiac, gastrointestinal, skeletal, and genitourinary systems. Cardiac defects are present in 23% of patients. The most common malformations are tetralogy of Fallot and interventricular septal defects. Chromosomal abnormalities such as trisomies 13, 21, and 18 also occur in association with CDH. The Morgagni type of CDH has been associated with trisomy 21 in several reports. Familial cases of CDH have a lower incidence of associated malformations.

Diagnosis

The sonographic diagnosis of CDH is based on these findings:[43,47]

1. Inability to demonstrate a normal fetal upper abdominal anatomy, particularly the inability to visualize the fetal stomach
2. Displacement of the fetal mediastinum
3. Presence of cystic or solid intrathoracic mass containing abdominal organs
4. Smaller than expected abdominal circumference
5. Polyhydramnios.

Once the diagnosis is suspected, a close examination of the fetal thorax in search of specific herniated abdominal contents should be undertaken. Left-sided CDHs are easier to diagnose; the echo-free fluid stomach and small bowel contrast with the more echogenic lung tissue,

and peristalsis may be observed. A useful hint in the diagnosis of CDH is the presence of abdominal contents in a transverse view of the fetal thorax, at the same level as the four-chamber view of the heart. Similarly, abdominal organs that are visualized cephalad to the inferior margin of the scapula are likely to be herniated. CDH is a dynamic process, and the abdominal herniated viscera move in and out of the fetal chest. When a sonographic diagnosis of CDH is highly suspected but not conclusive, amniography with or without computed tomography may be helpful. The diagnosis of CDH has been made as early as 18 weeks of gestation. Polyhydramnios, a diagnostic feature present in as many as 76% of cases, appears only late in pregnancy. Its presence has been related to upper gastrointestinal obstruction.

The antenatal differential diagnosis among the three types of CDH is difficult. Diaphragmatic eventration has the same features as a Bochdalek's hernia, but the abdominal circumference is usually normal. Morgagni's hernias are anteriorly located and may be accompanied by pericardial and pleural effusions.

The differential diagnosis of CDH includes other intrathoracic masses such as congenital cystic malformation of the lung, bronchogenic and enteric cysts, mediastinal cystic teratoma, pulmonary sequestration, bronchial atresia, and unilateral agenesis of the lung.

Prognosis

The prognosis of CDH is poor and has not changed much in recent years, in spite of advances in perinatal and postnatal care. The presence of associated anomalies is the most important prognostic factor. The association of central nervous system and cardiac anomalies has the worst prognosis. The presence of chromosomal abnormalities also compromises the prognosis and management. The mortality rate is also related to respiratory insufficiency caused by variable degrees of lung hypoplasia. The reported survival rate varies widely. Some estimates are as low as 10.5%. Others report 50% survival for fetuses who lived beyond delivery.

Other prognostic factors include the site of the fetal stomach when the diagnosis is initially made and the size and bilaterality of the diaphragmatic defect. Also, detection of early cardiac disproportion has a poor prognosis. The time of onset and degree of ventricular disproportion have been related to the degree of pulmonary hypoplasia. Polyhydramnios is a controversial sign of poor prognosis.

Management

Once the diagnosis of CDH has been made, an ultrasound level II study in search of associated anomalies and fetal echocardiography should be performed. Also, a cytogenetic study is warranted. If the diagnosis is made before viability, termination of pregnancy may be offered to the parents. In viable fetuses, the best approach is expectant management. The timing and mode of delivery must not be altered. The delivery must take place in a tertiary center where a team of pediatric surgeons and neonatologists can offer immediate assistance.

Therapeutic thoracentesis has been used in the third trimester to improve fetal cardiovascular dynamics. Successful in-utero surgery has been described. The procedure should be limited to fetuses with no associated abnormalities, a normal chromosomal study, and characteristics indicating a prediction that they will have a lethal outcome without antenatal repair. Unfortunately, it is not possible to identify such fetuses with accuracy. The techniques used are closure of the diaphragmatic defect and enlargement of the abdominal cavity with a patch to adequately accommodate the herniated contents.[48,49] In-utero surgery has significant complications including preterm labor, PROM, chorioamnionitis, and fetal death. The procedure is experimental, and further evaluation of the risks vs. the prognosis of a conservative approach will take place over the coming years.

◢ PLEURAL EFFUSION

Pleural effusion in the fetus may be primary or may be a component of generalized fetal hydrops. Primary pleural effusion is a relatively rare prenatal finding. It was first described as an isolated ultrasonic abnormality in 1978, and its association with pulmonary hypoplasia was first reported in 1981. The causes include chylothorax, intrauterine viral infections, congenital pulmonary lymphangiectasia, and Turner's and Down syndrome. Congenital chylothorax is by far the most common cause. This anomaly is associated with a high mortality rate, estimated between 15% and 57%.[50,51]

Diagnosis

The most important ultrasonic sign is an echo-free area between the lungs, chest wall, and dia-

phragm. Other findings include mediastinal shift and polyhydramnios. Approximately 67% of the cases have been initially diagnosed in the third trimester of pregnancy. Male infants are affected more than twice as often as females. Right-sided effusions are more common than left-sided, and a small number are bilateral (Figure 17-9).

Chylothorax, the most common cause of pleural effusion, can be diagnosed antenatally by demonstrating a predominance of lymphocytes on the differential cell count of the fluid. In the newborn it can be diagnosed by demonstrating chylomicrons in the pleural fluid after feeding the baby.

The most important differential diagnosis is with hydrops fetalis. In hydrops there are invariably other ultrasonic features including cutaneous edema, ascites, pericardial effusion, and placental enlargement.

Prognosis

The prognosis depends on the cause, associated anomalies, time of initiation of the effusion, and its evolution. Serial ultrasound should be performed to define persistence, resolution, or worsening of the lesion. Several studies have demonstrated spontaneous resolution of pleural effusion in utero. The presence of pulmonary hypoplasia and associated abnormalities is a major adverse prognostic factor. Unilaterality and absence of hydrops are good prognostic signs.

Management

Because of the recognized association between congenital pleural effusion and Down syndrome, amniocentesis should be performed to rule out chromosomal abnormalities. Sonography should be performed at intervals of 2 to 3 weeks to follow the course of the disease.

Intrauterine thoracentesis for decompression is impractical, other than immediately before delivery, because the fluid reaccumulates in the fetus within 6 to 48 hours after aspiration. Prepartum aspiration of fetal hydrothorax seems to facilitate neonatal resuscitation. Long-term drainage using pleuroamniotic shunts seems a good alternative during second trimester, in fetuses with normal chromosomes and no associated life-threatening abnormalities.[52] This procedure has been successful and prevented the development of pulmonary hypoplasia. In cases diagnosed late in pregnancy, expectant management is the best approach when the hydrothorax is small and unilateral. When the effusion is large

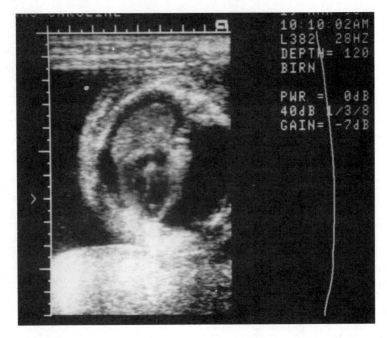

FIGURE 17-9 ◪ Bilateral pleural effusion. Pleural effusion is more prominent on the left side. The mediastinum and the heart are deviated toward the right. The heart shows four chambers, and there is no pericardial effusion. The right lung is posterior to the heart.

and its duration unknown, it may be preferable to place a pleuroamniotic shunt and decompress the lungs for several days before delivery. Delivery should take place in a tertiary center where aggressive neonatal support can be offered.

◪ GASTROSCHISIS

Gastroschisis is a paraumbilical defect of the anterior abdominal wall, through which abdominal viscera herniate. The defect is usually located at the right side of the cord insertion and compromises the full thickness of the abdominal wall. There is no sac or membrane covering the herniated organs. The incidence of gastroschisis is approximately 1 per 12,000 live births. Gastroschisis appears to be a sporadic event with no genetic association or recurrence risks.

The defect is usually small and located to the right of the umbilical cord insertion. The herniated organ is usually the bowel, and very rarely are other structures involved. Since there is no membrane covering the defect, the herniated bowel is continuously exposed to the irritating effect of the amniotic fluid, which produces thickening and edema of the intestinal wall. The bowel may appear covered by an inflammatory exudate.

The physiopathology of gastroschisis is controversial. The defect seems to result from an ischemic event at an early embryonic stage, either caused by a disruption of the right omphalomesenteric artery or by an alteration in the normal involution of the right umbilical vein.

Associated anomalies

In contrast with omphalocele, gastroschisis rarely is associated with other congenital abnormalities. The most frequently associated anomalies are gastrointestinal in origin and are related to the same vascular embryologic problem that causes the gastroschisis. Intestinal atresia, or stenosis, is found in 7% to 30% of the cases. Cardiac malformations are found in 8% of the cases, and sporadic cases of diaphragmatic hernia have been reported in fetuses with gastroschisis. Gastroschisis is also associated with IUGR and preterm labor.

Diagnosis

The sonographic diagnosis of gastroschisis may be made incidentally during a routine sonographic study or after a patient is referred because of high alpha-fetoprotein titer. The diagnosis is based on the presence of a mass adjacent to

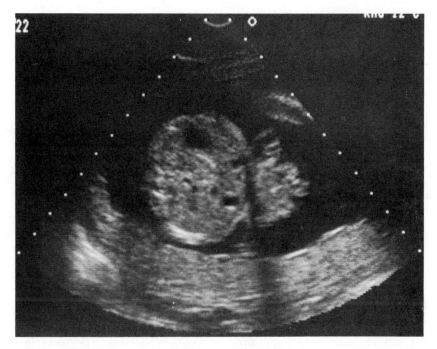

FIGURE 17-10 ◢ Gastroschisis. Loops of bowel are floating freely in the amniotic fluid in this transverse view of the fetal abdomen. The stomach and the liver are inside the abdomen.

the anterior abdominal wall[53] (Figure 17-10). The most valuable diagnostic findings that help to make a differential diagnosis with omphalocele are:

1. Presence of a normal cord insertion
2. Paraumbilical defect, usually on the right side
3. No evidence of membrane covering the defect, with the herniated organs floating in the amniotic fluid
4. Thickened bowel loops that are matted together

A differential diagnosis with omphalocele can be made in over 75% of the cases. This is important, since omphalocele has a much greater incidence of associated chromosomal and cardiac abnormalities and a worse prognosis. Other features that may help in the diagnosis of gastroschisis are the presence of polyhydramnios, which is not a constant finding, and the absence of multiple herniated organs.

Prognosis

The mortality is about 8% to 14%. This figure has been declining in the past few years because of advances in postnatal intensive care and surgery. The major causes of death are related to surgical complications, sepsis, and prematurity.

The sonographic appearance of the herniated bowel has been proposed as a prognostic factor. Thickening of the intestinal wall and small bowel dilation are considered by some as indicators of poor neonatal outcome. However, other studies have shown no clinical advantage in the use of these sonographic signs.

Management

After the diagnosis of gastroschisis has been made, it is necessary to perform a level II ultrasound examination to rule out the presence of other anomalies. A fetal echocardiogram and fetal karyotyping should also be performed.

Termination of pregnancy is an option that should be discussed when the diagnosis is made before viability. In the viable fetus, after the initial workup, serial sonographic studies are indicated for the detection of complications such as IUGR, bowel obstruction, or polyhydramnios. Delivery should be performed once pulmonary maturity is confirmed to decrease the duration of exposure of the bowel to the extraabdominal environment.

The mode of delivery for these fetuses has been a controversial issue over the past few years.[54,55] Cesarean section was initially proposed as the ideal mode of delivery, because it was thought to decrease the risk of bowel trauma and contamination. However, several recent studies have failed to demonstrate any advantage of cesarean section over vaginal delivery. Therefore cesarean section should be reserved for obstetric indications and not made simply because of the diagnosis of gastroschisis.

Recently it has been proposed that babies with gastroschisis should be operated on immediately after birth. In this protocol, confirmation of lung maturity is followed by scheduled cesarean section and aseptic delivery of the neonate, who is immediately moved to an adjacent operating room to have the defect repaired by the pediatric surgeon.[56] The only advantage of this protocol over the traditional management is a shortened neonatal hospital stay.

◤ OMPHALOCELE

Omphalocele is a midline defect of the anterior abdominal wall, characterized by herniation of the abdominal viscera into the base of the umbilical cord. The protruding organs are typically covered by a thin amnioperitoneal membrane. The incidence of omphalocele is approximately 1 in 4000 to 1 in 5000 live births. It occurs more frequently in males than in females, with a ratio of 3:1. The recurrence risk for isolated omphalocele is less than 1%.

The cause of omphalocele is unknown. Most cases are sporadic. Chromosomal abnormalities, such as trisomies 13 and 18, are commonly associated with this defect. A familial occurrence, with a sex X-linked or autosomal pattern of inheritance, has also been reported.

Omphalocele is a defect of the umbilical ring, which results from a failure of the two lateral abdominal wall folds to migrate and fuse normally in the midline around the third or fourth week of intrauterine life. The defect is characteristically located at the base of the umbilical cord and may contain abdominal and sometimes thoracic structures. The herniated viscera are included in a sac, which is formed internally by the peritoneum and externally by Wharton's jelly and the amnion.

Some investigators give physiopathologic significance to the presence or absence of hepatic tissue in the sac. For them, an omphalocele that only contains bowel represents a persistence of the primitive body stalk beyond 12 weeks of gestational age. In contrast, an omphalocele that contains liver suggests a primary failure of the body wall closure because the liver is normally not found outside the abdominal cavity anytime throughout the embryonic development.

Classically, two syndromes have been described in association with omphalocele:

1. The pentalogy of Cantrell, which includes midline supraumbilical abdominal defects, defect of the lower sternum, anomalies of the diaphragmatic pericardium, abnormality of the anterior diaphragm, and cardiac anomalies
2. The Beckwith-Wiedemann syndrome, which is characterized by macrosomia, macroglossia, visceromegaly, pancreatic hyperplasia, diaphragmatic hernia, and several degrees of omphalocele

Associated anomalies

Associated anomalies are detected in 50% to 88% of the cases. The most common include cardiac malformations such as ectopia cordis, transposition of the great vessels, and ventricular septal defects; skeletal malformations, mainly scoliosis and xyphosis; gastrointestinal anomalies, including diaphragmatic hernia and ascites; genitourinary anomalies, such as renal dysplasia; and central nervous system anomalies, including holoprosencephaly, encephalocele, and cerebellar hypoplasia.

Chromosomal abnormalities have been reported in as many as 43% of fetuses with omphalocele, the most common being trisomies 13, 18, and 21 and Turner's syndrome. An abnormal karyotype has been strongly related to the presence of polyhydramnios or oligohydramnios and to the absence of liver in the herniated sac.

Diagnosis

The echographic diagnosis of omphalocele is made by visualization of a mass in close proximity to the anterior abdominal wall (Figure 17-11). The defect, which may vary in size, has several characteristic features such as a central location, umbilical cord inserted into the sac, and presence of a membrane limiting the herniated contents. These findings are useful in making a differential diagnosis with gastroschisis.

Omphalocele has a strong association with high levels of maternal serum alpha-fetoprotein. Spontaneous in-utero rupture of an omphalocele

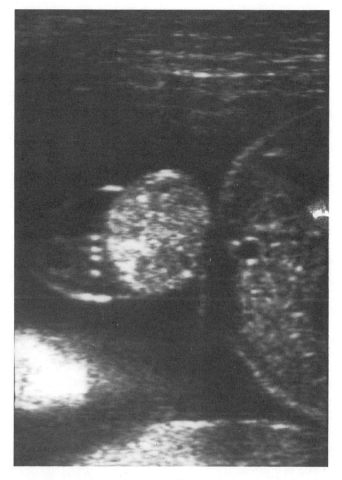

FIGURE 17-11 ◪ Omphalocele. A part of the fetal intestine has herniated through an anterior abdominal wall defect. The intestine is in close proximity to the umbilical vessels, and a membrane covers the herniated organ.

has been reported; in these cases a differential diagnosis with gastroschisis is difficult. Polyhydramnios is a frequent finding in patients with omphalocele.

Prognosis

The major prognostic factor in omphalocele is the presence of associated anomalies.[57] When they are present, the mortality may be as high as 80%. Mortality can be near 100% in the presence of major cardiovascular malformations. On the other hand, fetuses without additional malformations have a mortality of around 10%. The size of the omphalocele or the presence of ascites are not of prognostic importance. The presence of liver in the sac has been associated with normal fetal karyotype, whereas the absence of hepatic tissue has been associated with abnormal karyotype.[58] However, the information concerning the prognosis of fetuses with or without extracorporeal liver varies widely and is controversial.

Management

Once the diagnosis has been made, an ultrasound level II examination should be performed in search of associated anomalies. The fetal karyotype should be determined. Since cardiac anomalies are the most frequently associated abnormalities and possess a high prognostic value, an echocardiogram should always be practiced on these fetuses.

Termination of pregnancy is an option that should be discussed with the parents when the diagnosis is made before fetal viability. If the diagnosis is made late in pregnancy, the fetal karyotype is normal, and no life-threatening abnormalities are seen, expectant management is indicated. The pediatric surgeon and neonatologists should be notified and be ready for immediate postpartum evaluation and treatment.

The mode of delivery of these fetuses should not be altered by the presence of the defect. Several studies have demonstrated that vaginal delivery does not alter the prognosis.[52,59] Therefore cesarean section should only be performed for obstetric reasons or for fetuses with extracorporeal liver.

▰ RENAL CYSTIC DISORDERS

Fetal renal cystic disease encompasses a group of entities with varied clinical, sonographic, and pathologic manifestations. The disorders most commonly found are:

1. Infantile polycystic kidney disease
2. Multicystic dysplastic kidney disease
3. Adult polycystic kidney disease
4. Renal cystic displasia caused by obstructive uropathy

Infantile polycystic kidney disease

Infantile polycystic kidney disease (IPKD), also known as Potter's I, is a condition characterized by symmetric and bilateral enlargement of the kidneys resulting from a primary defect in the collecting tubules. The incidence of this problem is 1 in 6000 to 1 in 60,000 births.

IPKD is an autosomal-recessive condition with a 25% recurrence risk. The physiopathology of the disease has not been clearly established, but it seems to result from a hyperplasia of the renal collecting tubules. Medullary estasis produces innumerable 1- to 2-mm cysts that are radially arranged, extending from the renal cortex to the calices. There is no proliferation of connective tissue, and the calices, papillae, and renal pelvis are normal. Macroscopically, the kidneys are enlarged but maintain their reniform configuration. Cystic changes are also present in the liver, and there is portal and interlobular fibrosis with variable degrees of biliary duct hyperplasia. Fetuses with IPKD do not have an increased risk for other associated malformations.

IPKD has been classified into perinatal, neonatal, infantile, and juvenile depending on the time of diagnosis. The most common presentation is the perinatal variety, which unfortunately corresponds with a high mortality caused by pulmonary hypoplasia.

Diagnosis. The sonographic diagnosis of IPKD has been made as early as 16 weeks of gestation. The diagnosis relies on the visualization of bilateral enlarged hyperechogenic kidneys that retain their reniform shape.[60] The innumerable ectatic tubules provide a multitude of reflective interphases that explain this characteristic sonographic appearance. Other sonographic diagnostic features include an increase in the kidney-to-abdomen circumference ratio, oligohydramnios, and the impossibility of visualizing the bladder.

Although several studies report early diagnosis, IPKD is usually first apparent late in gestation. Hence fetuses at risk for the disease should be examined periodically throughout the pregnancy. When a fetus is first diagnosed, sonographic renal examination of the parents and other members of the family is warranted.

Obstetric management. The prognosis depends on the clinical variety of IPKD. As mentioned before, the most common presentation is the perinatal variety, which has a poor prognosis because it usually leads to stillbirth or to early neonatal death because of pulmonary hypoplasia. Other presentations lead to variable forms of renal insufficiency, with different prognoses.

Termination of pregnancy is an option to be considered when the diagnosis of IPKD is made before fetal viability. When the diagnosis is made late in gestation, the best course of action is expectant management. Rarely, enlarged kidneys can be a cause of dystocia.

Multicystic dysplastic kidneys

Multicystic dysplastic kidneys (MKD), also known as Potter's II, is a condition characterized by the presence of renal cysts resulting from dilation of the collecting tubules. It is considered to be the most common neonatal renal mass. The disorder is usually unilateral, but it can be bilateral or segmental. The approximate incidence is 1 per 10,000 live births, but many believe that this figure is an underestimation and that the real incidence is around 1 in 1000. MKD may represent as many as 10% of all fetal uropathies. MKD usually occurs as a sporadic condition; however, it may also be seen as part of the spectrum of a large variety of syndromes. In some studies MKD has been related to maternal diabetes mellitus.

The main alteration in MKD seems to be a disturbance in the differentiation of the nephrogenic tissue. Developmental failure of the mesonephric blastema to form nephrons and an early obstructive uropathy are the two types of insults that may initiate this process. Some authors believe that all developmental failures are caused by an obstructive process.

A classification of MKD has been proposed on the basis of an obstructive process as the primary cause, taking into consideration the macroscopic appearance of the kidneys. Two groups of patients are recognized:

1. *Patients with classic Potter's type II.* This abnormality is the result of pelvoinfundibular atresia and atresia of the proximal third of the ureter. The obstructive process occurs before 8 to 10 weeks. In these cases the cysts are randomly distributed and noncommunicating, and they grossly alter the normal architecture of the organ.

2. *Hydronephrotic variety.* This results from an obstructive event occurring after 10 weeks and leading to the same cystic changes observed in the Potter's type II form of disease, but with preservation of a normal renal pelvis and infundibulum. A differential diagnosis with obstructive uropathy is difficult to establish because the dilated renal pelvis communicates with the peripheral cysts and the normal reniform shape of the kidney is preserved.

Associated anomalies. The most common anomalies associated with MKD are malformations of the cardiovascular system, central nervous system, gastrointestinal tract, and chromosomal aberrations. In contrast with Potter's type I and type III diseases, MKD is not associated with cystic changes in other organs.

Diagnosis. The sonographic diagnosis of MKD has been made as early as 18 weeks of gestation. The typical sonographic appearance is that of a paraspinal mass with cystic changes. Characteristically, the cysts are noncommunicating, have a different size and shape, and are randomly distributed, resembling a "bunch of grapes."[61] The cystic images may change in size and position; these changes seem to be the result of residual renal function.

Prognosis and management. The prognosis depends on the severity of the process and the functional integrity of the contralateral kidney. Oligohydramnios is an important prognostic factor, and its presence is associated with an obscure prognosis. Up to 30% to 40% of cases have associated contralateral anomalies of the urinary tract. The contralateral kidney may be affected by MKD in 19%, renal agenesis in 11%, and ureteropelvic junction obstruction in 7% of the cases. The condition is lethal when complicated with the first two of these defects.

After the diagnosis is made, a complete workup, including genetic diagnosis and level II ultrasound, must be made. If bilateral MKD is diagnosed before viability, termination of pregnancy should be offered. If viability has been reached when the initial diagnosis is first made, a conservative approach should be followed. In cases of unilateral disease in the absence of other congenital anomalies and a normal karyotype, standard obstetric management should not be changed. In cases where MKD is associated with a contralateral obstructive process, delivery should take place as soon as lung maturity is confirmed.

Adult polycystic kidney disease

Adult polycystic kidney disease (APKD), also known as Potter's III, is an autosomal dominant disorder of unknown cause, characterized by multiple renal parenchymal cysts. The incidence is around 1 per each 1000 live births, but it may be as high as 1 in 500 in autopsy material.[62] The gene has a penetrance of 100%, but its expressivity varies widely, and the disease may manifest as a lethal neonatal condition or can be only an incidental finding during the autopsy of an adult.

APKD is the third most common cause of adult chronic renal failure. The disease is generally first diagnosed during the fourth decade of life, and neonatal and infantile presentations are rare. It is also rarely seen during fetal life. However, a recent study[63] demonstrated an increase in the prenatal and postnatal diagnosis of APKD with the wide use of high resolution ultrasound.

The characteristic feature of APKD is the coexistence of cysts and normal tissue. The cystic structures correspond to dilated collecting tubules and to other portions of the nephron. The renal compromise is almost always bilateral, with cystic structures of different size. Liver compromise in the form of periportal fibrosis occurs, but less frequently than in IPKD. APKD also has been associated with cystic lesions in the pancreas, lungs, spleen, and testes.

Diagnosis. The sonographic diagnosis of APKD has been made as early as 23 weeks of gestation. The most important diagnostic features include unilateral or bilateral kidney enlargement, seen in as many as 85% of the cases, increased renal echogenicity, and a normal amount of amniotic fluid.[60]

Prognosis and management. There are no adequate prognostic guidelines when the disease is diagnosed in utero because APKD is a chronic disease that can become symptomatic over a wide range of time and has varied degrees of renal involvement. When the diagnosis is made before fetal viability, termination of pregnancy is an option that may be considered. If it is made after viability, the diagnosis of APKD should not alter standard obstetric management.

Cystic dysplasia caused by obstructive uropathy

The term *obstructive uropathy* refers to a group of obstructive processes of the urinary tract that lead to progressive retrograde dilation of anatomic structures. The characteristics of each process varies widely, resulting in a broad spectrum of sonographic manifestations. Eventually, the obstruction may cause cystic dysplasia with irreversible damage of renal function.

The fetal urinary tract responds differently to obstruction depending on the gestational age. Whereas a urinary tract obstruction in the last half of pregnancy will cause hydronephrosis, the same phenomenon in the first half of pregnancy will produce dysplasia with formation of cysts in the renal parenchyma. Depending on the time of onset and the severity of the obstruction, the increased retrograde intraluminal pressure may lead to irreversible renal damage.

Cystic dysplasia, also known as Potter's IV, is mostly the result of posterior urethral valve (PUV) obstruction. Less frequent causes are ureteropelvic junction (UPJ) and ureterovesical junction (UVJ) obstruction.

Ureteropelvic junction obstruction. UPJ obstruction is a mechanical interruption of the urinary tract at the junction of the renal pelvis and the ureter. Its incidence has been estimated at 1 in 1258 live births. It is the most common congenital malformation of the urinary tract, representing approximately 40% of all obstructive uropathies, and 20% to 50% of all urologic congenital anomalies detected in utero.

Anatomic abnormalities such as adhesions, valves, and aberrant vessels have been described as causes of the obstruction. A peristaltic alteration of the ureter, caused by an abnormality in the arrangement of the longitudinal muscular layers, has also been proposed as an important etiologic factor.

UPJ is a unilateral defect in 70% of the cases, usually on the left side (Figure 17-12). Severe bilateral involvement is rare, and even in those cases the compromise is asymmetric and not necessarily fatal. Irreversible renal parenchymal damage is unusual, and in general, this entity has a good outcome. Prenatal identification may benefit the neonate by the adoption of measures to avoid the development of recurrent urinary infection.

Associated anomalies. Associated anomalies of the urinary tract are seen in 27% of the cases. These include vesicoureteral reflux, ureteral duplication, meatal stenosis, hypospadia, contralateral renal agenesis, and lower urethral obstruction.[64] Anomalies outside of the urinary system are seen in 19% of the cases and include Hirschsprung's disease, cardiovascular anomalies, neural tube defects, esophageal atresia, and congenital hip dislocation.

Diagnosis. The prenatal diagnosis of UPJ has improved dramatically in recent years with the advent of high resolution obstetric ultrasound.[65] Several criteria have been proposed for diagnosing UPJ. The most important is the demonstration of a dilated renal pelvis using the anteroposterior diameter of the pelvis or the pelvis-to-kidney diameter ratio.

The anteroposterior diameter is obtained on a transverse cross section of the abdomen. Values between 5 and 10 mm are considered a physiologic dilation. These fetuses should be managed expectantly, and in 97% of the cases, the condition will resolve spontaneously after birth. Patients with values between 10 and 15 mm are considered to have intermediate degrees of hydronephrosis and require close surveillance. Approximately 47% of these patients require postnatal surgery. Values greater than 15 mm with severe dilation of the calices are definitely abnormal, and in postnatal follow-up all these patients require surgical treatment.[66]

Other authors[61,67] have proposed as a marker of pathologic pelvic dilation a pelvis-to-kidney diameter ratio greater than 50%. Another important diagnostic feature is the visualization of dilated calices. This finding may be indicative of an obstructive process even if the pelvic-to-kidney diameter ratio is less than 50%.

The postnatal examination for hydronephrosis

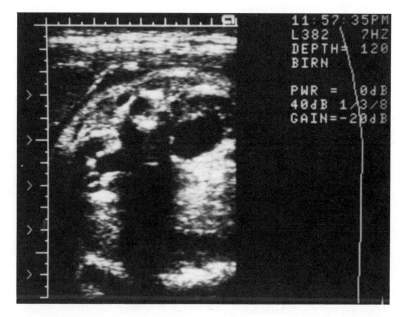

FIGURE 17-12 ▨ Unilateral renal pelvis dilation in a fetus with ureteropelvic junction (UPJ) obstruction. The prognosis for fetuses with unilateral UPJ obstruction is good. Bilateral UPJ obstruction is rare.

should be done 5 to 7 days after birth, when the muscle relaxant effect of maternal progesterone has completely disappeared.

Management. In cases of unilateral UPJ with contralateral normal kidney, there is no reason for altering the standard obstetric management. These patients have a good prognosis, and surgical correction is not an emergency even after birth. Rarely these fetuses develop huge pelvic dilations that may distend the abdomen and thorax and cause dystocia or pulmonary hypoplasia. These cases may require prenatal decompression. The most important factor in the follow-up of these patients is the amount of amniotic fluid. Oligohydramnios is a poor prognostic sign and suggests the possibility of contralateral renal agenesis or dysplasia.

Bilateral UPJ is quite rare. The management of these patients is complex and is reviewed later under treatment for bladder outlet obstruction.

Ureterovesical junction obstruction. UVJ is the second most common form of obstructive uropathy, accounting for approximately 23% of the cases. UVJ may result from an anatomic defect such as stenosis or fibrosis of the ureteral valves, from vesicoureteral reflux, in association with caudal regression syndrome, or from a

functional alteration of the normal ureteral musculature at the ureterovesical junction.

Associated anomalies. The most common anomalies associated with UVJ are contralateral renal agenesis, contralateral cystic dysplasia, and Hirschsprung's disease.

Diagnosis and management. The sonographic diagnosis of UVJ requires the demonstration of a dilated ureter or megaureter. Normal ureters are rarely seen through ultrasound examination. However, when dilated, they may be visualized as tortuous, fluid-filled hypoechogenic structures that can be traced to the renal pelvis. This visualization is not always easy to make, and often it is incomplete. Usually a normal size bladder is visualized in cases of UVJ with megaureter. However, megaureter associated with megacystis has been reported in cases of vesicoureteral reflux.

Unilateral megaureter does not require any specific prenatal therapy. Continuous monitoring for normal amount of amniotic fluid is warranted. Bilateral UVJ, with normal amount of amniotic fluid, should also be managed expectantly. The management of bilateral UVJ associated with oligohydramnios is reviewed in the following section.

Bladder outlet obstruction. Approximately 10% of all obstructive uropathies correspond to bladder outlet obstructions.[65] This term includes the following causes of urinary tract obstruction:

Posterior urethral valve syndrome

Urethral stricture

Urethral agenesis

Persistent cloaca with associated urethral agenesis or stenosis

Megacystis-microcolon-intestinal hypoperistalsis syndrome

Since posterior urethral valves (PUVs) account for the vast majority of cases of bladder outlet obstruction, we will analyze only this problem.

Posterior urethral valves. PUVs are a sporadic disorder that affects only male fetuses. They are membranous folds located in the posterior wall of the urethra, which have been classified as types I to III according to their localization and to their gross anatomic characteristics. Only types I and III have clinical relevance, type I being the most frequent.[64]

The obstruction of the lower urinary tract caused by PUVs is followed by a progressive retrograde dilation of the urinary tract. Depending on the severity and time of initiation of the obstruction, megacystis, megaureter, hydronephrosis, and eventually renal dysplasia or urinary tract rupture may develop.

Associated anomalies. Associated anomalies of the urinary tract include duplication of the urethra, megalourethra, cryptorchidism, and hypospadias. The most common extraurinary associated anomalies are cardiovascular anomalies, scoliosis, skeletal anomalies of the lower extremities, and rare chromosomal abnormalities.

Diagnosis. The sonographic diagnosis of PUV obstruction should be suspected in the presence of dilated bladder, dilated proximal urethra, megaureter, hydronephrosis, bladder wall hypertrophy, renal dysplasia, ascites, and oligohydramnios. Dilation of the renal pelvis is not a constant finding.

Prognosis and management. The prognosis for these fetuses depends on a series of factors: timing of the obstruction, severity of the process, associated anomalies, karyotype, and most important, the presence or absence of oligohydramnios. Abnormal karyotype has been found in 15% to 40% of fetuses with obstructive uropathy.[68]

The complete evaluation of fetuses with bladder outlet obstruction should include a level II ultrasound examination, echocardiography, fetal karyotyping, and in cases in which fetal surgery is considered, evaluation of renal fetal function. A frequent problem is the differentiation of obstructive hydronephrosis from multicystic dysplastic kidneys. Determination of urinary phosphate may be useful in these cases. In hydronephrosis urinary PO_4 is low (0.41 to 0.98 mg/dl), whereas it is higher (1.87 to 2.64 mg/dl) in MKD.

The evaluation of fetal renal function can be made by analysis of urine osmolarity and electrolytes by percutaneous aspiration. In a fetus with normal renal function, the urinary sodium must be less than 100 mEq/dl, the chloride less than 90 mEq/dl, and the osmolality less than 200 mOsm/L.[68,69] Lack of a drop in sodium concentration and osmolarity in repeated urine samples is more predictive than a single measurement.

Prenatal surgical treatment should be reserved for cases with bilateral obstruction, progressive and persistent oligohydramnios, preserved renal function, gestational age less than 30 to 32 weeks, normal karyotype, no sonographic evidence of renal dysplasia, and no other life-threatening anomalies.

The ideal surgical treatment for these patients is controversial. The most commonly used procedure between 26 and 30 weeks of gestation is shunting by means of a vesicoamniotic catheter.[70] However, there is no uniformity in shunt design, construction material, or method of shunting. The mortality rate caused by vesicoamniotic shunting is 4.7%. The most common complications are inadequate drainage, catheter displacement, premature labor, urinary ascites, and infection.

When a shunting procedure is done before 26 weeks and is intended to last for weeks or months, some favor open surgical decompression in the form of a vesicotomy or bilateral ureterostomies. The overall survival rate for surgically treated fetuses is around 45%. In-utero surgery must not be considered the panacea for the treatment of obstructive uropathy.[71] It is an alternative procedure, which when practiced rationally and under very precise indications, may be useful and life-saving.

◼ OSTEOGENESIS IMPERFECTA

The term *osteogenesis imperfecta* (OI) encompasses a heterogeneous group of inheritable connective tissue disorders. Although fractures and bone deformation are the main clinical landmarks of the disease, OI is a generalized metabolic disorder associated with multiple systemic manifestations such as blue sclerae, impaired hearing, dentinogenesis imperfecta, hypermetabolism, platelet dysfunction, loose jointedness, and shortened limbs.[72] The overall incidence of OI has been estimated at 1 in 20,000 to 1 in 60,000 live births. There is no preferential distribution of OI by gender, race, or ethnic group.

The cause of OI has been related to a disorder in the production of type I procollagen. OI has been classified into four types according to genetic and clinical criteria. These types are discussed below.

OI type I

OI type I is the mildest and probably the most common type of the disease. It is inherited as an autosomal-dominant trait and is characterized by the presence of blue sclerae, progressive presenile deafness, easy bruising, and skeleton fragility that may lead to deformity. It has been further subdivided into types IA and IB according to the absence or presence of dentinogenesis imperfecta, respectively.

OI type II

OI type II is the most severe form of the disease, being uniformly lethal for the fetus and the neonate. Although originally described as a recessive condition, more recent data suggest new dominant mutations.[72,73] The condition is characterized by very poor bone mineralization, which results in eggshell bone fragility and multiple in-utero fractures. The skull is usually large for the body size, the ribs are continuously beaded, and the long bones are bowed and/or deformed by fractures.

OI type III

OI type III is a severe recessive form of the disease, although compatible with a full life span. It is characterized by progressive deformity of the long bones and spine that leads to a deformed phenotype. At birth the presence of multiple fractures is common. Facies are quite characteristic, with a triangular appearance, and the skull is relatively large for the trunk size. Growth deficiency is also a common feature. The blue sclerae of infancy, characteristic of the disease, become progressively pale with age.

OI type IV

Type IV is the most rare presentation of OI. It is inherited as an autosomal-dominant disorder.

Its clinical features include normal sclerae, bowing of long bones, joint hyperextensibility, and moderate short stature. It has also been classified into types IVA and IVB according to the absence or presence of dentinogenesis imperfecta.[74] Patient's age at onset of fractures is variable and occasionally may show spontaneous improvement with adolescence.

Diagnosis

The sonographic diagnosis of OI type II has been made as early as 15 to 17 weeks of gestational age.[75] After this gestational age, a normal sonogram would exclude the diagnosis of this lethal condition. The sonographic diagnosis relies on the demonstration of deformed long bones with poor echogenic properties and a compressible thin skull with high sonographic transparency.

Other common ultrasonographic features include bone fractures, angulations, shortening, and localized thickening. Bowing of the limbs and hypoechogenicity of the skeleton often are not evident until after 24 to 32 weeks. Radiographic fetal studies may be helpful in a more precise evaluation of fetal limb growth and structure.[76] Prenatal diagnosis of other types of OI has been reported, although rarely. The differential diagnosis of OI includes hypophosphatasia and other forms of dwarfism.

Management

There is no treatment for the fetus with OI. If the diagnosis is made before viability, termination of pregnancy is an alternative that may be considered. If detection is made after viability, the only specific obstetric management deals with the mode of delivery. Cesarean section has been proposed as the ideal mode of delivery, since the risk for skull and/or body fractures could be avoided. However, there are no clinical data available to support this assumption.

▨ HETEROZYGOUS ACHONDROPLASIA

Heterozygous achondroplasia (HA) is a form of skeletal dysplasia characterized by rhizomelic shortening, megalencephaly, limb bowing, lordotic spine, depressed nasal bridge, and short proximal and middle phalanges.[77] The incidence of HA ranges from 1 in 10,000 to 1 in 30,000. However, these figures seem only an approximation, since until recently many short limb dysplasias were erroneously categorized as HA.

HA is caused by a retardation of endochondral

bone formation, which is transmitted in an autosomal-dominant pattern. However, in approximately 85% of cases, the parents are not affected, suggesting the occurrence of a new mutation. Advanced paternal age has been associated with nonfamiliar cases. Recurrence of the disease has been rarely reported.

HA is characterized by an abnormal cartilage growth followed by defective endochondral bone formation that causes the shortness of long bones characteristic of the disease. Other abnormalities include distal enlargement and bowing of long bones, caudally narrowed interpeduncular spaces of the spine, severe lordosis of the lumbar area, bulky head with shortened cranial base, flattened nasal bridge, square-shaped pelvic bones, and divergent third and fourth fingers (trident hand).

Diagnosis

The sonographic diagnosis of HA is based on the identification of a short femur in association with an enlarged biparietal diameter. Although some authors have reported diagnosing HA as early as 22 to 25 weeks of gestation, most studies agree that the entity is usually not detected before 27 weeks.[78]

Prognosis and management

Even though HA is a disease compatible with normal life span and intellectual capability, affected patients experience significant morbidity. Recurrent ear infections, dental malocclusion, short stature, mild hydrocephalus, and respiratory compromise are common problems in these patients.

There is no treatment for the fetus with HA.

◪ SACROCOCCYGEAL TERATOMA

Sacrococcygeal teratoma (ST) is a fetal tumor arising from pluripotent embryonic cells of the coccyx. Fetal teratomas are the most common congenital neoplasms, and ST is their most common form.[79]

ST is rare. Its incidence is approximately 1 in 40,000 live births. Although the majority of these tumors occur sporadically, a familial occurrence has been reported in association with an autosomal-dominant mode of transmission.[80] Females are affected 3 to 4 times more than males.

ST originates from an area in the caudal edge of the bilaminar embryonic disk known as the primitive, or Hensen's, knot. Pathologically, three grades have been described: benign, immature, and malignant. The first two are the most common varieties, accounting for 87% to 93% of all cases of ST. The malignant variety is rarely seen prenatally. It has only been reported in 7% to 13% of cases of ST. Benign forms usually are derived from all three germ layers, neuroglia being the most common element.[80]

The malignancy of the tumor has been related to the age at which the diagnosis is made. Whereas a prenatal diagnosis assures a low malignancy risk, a late postnatal diagnosis has a high correlation with the presence of malignant elements. The size and extension of the tumor also have been used as a form to classify ST. The disease has been divided into four types according to the internal or external components. Type I refers to an entirely external presentation of the tumor, whereas in type IV the tumor is entirely internal. In type II there is an intrapelvic component and in type III an intraabdominal extension.

Diagnosis

The initial sonographic diagnosis of ST is usually made when a patient is referred on the basis of a large-for-date uterus. The increased uterine size is the result of the size of the mass or of the association with polyhydramnios that exists in 70% of the cases. The cause of polyhydramnios is unclear, but its presence is not by itself a bad prognostic sign.

The sonographic appearance of ST is that of a mass attached to the fetal rump with alternating cystic and solid components. Fragments of bone, or other hyperechogenic images corresponding to dystrophic calcifications, are also visualized. The identification of intrapelvic or intraabdominal components of the teratoma are usually obvious in the sonographic study. Other less frequent sonographic findings are oligohydramnios and hydrops fetalis. The association with chromosomal abnormalities or other life-threatening congenital anomalies is rare.

The differential diagnosis of ST must be made with chordoma, neurogenic tumor, lipoma, hemangioma, and malignant melanoma if the mass is predominantly solid. If the main component is cystic, myelomeningocele must be specifically excluded.

Prognosis and management

Prognostic factors associated with a good outcome are external presentation of the mass, discovery after 30 weeks, and absence of placentomegaly, oligohydramnios, and hydrops.

Fetal surgery is the procedure of choice when the diagnosis is made early in gestation.[81] Because of the risk of avulsion with fatal fetal hemorrhage and/or dystocia, a cesarean section should be performed in cases with proven fetal lung maturity and a mass larger than 5 cm. Predominantly, cystic masses may be aspirated to facilitate delivery.

The delivery must take place in a tertiary center where a multidisciplinary team of neonatologist and pediatric surgeons are available for immediate evaluation.

■ **IMPORTANT POINTS** ◪

1. The most common maternal causes of polyhydramnios are diabetes and Rh isoimmunization. The most common fetal causes are congenital abnormalities. No etiologic factor will be identified in approximately 65% of the cases.

2. The most common causes of unexpected oligohydramnios in the second trimester are undetected PROM, severe fetal growth retardation, and fetal congenital abnormalities.

3. The most common causes of nonimmunologic fetal hydrops are cardiovascular malformations, chromosomal abnormalities, and hematologic and pulmonary problems.

4. Irregular rhythms account for over 85% of all fetal arrhythmias. Most irregular rhythms are caused by premature atrial contractions and resolve spontaneously during pregnancy or at delivery.

5. Spina bifida is the neural tube defect most difficult to diagnose by ultrasound. There are sonographic signs in the central nervous system useful in this diagnosis. They include the lemon and banana signs, obliteration of the cysterna magna, and hydrocephalus.

6. Recent studies have shown no benefit of abdominal over vaginal delivery in patients with spina bifida.

7. A transverse atrial diameter exceeding 10 mm is an early and accurate sign of fetal hydrocephalus.

8. The three main types of fetal hydrocephalus are aqueductal stenosis, communicating hydrocephalus, and Dandy-Walker malformation.

9. The most important factor in the prognosis of patients with hydrocephalus is the presence of associated anomalies.

10. The most common chromosomal abnormality associated with cystic hygroma is Turner's syndrome. Other conditions are trisomies 21 and 18 and mosaicisms.

11. The sonographic diagnosis of congenital diaphragmatic hernia is based on inability to visualize the fetal stomach, presence of a cystic or solid intrathoracic mass containing abdominal organs, mediastinal displacement, and smaller than expected abdominal circumference.

12. The mortality in fetuses with gastroschisis is between 8% and 14%. This figure has been decreasing in recent years because of advances in postnatal intensive care and surgery.

13. Several recent studies have failed to demonstrate any advantage of cesarean section over vaginal delivery in fetuses with gastroschisis. In these patients cesarean should be performed only for obstetric indications.

14. The major prognostic factor in fetuses with omphalocele is the presence of associated anomalies. They occur in 50% to 80% of the cases. Chromosome abnormalities have been reported in as many as 43% of the cases.

15. Fetal renal cysts are usually caused by multicystic dysplastic kidneys or obstructive uropathy.

16. Ureteropelvic junction obstruction is the most common congenital malformation of the urinary tract representing approximately 40% of all obstructive uropathies and 20% to 50% of all urologic congenital anomalies detected in utero.

17. A complete evaluation of the fetus with outlet bladder obstruction should include a level II ultrasound examination, echocardiography, karyotype, and evaluation of the fetal renal function.

18. The best index of fetal renal function is the determination of urinary sodium concentration.

19. Fetal surgery is the procedure of choice for sacrococcygeal teratoma when the diagnosis is made early in gestation.

REFERENCES

1. Queenan J and Gadow E: Polyhydramnios: Chronic versus acute. *Am J Obstet Gynecol* 1970;108:349.
2. Chamberlain PF, Manning FA, Morrison I, et al: Ultrasound evaluation of amniotic fluid volume. II: Relationship of increased amniotic fluid volume to perinatal outcome. *Am J Obstet Gynecol* 1984;150:250.
3. Carlson D, Platt L, Medearis A, et al: Quantifiable polyhydramnios: Diagnosis and management. *Obstet Gynecol* 1990;75:989.
4. Lyndon M, Breckle R, Thomas M, et al: Polyhydramnios: Ultrasonically detected prevalence and neonatal outcome. *Obstet Gynecol* 1987;69:21.
5. Cardwell M: Polyhydramnios: A review. *Obstet Gynecol Surv* 1987;42:10; 62.
6. Cabrol D, Landesman R, Muller J, et al: Treatment of polyhydramnios with prostaglandin synthetase inhibitor (indomethacin). *Am J Obstet Gynecol* 1987;157:422-426.
7. Kirshon B, Mari G, Moise K, et al: Effect of indomethacin on the fetal ductus arteriosus during treatment of symptomatic polyhydramnios. *J Reprod Med* 1990;35:529-532.
8. Mercer LJ, Brown LG, Petres RE, et al: A survey of pregnancies complicated by decreased amniotic fluid. *Am J Obstet Gynecol* 1984;149:355-361.
9. Shenker L, Reed KL, Anderson CF, et al: Significance of oligohydramnios complicating pregnancy. *Am J Obstet Gynecol* 1991; 164:1597-1600.
10. Queenan J Jr, Queenan J: Immune and nonimmune hydrops fetalis. *Postgrad Obstet Gynecol* 1990;10:1-5.
11. Hallac M, Donnenfeld A: Nonimmune hydrops fetalis. *Postgrad Obstet Gynecol* 1990;10:15.
12. Jauniaux E, Van Maldergen L, DeMunter C, et al: Nonimmune hydrops fetalis associated with genetic abnormalities. *Obstet Gynecol* 1990;75:568.
13. Carlton D, McGillivray B, Schreiber M: Nonimmune hydrops fetalis: A multidisciplinary approach. *Clin Perinatol* 1989;16:4.
14. Meisel RL, Alvarez M, Lynch L, et al: Fetal cytomegalovirus infection: A case report. *Am J Obstet Gynecol* 1990;162:663-664.
15. Fadel H, Ruedrich D: Intrauterine resolution of nonimmune hydrops associated with cytomegalovirus infection. *Obstet Gynecol* 1988;71:1003.
16. Reed K: Fetal arrhythmias: Etiology, diagnosis, pathophysiology, and treatment. *Semin Perinatol* 1989;13:294-304.
17. Kleinman CS, Copel J, Weinstein E, et al: In utero diagnosis and treatment of fetal supraventricular tachycardia. *Semin Perinatol* 1985;9:113.
18. Cameron A, Nicholson S, Nimrod C, et al: Evaluation of fetal cardiac dysrhythmias with two-dimensional M-mode and pulsed Doppler ultrasonography. *Am J Obstet Gynecol* 1988;158:286.
19. Bergmans M, Jonker G, Kock H: Fetal supraventricular tachycardia: Review of the literature. *Obstet Gynecol Surv* 1985;40:61-67.
20. Chervenak F, Isaacson G, Mahoney M: Advances in the diagnosis of fetal defects. *N Engl J Med* 1986;315:305.
21. Goldstein R, Filly R: Prenatal diagnosis of anencephaly: Spectrum of sonographic appearances and distinction from the amniotic band syndrome. *AJR* 1988;151:547.
22. Chervenak F, Farley M, Walters L: When is the termination of pregnancy during the third trimester morally justifiable? *N Engl J Med* 1983;309:822.
23. Stone D: The declining prevalence of anencephalus and spina bifida: Its nature, causes, and implications. *Dev Med Child Neurol* 1987;29:541.
24. Chervenak F, Duncan CH, Ment L, et al: Perinatal management of meningomyelocele. *Obstet Gynecol* 1984;63:376.
25. Nicolaides K, Campbell J, Gabbe S, et al: Ultrasound screening for spina bifida: Cranial and cerebellar signs. *Lancet* 1986;1:72.
26. Van den Hoff M, Nicolaides K, Campbell J, et al: Evaluation of the lemon and banana sign in one hundred thirty fetuses with open spina bifida. *Am J Obstet Gynecol* 1990;162:322.
27. Benaceraff B, Stryker J, Frigoletto F: Abnormal US appearance of the cerebellum (banana sign): Indirect sign of spina bifida. *Radiology* 1989;171:151.
28. Bensen J, Dillard R, Burton B: Open spina bifida: Does cesarean section delivery improve prognosis? *Obstet Gynecol* 1988;71:532.
29. Vintzileos A, Ingardia CH, Nochimson D: Congenital hydrocephalus: A review and protocol for perinatal management. *Obstet Gynecol* 1983;62:539.
30. Benacerraf B, Birnholz J: The diagnosis of fetal hydrocephalus prior to 22 weeks. *J Clin Ultrasound* 1987;15:531.
31. Cardoza J, Goldstein R, Filly R: Exclusion of fetal ventriculomegaly with a single measurement: The width of the lateral ventricular atrium. *Radiology* 1988;169:711.
32. Hossam F: Antenatal diagnosis of fetal intracranial anomalies. *J Child Neurology* 1989;4:S107.
33. Hirsh J, Khan P, Renier D, et al: The Dandy-Walker malformation. *J Neurosurg* 1984;61:515.
34. Nyberg D, Mack L, Hirsh J, et al: Fetal hydrocephalus: Sonographic detection and clinical significance of associated anomalies. *Radiology* 1987;163:187.
35. Chervenak F, Berkowitz R, et al: The management of fetal hydrocephalus. *Am J Obstet Gynecol* 1985;151:933.
36. Pinckert TH, Golbus M: Fetal surgery. *Clin Perinatol* 1988;15:4.
37. Chervenak F, Isaacson G, Blakemore K, et al: Fetal cystic hygroma. *N Engl J Med* 1983;309:822.
38. Bronshtein M, Rottem S, Yoffe N, et al: First trimester and second trimester diagnosis of nuchal cystic hygroma by transvaginal sonography: Diverse prognosis of the septated from the nonseptated lesion. *Am J Obstet Gynecol* 1989;161:78.
39. Langer J, Fitzgerald P, Desa D, et al: Cervical cystic hygroma in the fetus: Clinical spectrum and outcome. *J Pediatr Surg* 1990;25:1.
40. Bernstein HS, Filly RA, Goldberg J, et al: Prognosis of fetuses with a cystic hygroma. *Prenat Diagn* 1991; 11:349-355.
41. Shokeir MH: Hypoplastic left heart. *Birth Defects* 1974;10:223-230.
42. Copel JA, Pilu G, Green J, et al: Fetal echocardiographic screening for congenital heart disease: The importance of the four-chamber view. *Am J Obstet Gynecol* 1987;157:648-655.
43. Morris CD, Outcalt J, Manashe VD: Hypoplastic left heart syndrome: Natural history in a geographically defined population. *Pediatrics* 1990;85:977-983.
44. Harrison M, Adzick S, Nakayama D, et al: Fetal diaphragmatic hernia: Pathophysiology, maternal history, and outcome. *Clin Obstet Gynecol* 1986;29:490-501.
45. Crawford D, Wright V, Drake D, et al: Fetal diaphragmatic hernia: The value of echocardiography in the pre-

diction of postnatal outcome. *Br J Obstet Gynaecol* 1989;96:705-710.

46. Hertzberg B, Bowie J: Fetal gastrointestinal anomalies. *Radiol Clin North Am* 1990;28:110-111.

47. Benacerraf B, Adzick S: Fetal diaphragmatic hernia: Ultrasound diagnosis and clinical outcome in 19 cases. *Am J Obstet Gynecol* 1987;156:573-576.

48. Harrison M, Adzick S, Longaker M, et al: Successful repair in utero of a fetal diaphragmatic hernia after removal of herniated viscera from the left thorax. *N Engl J Med* 1990;322:1582-1584.

49. Harrison M, Langer J, Adzick S, et al: Correction of congenital diaphragmatic hernia in utero. V: Initial clinical experience. *J Pediatr Surg* 1990;25:47-57.

50. Castillo R, Devoe L, Falls G, et al: Pleural effusions and pulmonary hypoplasia. *Am J Obstet Gynecol* 1987; 157:1252-1255.

51. Adams H, Jones A, Hayward C: The sonographic features and implications of fetal pleural effusions. *Clin Radiol* 1988;39:398-401.

52. Rodeck CH, Fisk N, Fraser D, et al: Long term in utero drainage of fetal hydrothorax. *N Engl J Med* 1988;319:1135-1137.

53. Sermer M, Benzie R, Pitson L, et al: Prenatal diagnosis of congenital defects of the anterior abdominal wall. *Am J Obstet Gynecol* 1987;156:308-312.

54. Bethel C, Seashore J, Touloukian R: Cesarean section does not improve outcome in gastroschisis. *J Pediatr Surg* 1989;24:1-4.

55. Lewis D, Towers C, Garite TH, et al: Fetal gastroschisis and omphalocele: Is cesarean section the best mode of delivery? *Am J Obstet Gynecol* 1990;163:773-775.

56. Fitzsimmons J, Nyberg D, Cyr D, et al: Perinatal management of gastroschisis. *Obstet Gynecol* 1988;71:910.

57. Tucci M, Bard H: The associated anomalies that determine prognosis in congenital omphaloceles. *Am J Obstet Gynecol* 1990;163:1646-1649.

58. Nyberg D, Fitzsimmons J, Mack L, et al: Chromosomal abnormalities in fetuses with omphalocele: Significance of omphalocele contents. *J Ultrasound Med* 1989;8:299-308.

59. Sermer M, Benzie R, Pitson L, et al: Prenatal diagnosis and management of congenital defects of the anterior abdominal wall. *Am J Obstet Gynecol* 1987;156:308-312.

60. Habif VD, Berdon WE, Yeh MN: Infantile polycystic kidney disease: In utero sonographic diagnosis. *Radiology* 1982;142:475-477.

61. Rizzo N, Gabrielli S, Pilu G, et al: Prenatal diagnosis and obstetrical management of multicystic dysplastic kidney disease. *Prenat Diagn* 1987;7:109-118.

62. Avni F, Thoua Y, Lalmand B, et al: Multicystic dysplastic kidney: Natural history from in utero diagnosis and postnatal followup. *J Urol* 1987;138:1420-1424.

63. Pretorious D, Lee E, Manco-Johnson M, et al: Diagnosis of autosomal dominant polycystic kidney disease in utero and in the young infant. *J Ultrasound Med* 1987;6:249-255.

64. Patten R, Mack L, Wang K, et al: The fetal genitourinary tract. *Radiol Clin North Am* 1990;28:1115-1128.

65. Brown T, Mandell J, Lebowitz R: Neonatal hydronephrosis in the era of sonography. *AJR* 1987;148:959-963.

66. Grignon A, Filion R, Filiatrault D, et al: Urinary tract dilatation in utero: Classification and clinical applications. *Radiology* 1986;160:645-647.

67. Arger P, Coleman B, Mintz M, et al: Routine fetal genitourinary tract screening. *Radiology* 1985;156:485-489.

68. Evans M, Drugan A, Manning FA, et al: Fetal surgery in the 1990s. *Obstet Gynecol Surv* 1990;45:614.

69. Manning F: Fetal surgery for obstructive uropathy: Rational considerations. *Am J Kidney Dis* 1987;10:259-267.

70. Pringle K: Fetal diagnosis and fetal surgery. *Clin Perinatol* 1989;16:13-22.

71. Elder J, Duckett J, Snyder H: Intervention for fetal obstructive uropathy: Has it been effective? *Lancet* 1987, 2:1007-1010.

72. Marini J: Osteogenesis imperfecta. *Am J Obstet Gynecol* 1982;143:228-230.

73. Merz E, Goldhofer W: Sonographic diagnosis of lethal osteogenesis imperfecta in the second trimester: Case report and review. *J Clin Ultrasound* 1986;14:380-383.

74. Chervenak F, Romero R, Berkowitz R, et al: Antenatal sonographic findings of osteogenesis imperfecta. *Am J Obstet Gynecol* 1982;143:228-230.

75. Brons J, Van der Harten H, Wladimiroff J, et al: Prenatal ultrasonographic diagnosis of osteogenesis imperfecta. *Am J Obstet Gynecol* 1980;159:176-181.

76. Robinson P, Worthen N, Lachman R, et al: Prenatal diagnosis of osteogenesis imperfecta type III. *Prenat Diagn* 1987;7:7-15.

77. Donnenfeld A, Mennuti M: Second trimester diagnosis of fetal skeletal dysplasias. *Obstet Gynecol Surv* 1987;42:4.

78. Pretorius D, Rumack C, Manco-Johnson M, et al: Specific skeletal dysplasias in utero: Sonographic diagnosis. *Radiology* 1986;159:237-242.

79. Teal L, Angtuaco T, Jimenez J, et al: Fetal teratomas: Antenatal diagnosis and clinical management. *J Clin Ultrasound* 1988;16:329-336.

80. Sheth SH, Nussbaum A, Sanders R, et al: Prenatal diagnosis of sacrococcygeal teratoma: Sonographic-pathologic correlation. *Radiology* 1986;169:131-136.

81. Flake A, Harrison M, Adzick S, et al: Fetal sacrococcygeal teratoma. *J Pediatr Surg* 1986;21:563-566.

18

CONGENITAL INFECTIONS

Congenital infections are an important cause of fetal and neonatal mortality and morbidity. They may occur at any time during gestation, and their severity will vary depending on the virulence of the agent, the susceptibility and gestational age of the fetus, and the route of the infection.

The most common and important congenital infections caused by bacterial, viral, and protozoan agents are discussed in this chapter.

◢ GROUP B STREPTOCOCCAL INFECTION

Group B streptococcus (GBS) is the cause of a severe congenital infection that affects 1 to 4 neonates in every 1000 live births, or 12,000 to 15,000 babies every year in the United States.[1] It also causes chorioamnionitis, postpartum endometritis, wound infection, and sepsis in the mother and is an important cause of intrauterine asphyxia.[2] The cost of this disease to the health care system was calculated at $726 million in 1985.[3]

There are two types of GBS neonatal infection: early-onset and late-onset. Early-onset infection is usually evident during the first hours of life, is caused by any of the five GBS serotypes, and has the clinical characteristics of an overwhelming sepsis. Late-onset infection usually appears 5 or more days after birth; 90% of the cases are caused by GBS type III; and the

predominant manifestation is meningitis. Mortality of early-onset disease in preterm infants is 70% to 80%, and 50% overall. Mortality is 15% to 30% with late-onset disease, but the incidence of long-term neurologic sequelae is high.

In this chapter the focus is on the early-onset disease because it is acquired by vertical transmission from mother to fetus. The mechanism of transmission of late-onset disease is different, and nosocomial or community acquisition are predominant.

Description of the organism

Group B streptococcus, or *Streptococcus agalactiae,* is a gram-positive organism that is beta hemolytic on blood agar plates. GBS differs from group A streptococcus, or *Streptococcus pyogenes,* by having a specific carbohydrate antigen on the cell wall. GBS also produces type-specific polysaccharides antigens that encapsulate the organism and allow its classification into five serotypes: Ia, Ib, Ic, II, and III. All the capsular polysaccharides have a terminal sialic acid side chain that is their major antigenic determinant.

Maternal and neonatal colonization and infection

GBS colonizes the genitourinary tract of 10% to 35% of women of childbearing age. The incidence of colonization varies among different populations and is higher when selective broth rather than agar plates are used as culture media and when samples are taken from the lower third of the vagina and the rectum. The rectal sample is of particular importance because colonization of the birth canal is secondary to colonization of the anorectal region, which is the major locus for the bacteria. The distribution of serotypes of group B streptococci isolated from vaginal cultures reveals that approximately one third are types Ia, Ib, or Ic; one third type II; and one third type III. On the average about 15% of all women will be colonized at the time of delivery. However, only a few of them will have intrapartum or postpartum infections caused by GBS.

Antepartum cultures are predictive of intrapartum colonization only if they are obtained within 6 weeks of delivery. Boyer et al.[4] found 100% predictability of intrapartum colonization if the antepartum cultures were obtained less than 6 weeks before delivery, 72% if they were obtained 6 to 10 weeks before, 66% if they were obtained 11 to 30 weeks before, and 43% if they were obtained more than 30 weeks before delivery. Also, the predictability of colonization at delivery is 100% for patients found to be heavily colonized 1 week before parturition.[5] Patients that are heavily colonized can be easily identified because they will give positive results with rapid screening tests.

Between 40% and 50% of infants born to women with positive intrapartum cultures for group B streptococcus will be colonized at the time of delivery and exhibit positive surface cultures for the same maternal GBS serotype.[6] The attack rate is only a fraction of the colonization rate and is directly related to the severity of the colonization. According to Dillon et al.,[7] the incidence of early-onset infection is 4 per 1000 in lightly colonized patients and 50 per 1000 when colonization is heavy. The overall early-onset infection rate in colonized newborns is less than 1%. This low attack rate is surprising in view of the fact that 81% to 86% of vaginal carriers have positive amniotic fluid cultures for GBS at the time of labor.[8] Early-onset disease is often associated with risk factors,[9] especially premature labor, rupture of the membranes more than 12 hours before delivery, and development of fever during labor (Box 18-1).

Diagnosis

The best approach for the diagnosis of antepartum maternal colonization is to obtain samples from the lower third of the vagina and the anorectal region for culture in enriched broth medium. The problem with cultures is that it takes 24 to 48 hours to obtain results, and this is inadequate for intrapartum screening.

One approach for rapid diagnosis of patients in labor or at risk of delivering shortly after the culture is obtained is to acquire an additional sample from the vagina for rapid testing. There are several available commercial kits for rapid identification of GBS antigen. They identify approximately 60% of all colonized women. The other 40% have colony counts less than 10^5 and will be identified only by cultures in enriched broth. Because of this poor sensitivity, rapid tests for GBS detection are useful only if they are positive because they detect heavily colonized patients who are at high risk for early-onset neonatal sepsis and who need immediate treatment.

Another approach for the rapid identification of GBS in the vagina is the Gram stain. The problem with this technique is that it requires an experienced microbiologist to obtain adequate interpretation of the smear. Also, the sensitivity is low, 25%, and the positive-predictive value is only 44%.[10]

Prevention

Active immunization against GBS using a vaccine should potentially result in the eradication of this perinatal problem. A caveat is that women who deliver newborns who develop early-onset disease seem to be unresponsive to the immunologic challenge posed by the GBS infection[11] and may not respond to vaccination. The results of vaccination trials have been disap-

---

BOX 18-1

Risk Factors for Early-Onset GBS Infection

Preterm delivery
Term or preterm ruptured membranes at least 1 hour before the onset of contractions
Heavy maternal colonization
Multiple birth
Intrapartum fever
Urinary infection by GBS
Prolonged induction
Multiple pelvic examinations during labor
Prior baby with GBS sepsis
Chorioamnionitis

pointing, and only 57% of vaccinated pregnant women have an adequate serum antibody response.[12] The design of vaccines capable of eliciting a stronger induction of antibodies is an area of active research at the present time.

Management

There are three potential approaches for the management of congenital infection by GBS: antepartum treatment of colonized women, universal or selective intrapartum treatment, and treatment of the neonate. Each one of these strategies has advantages and disadvantages.

Screening the overall obstetric population, followed by antibiotic treatment of women colonized with GBS, is an approach with little or no value for the following reasons:

1. The correlation of antepartum and intrapartum colonization is not perfect. Approximately 4% to 9% of women who will test negative in antepartum screening will be colonized at the time of delivery and at high risk for neonatal infection. Approximately 33% to 43% of women testing positive for GBS before labor begins will not be colonized at the time of delivery, thereby receiving unnecessary treatment.
2. Antepartum screening later in pregnancy excludes patients delivering preterm, the group at highest risk.
3. Antepartum treatment of colonized women is ineffective because the rate of spontaneous recolonization is high.

Treatment of all neonates born to colonized women or to women at high risk is not effective because 40% of infected babies are bacteremic at birth, and many have severe infections unresponsive to treatment.

Intrapartum treatment of colonized women is an ideal approach to the prevention of early-onset GBS infection. The problem with this plan is the lack of adequate methods to accurately detect intrapartum colonization.

We are left with selective intrapartum treatment as the best approach to deal with this problem. There are multiple variations of this approach. The most comprehensive indicates intrapartum treatment of:

1. All women with colonization detected by universal screening within 6 weeks of delivery

2. All women who tested negative in the universal screening or who were not screened and have at least one of the risk factors described in Box 18-1

The defects of this comprehensive approach are that it requires universal screening within 6 weeks of delivery, will not identify 100% of colonized women at the time of delivery, will treat some patients unnecessarily, and will be expensive. Other approaches are:

1. No screening; treatment of high-risk patients only
2. No screening; treatment of all patients with preterm labor or preterm rupture of membranes before 37 weeks
3. Universal screening followed by intrapartum treatment of positive patients with additional risk factors

The problem of plans of management without universal screening is that 25% of all early-onset neonatal infections result from mothers with no risk factors. However, when universal screening is adopted, approximately 33% of patients testing positive in the screening will be negative at the time of delivery and will be treated unnecessarily. Also, approximately 8.5% of patients testing negative at the time of screening will be positive at the time of delivery, will not be treated, and will be at risk for neonatal early-onset GBS infection. Despite these problems, universal screening may be more advantageous than no screening.

Treatment

GBS is a beta lactam–sensitive organism that responds to penicillin treatment. However, ampicillin is the drug of first choice for treatment of pregnant women at risk because this drug is transported easily through the placenta into the fetus and the amniotic fluid (Box 18-2). This is important because as many as 81% of colonized mothers without signs of infection have GBS in the amniotic fluid, and two thirds of these babies will be colonized, although few will be infected. The usual dose is 2 g intravenously every 4 to 6 hours. The ampicillin should be given more than 1 hour before delivery because it takes 1 hour to reach adequate amniotic fluid levels.

An occasional management problem is the woman who has had a neonatal death caused by

---

> ## BOX 18-2
>
> ### Treatment for Women with GBS Infection
>
> **Urinary tract infection**
>
> Ampicillin, 500 mg orally 4 times daily for 7 days
>
> **Intrapartum colonization**
>
> Ampicillin, 2 g intravenously; initial dose at the onset of labor followed by 1 g every 4 hours until delivery

---

severe GBS infection and is found to be colonized early in the course of a subsequent pregnancy. These patients usually are carriers of the same serotype of GBS and are unable to produce an adequate immunologic response against the organism.[13] There is no universally accepted way of managing this situation, but treatment with ampicillin throughout gestation and at the time of labor seems to be an adequate alternative.

◪ SYPHILIS

The number of reported cases of primary and secondary syphilis in the United States has more than doubled between 1984 and 1990 to over 50,000 cases, and the rates of congenital syphilis are higher today than at any time since World War II. Most of the increased incidence of syphilis affects individuals under 25 years of age who are blacks or hispanics, unmarried, and living in large urban areas.[14] The infecting organism, *Treponema pallidum*, is a spirochete 6 to 15 μm in length and not visible by light microscopy, but readily identifiable by dark-field microscopy.

Maternal infection

In women syphilis is almost always acquired by sexual contact. The risk of acquiring the disease after exposure to an infected sexual partner is approximately 30%. The treponema enters the body through small abrasions of the skin or the genital mucosas, and after an incubation period of approximately 3 weeks, a primary chancre appears. The chancre is a painless, red, round ulceration with an indurated base and well-formed borders. Local, painless adenopathy is always present. If untreated, the chancre disappears

spontaneously in 3 to 8 weeks. However, the treponema spreads hematogenously through the body causing genital and extragenital lesions known as secondary syphilis. The occurrence of palmar and plantar targetlike lesions is a characteristic feature of secondary syphilis. Other lesions are cutaneous rash, mucous patches in the tongue or mouth, condyloma latum of the genitalia, and generalized lymphadenopathy. Although neurosyphilis is characteristically a tertiary lesion, central nervous system involvement is found in approximately one third of patients with secondary syphilis. Untreated secondary syphilis lasts 3 to 12 weeks, and latent syphilis then begins. This stage is characterized by serologic evidence of syphilis without signs or symptoms of primary or secondary disease. Latent syphilis is called early when it has less than a 1-year duration and late when it has lasted more than 1 year. After several years of latent syphilis, approximately 30% of affected individuals develop tertiary syphilitic lesions that predominantly affect the central nervous and cardiovascular systems, the bones, and other visceras.

Serology

Syphilis causes distinctive serologic reactions that are used to confirm the presence of the disease. Some of these reactions are nonspecific and caused by anticardiolipin antibodies. The most common tests using nonspecific antibodies are the rapid plasma reagin (RPR) and the Venereal Disease Research Laboratory (VDRL). Specific serologic reactions for syphilis are the fluorescent treponemal antibody absorption (FTA-ABS) test and the microhemagglutination assay for antibodies against *T. pallidum* (MHA-TP). These tests are positive in 80% of patients with primary syphilis and in almost all patients with secondary and early latent disease.

Approximately 1% to 5% of positive RPR and VDRL results are false positive, as demonstrated by negative-specific antibody testing with FTA-ABS. False-positive results usually have low titers and suggest the possibility of autoimmune disease, particularly antiphospholipid antibody syndrome.

Congenital syphilis

T. pallidum can cross the placenta and cause congenital fetal infection at any time during pregnancy. In addition to congenital infection, the organism may cause stillbirth, preterm labor,

---

BOX 18-3

Manifestations of Congenital Syphilis

Most infants look healthy at birth. A few have vesicular-bullous eruptions, usually on palms and soles.

From 4 days to 3 weeks of life, symptoms may begin and may be grouped as follows:

Flulike syndrome

Meningeal signs

Lacrimation (iritis)

Nasal discharge; mucous membranes red, swollen, eroded, loaded with *Treponema pallidum*

Sore throat—pharynx with mucous patches

Generalized arthralgia—splinting of arms and legs; osteochondritis on x-ray film; often periostitis, particularly of tibia (saber shin)

Generalized lymphadenopathy

Cervical, epitrochlear, inguinal, axillary, popliteal

Hepatosplenomegaly—if severe, probability of anemia, purpura, jaundice, edema, hypoalbuminemia

Rash

Maculopapular, papular, and bullous eruptions may all appear together

Occasionally papular lesions may coalesce to form condyloma latum

---

growth retardation, fetal hydrops, and neonatal infection.

Congenital syphilis is a multisystem disease that has a wide range of severity and different forms of presentation.[15] The manifestations, as anticipated, resemble those of adult secondary syphilis, since in congenital syphilis the treponemas obtain direct access to the bloodstream, but unlike secondary syphilis, frequently there is skeletal involvement such as osteomyelitis, osteochondritis, or periostitis. A list of the most common manifestations of congenital syphilis is shown in Box 18-3.

Examination of the placenta is often helpful in making the diagnosis of congenital syphilis. On gross examination the placenta is large, pale, and edematous. Microscopically, the *T. pallidum* can often be identified with silver stain. The villae are often immature, enlarged, and have bullous projections, and the vessels have endovascular and perivascular proliferation.

A principle of congenital syphilis is that the more recent the maternal infection, the more severe the congenital disease. The incidence of preterm delivery is 50% in mothers with primary and secondary infections, 20% in mothers with latent syphilis, and 9% in patients with late syphilis. Congenital syphilis will be present in 50% of the offspring of mothers with primary and secondary syphilis, and the other 50% will have neonatal disease, whereas only 40% of newborns from patients with early latent disease and 10% of newborns from patients with late latent syphilis exhibit congenital syphilis.[15]

The severity of congenital syphilis is also related to the gestational age of the fetus at the time of infection. Fetal morbidity will be severe when the infection occurs in the first or second trimesters, whereas many fetuses infected in the third trimester will be asymptomatic and will have negative serology.[16]

It has long been held that the placenta, via Langhans' cells, acts as a barrier for the first 16 to 18 weeks of pregnancy and protects the fetus from early infection. However, Harter and Benirschke[17] have clearly identified *T. pallidum* in first-trimester abortuses of women with recent syphilitic infections.

Diagnosis

The diagnosis of maternal syphilis is based on the type of lesions present. The test of choice for primary infection is a dark-field examination of secretions from the chancre. To perform this test, it is necessary to remove exudate from the chancre and place it on a glass slide, add saline, and examine it with a dark-field microscope. This technique is also applicable for secondary lesions.

Serologic tests are necessary to confirm the diagnosis in patients with secondary and latent syphilis. The VDRL and RPR tests are used for rapid screening. These tests are accurate in pregnancy. Their false-positive and false-negative rates are no different in pregnancy than in the nonpregnant status. The FTA-ABS test and the MHA-TP tests are specifically used to verify a positive screening test.

False positives in the screening tests are a significant problem. Their incidence is directly related to the prevalence of syphilis in the population: the lower the risk of syphilis, the higher the rate of false positives. Box 18-4 lists some causes of false-positive VDRL results. Women who have persistent unexplained false-positive VDRL results are at high risk for antiphospholipid antibody syndrome.

Patients with secondary, latent, and tertiary syphilis need cerebrospinal fluid examination to rule out central nervous system infection. A recent study[18] demonstrated that 40% of patients with untreated secondary and latent syphilis have asymptomatic neurosyphilis and need more intensive therapy for a cure.

Treatment

Box 18-5 shows the 1985 treatment guidelines recommended by the Centers for Disease Control (CDC). These guidelines are based on the use of penincillin and should not be used in patients allergic to this antibiotic. Unfortunately, there are occasional treatment failures even when these guidelines are applied, and they must be viewed as a minimum treatment that may be modified according to the specific circumstances of each individual patient.

Management of the penicillin-sensitive patient. The penicillin-sensitive gravida poses a major dilemma in intrauterine therapeutics. Maternal and fetal toxicity, poor placental transmission, and low fetal tissue penetration cause many otherwise satisfactory treatment alternatives to be undesirable in pregnancy. At present there is no drug that can be recommended with experience. The best approach is to perform skin testing to document serious allergy and desensitize the patient following established protocols (Table 18-1).

Box 18-6 lists possible therapeutic options for pregnant women with documented allergy to

---

BOX 18-4

Frequent Causes of False-Positive Syphilis Tests (RPR, VDRL)

Autoimmune disease (antiphospholipid antibody syndrome)
Febrile illness
Intravenous drug abuse
Immunization
Laboratory error

BOX 18-5

CDC Recommendations for the Treatment of Syphilis in Pregnant Patients Not Allergic to Penicillin

Early syphilis (less than a 1-year duration)
Benzathine penicillin G, 2.4 million units intramuscularly in a single dose

Late syphilis (more than a 1-year duration)
Benzathine penicillin G, 2.4 million units intramuscularly weekly for 3 consecutive weeks

Neurosyphilis
Aqueous procaine penicillin G, 2.4 million units intramuscularly daily, plus probenecid, 500 mg orally 4 times daily, both for 10 days, *or*
Aqueous penicillin G, 2.4 million units every 4 hours for 10 days, followed by benzathine penicillin G, 2.4 million units intramuscularly weekly for 3 weeks

---

BOX 18-6

Syphilis Treatment in Patients Allergic to Penicillin

Recommended treatment
Desensitization followed by appropiate penicillin dosage for stage of syphilis

Alternative treatments
Erythromycin, 500 mg orally 4 times daily for 15 days (early syphilis)
Tetracycline, 500 mg orally 4 times daily for 15 days (early syphilis)
Nonpenicillin therapy for disease of greater than a 1-year duration is NOT recommended

From Wendel GD: Gestational and congenital syphilis. *Clin Perinatol* 1988;15:287-303.

TABLE 18-1 ◪ Penicillin desensitization protocol

Dose number	Phenoxymethyl penicillin suspension (units/ml)	Penicillin amount (units)	Cummulative dose (units)
1	1000	100	100
2	1000	200	300
3	1000	400	700
4	1000	800	1500
5	1000	1600	3100
6	1000	3200	6300
7	1000	6400	12,700
8	10,000	12,000	24,700
9	10,000	24,000	48,700
10	10,000	48,000	96,700
11	80,000	80,000	176,700
12	80,000	160,000	336,700
13	80,000	320,000	656,700
14	80,000	640,000	1,296,700

From Wendel GD: Early and congenital syphilis. *Obstet Gynecol Clin North Am* 1989;16:479-494.

Observe for 30 minutes before administering penicillin.

Interval between doses: 15 minutes.

Elapsed time: 3 hours 45 minutes.

penicillin. Any infant born to a mother who receives one of these alternative treatments is suspect and should be treated with a full course of penicllin neonatally.

Serologic follow-up

Serologic follow-up of treatment is important for identifying therapeutic success and reinfection. Most commonly, the FTA-ABS test result remains positive for the lifetime of the patient, whereas reaction to the VDRL test progressively declines and becomes negative. If the disease has already entered the latent phase before treatment, a large percentage of patients may never attain a completely negative VDRL result; these patients are called sero-fast.

◪ CYTOMEGALOVIRUS INFECTION

Cytomegalovirus (CMV) is the most common congenital infection and the most important infectious cause of mental retardation and congenital deafness in the United States. CMV affects 1% to 2% of all pregnancies. About 10% of infected babies will be symptomatic at birth, and

5% to 25% of them may have sequelae, particularly deafness, later in life.[19] In many countries CMV is acquired in the infant years. In addition to the 1% of newborns that are infected in utero, 10% to 15% more acquire the infection in the perinatal period. However, the highest infection rate occurs during the second and third years of life when as many as 50% of children become infected. Another period of seroconversion occurs in the adolescent years.

Description of the organism

CMV is a icosahedric, enveloped, double-stranded DNA virus, a member of the herpes family. Histologic evaluation of cells infected with CMV reveals large intranuclear inclusions, leading to the alternate name, *cytomegalic inclusion disease.*

Similar to other members of the herpesvirus family, CMV has the ability to become latent following an acute attack and reactivate at a later time. A special feature of the CMV virus is the persistency of viral shedding. Children shed the virus for years, and adults for months following infection.

Replication of the CMV virus is slow, taking 48 to 72 hours. The viral particles are assembled in the nucleus of the infected cell in a rather inefficient manner, and the result is that infected cells contain more incomplete than complete viruses, making the yield of conventional cultures low.

Transmission

CMV is excreted in urine, semen, cervical secretions, and saliva, and the route of transmission, therefore, may be sexual or respiratory or by contact with infected urine or saliva. The risk of primary CMV infection in seronegative women during pregnancy is approximately 1%. The most common source of maternal infection is children who attend day-care centers.[20] The risk increases with the presence of high-risk factors such as age less than 25 years, white race, upper socioeconomic status, promiscuity, and exposure to young children at home or at work.

Patients with primary infections may show a mononucleosis-like syndrome of malaise, lymphadenopathy, and hepatosplenomegaly. However, fatigue is the most impressive symptom. Many patients are asymptomatic during primary and recurrent infections.

A primary maternal infection in any trimester

has the potential for congenital transmission. Congenital transmission appears to occur trans-placentally. Studies by Monif et al.[21] and Stern and Tucker[22] have shown that maternal infections in any trimester can lead to fetal infection. In the study by Monif et al.[21] more severely affected infants were born to mothers who developed infections during the second rather than during the third trimester. The risk of intrauterine infection following primary CMV infection in pregnancy is 30% to 40%, as determined by neonatal urine cultures.[23]

CMV infection can be acquired at the time of vaginal delivery.[24] This is not surprising because the frequency of viral shedding from the cervix increases from 5% to 15% in the nonpregnant status to as much as 28% at some point in gestation. Another common route of infection is breastfeeding. The virus is transmitted in the breast milk of 25.7% of women with serologic evidence of CMV infection.[25] Indeed, breastfeeding may account for the frequent seroconversion that occurs during infancy. Another potential but rare source of infection is introduction of the virus into the fetal bloodstream or the amniotic fluid during intrauterine transfusion or amniocentesis.

There is variation in the frequency and severity of the congenital infection depending on the nature of the maternal infection. When the maternal infection is primary, 30% to 40% of the neonates will be infected, and 10% of them will exhibit overt CMV disease. The risk is less when the infection is recurrent, and only 2% to 3% of the babies will be infected. Also, maternal immunity reduces the virulence of the fetal infection, and there are no reports of symptomatic babies born to mothers with CMV IgG antibodies.

Severe congenital infection

Infants born with severe congenital infection, or CMV disease, often exhibit hepatosplenomegaly, thrombocytopenia with petechiae and purpura, hepatitis associated with icterus, pneumonitis, and chorioretinitis. Abnormalities that result from faulty neurologic development include microcephaly, optic atrophy, aplasia of various parts of the brain, and microphthalmia. The incidence of fetal growth retardation is 30% to 40%. The presence of intracranial calcifications is an indication that the infant will have at least moderate-to-severe retardation. Half of infants with

severe congenital infection will die in the neonatal period. Most asymptomatic infected newborns will be undetected.

Late sequelae

Follow-up studies of infants with congenital CMV infections indicate that the most significant sequelae are the result of central nervous system infection. Auditory deficiencies are the most common handicap affecting 25% of congenitally infected newborns. Mental retardation affects 93% of newborns with severe infection and also 20% of those who are asymptomatic at birth. Visual difficulties affect 25% of newborns with symptomatic infection and include chorioretinitis, optic neuritis, optic atrophy, cataracts, and microphthalmia. In one study,[26] 44 of these infants were examined at 2 and 7 years of age. The infected group's mean IQ was 102.5, whereas the matched control group's mean IQ was 117. Bilateral hearing loss was present in 5 of 40 infected infants versus 1 in 44 in the control group. Three of the infected children had profound deafness.

Diagnosis

The gold standard for the diagnosis of CMV infection is the viral culture. The virus can be cultured by conventional techniques or by the shell vial method. In the latter method the sample is inoculated into vials containing coverslips seeded with tissue culture cells. After centrifugation and incubation for 24 to 48 hours, the coverslip is stained with fluorescein-tagged monoclonal antibodies to CMV antigens.

During acute infections the CMV virus may be recovered from the urine, throat, and blood. The most dependable source is a sample of the first urine voided in the morning. When blood samples are used for the diagnosis of acute infection, the yield is not as good as with the urine culture.

Serologic studies may also be useful in the diagnosis of acute infection. The primary infection is characterized by the appearance of specific IgM antibodies. These antibodies may persist for 6 to 9 months, complicating the interpretation of serologic evaluations during pregnancy. Recurrent infections will be characterized by at least a fourfold increase in IgG titers.

Isolation of the virus from amniotic fluid is the method of choice for the diagnosis of congenital infection.[27,28] Cordocentesis is not justified in these cases because fetal blood cultures and CMV-specific IgM antibodies are frequently negative in umbilical blood samples. Also, the diagnosis can be made with less invasive procedures. Ultrasound is also useful in the diagnosis of congenital CMV infection, but positive sonographic findings are limited to those fetuses with severe syndromes.

Prevention

There is no vaccination available for CMV. The only preventative measure available is to investigate the CMV immunity of new employees in high-risk places such as mental institutions, neonatal intensive care units, dialysis units, and day-care centers. Those who are not immune should be informed of the high risk of acquiring CMV and the effects of the infection in pregnancy so they can make a decision about occupational change.

Treatment

The antiviral agent gancyclovir is a potent inhibitor of CMV replication with potential use in congenital CMV infection.[29] This medication is available only for intravenous administration and has significant hematologic toxicity. The only approved indication for this agent at the time of this writing is the treatment of CMV retinitis in immunocompromised hosts. There are no published trials on the use of this drug during pregnancy. Acyclovir is not useful because the virus does not induce its own thymidine kinase.

◪ RUBELLA

Rubella was considered an inconsequential disease until 1941 when Gregg described the association between maternal rubella and congenital cataracts. In 1962 the virus was cultivated in cell culture, and in 1969 the first vaccine was licensed in the United States. The history of neonatal rubella infection is not unlike the history of Rh isoimmunization. In a relatively short time the cause of the disease was identified, the pathogenesis explained, a preventive measure created, and then public health measures markedly reduced the incidence of the disease. However, 15% to 20% of the U.S. population are not immune, and the incidence of congenital rubella syndrome has been increasing in the last few years. In 1988, 225 cases of congenital rubella syndrome were reported in the United States. This number doubled in 1989, and in 1990 it tripled to 1093 cases.

Signs and symptoms

The wild rubella virus is highly contagious, with only minimal contact necessary for transmission. Rubella occurs predominantly in young children and adolescents, most commonly in springtime. Rubella causes a usually mild exanthematous disease in children (fever, malaise, and lymphadenopathy) and a somewhat more severe form of the illness in young adults. Characteristic of the disease are a facial rash, postauricular adenopathy, flulike symptoms, and arthralgia or arthritis. The symptoms of arthralgia and arthritis occur largely in women and more commonly involve the smaller joints. Transmission usually occurs by contact with nasopharyngeal secretions.

Rubella has a typical time relationship between clinical signs, virus shedding, and antibody development that is important in the evaluation of potential exposures. When a person first contracts rubella, the virus enters through the upper respiratory tract, multiplies, invades the cervical lymph nodes, and after 7 to 10 days enters the bloodstream and has widespread dissemination. The viremia continues until antibodies appear, generally in another 7 days. The virus is present in blood for several days before the facial rash appears and is shed from the nasopharynx after the appearance of the rash. The total incubation time (exposure to symptoms) is 14 to 21 days, most commonly 16 to 18 days.

Immunity to rubella

Hemagglutination-inhibition (HI) antibodies begin to rise with the onset of symptoms, peak in 1 week, and remain elevated for 3 to 4 weeks. Complement-fixing (CF) antibodies begin to rise 1 week after the cutaneous rash and reach their maximum approximately 1 to 2 weeks after the peak of the HI antibodies. The rubella-specific IgM antibody appears shortly before the onset of symptoms, peaks approximately 1 week later, and disappears approximately 1 month after the onset of the disease.[30]

Acquired immunity is lifelong. However, rubella may occur again after natural infection and after vaccination.[31] Second infections occurring during pregnancy are not associated with congenital infections.

Congenital rubella

Rubella is a teratogenic virus. Most of the information about congenital rubella syndrome (CRS) is a product of observations made during the U.S. rubella epidemic of 1964. This epidemic made it possible to perform a large amount of clinical, serologic, and virologic research on this congenital infection.

Both clinically apparent and totally silent maternal infection can result in fetal infection. The fetus is at risk of CRS only during a primary infection. The possibilities of fetal infection are 61% when maternal transmission occurs during the first 4 weeks after conception, decrease to 26% during weeks 5 to 8, and decrease further to 8% during weeks 9 to 12. After 12 weeks the risk of congenital infection is less than 5%. Therefore the fetal consequences of first-trimester rubella may be no infection, unapparent infection with no clinical consequence, single-organ involvement (typically the ear), or multiple-organ involvement with mild-to-severe damage. Infection in the first weeks of gestation is associated with a doubling of the spontaneous abortion rate.

The most common abnormalities associated with first-trimester infection are hearing loss in 60% to 75%, eye defects in 50% to 90%, heart disease in 40% to 85%, and psychomotor retardation in 25% to 40% of affected infants. Other abnormalities are fetal and neonatal growth retardation and hepatosplenomegaly. Less frequently found are thrombocytopenia, meningoencephalitis, radiolucency of the long bones, and myocardial necrosis. Rarely found are microcephaly, brain calcifications, and hepatitis. Late-onset features appearing after 3 to 12 months include interstitial pneumonitis, chronic rubella-like rash, recurrent infections, hypogammaglobulinemia, chronic diarrhea, diabetes mellitus, and progressive central nervous system deterioration.

The sequelae of rubella are significant. Of those infants affected, 50% will attend schools for the deaf, and 25% will require special schooling because of hearing problems. Several will develop diabetes resulting from pancreatic infection, and some will develop subacute sclerosing panencephalitis.

Diagnosis

The cornerstone for the diagnosis of maternal infection is serologic testing. The most widely used test is the hemagglutination-inhibition (HI) test. In this test the presence of rubella antibodies impedes the agglutination of chick red cells by rubella virus. The HI test is time-consuming and technically complex and is being rapidly replaced by other techniques that are faster and less dependent on adequate technique. Among the new methods are solid-phase enzyme-linked immunosorbent assay (ELISA), passive agglutination (PHA) test, immunofluorescent assay (IFA), radioimmunoassay (RIA), and radial immunodiffusion test. Demonstration of rubella antibodies by any of these techniques constitutes proof of immunity, and demonstration of seroconversion implies recent infection. Recent infection can also be confirmed by demonstrating the presence of rubella IgM antibodies in maternal serum.

The fetal infection can be diagnosed by detection of rubella-specific IgM in fetal blood obtained by cordocentesis[32] or by fetoscopy,[33] provided that the fetus is more than 22 weeks old. Before this gestational age the fetus does not synthesize a significant amount of IgM antibodies.

Management

Every pregnant woman should have rubella immunity testing at her first prenatal visit. A history of prior infection or vaccination is often misleading because it may not have resulted in adequate immunization. The HI test is the most common screening test to assess immunity. A titer of 1:16 or 1:20 is conclusive evidence of immunity. Titers of 1:8 or 1:10 are more difficult to interpret. In one study,[34] up to 17% of these patients lacked antibodies when tested with RIA. These false-positive results are probably the result of incomplete removal of nonspecific inhibitors present in all human sera. Seronegative pregnant women should be counseled to avoid exposure to individuals with erythemas.

The most common problem faced by the obstetrician with respect to rubella infection is the evaluation of pregnant women potentially or actually exposed to an exanthematous illness. To evaluate a person seen 7 days or fewer after exposure, a sample for the HI test is drawn or, if available, the results of the test performed at the first prenatal visit are referred to. The titer may be as high as 1:256 in up to 15% of the normal immune population, and if the test has been obtained within 7 days after exposure, it does not indicate infection. If the patient is not immune (titer <1:10) or the titer is high (>1:256), the HI test should be repeated 2 to 3 weeks later. If the second HI titer shows a similar value or an insignificant variation (less than two dilutions) in relation to the first sample, infection has not occurred. The repeat titer in 2 to 3 weeks should show at least a fourfold rise if an infection has occurred. Rubella-specific IgM antibody titers rise rapidly after a recent infection and disappear after 4 to 5 weeks. A positive rubella-specific IgM is the most specific test indicating recent rubella infection and should be done in every case in which infection is suspected.

When the patient is seen 1 to 5 weeks after exposure or up to 3 weeks after the onset of a rash, serum HI and CF antibody levels should be obtained immediately and again 2 weeks later. A fourfold increase in either antibody will be evidence of acute infection. Absence of CF antibody in both specimens will rule out acute infection. Stable, elevated positive titers for both HI and CF antibodies will require determination of rubella-specific IgM to confirm the diagnosis of infection.

Vaccination

In 1969 two vaccines were licensed in the United States, the HPV77-DE5 and the Cendenhill strain. HPV77 was the most commonly used vaccine until its replacement by RA 27/3 in 1979. RA 27/3 mimics natural rubella better and more consistently than the other vaccines. The vaccines produce seroconversions in 95% to 98% of susceptible individuals and cause symptoms resembling mild rubella in 10% to 15% of recipients. Transient arthralgias and arthritis are particularly common in adult women receiving the vaccine; in those over 20 years of age, up to 20% to 30% may experience joint involvement.

The major problem with the earlier vaccines was that they were not as immunogenic as the natural virus. Several recent studies have shown absent HI antibody titers in long-term follow-up in an alarming 10% to 25% of individuals vaccinated earlier, whereas the RA 27/3 vaccine has had a serologic failure rate in 4 to 5 years of follow-up of only 3%.[35] However, there is some evidence that patients with absent titers after vaccination still have some protection against viremia. Their serologic response to reimmunization resembles a "booster" response more closely than a primary one.

With the decrease in the number of cases of congenital rubella, public concern about the need for vaccination has fallen so that at the present time only 65% to 70% of children have been immunized. Consequently, there has been a dramatic shift in the age at which a person gets rubella, and most of the reported cases are in persons 15 years of age or older. Another conse-

quence of the lack of immunity is dramatized by outbreaks of rubella in hospitals in New York and California. In the New York incident[36] a male obstetrics house officer exposed 170 persons to the disease, including susceptible pregnant patients. A similar report concerning a private obstetrician in Texas[37] again highlights the need for health personnel to be vaccinated.

Selective immunization of women of childbearing age has been difficult and incomplete at best. Several studies have shown that even when physicians obtain routine serologic tests of women, the results are rarely acted upon.[38] Just as prenatal serologic testing has become commonplace in the United States, so should postnatal immunization of all susceptible patients. The newly vaccinated woman is not contagious to other pregnant women in the hospital, nor is her baby at risk even if she breastfeeds. Despite extensive testing, there is no documentation of spread of rubella vaccine virus from a vaccinated person to a susceptible contact. Therefore it is not necessary to vaccinate susceptible household members of a pregnant woman vaccinated after delivery.

Rubella vaccine is contraindicated in pregnancy, as are the other live attenuated vaccines. However, the risk of fetal infection is not nearly as great as with the wild virus. The CDC have reviewed their data and estimated that the maximum risk of fetal infection after vaccination is between 3% and 5%.[39] To date there has not been a reported live birth with the congenital rubella syndrome after immunization of the mother during pregnancy with HPV77, Cendenhill, or RA 27/3 vaccines.

The role of immune globulin for exposed first-trimester mothers remains controversial. Some investigators recommend its use in infected patients who refuse termination of pregnancy. However, the CDC do not recommend its use; preparations of immune globulin vary greatly in their rubella-antibody content, and to be effective, the immune globulin needs to be given at the time of exposure before viremia occurs. Thus immune globulin is an uncertain option of controversial benefit that should be offered only to a small number of women in special circumstances.

◢ HUMAN IMMUNODEFICIENCY VIRUS INFECTION

The human immunodeficiency virus (HIV) is the cause of the acquired immune deficiency syndrome (AIDS), a condition that affects hundreds of thousands of individuals in the United States and many more throughout the world. The demographics of this disease are changing, and HIV is infecting a growing number of women of reproductive age. As a consequence, the number of infants born to HIV-infected mothers is also rapidly increasing.

Virology

There are five known human retroviruses (HIV-1, HIV-2, HIV-I, HIV-II, and HIV-IV), and three of them are associated with human disease. HIV-1 and HIV-2 cause AIDS, and HIV-I most probably is the causal agent of T-cell leukemia/lymphoma. HIV-1, the most common cause of AIDS in the United States, has an envelope formed by three glycoproteins (gp160, gp120, and gp41) surrounding a core that contains other proteins (p55, p40, p24, p17), reverse transcriptase, and endonucleases.

Attachment of the virus to the host cell is a critically important step in the mechanism of infection. The virus only infects susceptible cells that express in their surface a glycoprotein called CD4. CD4 is recognized by the glycoprotein gp120 that is present in the viral envelope. The best-known susceptible cell in humans is the CD4 or T4 helper-inducer T lymphocyte. Invasion and eventual destruction of these cells by the HIV-1 virus will cause the profound alteration in the immune system that is characteristic of AIDS.

Once inside the cell, retroviruses follow a unique reproductive cycle that involves reverse transcription of their ribonucleic acid (RNA) into deoxyribonucleic acid (DNA), incorporation of the newly synthesized DNA into a host cell DNA, transcription of the viral DNA into RNAs, and translation of the RNA into viral components. The viral DNA may remain incorporated into the host cell DNA for prolonged latent periods until viral synthesis is activated. What conditions initiate viral activation is unclear.

Maternal infection

Women account for approximately 10% of AIDS cases. The large majority of them are black or hispanic and between 15 and 35 years of age. Most of them are intravenous drug abusers, have multiple sexual partners, and have intercourse with partners at high risk.

Maternal HIV is acquired primarily by sexual contact or by parenteral exposure to blood or blood products. Most sexual transmission is the result of receptive vaginal or anal intercourse with infected partners. Transmission by exposure to blood or blood products is usually the result of needles or syringes being shared between intravenous drug abusers. Rarely, maternal infection results from the administration of blood or blood products, especially if they were received before April 1985 when individuals from high-risk groups were not excluded as donors.

The initial infection with HIV is asymptomatic. Serologic evidence that infection has occurred may be obtained 2 to 8 weeks after the initial infection, but in some cases it takes up to 6 months before an antibody response is present. Then infected individuals undergo a prolonged period without symptoms, during which they are shedding virus into most body fluids and are infective. Most pregnant women with HIV infection are in this phase of asymptomatic carriers. At some point in the evolution of the disease, infected individuals develop symptoms and signs called AIDS-related complex, or ARC. ARC is characterized by generalized lymph node enlargement, fever, night sweats, weight loss, and unusual recurrent infections such as herpes or candidiasis. ARC is followed by the final stage of the disease, or AIDS, that is a condition characterized by the consequences of a severe dysfunction of the immune system. Patients with AIDS develop a series of systemic or local infections by opportunistic organisms such as candidiasis, cytomegalovirus, herpes, histoplasma, cryptococcus, and *Pneumocystis carinii* or develop Kaposi's sarcoma, lymphoma of the brain, or multiple recurrent bacterial infections.

Prospective studies have demonstrated that maternal HIV infection does not affect the outcome of pregnancy.[40,41] However, since a significant number of infected mothers are IV drug abusers, they are at increased risk for preterm delivery and low birth weight infants. Also, there is no evidence that pregnancy accelerates the progression of HIV infection.

Diagnosis

The diagnosis of HIV infection is serologic, by virus culture or by detection of viral DNA or RNA using polymerase chain reaction (PCR). The screening procedure is an ELISA test that is extremely sensitive, specific, inexpensive, and easy to perform. The ELISA test may produce false-positive results, and all positive tests should be followed by Western blot analysis. Western blot detects antibodies against glycoproteins p24, p31, gp41, and gp160. The presence of antibodies against these structural and envelope proteins is a reliable indication of infection. Results of the Western blot are given as positive, negative, or undetermined. The probability of a false-positive diagnosis is almost nil if two ELISAs and one Western blot are positive. Once the presence of infection has been demonstrated, it is possible to use determination of CD4 cells to assess the severity of the immunologic dysfunction.

Viral cultures and PCR may be used for diagnosis of HIV under special circumstances. Cultures are labor intensive, expensive, and less sensitive than serologic testing. PCR is a very sensitive technique that has the potential to become the test of choice for the diagnosis of HIV infection.

Fetal transmission

Approximately 24% of infants born to HIV-infected mothers will demonstrate the presence of the disease by 1 year of age.[42] It is not clear if the infection is transmitted during pregnancy, during delivery, or shortly after birth, although there is evidence that fetal infection may occur by transplacental transmission, by contact with infected secretions, and through breastfeeding.

Significant effort has been directed to the identification of factors predictive of fetal infection. One of these factors is the previous birth of an infected child. Another is severely depressed immune function as shown by low CD4 counts.[43] The presence of maternal antibodies against certain epitopes or against the principal neutralizing domain of the envelope protein gp120 is also predictive of the absence of newborn infection.[44-46]

The majority of babies born to HIV-positive mothers have no physical signs of infection. A few of them may exhibit the so-called HIV embryopathy characterized by growth retardation, microcephaly, and craniofacial abnormalities. All infants of HIV-infected mothers have positive HIV serology as a consequence of passive transfer of maternal antibodies. Levels of these antibodies decline gradually, and by 6 months of age, most noninfected newborns will be seronegative. The presence of positive serology resulting from passive transmission of antibodies makes difficult the diagnosis of HIV infection in the newborn. In this situation viral cultures and PCR testing should be done to confirm or rule out infection.

Management of HIV-infected pregnant women

Detection. The first issue in the management of HIV infection during pregnancy is detection. The dismal prognosis of affected individuals and the fear of acquiring the disease has generated a demand for universal screening. However, this measure is controversial, especially as it relates to the issue of confidentiality, and in many states is the subject of specific legal requirements. Everybody agrees that screening should be selectively offered to high-risk patients (Box 18-7), and some believe that it should be universal if the prevalence of the disease in a particular community is greater than 1%. When the test is strongly recommended by a physician, it will be accepted by 70% to 80% of the patients.

To induce patients to be tested, some institutions have developed specific protocols that include giving to all pregnant patients a pamphlet containing information about AIDS. This booklet identifies patients at high risk (Box 18-7) and suggests taking the test if the patient feels that she belongs to one of those groups.[47] Patients requesting HIV testing should be counseled, and written informed consent should be obtained before the test. If the patient is HIV negative, the test should be repeated in the third trimester to detect patients that seroconvert between the first test and delivery.

Antepartum care. Pregnant patients with positive HIV serology should be counseled, including the option of abortion if the pregnancy is less than 22 weeks. If the patient decides to con-

---

BOX 18-7

Individuals at High Risk for HIV Infection

Prostitutes
IV drug abusers
Women whose partners are:
   HIV positive
   IV drug abusers
   Hemophiliacs
   African or Haitian immigrants who arrived after 1975
Women whose partners have had:
   Homosexual experiences
   Blood transfusions between 1977 and 1985

BOX 18-8

Antepartum Management of the HIV-Infected Patient

- Evaluate for other sexually transmitted diseases
- Perform serial ultrasounds to follow fetal growth
- Perform weekly nonstress tests after 32 weeks
- Measure CD4 cell count every trimester
- If the CD4 cell count is greater than 500, provide regular obstetric care
- If the CD4 cell count is less than 500, start therapy with azidothymidine (AZT), 100 mg 5 times daily
- If the CD4 count is less than 200, start prophylaxis for *Pneumocystis carinii* infection, using trimethoprim-sulfamethoxazole, double-strength, two tablets twice daily, 3 times every week
- Obtain infectious disease consultation if any opportunistic infection develops
- Coordinate participation in patient's care of other services such as nutrition, pediatrics, social services

---

BOX 18-9

Intrapartum Measures for HIV-Infected Patients

- Health care personnel should use protective barriers, including protective eyeglasses, impermeable gowns, and double gloves
- Handle blood, amniotic fluid, and other secretions and body fluids as if they were infected
- Properly handle needles and scalpels
- Nasopharyngeal secretions of the neonate should be removed using wall suction with a device that will keep the pressure below 140 mm Hg; oropharyngeal secretions should be removed with bulb or with wall suction

---

tinue with the pregnancy, her antepartum management should include the measures described in Box 18-8.

Intrapartum management. At the time of delivery, special precautions should be taken to avoid contact of the health-care personnel with body fluids of the HIV-infected patients. The pediatric service should be notified in advance so they will be present at the time of delivery and provide adequate follow-up of the infant.

Most investigators have the opinion that cesarean section plays little or no role in the prevention of HIV perinatal infection. However, if evidence that exposure to vaginal secretions may be harmful to the fetus continues to accumulate, the role of cesarean delivery will be reevaluated. To avoid contact between the vaginal secretions and the fetal blood, it is recommended that the use of fetal scalp electrodes and fetal blood sampling be avoided.

At the time of delivery it is important to take measures to avoid transmission of HIV to the health care providers. These measures are shown in Box 18-9.

Postpartum care. Universal precautions should continue in the postpartum period. The mother should be instructed to avoid breastfeeding. Medical and pediatric follow-up for mother and baby are extremely important.

◼ GENITAL HERPES

The herpes simplex virus (HSV) is of major obstetric interest because along with gonorrhea and chlamydia, it is one of the most common sexually transmitted diseases and because of its potential to cause severe fetal and neonatal infection.

Description of the organism

HSV belongs to the herpesvirus family, a large group of DNA viruses that includes at least three other human viruses—cytomegalovirus, varicella-zoster, and Epstein-Barr virus. These viruses have the ability to persist throughout the life of their hosts, to produce recurrent infections, and to induce intranuclear inclusions in infected cells.

There are two main antigenic types of HSV: HSV-1 and HSV-2. Although there is a 50% concordance in DNA sequences, several biologic and biochemical differences between HSV-1 and HSV-2 have been identified. Both types of HSV can affect the genital areas, and both can lead to neonatal infections of equal severity. Approximately three fourths of neonatal HSV infections are of type 2 and one fourth of type 1.

Maternal infection

Genital HSV infections have been detected in 1% to 2% of low-income pregnant patients surveyed by cytologic or viral screening. The incidence of positive studies at the time of delivery is lower, approximately 1 case in 250 as determined by viral cultures.[48] Women of higher socioeconomic status and nonpregnant women have lower infection rates.

Women affected with primary or recurrent infections usually show characteristic lesions in the external genitalia and have nonspecific manifestations of genital infection, including cervical inflammation, dysuria, hematuria, leukorrhea, and pelvic pain. However, approximately 43% of patients with positive cultures are asymptomatic at the time of diagnosis. Asymptomatic shedding occurs between 1 week and 3 months after an infection, most commonly from 1 to 3 weeks. Shedding tends to be longer with primary infections. The rate of asymptomatic shedding during pregnancy is between 0.2% and 7.4%, and at the time of delivery between 0.1% and 1.4%.

Hematogenous transmission

Women with genital HSV infections during the first half of pregnancy have a 50% incidence of spontaneous abortions.[49] The risk of abortion seems to be higher in those with primary infections. The HSV has been isolated from abortus material, but it is unclear whether the increased abortion rate results from generalized maternal toxicity or whether it is related to the fetal infection.

Transplacental intrauterine herpes infections are infrequent. However, their occurrence has been well documented, and these babies show skin lesions and scars at birth, microcephaly, microphthalmia, and hydranencephaly, as well as positive HSV-2 cultures.[50]

Maternal infection after 20 weeks of gestation is associated with an increased incidence of preterm delivery. In the study of Nahamias et al.,[49] 35% of a group of women experiencing primary infections after 20 weeks of gestation delivered prematurely, as compared to 14% of women of similar gestational age affected by recurrent infections. Other investigations in women with recurrent infections have not confirmed this observation.[51] It seems that the risk of preterm delivery is most pronounced in women experiencing primary HSV infections.

Transmission at delivery

The most important source of infection to the neonate is the mother's genital tract at the time of delivery. Passage through virus-containing ma-

ternal secretions during the second stage of labor allows HSV to enter the infant via the eyes, upper respiratory tract, scalp (especially if internal fetal monitoring devices were used), and cord. Prolonged rupture of the membranes has also been associated with neonatal infections, suggesting an ascending spread of infection.

When an infant is delivered vaginally from a mother affected by primary HSV genital infection, the risk of acquiring the infection is 40% to 60%.[51] This risk is less than 5% if the mother is affected by a recurrent infection, because in these patients the immune response limits the infection and has a protective effect on the fetus.

The risk of neonatal infection in patients with active genital herpes at the time of delivery is markedly decreased if the infant is delivered by cesarean section. If the infant is delivered by cesarean section more than 4 hours after rupture of the membranes, it does not necessarily develop infection. Grossman et al.[52] reported that of 58 pregnancies complicated by HSV infection, 6 infants were delivered by cesarean section more than 4 hours after rupture of the membranes, and none of them became infected.

The risk of acquiring HSV infection appears to be similar whether the infant is term or preterm. Transplacentally acquired antibodies against HSV may protect the infant from disseminated HSV infection but do not protect against localized disease, which may be fatal.[53]

Newborns with herpes may have disseminated disease, central nervous system infection, or local infection in skin, eyes, or mouth. Babies with disseminated herpes infection usually have unspecific symptoms such as lethargy, irritability, and apnea between 9 and 11 days of age. This is followed within 24 hours by seizures, coagulopathy, cardiovascular compromise, liver involvement, and death. Visintine et al.[54] reviewed the clinical course of 324 infants with HSV infections and found that the disseminated form of HSV infection in the neonate involves primarily the liver and adrenal glands. Other organs frequently involved include the larynx, trachea, lungs, esophagus, stomach, intestines, spleen, and heart. If the infant does not die early from visceral involvement, central nervous system disease is often manifest. Skin, oral, or ocular lesions are often associated with disseminated disease.

Encephalitis may occur as a part of disseminated herpetic infection or as the predominant manifestation. It is characterized by nonfocal, intractable seizures. Most of the survivors have neurologic sequelae.

Almost 50% of newborns with neonatal herpes have disease localized to the skin, mouth, or eye. Also, several cases have been reported in which pneumonia, appearing between days 3 and 14 of life, is the most prominent feature of the infection.

Diagnosis

Viral isolation is the most definitive means of establishing HSV infections. Specimens are obtained from any active lesions and from the cervix and vagina. If not tested within a few hours, the specimen should be frozen at $-70°$ C or in dry ice or stored in a Leibovitz-Emory transport medium. A tentative diagnosis can usually be obtained by the viral laboratory in 1 to 3 days.

Serologic tests are of limited value because of the cross reactivity of HSV-1 and HSV-2. However, if an individual is seronegative, acute and convalescent titers can define a primary infection.

Cytologic techniques are a readily available, rapid means of identifying HSV infections. Cell scrapings are obtained from the base of lesions and from the cervix; they are smeared, fixed in alcohol, and then stained with Papanicolaou's stain. The typical morphologic findings include intranuclear inclusions and multinucleated giant cells. In skilled hands, cytologic techniques will identify 60% to 80% of HSV infections.[28]

Management

A careful history of prior HSV infections, both genital and labial, and of exposure to the virus is useful during an initial evaluation. Any suspicious lesions should be cultured and smeared for cytologic evaluation. If the patient has no history of prior genital or labial HSV infections, acute and convalescent serologic titers may be helpful.

It is unnecesary to obtain cervical cultures from patients with recurrent infections in attempts to document HSV infection before delivery.[55] Cultures are useless[56] because:

1. Their predictive value for viral shedding during labor is very poor.
2. Most babies with herpes infections are born to mothers with no history of herpes.
3. Culture results are frequently not available in adequate time to allow proper clinical decisions.

4. Cultures are focused on women with recurrent infections who have protective antibodies and are at relatively low risk of having neonates with disseminated infections.[57]

The present recommendation for the prevention of neonatal herpes is to inspect the vulva, vagina, and cervix for herpes infections at the time of labor. If herpetic lesions are present, they should be cultured to confirm the diagnosis, and the patient should be delivered by cesarean section. Cesarean is justified even if the infected woman has had ruptured membranes for more than 4 hours. If no herpetic lesions are present, cultures are unnecessary, and the patient should be allowed to deliver vaginally. Because of the very low incidence of early congenital infections leading to affected infants, amniocentesis is not indicated.

There is considerable controversy regarding isolation policies for both mother and infant who may have HSV infection. Also, there are no defined policies with respect to herpes labialis, which puts infants at greater risk, since it is almost impossible for mothers and nurses with "cold sores" to keep their hands from their face, and the virus may be transferred to the hands and then to the baby. In general, as long as the mother maintains scrupulous handwashing after personal hygiene care, there is no increased risk of transmission of genital or labial HSV to other patients or to the baby. A recent review article set forth some useful recommendations for the care of mothers with both genital and nongenital HSV infections.[58] These recommendations are summarized in Boxes 18-10 and 18-11.

In cases of both genital and nongenital infections, standard operating room technique and proper cleaning of labor and delivery rooms should be sufficient to prevent transmission of HSV infection in these areas.

Treatment

HSV infections in nonpregnant individuals can be successfully treated with acyclovir (ACV). This drug is a synthetic purine nucleoside analogue that is metabolized only in cells infected with HSV. After entering the infected cell, ACV is phosphorylated by a thymidine kinase produced by the virus and converted into ACV-monophosphate. This is followed by another phosphorylation step, this time carried out by host cell enzymes, which results in the formation

---

BOX 18-10

Care of Mother with Proven or Clinically Suspected Genital HSV Infection

- Mother should be in private room
- All personnel having direct contact with the patient or with contaminated articles should wear gown and gloves
- Perineal pads and other genital dressings and bed linen should be handled as if infected (i.e., double-bagged)
- Mother may handle and feed her infant if:
  1. She is not in bed and has washed her hands carefully (For mother-newborn contact this is preferable to wearing gloves)
  2. She puts on a clean gown before the baby is brought to her from the nursery
- Mother may leave room after washing her hands and view baby through nursery windows

---

BOX 18-11

Care of Mother with Active Nongenital HSV Infection

- Mother should be in a private room
- All personnel having direct contact with patient or contaminated articles should wear gown and gloves
- Bed linen and dressings covering lesions should be handled as if infected (i.e., double-bagged)
- Attempts should be made to expedite crusting of lesions by applying drying agents such as providone-iodine (Betadine), benzoin, or ethyl ether
- Once lesions are crusted (generally after 2 to 3 days), mother may handle infant as described for mother with genital HSV infection, except she should wear a face mask

---

of ACV-triphosphate. The latter compound is a substrate and a competitive inhibitor of the HSV DNA polymerase and effectively stops viral replication.

ACV has little toxicity, but its use in pregnancy is not recommended because of potential unknown effects on the fetus. However, the medication has been used during pregnancy for the treatment of disseminated HSV infection without fetal effects.[59,60] A registry of patients taking ACV during pregnancy had 312 exposed pregnancies through June 30, 1990, without evidence of harmful fetal effects.[61] In view of this preliminary information about ACV safety, trials of the drug for patients with genital infection and labor or ruptured membranes are fully justified.

◪ VARICELLA

Varicella (chicken pox) is a highly contagious disease, usually contracted by children, that may occur in a pregnant woman and cause significant maternal and fetal morbidity and mortality. Since varicella is a common infection in children and confers a lifelong immunity, it is not surprising that approximately 95% of women of reproductive age in the United States are immune.[62] Therefore the incidence of varicella in pregnant women is low, approximately 5 per 10,000.[63]

Description of the organism

The varicella-zoster virus is a member of the herpesvirus family. It measures approximately 200 nm in diameter, is enveloped, and its genetic material is double-stranded DNA.

Transmission

The varicella virus is transmitted usually by the respiratory route. It also can be transmitted from pregnant women to their fetuses by the hematogenous transplacental route.

Maternal infection

The incubation period of varicella is, on the average, 11 days. The first symptoms are fever, malaise, myalgias, and headaches. These symptoms are followed within 1 day by the onset of a maculopapular rash on the skin and mucosal membranes that rapidly transforms into vesicles that are extremely pruritic. The vesicles progress rapidly to pustules and then scabs. Characteristically, new crops appear for 3 to 4 days, and all stages of the cutaneous lesion are present at the same time. All skin lesions crust by the tenth day after the rash starts. The disease is self-limited, and if there are no complications, the process ends in 2 to 4 weeks.

Varicella infection is more severe in adults than in children. When varicella occurs in pregnancy, maternal morbidity and mortality are increased, and there are potentially severe fetal complications. The most serious maternal complication is the development of pneumonia, a problem that affects approximately 10% of pregnant patients.[64] Pneumonia usually occurs 1 or 2 days after the appearance of the cutaneous lesions. The initial symptoms are shortness of breath, pleuritic pain, and cough. The chest x-ray will show characteristic pneumonic infiltrates. Many patients develop severe adult respiratory distress syndrome (ARDS), and the mortality varies between 10% and 35%.[65,66] Another serious, albeit rare, maternal complication is encephalitis. More common are preterm labor, preterm delivery, and herpes zoster.

Fetal infection

Congenital varicella is diagnosed when the disease occurs before the tenth day of life or when the baby is born with the developmental abnormalities associated with varicella infection. Postnatal varicella that begins between 10 and 28 days after birth usually has a mild course. The pattern of fetal disease will depend on the gestational age of the fetus at the time of infection. When fetal disease occurs within the first 15 weeks of gestation, approximately 2% to 10% of the newborns will be affected by varicella embryopathy.[40,67] This syndrome is characterized by low birth weight, ophthalmologic lesions, neurologic symptoms, hypotrophic limbs, skin scars, and psychomotor retardation.

Another serious perinatal problem occurs when the mother acquires varicella late in the third trimester of pregnancy, because 25% to 50% of the newborns will develop a severe form of varicella that has a 30% mortality rate. Neonatal varicella is characterized by pneumonitis, hepatitis, and disseminated intravascular coagulation. The severity of the neonatal infection is directly related to the presence of maternal antibodies in the newborn circulation.

Of particular interest is the period between 5 days before and 10 days after delivery. The mother starts to produce and transfer to the fetus protective antibodies approximately 5 days after the onset of her disease. Thus babies born 5 days or more after the beginning of the maternal disease will be protected. Babies that develop neonatal varicella between birth and 5 days of age also will be protected. In contrast,

TABLE 18-2 ◪ Deaths from congenital varicella in relation to date of onset of rash in mother or neonate

	Neonatal deaths	Neonatal cases	Mortality (%)
Day of onset of rash in neonate			
0 to 4	0	22	0
5 to 10	4	19	21
Onset of maternal rash, days antepartum			
0 to 4	4	13	31
>5	0	23	0

From Gershon AA: Chickenpox, measles, and mumps, in Remington JS, Klein JO (eds): *Infection diseases of the fetus and newborn infant.* Philadelphia, WB Saunders, 1990, p 413.

mortality will be elevated if the neonatal rash appears between days 5 and 10 (Table 18-2). Neonatal infection after day 10 is usually mild.

The fetus also may develop varicella in utero that is healed at the time of birth. These babies are carriers of the virus and will develop herpes zoster during childhood.

Diagnosis

The diagnosis of maternal varicella is primarily clinical. However, the presence of the disease may be documented by viral culture or by serologic seroconversion. The main serologic tests are the fluorescent antibody to membrane antigen (FAMA), the enzyme immunoassay (EIA), and the complement fixation (CF).

Management

The most common problem related to varicella that the obstetrician finds in practice is the pregnant patient with a history of exposure to a child with varicella and who does not know whether she had the illness during childhood. This is a relatively simple problem. The patient immunity should be determined with a FAMA test.[68] If the patient is immune, no treatment will be necessary. If the patient is not immune, she should be treated with varicella-zoster immune globulin (VZIG) in a single dose, intramuscularly, ideally no later than 96 hours after exposure. VZIG comes in vials containing 125 units per vial with a volume of approximately 1.25 ml. The recommended dose is 125 units per each 10 kg of body weight up to a maximum of 625 units. VZGI is effective in preventing and attenuating maternal disease.[69]

Maternal varicella may appear before the last weeks of the third trimester. These patients require special attention because they are prone to have a difficult course and develop serious complications. The biggest fear is the development of pneumonia. If this occurs, the patient should be admitted to the hospital. To avoid nosocomial spread of the infection, the patient should be in respiratory isolation, and her care should be given only by individuals with known varicella immunity. Treatment should start immediately using acyclovir, 500 mg/m^2 (10 to 15 mg/kg) intravenously, every 8 hours for 7 days.[70] Mechanical ventilation should be used aggressively if necessary. Another antiviral drug that may be used in pregnant patients with varicella is vidarabine (Ara-A), in doses of 10 ml/kg over a 12-hour period, every day for 5 days.[71]

Pregnant patients with varicella in the last weeks of the third trimester should be monitored for uterine contractions and treated with tocolytic agents if they develop excessive uterine activity. The objective of the treatment is to delay delivery for at least 5 days after the onset of maternal symptoms so the fetus has the protection of passively transmitted maternal antibodies.

Although the present recommendation is to give acyclovir only if pneumonia, encephalitis, or other complications develop, an argument can be made about the potential advantages of giving acyclovir to *all* pregnant women that develop varicella at any time during pregnancy. Studies are necessary to determine whether the course of maternal and fetal disease is modified and complications are avoided by administering acyclovir before complications appear.

◪ HEPATITIS B

There are at least six different types of viral hepatitis. They include hepatitis A, B, D, E, and at least two subtypes of non-A, non-B. Hepatitis A is not transmitted vertically to the fetus. Hepatitis B may be transmitted to the fetus and is the main concern of the obstetrician. Hepatitis D has similar characteristics to and requires concomitant infection with hepatitis B. Hepatitis E has characteristics similar to hepatitis A, but is a more serious condition. It has caused large epidemics of acute viral hepatitis in developing countries, with significant mortality in pregnant women. The non-A, non-B hepatitis is caused by several distinct agents, the most commonly recognized being the hepatitis C virus and the enterically transmitted form.

Hepatitis B virus

The hepatitis B virus (HBV) is the cause of 40% to 45% of all cases of hepatitis found in the United States. It occurs de novo in approximately 1 or 2 of every 1000 pregnancies, and the frequency of asymptomatic carriers is 6 to 10 per 1000 pregnancies for a total prevalence of 7 to 12 per 1000 pregnancies.

The HBV, or Dane particle, is a DNA virus with a diameter of 42 nm, formed by a nucleocapsid containing the core antigen (HBcAg) surrounded by inner and outer envelopes. The surface antigen (HBsAg) and the e antigen (HBeAg), which is a soluble polypeptide, are part of the viral envelope. The HBsAg is the marker of ongoing HBV infection and is found not only in the 42-nm intact virion or Dane particle, but also in incomplete viral surface capsule particles devoid of DNA, one of them spherical and measuring 20 nm and another long and filamentous, measuring up to 200 nm in length. The genetic material of HBV is a long, circular DNA molecule that is partially double stranded.

Transmission

The HBV is highly infectious and can be transmitted by the parenteral route, by sexual intercourse, and by vertical transmission to the fetus. There are certain groups of individuals that are at high risk of being chronic carriers of HBV (Box 18-12). In some places in the world with high prevalence of HBV infection, perinatal transmission from chronic carriers is responsible for 35% to 50% of all new infections.

Maternal infection

Pregnant women are affected by acute HBV infection or have chronic infections. The acute infection is manifested by flulike symptoms in approximately 25% of the patients and is asymptomatic in the rest. The majority of patients do not develop jaundice, and fever is uncommon. Approximately 90% of these individuals have spontaneous complete resolution of the acute in-

BOX 18-12

Individuals at High Risk of Being Hepatitis B Chronic Carriers

- Intravenous drug abusers
- Individuals that work in hemodialysis units
- Household contacts of HBV carriers
- Immigrants from Asia, the Pacific basin, sub-Saharan Africa, the Caribbean, and Central and South America and Alaskan Eskimos
- Clients or staff of institutions for the mentally retarded
- Prostitutes
- Sexual partners of IV drug users, hemophiliacs, or bisexual individuals
- Multiple blood transfusion recipients
- Individuals with acute or chronic liver disease
- Professional exposure to blood or blood products

fection, fewer than 1% will die of fulminant hepatitis, and 5% to 10% will become chronic carriers manifested by the continuous presence of HBsAg in their serum.

Seven of each 10 chronic HBV carriers have chronic persistent hepatitis (CPH), and the other 3 have chronic active hepatitis (CAH). In individuals with CPH, the disease does not progress, and liver enzymes are normal. Patients with CAH follow a different course and frequently develop cirrhosis, hepatic failure, and primary hepatocellular carcinoma. Also, about 50% of CAH patients of Mediterranean origin are simultaneously infected with the delta virus agent of hepatitis D, suffer recurrent attacks of acute hepatitis, and die of cirrhosis and liver failure.

Diagnosis

The diagnosis of acute HBV infection is made by detecting the presence of HBsAg early in the course of the disease, followed by the appearance of antibodies against the core (anti-HBc), the e (anti-HBe), and the surface (anti-HBs) antigens. The liver enzymes will be elevated during the initial phase of the disease.

The diagnosis of chronic carriers is more complex. Their serology marker is a persistence of HBsAg more than 6 months after the initial infection. The presence of a positive HBeAg indicates a highly infectious carrier. The presence of

anti-HBc is a marker for prior disease. The presence of anti-HBe antibody and the absence of HBV DNA in the patient serum indicate the end of the active liver disease, even if the HBsAg is still positive.

Approximately 10% to 40% of chronic HBV carriers with positive HBsAg have detectable anti-HBs antibodies. In these cases the antibodies are probably against a different viral genome having as little as a single amino acid substitution in the surface antigen.

Management

All pregnant women should be screened for HBV infection.[72] Selective screening of high-risk groups has failed to identify a high number of infected individuals. Screening is usually made during the first prenatal visit and should be repeated during the third trimester in high-risk patients. The screening test is a determination of HBsAg.

Neonatal transmission

Most newborn infections are the result of vertical transmission from chronic carriers or occur after acute infection in the last trimester of pregnancy. Mothers with acute infection during the first and second trimesters transmit the infection to approximately 10% of their newborns. When the acute infection occurs in the third trimester, 80% to 90% of the newborns will be infected.

The higher risk for vertical transmission is attributed to chronic carriers with positive HBeAg. These patients are highly infective, and as many as 90% of their newborns will be infected. Mothers with positive anti-HBe antibody have a 25% probability of transmitting the infection. If both HBeAg and anti-HBe are not present, there is a 10% probability of neonatal infection.

The relative contribution to neonatal infection of hematogenous infection and the contact with maternal blood and vaginal secretions during delivery has not been completely elucidated. For that reason the use of cesarean delivery for the prevention of neonatal infection in HBV carriers is controversial. Some studies have shown no advantage in cesarean delivery, whereas others have shown a reduction in neonatal infection from 24.9% in infants delivered vaginally to 10% in infants delivered by cesarean.[73]

Infants born to HBsAg-positive mothers do not need to be isolated at birth. However, the mother's secretions should be considered potentially infected and managed with universal precautions. Breastfeeding should be discouraged.

Prevention of neonatal hepatitis

The current recommendation for prevention is to administer HBV immune globulin (0.5 ml intramuscularly) within 12 hours of birth, followed by hepatitis B vaccine (0.5 ml intramuscularly) within 12 hours of birth and again 1 and 6 months later. The efficacy of combined passive and active immunization in preventing perinatal transmission of HBV ranges between 85% and 95%.[74]

■ PARVOVIRUS B19 INFECTION

Parvovirus B19 is a single-stranded DNA virus that requires rapidly dividing cells for replication. Parvoviruses are small (20 to 25 nm), nonenveloped, and structurally simple, being able to code for only a few proteins.

Parvovirus B19 is the cause of erythema infectiosum, or fifth disease, a condition characterized by diffuse erythema of the cheeks (slapped-cheek disease) that usually affects elementary school children. The organism is also responsible for arthralgias in the adult and may have a role in the development of rheumatoid arthritis. Also, it causes aplastic anemia crisis in patients with sickle cell disease and other hemolytic anemias and is a cause of chronic anemia in immunologically deficient patients. The virus is of interest to the obstetrician because infected mothers can transmit the organism to the fetus causing nonimmune fetal hydrops and death.

Maternal infection

Approximately 50% of women of childbearing age are seronegative for parvovirus B19 and susceptible to infection during pregnancy. The virus can be transmitted to a pregnant woman in several ways, including parenterally and through contact with contaminated plates and eating utensils, but the primary mechanism is person-to-person via the oropharyngeal route. Maternal infection is usually asymptomatic. A few patients complain of arthralgias, rash, and low-grade fever.

Studies have demonstrated that the risk of becoming infected is job related, with individuals working in school cafeterias and day-care centers and school teachers having the highest infection rate.[75] The risk of infection for susceptible seronegative individuals during a school outbreak of erythema infectiosum is approximately 6% for women in the community, 20% for teachers, 30% for day-care personnel, and 50% for school cafeteria workers. For susceptible teachers the rate of infection will be increased if they are exposed to a large number of children with the disease.

Fetal transmission

The initial studies indicated a high rate of fetal transmission. This has been proven incorrect, and the large majority of infected mothers (84%) will go to term and deliver normal newborns.[76] Of the fetal losses, only 9% have positive virologic findings in the fetus. Other studies have suggested an even lower rate of fetal transmission, less than 5%.[77] The rate of fetal loss is higher when the infection occurs in the first 20 weeks of pregnancy. It is not known what proportion of those fetuses that become infected develop aplastic anemia. There is evidence that infected fetuses may tolerate the disease and be born without sequelae. Woernle et al.[78] described four women with parvovirus B19 infection. One delivered a stillborn hydropic fetus. The other three delivered at term. One of these normal term infants had serologic evidence of intrauterine infection. Chao[79] described a fetus that developed hydrops at 17 weeks and had parvovirus B19 IgM detected in pleural effusion fluid. This fetus had spontaneous resolution of the hydrops followed by development of growth retardation. The fetus was delivered at 35 weeks and had an uneventful course in the nursery.

Fetal infection is characterized by the presence of nonimmunologic fetal hydrops. These fetuses have ascites, pleural and pericardial effusions, and subcutaneous edema. Most likely the cause of the hydrops is fetal aplastic anemia caused by destruction of erythroid precursor cells by the virus. Also, the myocardial cells may become infected and the hydrops aggravated by congestive heart failure.[79,80]

Diagnosis

Parvovirus B19 does not grow in cell cultures, and the diagnosis of the infection is based on serology and the use of DNA probes.

Management

The most common problem that the obstetrician faces in relation to parvovirus B19 infection is assessment of the risk of becoming infected in pregnant women that actually or potentially are exposed to affected children during an outbreak of fifth disease. Unfortunately, there is no rapid test to assess the patient's immunity, and B19 antibody testing is restricted to a few places in the United States. Under these circumstances, calculation of the probability of infection should be based on the prevalence of seronegativity in the reproductive-age population (50%), occupational risk for infection (20% for teachers, 30% for day-care center personnel), and the risk of fetal infection if the mother develops the disease (10%). The overall risk will be 1 to 5 in 1000.

In these cases the mother should be followed with maternal serum alpha-fetoprotein (MSAFP) determinations. This substance seems to be a marker for the development of fetal hydrops.[81,82] If the MSAFP increases or the mother develops symptoms of infection, it is important to follow the fetal situation with weekly ultrasound examinations to detect the appearance of hydrops. If the fetus develops hydrops, direct intravascular intrauterine transfusion is the treatment of choice.

▰ TOXOPLASMOSIS

Approximately 3300 infants born every year in the United States are congenitally infected with toxoplasmosis. Most of these infants are asymptomatic during the neonatal period, but many subsequently develop adverse sequelae. Early treatment—maternal or neonatal—may reduce the severity of the sequelae. The main challenge lies in the early diagnosis of the asymptomatic infected gravidas and neonates.

Description of the parasite

Toxoplasma gondii exists in three forms: the trophozoite, tissue cysts, and oocysts. The trophozoite requires an intracellular habitat to survive and multiply. Reproduction is endogenous (internal budding). During the acute phase of an infection, the trophozoite invades virtually every type of cell. After invasion the organisms multiply until the cell cytoplasm is so filled that the cell is disrupted.

The second form of the parasite, tissue cysts, are formed within the host cell as early as the eighth day of an acute infection and probably persist throughout the life of the host. The skeleton, heart muscles, and brain are the most common sites for latent infections.

The oocysts are produced in the small intestine of the cat. Once shed, the oocyst sporulates in 1 to 5 days and becomes infectious. Under appropriate conditions (warm moist soil), it may re-main infectious for more than 1 year. The parasite, in addition to being transmitted by direct handling of contaminated soil and cat feces, can be transmitted to food via insect vectors.

All forms of the parasite are destroyed by adequate freezing and heating. Tissue cysts and oocysts are resistant to stomach and small bowel digestion and destruction.

Maternal infection

Transmission of *Toxoplasma* to humans commonly occurs through the ingestion of undercooked meat (pork or lamb and occasionally beef) and through other foods contaminated with oocysts. Isolated cases have been transmitted by the transfusion of whole blood.

Most maternal infections with *Toxoplasma* are mild or asymptomatic. The commonly recognized clinical signs are adenopathy and fatigue without fever. The groups of nodes most often involved are the cervical, suboccipital, supraclavicular, axillary, and inguinal nodes. The adenopathy may be localized in one node or diffused. Retroperitoneal and mesenteric nodes may also be involved, as well as the spleen and liver. Occasionally there may be a fever or exanthem. Chorioretinitis rarely occurs in the acute infection, but several cases have been documented.

Congenital transmission

Of major obstetric concern is the congenital transmission of the parasite. With very rare exceptions, congenital transmission occurs only during an acute infection acquired during pregnancy. Most fetal transmission appears to be transplacental and usually occurs before labor as evidenced by cord antibody titers. *Toxoplasma* is rarely transmitted to the fetus when the acute infection occurs at conception or during the first 2 months of gestation. During this time the placenta appears to serve as a "barrier" to fetal infection more effectively than later in gestation and provides nearly 80% protection. Although the placenta is infected with *Toxoplasma*, there is evidence that, in some cases, transmission to the infant does not occur until labor begins.[83] Occasionally women secrete *Toxoplasma* in their vaginal fluids, and exposure to the infant may be through vaginal delivery.

The relative risk of acquiring toxoplasmosis during pregnancy is related in part to the overall incidence of the disease in each community. Studies of U.S. citizens reveal a wide variation of antibody positivity ranging from 13% to 67% and tending to increase with age. Studies of pregnant women with toxoplasmosis in the United States have been few. In one study in New York City of over 4000 pregnant women,[31] the overall incidence of positive *Toxoplasma* antibodies was 31%. Women who were older, more affluent, and white had the highest incidence of prior infection. The higher-income white patients also had the greatest risk of acquiring toxoplasmosis acutely during pregnancy; in this group, 3 of 189 women seroconverted during gestation.

Studies uniformly have shown that toxoplasmosis is transmitted to the fetus in less than 50% of the acute cases. Transmission to the fetus is lower in the first trimester (15%) than in the third (60%), but the severity of the infection is greater when it occurs in early pregnancy. Multiple prospective studies have been done in France where the incidence of toxoplasmosis is high and seroconversion during pregnancy frequent (6.3% risk in each pregnancy). In one group of 183 women who seroconverted during pregnancy, the results were an overall vertical transmission rate of 33% to 39%, resulting in 11 abortions, 7 stillbirths or immediate newborn deaths, and 59 infants born with congenital toxoplasmosis.[84] Of the 59 infected infants, 9 were severely affected, 11 were mildly affected, and 39 had subclinical disease at birth. The severely infected infants all acquired their infections during the first two trimesters of pregnancy. Third-trimester transmission resulted only in subclinical infection. None of the infants of 195 mothers with elevated antibody titers suggesting infection before gestation were infected.

Congenital infection

Infants with congenital toxoplasmosis may be stillborn, may be obviously affected at birth, gradually develop symptoms in the first months of life or even later, or remain asymptomatic. The *classic triad* of congenital toxoplasmosis includes hydrocephalus, chorioretinitis, and intracranial calcifications. Many affected infants have other symptoms including hydrops fetalis or erythroblastosis, hepatosplenomegaly, and abnormal cerebrospinal fluid.

One prospective 5-year study of infants who had toxoplasmosis as neonates revealed that 85% of them were mentally retarded; 75% developed seizures, spasticity, or other major motor defects; 50% had severely impaired vision; and 15% had significant hearing impairment. Even more wor-

risome are follow-up studies of infants detected by serologic screening who were completely asymptomatic at birth. A high percentage of these infants develop significant visual impairment, mental retardation, and other neurologic sequelae later in life.[85] In one study,[86] 20 of 23 asymptomatic infants developed significant visual impairment, with 6 becoming blind in both eyes and 5 more becoming blind in one eye. The mean IQ in this group was 89.4, with 5 children having IQs below 80. It is unclear whether early treatment of such infants reduces the incidence and severity of sequelae, although in preliminary studies treated infants appear to have done better than their untreated cohorts.[87]

Toxoplasma cysts can be isolated from the myometrium, endometrium, and vaginal secretions of chronically infected women who have stable low antibody titers. Likewise, the organism has been isolated from aborted products of conception. Data indicate, however, that although chronic toxoplasmosis is associated with abortion, it is not a common event.

Diagnosis

A number of serologic tests have been developed for the diagnosis of toxoplasmosis. The two most helpful tests for the obstetrician are the Sabin-Feldman dye test and the IgM-indirect fluorescent antibody (IgM-IFA) test.

The Sabin-Feldman dye test rises relatively slowly following an acute infection, frequently taking 2 months to attain maximum levels, which are generally greater than 300 IU/ml and may be as high as 3000 IU/ml or more. High titers persist for months to years. Low titers almost always persist for life.

The IgM-IFA test becomes positive early in the course of an infection and may be the first serologic test to detect *Toxoplasma* antibodies. Titers in patients with an acute acquired infection vary widely, ranging from 1:10 to 1:1000. High titer persists for several years, and its presence does not necessarily indicate recent primary infection. In most cases the test becomes negative 3 to 4 months after infection.

The most common situation faced by the obstetrician is that of determining the implications of a positive dye test for *Toxoplasma* done on a routine basis or at the patient's request. The following guidelines for interpretation of the test are useful, but it must be clearly understood that they are not absolute:

1. If the dye test is negative, the patient is not immune and is at risk of seroconversion during pregnancy.
2. If the dye test is positive, it is necessary to obtain a IgM-IFA test. If the IgM-IFA test is negative, the patient had infection months or years before pregnancy, and the possibility of congenital infection is excluded.
3. If the dye test is less than 300 IU/ml and the IgM-IFA is positive, the dye test should be repeated 3 weeks later. If there is an increase in the dye titer, the infection probably was acquired within the last 2 months, and the possibility of congenital infection will depend on the gestational age at the presumed time of maternal infection.
4. If the dye test is above 300 IU/ml and the IgM-IFA is positive, there is a possibility that the mother has active toxoplasmosis, and the fetus may become infected.

Congenital infection may be diagnosed: (1) by isolating *Toxoplasma* from the amniotic fluid[88] or fetal blood;[89] or (2) by determination of specific IgM antibody and gamma-glutamyltransferase levels in fetal blood obtained by cordocentesis after 22 weeks.[89] Ultrasound also may be valuable for determining the presence of lesions, especially hydrocephaly, in fetuses known to be infected.[90]

Unfortunately, fetal IgM antibodies are found only after 22 weeks and only in 21% of affected fetuses.[91] The results of mouse inoculation take 4 to 5 weeks and are positive in 64% of infected fetuses when fetal blood is used for inoculation. With the use of multiple tests in fetal blood and amniotic fluid, the specificity of the antenatal diagnosis reaches 90%. Another diagnostic method is that of immunofluorescence of the parasite in in vitro cultures of chorionic villi using monoclonal antibodies.[92]

Management

Treatment during pregnancy attempts to decrease both the incidence and the severity of congenital infection. A combination of sulfadoxine or sulfadiazine and pyrimethamine have been used, although, because of possible teratogenic effects, pyrimethamine was not given during the first 12 to 14 weeks of pregnancy. With this treatment a definite reduction was noticed in the incidence of congenitally infected infants born to treated mothers (5% versus 16.6% for untreated mothers). In France women who seroconverted during pregnancy are treated with spiramycin, which is available in the United States only by request to the U.S. Food and Drug Administration. The treated French women had significantly fewer infants who were congenitally infected (24% versus 45% in untreated mothers), although the incidence of clinically obvious infection was similar (11%) in both groups.[93] Thus treatment of mothers who seroconvert during pregnancy appears helpful. Data are insufficient to recommend therapy of women with chronic infections.

Prevention

Heating meat thoroughly to 66° C (150° F) or having meat smoked or cured eliminates tissue cysts. Pregnant women should thoroughly wash their hands after handling raw meats. If at all possible, seronegative pregnant women should avoid handling cat litter or soil contaminated with cat feces. Cat litter should be flushed away daily. To destroy viable oocysts, the empty litter pan can be filled with nearly boiling water for 5 minutes daily. Gloves should be worn when working in contaminated soil, and hands should be washed carefully.

Recommendations

Because of the relatively low incidence of acute toxoplasmosis during pregnancy in this country and the mixed reliability of serologic tests, routine serologic screening is generally not performed. However, experts are urging that regional screening programs be developed.[94] Patients at high risk for toxoplasmosis, such as women working in veterinary clinics, cat owners, and raw and rare meat eaters, should have screening with a dye test and, if possible, the IgM-IFA test. Similarly, any woman who develops adenopathy during pregnancy should be screened and have follow-up serologic testing.

Any woman who develops acute toxoplasmosis during pregnancy should be counseled, including the possibility of legal abortion. Inasmuch as congenital toxoplasmosis is limited almost exclusively to women with acute infections, reassurances can be made regarding future pregnancies. It should be emphasized during counseling that the risk of fetal infection appears minimal if the mother's infection occurred during the first 2 months of gestation, but the risk is significant, although less than 50%, later in gestation.

Women with acute toxoplasmosis who elect not to terminate their pregnancies or who are gestationally too far advanced for an abortion may benefit from treatment. In the United States one reasonable regimen includes pyrimethamine (15 mg/m^2 per day) and sulfadiazine (1 to 3 g/day) for 3 weeks. Before using these potentially toxic medications, the reader should see the report of Remington and Desmonts[95] on therapy. When spiramycin is approved in this country, it should provide an easier, safer regimen. It is important to alert the pediatrician, so that evaluation of the infant and treatment are begun shortly after birth.

◼   IMPORTANT POINTS   ◼

1. Group B streptococcus colonizes the genital tract of 10% to 35% of women of childbearing age. Between 40% and 50% of infants born to women who are colonized at the time of delivery also will be colonized. Less than 1% of these colonized newborns will develop early-onset GBS septicemia. Thus the overall risk for any newborn baby of developing early-onset GBS infection is approximately 1 in 1000.

2. The current approach for the prevention of early-onset GBS infection is selective intrapartum treatment of patients at high risk, such as patients with preterm rupture of membranes, patients colonized within 6 weeks of delivery, and patients with intrapartum fever. Approximately 300 women at high risk need to be treated to prevent one neonatal GBS septicemia.

3. Antepartum cultures for group B streptococcus are predictive of intrapartum colonization only if they are obtained within 6 weeks from delivery. Cultures should be obtained from the rectum and the lower third of the vagina.

4. Traditionally neurosyphilis has been considered a manifestation of tertiary syphilis. However, central nervous system involvement can be demonstrated by cerebrospinal fluid analysis in a high number of patients with secondary and early-latent syphilis.

5. Neonatal syphilis will occur more frequently and will be more severe in mothers with primary or secondary syphilis than in patients with latent syphilis. The severity of neonatal infection is also related to gestational age,

and fetal morbidity will be more severe if the infection occurs in the first or second rather than in the third trimester.

6. Approximately 25% of all pregnant women in the United States are seronegative for CMV, and their risk for primary infection is approximately 1%. Only 10% of the newborns from mothers with primary CMV infection will have severe congenital infection. Therefore the risk for a pregnant woman of unknown CMV immunity to have a baby with overt CMV infection is 1 in 4000. The risk for the same woman of having a child asymptomatic at birth that will develop hearing problems as a sequela of congenital CMV infection is 1 in 1300.

7. Specific CMV IgM antibodies persist for several months after the primary infection. Therefore the presence of CMV IgM antibodies is not necessarily evidence of recent infection. The best evidence of primary maternal CMV infection is seroconversion or isolation of the virus from urine or blood. The diagnosis of fetal CMV infection requires viral culture of the amniotic fluid.

8. The best contribution of the obstetrician to the prevention of congenital rubella is postpartum vaccination of nonimmune patients.

9. The diagnosis of HIV infection can be made by serology, by viral culture, or by detection of viral RNA or DNA. The procedure most commonly used for screening purposes is the ELISA test. All positive ELISA tests require confirmation by Western blot analysis.

10. HIV screening should be offered to all pregnant patients at high risk for this infection, such as prostitutes and intravenous drug abusers. When the test is strongly recommended by a physician, the acceptance rate is greater than 70%.

11. The practice of obtaining weekly herpes cultures from the cervix during the last 4 weeks of gestation in patients with a history of genital herpes should be abandoned because most babies with neonatal herpes are born to mothers with no history of herpes, and because the predictive value of these cultures for viral shedding during labor is very poor.

12. Varicella (chicken pox) during pregnancy is rare. However, the potential maternal and fetal consequences of this disease are very

serious. The maternal mortality when pneumonia complicates varicella during pregnancy is between 10% and 35%. The mortality rate of neonatal varicella is approximately 30%.

13. Pregnant women exposed to varicella should have their immunity evaluated with a FAMA test. If the patient is not immune, she should be treated immediately with varicella-zoster immune globulin (VZIG).

14. Chronic carriers of hepatitis B are identified by the serologic persistence of HBsAg more than 6 months after the initial infection. The presence of HBe indicates a highly infectious carrier, and the possibility that the newborn will be infected is 90%.

15. The current recommendation for preventing neonatal hepatitis is to administer HBV immune globulin and hepatitis B vaccine within 12 hours of birth to every infant born to a mother with positive HBsAg.

16. The possibility of fetal parvovirus B19 infection developing in a schoolteacher following an outbreak of erythema infectiosum is approximately 5 in 1000. The probability for a pregnant woman that does not work at the school and is exposed to one child with the disease is approximately 1 in 1000.

17. Congenital transmission of toxoplasmosis occurs only during an acute infection. Transmission is lower in the first trimester (15%) than in the third (60%), but the severity of the fetal infection is greater when the infection occurs early in pregnancy.

18. Congenital *Toxoplasma* infection can be diagnosed in more than 90% of the cases using a combination of tests in the amniotic fluid and in fetal blood obtained by cordocentesis.

19. Because of the low incidence of acute toxoplasmosis during pregnancy in the United States and the unreliability of serologic tests, routine serologic screening for toxoplasmosis during pregnancy is not recommended.

REFERENCES

1. Baker CJ: Summary of the workshop on perinatal infections due to group B streptococcus. *J Infect Dis* 1977;136:137.
2. Peevy KJ, Chalhub EG: Occult group B streptococcal infection: An important cause of intrauterine asphyxia. *Am J Obstet Gynecol* 1983;146:989-990.
3. Boyer KM: Maternal screening in prevention of neonatal infections: Current status and rationale for group B streptococcal screening. *J Hosp Infect* 1988;11:328.
4. Boyer KM, Gadzala CA, Kelly PD, et al: Selective intrapartum chemoprophylaxis of neonatal group B streptococcal early-onset disease: II. Predictive value of prenatal cultures. *J Infect Dis* 1983;148:810.
5. Morales WJ, Lim DV, Walsh AF: Prevention of neonatal group B streptococcal sepsis by the use of a rapid screening test and selective intrapartum chemoprophylaxis. *Am J Obstet Gynecol* 1986;155:979.
6. Antony BF, Okada DM, Hobel CJ: Epidemiology of group B streptococcus: Longitudinal observations during pregnancy. *J Infect Dis* 1977;137:524.
7. Dillon HC, Khare S, Gray BM: Group B streptococcal carriage and disease: A 6-year prospective study. *J Pediatr* 1987;110:31-36.
8. Matorras R, Garcia-Perea A, Undizaga JA, et al: Natural transmission of group B streptococcus during delivery. *Int J Gynecol Obstet* 1989;30:99-103.
9. Boyer KM, Gadzala CA, Burd LI, et al: Selective intrapartum chemoprophylaxis of neonatal group B streptococcal early-onset disease: I. Epidemiologic rationale. *J Infect Dis* 1983;148:795-801.
10. Lugenbill C, Clark RB, Fagnant RS, et al: Comparison of the cervicovaginal Gram stain and rapid latex agglutination slide test for identification of group B streptococcus. *J Perinatol* 1990;10:403-405.
11. Christensen KK, Christensen P, Lindberg A, et al: Mothers of infants with neonatal group B streptococcal septicemia are poor responders to bacterial carbohydrate antigens. *Int Arch Allergy Appl Immunol* 1982;67:7-12.
12. Baker CJ, Rench MA, Edwards MS, et al: Immunization of pregnant women with a polysaccharide vaccine of group B streptococcus. *N Engl J Med* 1988;319:1180-1185.
13. Dykes AK, Christensen KK, Christensen P: Chronic carrier state in mothers of infants with group B streptococcal infections. *Obstet Gynecol* 1985;66:84-88.
14. Mascola L, Pelosi R, Blount JH, et al: Congenital syphilis: Why is it still occurring? *JAMA* 1984;252:1719-1722.
15. Fiumara NJ: Syphylis in newborn children. *Clin Obstet Gynecol* 1975;18:183.
16. Dorfman DH, Glaser JH: Congenital syphilis presenting in infants after the newborn period. *N Engl J Med* 1990;323:1299-1302.
17. Harter CA, Benirschke K: Fetal syphilis in the first trimester. *Am J Obstet Gynecol* 1976;124:705.
18. Lukehart SA, Hook EW, Baker-Zander SA, et al: Invasion of the central nervous system by *Treponema pallidum:* Implications for diagnosis and treatment. *Ann Intern Med* 1988;109:855.
19. Stagno N, Whitley RJ: Herpes virus infection in pregnancy: I. Cytomegalovirus and Epstein-Barr virus infection. *N Engl J Med* 1985;313:1270-1274.
20. Pass RF, Little EA, Stagno S, et al: Young children as a probable source of maternal and congenital cytomegalovirus infection. *N Engl J Med* 1987;316:1366-1370.
21. Monif GRG, Egan EA, Held B, et al: The correlation of maternal cytomegalovirus infection at varying stages in gestation with neonatal involvement. *J Pediatr* 1972; 80:17.
22. Stern H, Tucker SM: Prospective study of cytomegalovirus infection in pregnancy. *Br Med J* 1973;2:268.
23. Stagno S, Pass RF, Cloud G, et al: Primary cytomegalovirus infection in pregnancy: Incidence, transmission to

the fetus, and clinical outcome. *JAMA* 1986;256:1904-1908.

24. Reynolds DW, Stagno S, Hosty TS, et al: Maternal cytomegalovirus excretion and perinatal infection. *N Engl J Med* 1973;289:1..

25. Stagno S, Reynolds DW, Pass RF, et al: Breast milk and the risk of cytomegalovirus infection. *N Engl J Med* 1980;302:1073.

26. Hanshaw JB, Scheiner AP, Moxley AW, et al: School failure and deafness after "silent" congenital cytomegalovirus infection. *N Engl J Med* 1976;295:468.

27. Lynch L, Daffos F, Emmanuel D, et al: Prenatal diagnosis of fetal cytomegalovirus infection. *Am J Obstet Gynecol* 1991;165:714-718.

28. Hohlfeld P, Vial Y, Maillard-Brignon C, et al: Cytomegalovirus infection: Prenatal diagnosis. *Obstet Gynecol* 1991;78:615-618.

29. Fan-Havard P, Nanata MC, Brady MT: Gancyclovir—a review of pharmacology, therapeutic efficacy, and potential use for treatment of congenital cytomegalovirus infection. *J Clin Pharm Ther* 1989;14:329-340.

30. Sever JL: Pattern of development of rubella antibody levels. *Clin Perinatol* 1979;6:347.

31. Das BD, Lakhani P, Kurtz JB, et al: Congenital rubella after prior maternal immunity. *Arch Dis Child* 1990;65:545-546.

32. Daffos F, Forestier F, Grangeot-Keros L, et al: Prenatal diagnosis of congenital rubella. *Lancet* 1984;2:1-3.

33. Morgan-Capues D, Rodeck CH, Nicholaides KH, et al: Prenatal detection of rubella specific IgM in fetal sera. *Prenat Diag* 1985;5:21-26.

34. Harris RE, Smith KO, Gehle WD, et al: Rubella immunity: Comparison of hemaglutination inhibition and radio immunoassay antibody methods. *Obstet Gynecol* 1980;55:603.

35. Balfour HH: Rubella reimmunization now. *Am J Dis Child* 1979;133:1231.

36. McLaughlin MC, Gold LH: The New York rubella incident: A case for changing hospital policy regarding rubella testing and immunization. *Am J Public Health* 1979;69:287.

37. McCubbin JH, Smith JS: Rubella in a practicing obstetrician: A preventable problem. *Am J Obstet Gynecol* 1980;136:1087.

38. Cheldelin LV, Francis DP, Tilson H: Postpartum rubella vaccination: A survey of private physicians in Oregon. *JAMA* 1973;225:158.

39. Preblund SR, Stetler HC, Frand JA, et al: Fetal risks associated with rubella vaccine. *JAMA* 1981;246:1413-1417.

40. Minkoff H, Nanda D, Menez R, et al: Pregnancies resulting in infants with acquired immunodeficiency syndrome or AIDS-related complex: Follow-up of mothers, children, and subsequently born siblings. *Obstet Gynecol* 1987;69:288.

41. Selwyin PA, Schoenbaum EE, Davenny K, et al: Prospective study of human immunodeficiency virus infection and pregnancy outcome in intravenous drug users. *JAMA* 1989;261:1289.

42. The European Collaborative Study: Mother-to-child transmission of HIV infection. *Lancet* 1988;2:1039-1042.

43. Ryder RW, Nsa W, Hassig SE, et al: Perinatal transmission of the human immunodeficiency virus type 1 to infants of seropositive women in Zaire. *N Engl J Med* 1989;320:1637.

44. Padian N, Marquis L, Francis DP, et al: Male-to-female transmission of human immunodeficiency virus. *JAMA* 1987;258:788.

45. Rossi P, Moschese V, Broliden P: Presence of maternal antibodies to human immunodeficiency virus 1 envelope glycoprotein gp120 epitopes correlates with the uninfected status of children born to seropositive mothers. *Proc Natl Acad Sci U S A* 1989;86:8055-8058.

46. Devash Y, Calvelli T, Wood D, et al: Vertical transmission of human immunodeficiency virus is correlated with the absence of high-affinity maternal antibodies against the gp120 principal neutralizing domain. *Proc Natl Acad Sci U S A* 1990;87:3445-3449.

47. Sachs BP, Tuomala R, Frigoletto F: Acquired immunodeficiency syndrome: Suggested protocol for counseling and screening in pregnancy. *Obstet Gynecol* 1987;70:408-411.

48. Tejani M, Klein SW, Kaplan M: Subclinical herpes simplex genitalis infections during the perinatal period. *Am J Obstet Gynecol* 1979;135:547.

49. Nahamias AJ, Josey WE, Naib ZM, et al: Perinatal risk associated with maternal genital herpes simplex infection. *Am J Obstet Gynecol* 1971;110:825.

50. Hutto C, Arvin A, Jacobs R, et al: Intrauterine herpes simplex virus infections. *J Pediatr* 1987;110:97-101.

51. Brown ZA, Berry S, Vontver LA: Genital herpes simplex virus infections complicating pregnancy: Natural history and peripartum management. *J Reprod Med* 1986;31:420.

52. Grossman JH, Wallen WC, Sever JL: Management of genital herpes simplex virus infection during pregnancy. *Obstet Gynecol* 1981;58:1.

53. Amstey MS, Monif GRG, Nahmias Aj, et al: Cesarean section and genital herpes virus infection. *Obstet Gynecol* 1979;53:641.

54. Visintine AM, Nahamias AJ, Josey WE: Genital herpes. *Perinat Care* 1978;2:32.

55. Gibbs RS, Amstey MS, Sweet RL, et al: Management of genital herpes infection in pregnancy. *Obstet Gynecol* 1988;71:779.

56. Arvin AM, Hensleigh PA, Prober CG, et al: Failure of antepartum maternal cultures to predict the infant's risk for exposure to herpes simplex virus at delivery. *N Engl J Med* 1986;315:796-800.

57. Prober CG, Sullender WM, Yasukawa LL, et al: Low risk of herpes simplex infections in neonates exposed to the virus at the time of vaginal delivery to mothers with recurrent genital herpes simplex virus infections. *N Engl J Med* 1987;316:240-244.

58. Kibrick S: Herpes simplex infections at term: What to do with mother, newborn, and nursery personnel. *JAMA* 1980;243:157.

59. Lagrew DC, Furlow TG, Hager D, et al: Disseminated herpes simplex virus infection in pregnancy: Successful treatment with acyclovir. *JAMA* 1984;252:2058-2059.

60. Klein NA, Mabie WC, Shaver DC, et al: Herpes simplex virus hepatitis in pregnancy: Two patients successfully treated with acyclovir. *Gastroenterology* 1991;100:239-244.

61. Andrews EB, Yankaskas BC, Cordero JF, et al: Acyclovir in pregnancy registry: Six years experience. *Obstet Gynecol* 1992;79:7-13.

62. Gershon AA, Raker R, Steinberg S, et al: Antibody to varicella-zoster virus in parturient women and their offspring during the first year of life. *Pediatrics* 1976;58:692.

63. Sever JL: Infections in pregnancy: Highlights from the collaborative perinatal project. *Teratology* 1982;25:227.

64. Paryani SG, Arvin AM: Intrauterine infection with varicella-zoster virus after maternal varicella. *N Engl J Med* 1986;314:1542-1546.

65. Guess HA, Broughton DD, Melton LJ, et al: Population-based studies of varicella complications. *Pediatrics* 1986;78:723.

66. Preblud SR: Varicella: Complications and cost. *Pediatrics* 1986;78:728.

67. Fucillo DA: Congenital varicella. *Teratology* 1978;15: 329.

68. McGregor JA, Mark S, Crawford GP, et al: Varicella zoster antibody testing in the care of pregnant women exposed to varicella. *Am J Obstet Gynecol* 1987;157:281-284.

69. Enders G: Management of varicella-zoster contact and infection in pregnancy using a standarized varicella-zoster ELISA test. *Postgrad Med J* 1985;61:23.

70. Smego RA, Asperilla MD: Use of acyclovir for varicella pneumonia during pregnancy. *Obstet Gynecol* 1991;78: 1112-1115.

71. Cox SM, Cunningham FG, Luby J: Management of varicella pneumonia complicating pregnancy. *Am J Perinatol* 1990;7:300-301.

72. Cruz AC, Frentzen BH, Behnke M: Hepatitis B: A case for prenatal screening of all patients. *Am J Obstet Gynecol* 1987;156:1180-1183.

73. Lee S-D, Lo K-J, Tsai Y-t, et al: Role of cesarean section in prevention of mother-infant transmission of hepatitis B virus. *Lancet* 1988;1:833-834.

74. Stevens CE, Toy PA, Tong MJ, et al: Perinatal hepatitis B virus transmission in the United States. Prevention by passive-active immunization. *JAMA* 1985;253:1740-1748.

75. Gillespie SM, Cartter ML, Asch S, et al: Occupational risk of human parvovirus B19 infection for school and day-care personnel during an outbreak of erythema infectiosum. *JAMA* 1990;263:2061-2065.

76. Public Health Laboratory Service Working Party on Fifth Disease: Prospective study of human parvovirus (B19) infection in pregnancy. *Br Med J* 1990;300:1166.

77. Rodis JF, Quinn DL, Gary WG, et al: Management and outcomes of pregnancies complicated by human B19 parvovirus infection: A prospective study. *Am J Obstet Gynecol* 1990;163:1168-1171.

78. Woernle CH, Anderson LJ, Tattersall P et al: Human parvovirus B19 infection during pregnancy. *J Infect Dis* 1987;156:17-20.

79. Chao WT: Human parvovirus B19: Infection in pregnancy and fetal manifestations. *Res Med* 1990;5:28-32.

80. Naides Sj, Weiner CP: Antenatal diagnosis and palliative treatment of non-immune hydrops fetalis secondary to fetal parvovirus B19 infection. *Prenat Diagn* 1989;9:105-114.

81. Carrington D, Gilmore DH, Whitle MJ, et al: Maternal serum alpha-fetoprotein: A marker of fetal aplastic crisis during intrauterine human parvovirus infection. *Lancet* 1987;1:433.

82. Bernstein IM, Capeless EL: Elevated maternal serum alpha-fetoprotein and hydrops fetalis in association with parvovirus B19 infection. *Obstet Gynecol* 1989;74:456.

83. Kimball AC, Kean BH, Fuchs F: Toxoplasmosis: Risk variations in New York City obstetric patients. *Am J Obstet Gynecol* 1974;119:208.

84. Desmonts G, Couvreur J: Congenital toxoplasmosis: A prospective study of 378 pregnancies. *N Engl J Med* 1974;290:1110.

85. Koppe JG, Lower-Sieger DH, Roever-Bonnet H: Results of 20- year follow-up of congenital toxoplasmosis. *Lancet* 1986;1:254-256.

86. Wilson CB, Stagno S, Remington JS: Follow-up of children with subclinical toxoplasmosis. *Pediatr Res* 1979; 13:471.

87. Saxon SA, Knight W, Reynolds DW, et al: Intellectual deficits in children born with subclinical congenital toxoplasmosis: A preliminary report. *J Pediatr* 1973;82:792.

88. Teutsh SM, Sulzer AJ, Ramsey JE, et al: *Toxoplasma gondii* isolated from amniotic fluid. *Obstet Gynecol* 1980;55:2S.

89. Desmonts G, Daffos F, Forestier F, et al: Prenatal diagnosis of congenital toxoplasmosis. *Lancet* 1985;1:500-504.

90. Hohlfeld P, MacAleese J, Capella-Pavloski M, et al: Fetal toxoplasmosis: Ultrasonographic signs. *Ultrasound Obstet Gynecol* 1991;1:241-244.

91. Daffos F, Forestier F, Capella-Pavloski M, et al: Prenatal management of 746 pregnancies at risk for congenital toxoplasmosis. *N Engl J Med* 1988;318:271-275.

92. Foulon W, Naessens A, de Catte L, et al: Detection of congenital toxoplasmosis by chorionic villus sampling and early amniocentesis. *Am J Obstet Gynecol* 1990;163: 1511-1513.

93. Desmonts G, Couvreur J: Congenital toxoplasmosis: A prospective study of 378 pregnancies. *N Engl J Med* 1974;290:1110.

94. Wilson CB, Remington JS: What can be done to prevent congenital toxoplasmosis? *Am J Obstet Gynecol* 1980; 138:357.

95. Remington JS, Desmonts G: Toxoplasmosis, in Remington JS, Klein JO (eds): *Infectious Diseases of the Fetus and Newborn Infant*. Philadelphia, WB Saunders 1976, pp 191-332.

PART FIVE

Intrapartum Problems

19

ABNORMAL LABOR
AND DELIVERY

Labor and delivery is a complex physiologic process causing the expelling of the products of conception from the uterus into the outside world. This process is characterized by increased frequency, intensity, and duration of uterine contractions, by progressive effacement and dilation of the cervix, and by descent of the fetus through the birth canal.

◼ A GRAPHIC REPRESENTATION OF LABOR: THE FRIEDMAN CURVE

Most of the present understanding of labor and its abnormalities is based on the work of Emanuel A. Friedman. Friedman found that it is possible to construct a graphic representation of labor by plotting cervical dilation and descent of the presenting part against time. During normal labor, cervical dilation follows a sigmoid-shaped curve (Figure 19-1, *line A*) with three distinct parts: (1) the initial part where there is little progression in cervical dilation, the latent phase; (2) the part of the curve where there is a fast progression in dilation, the active phase; and (3) the final part of the sigmoid where the rate of cervical dilation becomes slow again, the deceleration phase. Descent of the presenting part (Figure 19-1, *line B*) follows a hyperbolic-shaped curve

with little initial change, followed by rapid progress at the beginning of the deceleration phase.

◼ LABOR ABNORMALITIES

The abnormalities of labor may be classified according to the period of labor in which they occur. The latent phase of labor has only one abnormality, prolonged latent phase. The abnormalities of the active phase of labor are protracted active phase, secondary arrest of dilation, and prolonged deceleration phase. The abnormalities of the second stage of labor are failure of descent, protracted descent, and arrest of descent. Finally, there is an abnormality characterized by a rapid labor, precipitate labor. These abnormalities are easily recognized by using the Friedman's curve. Their diagnosis in the absence of a graphic analysis of labor is imprecise and frequently in error. A summary of the abnormalities of labor and the criteria for their diagnosis is shown in Table 19-1.

Causes

Identification of labor abnormalities by means of the Friedman's curve is only the first step in the analysis of the problem. Labor abnormalities

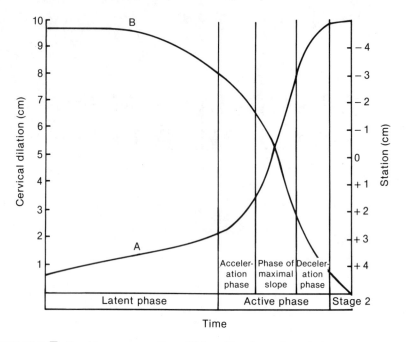

FIGURE 19-1 ◪ Graphic representation of labor (Friedman Curve). *Line A,* progress in cervical dilation with time, and *line B,* descent of the presenting part with the progression of labor.

have their origin in conditions affecting the *power* of the expulsive forces, the fetal *passenger,* or the maternal *pelvis.*

Expulsive forces. During normal labor the uterus contracts every 3 to 4 minutes, and each contraction increases the intrauterine pressure 25 to 75 mm Hg above a baseline of 5 to 20 mm Hg. Uterine work can be expressed as Montevideo units by subtracting the baseline pressure of each contraction from the peak pressure and adding the results of all the contractions occurring in 10 minutes. Most women in spontaneous labor will have three contractions in 10 minutes and will produce approximately 100 to 200 Montevideo units. A patient having strong contractions every 2 minutes will generate more than 300 Montevideo units. In the second stage of labor, the uterine work is complemented by maternal expulsive efforts that become an important part of the power required to achieve vaginal delivery.

Abnormalities of uterine work and maternal expulsive efforts are a common cause of aberrant labor patterns. The most common abnormalities are hypotonic dysfunction, hypertonic dysfunction, and inadequate maternal pushing efforts.

Hypotonic dysfunction is characterized by a decrease in the frequency and intensity of uterine contractions. In some instances hypotonic labor is manifested by biphasic contractions that are another sign of ineffective uterine work.[1] It may be primary when it is caused by an intrinsic failure of the uterine muscle or secondary when it results from pharmacologic intervention such as excessive sedation or regional anesthesia. Hypertonic dysfunction is characterized by frequent, intense, and painful contractions having no effect on cervical dilation or effacement. Inadequate maternal pushing efforts are usually the result of maternal disease or of epidural anesthesia.

To have a quantitative measurement of the power of the uterus, it is necessary to use an intrauterine pressure catheter. External monitoring with tocodynamometer or with palpation is inaccurate.

Fetal passenger. Evaluation of the fetal passenger is also important in labor abnormalities assessment. The most important variables are fetal size, presentation, position, and attitude.

Fetal macrosomia is a relatively frequent finding in patients with abnormal labor. Unfortunately, the ability to determine the fetal size at term clinically and by ultrasound is limited. Abnormal fetal presentations (brow, shoulder, face), positions (occiput posterior, occiput transverse), and attitude (extension, asynclitism), are important causes of abnormal labor. They are relatively easy to diagnose with careful pelvic and ultrasound examination.

Fetal abnormalities such as hydrocephaly, fetal ascites, and fetal tumors may be a cause of abnormal labor. Most patients have one or more ultrasound examinations during pregnancy, and these gross abnormalities have been ruled out. It is a good idea to do a rapid fetal survey with ultrasound to rule out malformations in the rare patient with abnormal labor that had no ultrasound examinations during pregnancy.

Pelvic abnormalities. Abnormalities of the pelvis are a rare cause of abnormal labor. However, the presence of a disparity between the diameters of the fetal head and the dimensions of the maternal pelvis (cephalopelvic disproportion or CPD) is a frequent and serious cause of abnormal labor. The American College of Obstetricians and Gynecologists is encouraging the use of the term *dystocia* instead of CPD.[1]

CPD may be *absolute* if the disparity between head and pelvis exists when optimal fetal head diameters are present or *relative* when an abnormal position of the fetal head results in the presentation of a head diameter too large to pass through the pelvis.

CPD should not be confused with *lack of progress* or *failure to progress* in labor, expressions that are frequently used as an indication for cesarean delivery. Failure to progress in labor has multiple causes, and the use of this or similar terms as an indication for cesarean should be strongly discouraged.

The diagnosis of CPD is important because it does indicate the need for cesarean delivery. For that reason a significant part of the evaluation of patients with abnormal labor patterns is directed toward ruling out CPD. Unfortunately, there are no objective and precise methods for assessing the fetopelvic relationship, and it is necessary to rely on indirect signs (Box 19-1) and on the results of clinical pelvimetry (Box 19-2).

TABLE 19-1 ■ Abnormalities of labor

Abnormality	Criteria for diagnosis
Prolonged latent phase	
Nulliparas	>20 hours
Multiparas	>14 hours
Protracted active phase	
Nulliparas	<1.2 cm/hr
Multiparas	<1.5 cm/hr
Secondary arrest of dilation	
	Cessation of dilation for 2 or more hours
Prolonged deceleration phase	
Nulliparas	>3 hours
Multiparas	>1 hour
Failure to descend	
	No descent
Protracted descent	
Nulliparas	<1 cm/hr
Multiparas	<2 cm/hr
Arrest of descent	
	Cessation of descent for 1 hour or more
Precipitate labor	
Nulliparas	Dilation and descent >5 cm/hr
Multiparas	Dilation and descent >10 cm/hr

BOX 19-1

Signs of CPD

Abdominal examination
Large fetal size
Fetal head overriding the pubic symphysis

Pelvic examination
Cervix shrinking after amniotomy
Edema of the cervix
Head not well applied against the cervix
Head not engaged with leading point at −2 station
Caput formation
Molding (cranial bones overlapping)
Deflexion (anterior fontanelle easily palpable)
Asynclitism (sagittal suture is not in the middle of the pelvis)

Other
Maternal pushing before complete dilation
Early decelerations
Negative Hillis-Müller test
Reverse Hillis-Müller test

BOX 19-2

Clinical Pelvimetry Findings Suggestive of CPD

Narrow subpubic arch
Biischial diameter less than 8 cm
Prominent ischial spines
Flat sacrum
Diagonal conjugate diameter less than 11.5 cm

BOX 19-3

Causes of Labor Abnormalities

Power
Hypotonic dysfunction
Hypertonic dysfunction
Poor maternal expulsive efforts

Passenger
Size
Presentation
Position
Attitude
Congenital abnormalities

Pelvis
CPD
    Absolute
    Relative

The most important clinical maneuver for evaluating the fetopelvic relationship is the Hillis-Müller test. It is performed during a pelvic examination. When a contraction is at its peak, an attempt is made to push the presenting part into the pelvis by pressing on the uterine fundus with the free hand. The hand in the vagina is used to determine whether or not there is downward mobility of the presenting part. If the presenting part does not move or moves very little, the possibility of CPD is high. If the presenting part moves easily into the pelvis, the possibility of disproportion is low.

Radiographic pelvimetry is not used anymore in the evaluation of abnormal labor patterns. This technique is not accurate in predicting the patient's ability to deliver vaginally,[2] and there is concern about unnecessary fetal exposure to x-ray. Evaluation of the maternal pelvis in present-day obstetrics is based on clinical pelvimetry.

A summary of the causes of labor abnormalities is shown in Box 19-3.

Prolonged latent phase

Definition. The latent phase is the interval from the onset of labor to the beginning of the active phase. Its mean duration is 8.6 hours in the nullipara and 5.3 hours in the multipara. A prolonged latent phase exists when its duration exceeds 20 hours in the nullipara and 14 hours in the multipara.

Diagnosis. The diagnosis of prolonged latent phase is made by observation of the Friedman's curve (Figure 19-2) showing little progress in cervical dilation for several hours. The most common problem with this diagnosis is the difficulty in defining the beginning of labor. In most patients, estimation of the onset of labor depends on the maternal perception of when regular contractions started. The lack of an objective

marker of the beginning of labor introduces an error in the measurement of the latent phase.

More common than the diagnosis of prolonged latent phase is the need to differentiate whether a patient is in false labor or in the latent phase. This differentiation may be achieved by continuous observation of the patient for a period of at least 2 hours. Patients in false labor will show a pattern of irregular contractions that eventually decrease in frequency and intensity, and there are no cervical changes during the observation period. Patients in latent phase will show persistent regular uterine contractions that usually increase in intensity and frequency. In addition, patients in latent phase will show some cervical changes.

A second method used to differentiate false labor from the latent phase of labor is *therapeutic rest*. For this purpose, the patient is given a 15-mg dose of morphine sulfate. Patients in false labor sleep for a few hours and awake without contractions. Patients in latent phase continue with contractions and show cervical changes after the sleeping period.

The second most common practical problem related to the latent phase of labor occurs when patients have 3 or 4 cm of cervical dilation and regular uterine contractions, and no progress is observed during the following few hours. These patients may be in a late stage of their latent phase or may have an early secondary arrest of dilation. This differential diagnosis is important

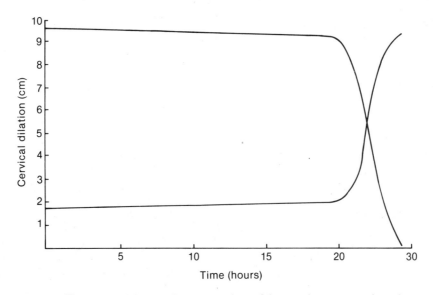

FIGURE 19-2 ◪ Prolonged latent phase. A prolonged latent phase exists when the interval between the beginning of labor and the upswing of the cervical dilation curve exceeds 20 hours in the nullipara and 14 hours in the multipara.

because the first is a benign condition, whereas the latter implies a significant risk of CPD.

To distinguish between late latent phase and early secondary arrest, it is necessary to take into consideration the patient's parity. A multipara making little progress at 4 cm of dilation most likely will be in latent phase. A nullipara under the same circumstances most likely will be in early secondary arrest. The degree of cervical dilation is also important: 60% of the patients will be in active phase if the cervix is 4 cm dilated, and 90% if it is 5 cm.[3] Finally, cervical effacement is a good criterion for recognizing patients in active phase. Most patients will be in active phase if their cervix is dilated 3 cm or more and 100% effaced. If effacement is 50% or less, most likely they are in latent phase.[4]

Frequency. Prolonged latent phase is not a common event. According to Friedman and Sachtleben,[5] it affects 1.45% of nulliparas and 0.33% of multiparas. However, when cases of prolonged latent phase alone and combined with other labor disorders are put together, the incidence increases to 2.31% in nulliparas and 0.44% in multiparas. In the study of Sokol et al.,[6] this disorder affected 3.6% of nulliparas and 4.2% of multiparas. However, these investigators did not differentiate between prolonged latent phase alone and combined with other disorders.

Etiology. In most nulliparous patients the cause of prolonged latent phase is an unripe cervix at the beginning of labor. The most common cause of prolonged latent phase in multiparas is false labor, which is the final diagnosis in more than 50% of patients initially diagnosed as having prolonged latent phase.

Management. There are two modes of management for patients with a prolonged latent phase: therapeutic rest and oxytocin stimulation. Both methods have approximately the same effectiveness and are capable of eliminating the labor abnormality in about 85% of the cases. The selection of the type of management should be based on considerations such as the state of fatigue and anxiety of the patient, the cause of the problem, and the convenience of the patient and the obstetrician.

If rest is chosen as the mode of management, 15 mg of morphine should be given intramuscularly. The majority of patients are asleep within 1 hour and awake 4 to 5 hours later in active labor or in no labor. There are two possible problems with this approach. The first is the possibility of giving this dose of narcotic to a patient who in reality is in the active phase of labor. This problem can be avoided by careful evaluation of the patient before administering the drug. If it occurs, the pediatrician should be notified and be

---

BOX 19-4

Oxytocin Administration for Induction or Augmentation of Labor

- Dilute 10 U of oxytocin in 1000 ml of normal saline.
- Use continuous IV piggyback administration with Harvard pump or similar device.
- If the cervix is already dilated, monitor with pressure catheter and scalp electrode.
- Initiate oxytocin infusion at 0.5 to 1.0 mU/min.
- Increase the dose by 1 U every 40 to 60 minutes, until an adequate pattern of contractions is achieved.

---

ready to administer adequate treatment if the baby is sleepy after birth. The second problem is that administration of morphine may cause further prolongation of the latent phase.

If oxytocin stimulation is chosen as the mode of treatment, the medication must be started at 0.5 to 1.0 mU/min and increased gradually at 40- to 60-minute intervals (Box 19-4). These patients usually do not need a large amount of medication to develop adequate contractions. The majority of them respond to dosages less than 8 mU/min. The main problem with this approach is that induction is usually long, especially if the cervix is unripe. The long latent phase and the long induction combine to produce patient fatigue and anxiety.

Amniotomy is not useful and should be avoided in patients in prolonged latent phase. Also, since the prognosis of this labor abnormality is benign, there is no indication for cesarean section.

Prognosis. Prolonged latent phase is an abnormality of labor that entails little or no risk for mother and baby. Approximately 75% of these patients will have a normal labor and deliver vaginally. Some will develop other labor abnormalities such as protracted active phase or secondary arrest of cervical dilation, and in that case their prognosis is not benign.

Protracted active phase

Definition. A protracted active phase is characterized by a rate of cervical dilation in the active phase of labor that is less than 1.2 cm/hr in the nullipara and 1.5 cm/hr in the multipara (Figure 19-3, *line A*).

Diagnosis. The diagnosis of protracted active phase has the following requirements:

1. The patient must be in the active phase of labor. Patients with 3 or 4 cm of cervical dilation may be erroneously diagnosed as having protracted active phase when in fact they still are in the latent phase.
2. Protracted active phase should not be confused with prolonged deceleration phase. In prolonged deceleration the slow rate of cervical dilation occurs at the end of the active phase, whereas in protracted active phase the slow progress in cervical dilation affects the whole length of the active phase.
3. The diagnosis requires a minimum of two pelvic examinations at least 1 hour apart. The diagnosis is more precise if the slope of cervical dilation is calculated from the findings in three or four pelvic examinations carried out during a 3- to 4-hour period.

Frequency. Protracted active phase is present in about 2% to 4% of all labors. In more than 70% of the cases, this abnormality occurs in combination with arrest disorders or with prolonged latent phase.

Etiology. Fetal malpositions, CPD, hypotonic contractions, and conductive anesthesia are the most common etiologic agents. Occiput transverse (OT) and occiput posterior (OP) positions are found in 70.6% of the cases.[6] CPD is present in 28.1% of the cases.

Management. The treatment of protracted active phase depends on the cause of the disorder. Since the frequency of CPD is high, an evaluation of the fetopelvic relationship must precede any therapeutic procedure (see Boxes 19-1 and 19-2). The possibility of an abnormal fetal position is the next factor to consider.

In some patients protracted active phase is the consequence of inadequate uterine work. In these cases an intrauterine pressure (IUP) catheter should be inserted to obtain a precise evaluation of uterine contractility. If the contractions are more than 3 minutes apart, last less than 40 seconds, and provoke a rise in IUP less than 50 mm Hg, or if the patient is generating less than 100 Montevideo units per 10 minutes in the previous hour of labor, it is proper to assume that a deficiency in the expulsive power of the uterus is the cause of the problem, and stimulation with oxytocin is in order. If contractions are adequate, no benefit will be obtained from oxytocin augmentation, amniotomy, rest, or sedation, and

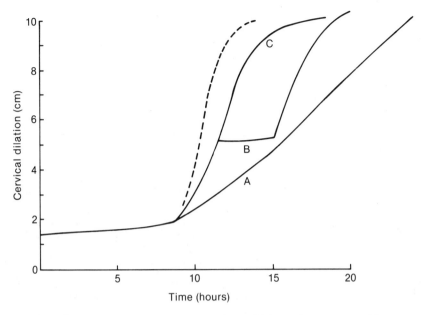

FIGURE 19-3 ◪ Abnormalities of the active phase of labor. The *interrupted line,* a normal pattern of cervical dilation during the active phase of labor. *Line A,* cervical dilation in a patient with protracted active phase dilation. *Line B,* cervical dilation in a patient with secondary arrest of cervical dilation; the postarrest slope of the dilation curve is normal. *Line C,* the cervical dilation pattern of a patient in a prolonged deceleration phase; in these cases dilation is normal until it reaches 8 or 9 cm, then it becomes abnormally slow.

these patients will continue with their slow progress in cervical dilation until delivery.

If CPD is present, cesarean delivery is indicated. If a fetal malposition is found, the patient should be supported and reassured. If excessive sedation or regional anesthesia are the causal agents, waiting for spontaneous abatement of the labor-inhibiting factors is the adequate course of action.

Prognosis. Almost 70% of patients in protracted active phase subsequently develop arrest of cervical dilation or arrest of descent. The other 30% continue with their slow progress, and the maternal and fetal prognosis is good as long as the delivery is atraumatic.

The prognosis for patients who develop arrest patterns after protracted active phase is guarded. According to Friedman and Sachtleben,[7] 42% require cesarean, and 20% have midforceps deliveries. Also, combined disorders have a poor prognosis, especially when they are diagnosed before the cervix reaches 6 cm of dilation. Another important factor in the prognosis is the patient's parity: 83.3% of multiparas with combined protraction and arrest disorders respond

to therapy and dilate further, whereas most nulliparous patients fail to respond to treatment.

Secondary arrest of cervical dilation

Definition. Secondary arrest of cervical dilation occurs when the dilation of the cervix stops for 2 or more hours during the active phase of labor (Figure 19-3, *line B*).

Frequency. Secondary arrest of dilation is the most common disorder of the active phase of labor. Sokol et al.[6] found this problem in 6.8% of nulliparas and in 3.5% of multiparas. These figures are lower than the 11.7% in nulliparas and 4.8% in multiparas found by Friedman and Kroll,[8] using the data of the Collaborative Perinatal Study. This labor abnormality is a frequent component of combined labor disorders.

Etiology. In 20% to 50% of the cases, the etiologic factor of secondary arrest of cervical dilation is CPD. This high incidence of disproportion makes it necessary to evaluate rigorously the fetopelvic relationship in every patient exhibiting this abnormality of labor.

In the original work of Friedman and Sachtleben,[9] 44.6% of all patients with secondary arrest of cervical dilation had CPD. A more recent overview of arrest disorders in labor demonstrated a much lower incidence.[10] Other prevalent causes are hypotonic labor, malposition of the fetal head, excessive sedation, and regional anesthesia. Frequently, patients are affected by a combination of two or more of these factors.

Management. The first thing to do after the diagnosis of secondary arrest of cervical dilation is to evaluate the fetopelvic relationship to determine if CPD is present. A search should be performed for clinical indicators of CPD (see Box 19-1), and clinical pelvimetry (see Box 19-2), including a Hillis-Müller test, should follow.

Patients without clinical signs of CPD, normal clinical pelvimetry, and adequate downward movement of the fetal head during the Hillis-Müller test may have poor uterine activity and require direct monitoring with IUP catheter and fetal scalp electrode. In these cases improvement of labor with intravenous oxytocin may overcome the arrest disorder. Oxytocin must be administered as shown in Box 19-4. In most cases the dose of oxytocin required to overcome arrest of dilation is not greater than 12 mU/min.

Friedman and Sachtleban,[11] found that 85% of patients in secondary arrest that respond to oxytocin do that within 3 hours. An adequate response consisted in an upswing of the cervical dilation curve. Therefore 3 hours of oxytocin augmentation constitute an adequate trial of labor. If no change in cervical dilation is observed after 3 hours, further attempts to achieve a vaginal delivery are unwarranted, and the patient should have a cesarean delivery.

In patients that respond positively to oxytocin augmentation, the slope of the postarrest curve of dilation is equal or larger than that observed before the arrest. In these cases the prognosis is good, and the chances for vaginal delivery are excellent. When the patient does not respond to oxytocin stimulation or the postarrest slope of cervical dilation is less than it was before the arrest, there is a strong possibility that CPD is present.

Some patients with secondary arrest of cervical dilation and normal clinical pelvimetry show adequate uterine contractions when the IUP catheter is applied. In these patients the uterus is working adequately, and further stimulation may be dangerous.

There are some differences in the nature and outcome of secondary arrest of cervical dilation

depending on how early the arrest occurs in the course of labor. Early arrests are often caused by CPD and require operative delivery more frequently than arrests occurring late in the active phase. The recurrence of a secondary arrest of cervical dilation must be treated by cesarean section. A summary of the management plan for secondary arrest is found in Figure 19-6.

Prognosis. The high incidence of CPD makes the prognosis of secondary arrest of dilation guarded.

Prolonged deceleration phase

Definition. The deceleration phase is difficult to detect unless frequent pelvic examinations are carried out at the end of the active phase. However, when an abnormality of the deceleration phase occurs, it usually is readily detectable. Under normal circumstances the mean duration of the deceleration phase is 54 minutes in the nullipara and 14 minutes in the multipara. Prolonged deceleration phase occurs when it lasts more than 3 hours in the nullipara or more than 1 hour in the multipara (Figure 19-3, *line C*).

Diagnosis. The diagnosis of a prolonged deceleration phase requires a minimum of two pelvic examinations, 3 hours apart in the nullipara and 1 hour apart in the multipara. Usually more than two pelvic examinations are carried out during the time required to establish the diagnosis.

In about 70% of the cases, prolonged deceleration is associated with protracted active phase or with arrest of descent. In some cases the diagnosis of prolonged deceleration is not made because more emphasis is given to the definition and management of associated disorders.

Frequency. Prolonged deceleration phase is the least frequent of all labor abnormalities. Sokol et al.[6] observed this abnormality in 0.8% of nulliparas and in 1.7% of multiparas. Friedman[12] found that up to 5% of all labors may be complicated by this disorder.

Etiology. The most common cause of prolonged deceleration phase is fetal malposition. In fact, 40.7% of multiparous patients with this labor abnormality have infants in the OP position, and 25.4% have infants in the OT position. In nulliparas 60% have infants in the OT position, and 26.3% in the OP position. CPD is the cause in about 15% of both nulliparas and multiparas. Prolonged deceleration is a frequent abnormality in labors complicated by shoulder dystocia.

Management. The management of prolonged deceleration depends primarily on the characteristics of the descent of the presenting part. If there is adequate descent, and especially if the presenting part is below the level of the spine, the possibility of CPD is small, and the prognosis for vaginal delivery is good. In contrast, if the prolonged deceleration phase occurs when the presenting part is at a high station, and especially if it is accompanied by arrest of descent, the condition is serious, and the possibility of CPD is large. When the arrest occurs at +1 or lower station, fetal malposition, poor uterine contractility, heavy sedation, or epidural anesthesia are the most frequent causes. In these cases gentle stimulation with oxytocin or waiting for the anesthetic block to abate are adequate management. In patients with the presenting part above 0 station, CPD is a strong possibility, and cesarean delivery may be the best management.

The patient's parity should not influence the management of prolonged deceleration phase. The incidence of cephalopelvic disproportion is similar for nulliparas (15.8%) and multiparas (15.3%) with this labor disorder.

Prognosis. More than 50% of nulliparas and about 30% of multiparas with prolonged deceleration phase require instrument delivery. In Friedman's study,[12] midforceps, usually forceps rotations, were necessary in 40% of nulliparas and in 16.9% of multiparas, and cesarean section was necessary in 16.7% of nulliparas and in 8.5% of multiparas. The difference in outcome between nulliparas and multiparas probably reflects more frequent and aggressive use of uterotonic stimulation in multiparas.

Failure of descent

Definition. The progressive caudal advancement of the presenting part is an important characteristic of normal labor. Descent usually starts during the phase of maximal cervical dilation and is easily observable during the deceleration phase and especially during the second stage of labor. In some patients descent does not occur at all, and this abnormality is named *failure of descent* (Figure 19-4, *line A*).

Diagnosis. The diagnosis of this abnormality requires documentation that descent has not occurred during the second stage of labor. In the

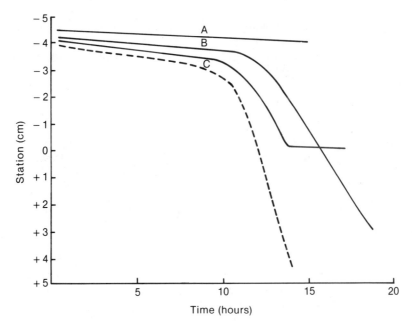

FIGURE 19-4 ◪ Abnormalities of the second stage of labor. The *interrupted line,* the descent of the presenting part during normal labor. *Line A,* failure of descent, a situation in which descent does not occur. *Line B,* protracted descent, a situation in which descent is abnormally slow. *Line C,* arrest of descent, a situation in which there is no progress in the movement of the fetus through the birth canal for at least 1 hour.

majority of cases, failure to descend is associated with other labor abnormalities: 94.1% of the patients have secondary arrest of cervical dilation, and 78.4% have associated protraction disorders. The diagnosis can be made with two vaginal examinations 1 hour apart during the second stage of labor.

Frequency. According to the study of Friedman and Sachtleben,[13] failure of descent affects 3.6% of all labors.

Etiology. The overwhelming majority of patients with failure of descent have CPD. According to Friedman,[12] disproportion can be documented radiologically in 54% of these patients and is present by clinical criteria in almost all cases.

Management. The patient with failure of descent must have immediate cesarean delivery.

Prognosis. Since cesarean section is required, the prognosis is guarded.

Protracted descent

Definition. Protracted descent is an abnormally slow rate of descent of the presenting part (Figure 19-4, *line B*). It occurs when the maximal slope of descent is 1.0 cm/hr or less in nulliparas or 2.0 cm/hr or less in multiparas. The normal slope of descent is 3.3 cm/hr for nulliparas and 6.6 cm/hr for multiparas.

Diagnosis. The slope of descent can be calculated from data collected in two pelvic examinations 1 hour apart, but the accuracy of the diagnosis increases if the observation period is 2 hours long and includes three pelvic examinations.

Frequency. According to Friedman and Sachtleben,[13] protracted descent occurs in 4.7% of all labors.

Etiology. CPD, hypotonic labor, excessive sedation, regional block anesthesia, and fetal malpositions are factors associated with protracted descent. CPD is present in 26.1% of nulliparas and in 9.9% of multiparas with this disorder of labor.

Protracted descent occurs frequently when the infant is macrosomic. In the Friedman and Sachtleben study,[13] 9% of the infants born to mothers with protracted descent weighed more than 4000 g as compared with 4.2% in patients without labor abnormalities. Fetal malpositions of no consequence in normal-size infants frequently represent the difference between vaginal and cesarean delivery in macrosomic babies.

Patients receiving epidural anesthesia during labor have more descent disorders and a higher incidence of operative vaginal deliveries than patients without epidural blocks.[14] This occurs because epidural blocks interfere with the bear down reflex and impair the ability of patients to push during the second stage of labor. On the other hand, epidural anesthesia is the best method to relieve pain during labor and has no deleterious effects on the baby.

Several of the disadvantages of traditional epidural blockade during labor are minimized by using a mixture of low-dose bupivacaine, fentanyl, and epinephrine for continuous epidural infusion. The analgesia achieved with this methodology is excellent, and there is minimal motor blockade with preservation of the patient's ability to push during second stage.[15]

The effect of epidural anesthesia on the duration of the second stage should be taken into consideration for the management of prolonged second stage of labor. As long as descent continues and fetal monitoring is reassuring, prolongation of the second stage beyond the classical limit of 2 hours for nulliparas and 1 one hour for multiparas is permissible for patients receiving epidural anesthesia.[16]

A frequent cause of protracted descent in the multipara is a decrease in the expulsive forces of the uterus during the second stage of labor. This can be documented by means of an IUP catheter.

Management. The first thing to do in the patient with protracted descent is to rule out obvious reasons for the problem, such as inadequate contractions, epidural anesthesia, excessive sedation, and fetal malposition. If these factors are not present, CPD should be suspected. In primiparas with this disorder, the incidence of CPD is about 30%. Also, CPD is the most likely diagnosis in patients with protracted descent and macrosomic infants.

Treatment must be directed toward the suspected etiologic agent: epidural block or excessive sedation must be managed with an abatement policy; CPD requires cesarean delivery; poor uterine contractility requires oxytocin stimulation. Cesarean delivery is the choice in cases of macrosomia combined with malposition.

Prognosis. The prognosis for patients with protracted descent depends to a large extent on the further development of an arrest pattern. Approximately 65% of patients that continue progressing, even if the descent is slow, will have uncomplicated vaginal delivery, and 25% will deliver vaginally with the help of forceps. In contrast, if an arrest develops, the prognosis becomes bleak: 43% incidence of cesarean section and 18% incidence of operative vaginal delivery.[17]

Arrest of descent

Definition. Arrest of descent is defined as no progress in movement of the fetus through the birth canal in the second stage of labor for 1 hour, as documented by appropriately spaced vaginal examinations (Figure 19-4, *line C*).

Diagnosis. The diagnosis of arrest of descent requires a minimum of two pelvic examinations 1 hour apart. The evaluation of the fetal descent is complicated by the development of molding and caput at the end of labor. In many cases a pelvic examination shows that progress is being made when in reality what has been felt as a positive change is caput formation. This error is so common that Friedman[12] recommends assessing the station of the presenting part by both abdominal and pelvic examinations in all cases of suspected abnormalities of descent.

To evaluate the descent of the presenting part by abdominal examination, the first and second Leopold's maneuvers should be carried out and the station assessed from −5 to 0 (Figure 19-5). This method is not as precise as station assessment by pelvic examination, but with the use of both methods, it is possible to avoid mistakes caused by caput formation during labor.

Frequency. Arrest of descent occurs in about 5% to 6% of all labors.

Etiology. There are four main causes for arrest of descent: inadequate uterine contractions, fetal malposition, CPD, and regional anesthesia. In the nullipara, CPD is the cause of more than 50% of the cases of arrest of descent. This incidence is larger when the arrest occurs at a high station or when the patient is receiving uterotonic stimulation. OT or OP malpositions were present in 75.9% of all patients with arrest of descent in Friedman and Sachtleben's series.[17] However, almost all nulliparas with fetal malposition have several factors operating simultaneously, and it is difficult to isolate the etiologic role of malposition alone. Epidural anesthesia was present in 80.6% of nulliparas with arrest of descent. This does not mean that the regional block was the cause of the problem, but indicates that it may be a contributory factor.

In multiparas with arrest of descent, the incidence of CPD is only 29.7%. The proportion of patients with fetal malpositions or under epidural anesthesia is similar to that found in nulliparas.

Management. The first step after making a diagnosis of arrest of descent is to search for etiologic factors. The presence of an obvious reason for the abnormality, such as epidural anesthesia or fetal malposition, must not distract the observer from ruling out the possibility of CPD. Clinical pelvimetry and a Hillis-Müller maneuver must be performed, and the assessment should be directed toward factors other than disproportion only if both are normal. If the Hillis-Müller test gives a negative result, the possibility

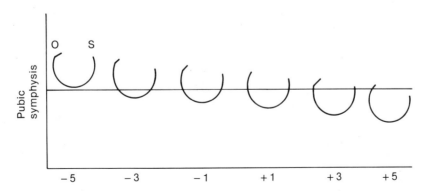

FIGURE 19-5 ◪ Assessing the station of the presenting part by abdominal examination. The graph shows the progressive descent of a fetal head (*O*, occiput; *S*, sinciput) through the pelvis. The head eventually crosses a line that represents the *pubic symphysis*. The station is evaluated using a range of −5 when the head is floating to +5 when the head is deep inside the true pelvis. (From Crichton D: *S Afr Med J* 1974;48:784.)

of CPD is high, and the pregnancy should be terminated by cesarean section.

Oxytocin augmentation is indicated if the uterine contractions seem to be inadequate as evaluated with the IUP catheter. Oxytocin must be administered starting at a dose of 0.5 to 1.0 mU/min with increases in doses separated by intervals of at least 40 minutes (see Box 19-4).

Abatement of regional anesthesia may be indicated after disproportion has been ruled out. If abatement of anesthesia or oxytocin stimulation is chosen as treatment, invasive monitoring with fetal scalp electrode and IUP catheter is mandatory because it has been shown that the fetus becomes progressively acidotic during the second stage.[18]

Most patients who respond to abatement of anesthesia or to oxytocin augmentation do so in 1 to 2 hours. If no response is noticed 3 hours after the beginning of oxytocin stimulation, the possibility of CPD is high, and the pregnancy should be terminated by cesarean section.

Prognosis. Patients with arrest of descent have a guarded prognosis. The reason for this is the high frequency of CPD. In Friedman and Sachtleben's study,[17] 30.4% of patients with arrest of descent required cesarean section, 37.6% were delivered with midforceps, 12.7% had forceps rotations, and 5.1% had failed forceps.

The most important prognostic indices in patients with arrest of descent are the fetal station at the time of arrest—the higher the station, the greater the possibility of disproportion; the duration of the arrest—the longer the duration, the greater the possibility of disproportion; and the characteristics of the postarrest progression. If the postarrest descent rate is equal to or larger than the prearrest slope, the prognosis for atraumatic vaginal delivery is good.

Arrest of descent is associated with significant maternal and fetal morbidity, independent of the need for operative intervention. Postpartum bleeding is common, occurring in 12.5% of the cases. Fetal distress, as evidenced by a low Apgar score, is also common, occurring in 21.9% of the cases. Shoulder dystocia with its associated morbidity occurs in 14.1% of the cases.

Precipitate labor

Definition. Precipitate labor is characterized by rates of dilation and descent greater than 5 cm/hr in nulliparas and 10 cm/hr in multiparas. According to Friedman,[12] the 95th percentile for the rate of dilation of the cervix during labor is 6.8 cm/hr in nulliparas and 14.7 cm/hr in multiparas. For the descent of the presenting part, these limits are 6.4 cm/hr and 14.0 cm/hr, respectively. In most cases precipitate dilation and descent occur simultaneously.

Diagnosis. The diagnosis of precipitate labor is usually made in retrospect when the labor curve of a patient who delivered after a fast labor is analyzed.

Etiology. Etiologic factors are unclear. Oxytocin stimulation may be a trigger for this disorder, although in the series of Friedman and Sachtleben,[11] only 11.1% of all patients with precipitate labor received oxytocin.

Management. If precipitate labor is diagnosed before delivery, and especially if there are electronic monitoring signs of fetal distress, labor should be inhibited with beta mimetic agents. Terbutaline (250 to 500 µg IV push) or ritodrine (300 µg/min IV) are effective drugs for decreasing the frequency and intensity of contractions. These drugs paralyze the uterus momentarily, and when labor restarts, the contraction pattern usually does not have a tumultuous character. Another useful medication is magnesium sulfate, 6 g initial dose, given IV piggyback in 30 minutes followed by 2 g/hr.

Prognosis. The prognosis for vaginal delivery is good. Occasionally labor is so fast that the patient has a precipitous delivery in bed. Following delivery the obstetrician must inspect the cervix for lacerations, since they occur frequently in these patients.

The fetal and neonatal prognosis is guarded. Frequently the fetus does not tolerate the hypoxic insult of the intense uterine contractions, and the result is intrapartum distress, neonatal depression, and hyaline membrane disease.

A summary of the management of abnormalities of the active phase and the second stage of labor is shown in Figure 19-6.

◪ CERVICAL RIPENING AND INDUCTION OF LABOR

The need to deliver patients with unripe cervix, to induce labor, and to increase the efficiency of labor are frequent problems for the obstetrician. There are several methods for the solution of these problems, but none of them produce good results with reliability.

Cervical ripening

The cervix undergoes a series of biochemical and physical changes at the end of the preg-

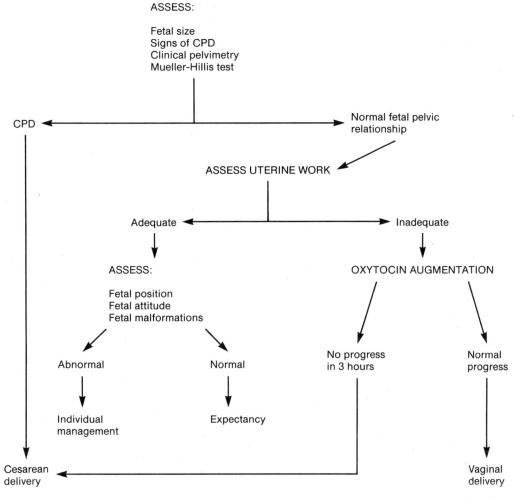

ASSESS:

Fetal size
Signs of CPD
Clinical pelvimetry
Mueller-Hillis test

CPD ← → Normal fetal pelvic relationship

ASSESS UTERINE WORK

Adequate ← → Inadequate

ASSESS: OXYTOCIN AUGMENTATION

Fetal position
Fetal attitude
Fetal malformations

Abnormal   Normal   No progress in 3 hours   Normal progress

Individual management   Expectancy

Cesarean delivery   Vaginal delivery

FIGURE 19-6 ◪ Management of abnormalities of the active phase and the second stage of labor.

nancy that are clinically recognized as *cervical ripening*. At the molecular level, the most striking finding is an increase in concentration and activity of collagenases. These enzymes transform the densely packed and rigid bundles of collagen present in the "unripe" cervix into loose fibers that allow tissue distensibility. For the physician, these changes are manifested as softening, shortening, and opening of the cervix. Unfortunately, in some patients cervical ripening has not occurred when delivery is necessary or when labor starts. In these cases, induction of labor is frequently unsuccessful, and the incidence of cesarean delivery is approximately 50%.

There are several methods available for promoting cervical ripening. The most frequently used are stripping of the membranes, osmotic dilators, mechanical dilators, estrogens, prostaglandin E_2, relaxin, and RU486.

Stripping the membranes. Stripping is an uncomfortable method for the patient, has questionable efficacy, and may generate some problems, but continues to be used frequently. It requires a cervix compliant enough to allow the introduction of one of the examiner's fingers, which is swept around the low uterine segment attempting to strip or detach the amniotic membrane from the uterus. This maneuver causes local release of prostaglandins that are responsible for the ripening effect.

The main problems associated with stripping the membranes are vaginal bleeding and chorioamnionitis. Vaginal bleeding is usually light and short-lasting, but it can be severe if the placental border or a succenturiate lobe is detached. Chorioamnionitis may occur secondary to the placement of a large inoculum of vaginal bacteria in the extraovular space. The efficacy of this procedure is unpredictable.

Osmotic dilators. There are two types of osmotic dilators for cervical ripening: laminaria tents and synthetic dilators. The first are obtained from the seaweed *Laminaria japonicum* and have been used for many years for first- and second-trimester abortions. The synthetic dilator Lamicel is made of synthetic polymers and magnesium sulfate. The polymer matrix will swell when water is drawn into the device because of the osmotic properties of magnesium sulfate. Another synthetic dilator, Dilapan, is a polymer of polyacrylonitrile.

The dilators are placed inside the endocervical canal, and two gauzes saturated with water are placed in the upper third of the vagina to facilitate the process. In 4 to 6 hours the dilators swell and cause cervical dilation. The treatment may be repeated using more dilators to achieve a larger degree of cervical ripening.

In a strict sense, osmotic dilators do not ripen the cervix. These devices open the endocervical canal and promote prostaglandin release, but in the majority of patients, the cervix is still uneffaced and hard in consistency at the end of the procedure. However, the dilators open the cervix to a point where amniotomy is feasible. The patient should be informed of the need for several hours of induction after the removal of the dilators. The treating physician should avoid confusing the dilated and unripe cervix with an early secondary arrest of dilation. The patient should have enough time after removal of the dilators and rupture of the membranes to complete the cervical changes necessary to initiate the active phase of labor.

The main concern with the use of osmotic dilators, particularly with the laminaria tents, is the possibility of chorioamnionitis.[19] This complication does not occur frequently, and its incidence decreases when patients are delivered within 24 hours of initiating the procedure.

Mechanical dilators. The most commonly used mechanical dilator is a Foley catheter with a 30-ml balloon. The catheter is introduced into the uterus and the balloon inflated. The catheter is pulled slightly so that the balloon is applied against the internal cervical os. Some investigators[20] use a continuous extraovular induction of normal saline through the Foley catheter, and others use the catheter alone. Some administer oxytocin while the balloon is inside the uterus. Others use the catheter overnight without concomitant oxytocin stimulation. After 3 to 12 hours the balloon usually is spontaneously passed into the vagina or is removed. The membranes occasionally rupture when the catheter is inserted.

Similar to osmotic dilators, the Foley catheter dilates the cervix 3 to 4 cm without adequate effacement. However, amniotomy for induction of labor can be easily performed once the catheter passes.

Failure to insert the Foley catheter occurs in approximately 5% of the cases. The Foley catheter is not better than traditional oxytocin induction for achieving vaginal delivery. Also, there is a theoretical risk of infection associated with this method.

Estrogen. The onset of parturition in the sheep is preceded by a significant elevation of estradiol plasma levels. Although a similar phenomenon has not been demonstrated in the human, many attempts have been made to ripen the cervix and induce labor using estradiol. The hormone seems to have an effect on the cervix when it is given in high doses intravenously or as an intracervical gel.[21] Inconsistencies in the cervical effects and fear of side effects in the fetus and mother have decreased the enthusiasm about the use of estradiol for cervical ripening.

Prostaglandin E_2. Prostaglandin E_2 (PGE_2) deposited in the posterior vaginal fornix or inside the cervical canal has been shown to be more effective than placebo in promoting cervical ripening. However, there are no commercially available PGE_2 preparations in the United States for use in the third trimester of pregnancy. For this reason most of the experience in this country has been with 20-mg PGE_2 vaginal suppositories mixed with methylcellulose gel to obtain doses of 0.5 mg for cervical and 2 to 5 mg for vaginal use.[23]

Most studies have failed in demonstrating a clear superiority of PGE_2 gel over oxytocin for ripening of the cervix and induction of labor.[24] The incidence of cesarean section is similar in patients induced with oxytocin or with PGE_2 gel. The reasons for the procedural failure and the inconsistency and irregularity of the response to

PGE_2 are many and include inadequate mixing of gel and PGE_2 resulting in variations in the potency from one preparation to the next, heat inactivation during preparation of the gel resulting in a lower dose of the active compound, and variations in patient sensitivity.

The main problem with PGE_2 vaginal gel, in addition to poor results, is the possibility of hyperstimulation. The majority of investigators define hyperstimulation as the occurrence of more than five uterine contractions in 10 minutes or two or more contractions lasting more than 2 minutes. This excessive uterine activity is frequently associated with fetal heart monitoring evidence of distress and occasionally requires emergency cesarean delivery. The best method for treating hyperstimulation is with an intravenous injection of 250 μg of terbutaline sulfate.

Oxytocin. Continuous intravenous administration of oxytocin in doses not exceeding 3 mU/min is an effective method of cervical ripening. The problem is that it takes, on the average, 72 hours to obtain results, and patients are reluctant to accept this extended procedure.

Relaxin. Relaxin is a polypeptide hormone produced by several tissues, particularly the corpus luteum and the decidua, that is effective in promoting cervical ripening. Relaxin activates the cervical collagenases and inhibits uterine contractions causing cervical ripening without hyperstimulation. Porcine relaxin induces ripening of the human cervix effectively.[25] Unfortunately, this compound is not available for clinical use.

RU-486. RU-486 is an antiprogestin derived from norethindrone that binds to the progesterone receptor with an affinity greater than the natural hormone and is used widely in France for first-trimester abortion. RU-486 also has a definite and marked effect on cervical ripening. This medication is not available in the United States.

Induction and augmentation of labor

The most commonly used methods of induction and augmentation of labor are amniotomy and intravenous oxytocin administration. These methods should not be used until all the requisites shown in Box 19-5 are completed.

Amniotomy. Amniotomy is an effective way to induce labor, especially when the cervix is ripe. Manipulation of the membranes causes prostaglandin release, uterine contractions, and

---

> **BOX 19-5**
>
> ### Conditions for Cervical Ripening, Induction, and Augmentation of Labor
>
> 1. A clear indication for the procedure
> 2. Vertex presentation
> 3. Bishop cervical score less than 4
> 4. Reactive nonstress test
> 5. No evidence of CPD
> 6. No placenta previa

---

cervical ripening. When the cervix is not ripe, the results of amniotomy are not good, and these patients frequently require cesarean section because of "lack of progress."

Amniotomy should be performed with discrimination. Before rupturing the membranes, it is necessary, in addition to a ripe cervix, to have a reactive fetal heart rate (FHR) monitoring tracing and to be certain that the head is well applied against the cervix.

Oxytocin. This hormone is an octapeptide synthesized in the neurons of the paraventricular and supraoptic nuclei of the hypothalamus and transported and stored in the neurohypophysis. It has a half-life of 3 to 10 minutes. In myometrial cells, oxytocin increases the activity of phosphodiesterases, bringing about a decrease in cyclic adenosine monophosphate concentration that in turn causes release of calcium from the endoplasmic reticulum. The increased concentration of free intracellular calcium activates the mechanism of muscular contraction. Oxytocin also promotes the formation of gap junctions necessary for the orderly propagation and synchronization of uterine contractions.

Because of its powerful effect on the myometrial cells, oxytocin is the medication most commonly used to stimulate uterine contractions and induce labor. The patient's response to oxytocin is directly related to the hormone plasma concentration and to the sensitivity of the myometrium. Plasma concentration, in turn, depends on the rates of administration and clearance. Myometrial sensitivity depends on the concentration and affinity of oxytocin receptors, which, to a large extent, are a function of the gestational age.

Oxytocin should always be given by continuous intravenous infusion using a pump capable of precisely delivering small amounts of medication. Until recently most methods of oxytocin administration used high doses of the hormone and short intervals for dose increase. This has changed dramatically after the work of Seitchik and Castillo[26] on the pharmacokinetics of oxytocin. These investigators demonstrated that steady-state plasma concentrations after initiation or after change in the rate of administration was achieved in 40 to 60 minutes. Therefore it is unnecessary to increase the dose of oxytocin at intervals less than 40 minutes. Several studies have corroborated these findings and demonstrated that increasing the dose at 15-minute intervals offers no advantages.[27-29]

The initial dose of oxytocin administration usually is 0.5 to 1.0 mU/min. A comparison of starting doses of 2, 5, and 10 mU/min found no differences in induction-delivery interval or in rate of vaginal delivery.[30] Therefore it is preferable to start at the lowest dose. The initial dose is increased by one milliunit per minute every 40 to 60 minutes until an adequate pattern of uterine contractility is achieved. An adequate pattern consists of contractions of good quality, 50 to 75 mm Hg above baseline, every 2 to 3 minutes, or in 150 to 250 Montevideo units per 10 minutes.

Approximately 75% of patients being augmented with oxytocin require 5 mU/min or less, and 95% require 10 mU/min or less. Most investigators agree that the dose of oxytocin should exceed 20 mU/min only in exceptional cases. A summary of the method usually followed for intrapartum administration of oxytocin is shown in Box 19-4. The most frequent indications for cervical ripening, induction, and augmentation of labor are shown in Box 19-6.

There is no need for changes in the method of oxytocin administration for patients undergoing induction rather than augmentation of labor. The only difference is that patients being induced require a larger amount of medication and more time to achieve an adequate pattern of contractions than patients being augmented.

The main problems associated with oxytocin administration are hyperstimulation and neonatal hyperbilirubinemia. Hyperstimulation is characterized by excessive frequency and intensity of contractions causing FHR abnormalities. This is an emergency situation requiring discontinuation of the oxytocin infusion, administration of oxygen to the mother, and treatment with intravenous terbutaline (250 μg intravenous [IV] push)

BOX 19-6

Common Indications for Cervical Ripening, Induction, and Augmentation of Labor

Maternal medical problems
Hypertension
Diabetes
Renal disease
Sickle cell disease

Obstetric complications
PROM
Postterm pregnancy

Fetal problems
Fetal demise
Fetal macrosomia
Suspected fetal jeopardy
Fetal growth retardation
Congenital abnormalities

Patient safety
Cervix dilated 4 cm or more
History of rapid labors

Patient convenience

---

to paralyze the uterus and allow fetal recovery. Neonatal hyperbilirubinemia results from osmotic swelling of the fetal erythrocytes, causing increased fragility and rapid destruction. This side effect is more pronounced when the total amount of oxytocin given to the mother is high, such as happens in prolonged inductions.

ABNORMAL FETAL PRESENTATIONS

The usual presentation at the time of parturition is vertex, and the usual mechanism of labor involves internal rotation of the vertex to an occipitoanterior position with subsequent delivery. Situations that deviate from this are known as abnormal fetal presentations, and they are a management problem for the obstetrician.

Breech presentation

Breech presentation occurs in 3% to 4% of all deliveries. Fetal and neonatal mortality and morbidity are considerably higher for the fetus in breech than for the fetus in vertex position. In one study[31] the overall fetal mortality for breech deliveries was 25.4% compared with 2.6% for nonbreech. In another study[32] breech deliveries were 3.3% of the total deliveries and accounted for 24.3% of the perinatal mortality. This poor fetal outcome persists when some factors such as prematurity and congenital abnormalities are excluded.[33,34]

Associated problems. A considerable part of the fetal and neonatal morbidity and mortality found in breech presentations is the result of associated factors. The most important of these factors are preterm delivery, congenital malformations, preterm rupture of membranes, placenta previa, and abruptio placentae.

Preterm delivery. The prevalence of preterm birth among infants delivered in breech presentation varies from 20.1%[35] to 41.6%.[36] Therefore a significant proportion of the morbidity and mortality associated with the breech presentation is a consequence of preterm birth. However, the perinatal outcome of the preterm infant delivered in a breech presentation is worse than could be expected on the basis of the prematurity alone.[37]

Congenital malformations. Congenital malformations occur more often in breech than in vertex presentations. In one study[38] the frequency of major congenital abnormalities for preterm breech and preterm vertex infants delivered vaginally was 6.2% and 2.3%, respectively. In another series[32] the incidence of congenital malformations was 10.2% for breech infants under 2500 g and 8.3% for those above 2500 g. In still another study[39] congenital abnormalities accounted for 23.6% of all perinatal deaths in a group of preterm single breech births. The chances of a major congenital malformation may be as high as 15% in breech infants of less than 1500 g.

The predominant major congenital malformations in breech infants involve the central nervous system (hydrocephaly, anencephaly, and meningomyelocele). The most common abnormality is, however, dislocation of the hip, a process that affects more females than males (ratio 3:1). Anomalies of the gastrointestinal, respiratory, cardiovascular, and urinary systems and multiple abnormalities are also relatively common. Many of these abnormalities can be detected by careful ultrasound evaluation.

Preterm rupture of membranes. There is no clear evidence that preterm rupture of the fetal membranes (PROM) occurs more often in breech than in vertex presentations. Brenner et al.[31] found that rupture of the membranes was significantly increased in breech presentations only after 36 weeks of gestation (25.1% in breech vs. 15.8% in nonbreech). Other investigators[36] found a 1.5% greater incidence of PROM in breech vs. nonbreech presentations, but no analysis was made of the statistical significance of this difference. The same authors also point out that 8 of 12 fetal deaths in patients with ruptured membranes and breech presentation were the result of intrauterine infection.

PROM is a cause of significant morbidity in breech presentation. Chorioamnionitis and cord prolapse are two of the complications frequently associated with PROM.

Placenta previa and abruptio placentae. In one study[36] the incidence of placenta previa in breech presentation was sevenfold higher than in vertex presentation. Other investigators[31] found an incidence of placenta previa and abruptio of 1.6% and 6.0% in breech presentations in contrast with incidences of 0.6% and 1.8% for vertex presentations, respectively. In these cases the complications associated with placenta previa or abruptio placentae are the determinants of the fetal outcome rather than the breech presentation.

Other causes of perinatal mortality and morbidity. Even if prematurity, congenital abnormalities, PROM, and placental abnormalities are taken out of consideration, mortality and morbidity in breech births are greater than in vertex presentations. This is caused by a series of problems, some of them occurring exclusively and others happening frequently in breech presentation.

Prolapse of the umbilical cord. Prolapse of the umbilical cord is a dangerous accident that occurs in about 6% of all breech deliveries and has a fetal mortality of 30% to 50%. Prolapse of the cord happens in about 1% of frank breech, 5% of complete breech, and 10% of footling breech deliveries. Fortunately, frank breech is the most common type of breech presentation (Box 19-7).

Entrapment of the fetal head. There is no adequate description in the literature of the incidence, methods of management, and outcome of infants when the fetal head is entrapped during a breech delivery. Several papers mention this complication, and every obstetrician who has delivered preterm breech infants has had the expe-

---

BOX 19-7

Frequency of Different Types of Breech Presentation

Frank breech	64%
Single footling	14%
Complete breech	12%
Double footling	10%

---

rience of the entrapped head. This complication is an important cause of fetal asphyxia, second only to prematurity as the leading factor in perinatal mortality for breech infants.

The reason for the occurrence of head entrapment has to do with the relative size of the fetal head and buttocks of the preterm infant. The smaller diameter of the pelvic pole makes it possible to deliver the pelvis and the body of a breech infant through a partially dilated cervix that does not permit the delivery of the larger cephalic pole. The consequences are delayed head delivery, fetal asphypxia, brain damage, and death. The problem occurs more often in the preterm infant because the difference between head and body diameters is larger than in term infants.

There is no accepted method to identify in advance the breech fetus who is going to have an entrapped head. The best policy is to assume that every preterm breech fetus has a significant chance of developing this complication. The risk increases with smaller infant size, nulliparity, and footling presentations.

The most rapid and effective approach for managing an entrapped fetal head is the use of Dührssen's incisions in the cervix. These incisions may extend into the lower uterine segment and cause cervical incompetence. Another approach is to use intravenous terbutaline (300 μg IV push) or intravenous diazoxide (300 mg IV push) to relax the cervix. Terbutaline has less pronounced cardiovascular effects than diazoxide. Another powerful uterine and cervical relaxant is halothane. However, its use requires general anesthesia with endotracheal intubation. Nitroglycerine has been used to relax the cervix in patients with retained placentas, but its use in breech infants with entrapped head has not been reported.

Fetal trauma. After prematurity and asphyxia, fetal trauma is the most frequent cause

of perinatal death in the breech baby. In one study[40] traumatic hemorrhage was the cause of death in 43.4% of breech infants.

Traumatic injury often affects the central nervous system. This occurs frequently in fetuses with hyperextended heads, a condition complicating about 5% of all term breeches. In one study[41] the perinatal mortality was 13.7%, and the incidence of medullar and vertebral injuries was 20.6% in vaginal deliveries of breech babies with hyperextended heads.

A large proportion of the traumatic injuries to the breech fetus is the result of manipulations by the obstetrician at the time of delivery. Occipital osteodiastasis (separation of the squamous and lateral portions of the occipital bone) is one injury that is usually caused by suprapubic pressure on the fetal head at the time of delivery. The separation of the bone causes tentorial tears and intraventricular and subdural hemorrhages.[42]

Erb's palsy and facial nerve paralysis also happen frequently during vaginal breech delivery. Muscle trauma is common and severe. In an autopsy study,[43] it was found that hemorrhages in the injured muscles of infants who died after breech delivery were equivalent to approximately 20% to 25% of the infants' total blood volume. The muscle damage was predominant in the lower limbs, genitalia, and the anal region. The liver, adrenal glands, and spleen may also suffer traumatic damage during breech delivery. One study[40] recorded 24 hepatic and 4 adrenal lethal injuries.

The mechanism of trauma during breech delivery is directly related to the amount of obstetric manipulation during delivery, which, in turn, is directly related to the difficulties encountered in that process. The maneuver most strongly associated with traumatic injury is total breech extraction. This procedure is only used in exceptional circumstances. Vaginal delivery of the breech fetus carries a considerable risk of traumatic injury under the following circumstances.

UNRECOGNIZED CEPHALOPELVIC DISPROPORTION. A condition often associated with fetal trauma during breech delivery is unrecognized CPD. The unmolded fetal head requires wide pelvic diameters to negotiate the bony pelvis. Multiparity does not guarantee the existence of adequate pelvic diameters for a nontraumatic breech delivery unless the birth weight of a previous infant was significantly larger than the size of the breech infant. Adequate evaluation of the maternal pelvis is an important prerequisite for the vaginal delivery of a breech infant. Difficult breech vaginal deliveries were as frequent in nulliparous as in multiparous patients in a large series.[37]

TRAPPING OF THE FETAL HEAD. This problem is discussed on p. 401. It is a complication that affects primarily the delivery of preterm breech infants.

EXTENSION OF THE FETAL ARMS. Delay in delivery of the head because of extension of the fetal arms is a complication mostly seen in cases of total or partial breech extraction. Pulling the baby's body during breech extraction causes extension of the fetal arms, and one or both of them is placed in apposition with the neck (nuchal arm). The result is an increase in the diameter of the cephalic pole and impossibility of delivering the baby's head unless the arms are displaced from the abnormal position. In some cases the arms can be displaced relatively easily; in other cases it is necessary to fracture the fetal humerus or clavicle; and in other cases, despite all efforts, there is considerable delay in delivering the infant's head with resulting asphyxia and death. Extension of the arms complicated 5.2% of nulliparous and 9.7% of multiparous full-term partial breech extractions in Kauppila's series.[37]

RAPID DELIVERY OF THE FETAL HEAD. Another situation with considerable risk of traumatic injury to the breech fetus is a rapid delivery of the fetal head. This problem may be decreased by using Piper's forceps. This instrument was originally designed to avoid delays in the delivery of the head. It has been demonstrated that Piper's forceps delivery of the head is safer than delivery without the instrument for infants weighing between 1000 and 3000 g.[44] The Piper's forceps is also useful in preventing trauma to the fetal mouth and throat during the Mauriceau maneuver, as well as preventing the intracranial bleeding associated with sudden "popping out" of the fetal head.

During the Mauriceau maneuver the middle finger of the obstetrician is introduced into the mouth of the infant while the body rests on the palm of the hand and the forearm. The index and the annular fingers are placed at each side of the baby's nose and press on the upper maxillary bone. Two fingers of the other hand are hooked over the infant's neck and used to apply downward traction. Sometimes voluntary or involuntary traction is exerted with the finger placed in the infant's mouth for the purpose of obtaining maximal flexion of the baby's head, and a frequent result is traumatic injury to the

baby's mouth and pharynx. Routine use of Piper's forceps eliminates this complication.

Management. Management of breech presentations is complex. Unfortunately, much of the information available for making decisions comes from retrospective and uncontrolled studies. The problem of what to do with a breech presentation usually occurs under two different sets of circumstances. One is when the patient has a persistent breech presentation in the last 6 weeks of gestation. The second situation is when a breech presentation is found unexpectedly at the time of labor.

Antepartum management. Although spontaneous rotation may occur during the last 4 to 6 weeks of gestation, the chances of it happening are small. In these cases serious consideration should be given to the performance of an external cephalic version.

EXTERNAL CEPHALIC VERSION. External version is usually performed at 36 weeks when the chances of spontaneous rotation decrease and the amount of amniotic fluid is at a peak. The first step is to find out whether it is feasible to perform the external version. The procedure can be performed if none of the conditions listed in Box 19-8 are present. Then, the following steps should be followed:

1. External version should be carried out in labor and delivery at 36 weeks of gestation. An ultrasound should be performed to assess the fetal position and rule out congenital abnormalities. A reactive nonstress test (NST) should precede the maneuver.
2. Start an intravenous infusion of terbutaline (5 to 8 μg/min) with the patient lying on her left side with her feet slightly elevated. The infusion needs to be continued for 15 minutes. Maternal pulse should be between 100 and 120 beats/min.
3. When the uterus is completely relaxed, the version should be begun by dislodging the breech from the pelvis using both hands. Then, the fetus is moved upward using manual pressure on the buttocks. Once the baby has reached a transverse position, the rotation is completed by pushing up the breech with one hand and pushing down the fetal head with the other hand. Fetal heart activity must be constantly monitored.
4. The procedure should be interrupted if: (1) the version is not easy, (2) the mother is in

---

BOX 19-8

Contraindications to External Version

Indicated cesarean delivery

Placenta previa
Contracted pelvis

Indicated vaginal delivery

Fetal death
Severe congenital abnormality (e.g., anencephaly)

Difficult procedure

Rupture of the membranes
Oligohydramnios
Lack of uterine relaxation (patient in labor)
Multiple pregnancy
Anterior placenta
Pregnancy close to term with engaged breech

Increased maternal or fetal risks

Sensitized Rh-negative mother°
Severe hypertension
Severe intrauterine growth retardation
Fetus with hyperextended head

°If the mother is nonsensitized, RhoGAM should be given after the procedure.

BOX 19-9

Indications for Cesarean Section in Patients in Labor with Breech Presentation

Fetal weight <2500 or >3500 g
Hyperextended fetal head
Previa or abruptio
Abnormal clinical pelvimetry
Suspected fetal jeopardy
Oligohydramnios
Footling breech
Complete breech

---

pain, (3) there is a marked increase or decrease in FHR or an irregular rhythm of the fetal heart.

5. A reactive NST should be obtained after completing the procedure. The patient should be allowed to walk and eat, and FHR monitoring should be continued for a short period before discharge.

6. If the mother is Rh negative, RhoGAM must be given.

Some investigators enthusiastically favor external version, and others find no advantage to its use. The reason external cephalic version is not universally accepted is the 1% to 4% possibility of complications, including fetal losses as high as 1.7%.[45] However, some investigators believe that cephalic version is a reasonable management alternative for most persistent breech presentations. This procedure reduces the incidence of cesarean deliveries as a consequence of breech presentations and is safe when performed without application of excessive force and with continuous fetal monitoring.

External version is facilitated greatly by the use of uterine relaxants. The fetal manipulation should be gentle, and the procedure must be stopped if the mother has pain or if there is more than a 15% increase or decrease in FHR frequency.

Intrapartum management. When a breech presentation is suspected or diagnosed in a patient in labor, the uterine contractions should be inhibited with a tocolytic agent (terbutaline, 250 µg IV push) to allow time for an evaluation of the situation. The first part of the evaluation involves searching for factors indicating the need for cesarean delivery (Box 19-9).

An ultrasound examination is valuable in determining the presence or absence of anencephaly, microcephaly, hydrocephaly, and limb-reduction defects. The ultrasound examination is also useful for ruling out other anomalies such as polycystic kidney disease, meningomyelocele, and fetal ascites.

Once fetal anomalies are ruled out, the next consideration is the fetal weight. For management purposes, the weight of the breech baby should be categorized into one of the following groups: (1) less than 2500 g, (2) between 2500 and 3500 g, and (3) larger than 3500 g.

If the estimated fetal weight is more than 3500 g, pregnancy should be terminated by cesarean section. As shown in Table 19-1, perinatal mortality increases above this birth weight. This is mainly the result of fetal asphyxia and fetal trauma caused by difficult vaginal deliveries.

If the fetal weight is less than 2500 g, the perinatal mortality associated with vaginal delivery is high, and the breech should be delivered by cesarean section. A large part of the perinatal morbidity and mortality associated with vaginal delivery of preterm breech infants is a consequence of prematurity, congenital abnormalities, maternal disease, and placental complications.[46] These causes of perinatal mortality are not preventable by cesarean delivery. Other causes of perinatal mortality and morbidity in the preterm breech infant, such as prolapse of the cord, entrapment of the fetal head, and fetal trauma during vaginal delivery, are preventable by surgical intervention.

A fetal weight between 2500 and 3500 g is adequate for a vaginal breech delivery as long as the fetal head is not hyperextended and the baby is a frank breech. Hyperextension of the fetal head is a clear indication for cesarean delivery of a breech even in situations looking extremely favorable for vaginal delivery. Also, since vaginal deliveries of nonfrank breech presentations are frequently associated with umbilical cord accidents, these pregnancies should be delivered by cesarean section. Therefore the best fetal conditions for vaginal delivery are frank breech presentation, head well flexed, and birth weight between 2500 and 3500 g.

The next step is to decide whether the maternal pelvis is adequate for a breech delivery. The criteria for judging pelvic adequacy for breech delivery should be more stringent than those used for vertex delivery. The reason is that during a vertex delivery the fetal head suffers a process of accommodation to the maternal pelvis that may allow vaginal delivery despite marginal pelvic diameters. In contrast, during breech delivery the fetal head should rapidly pass through the pelvis without a previous accommodation process. The minimal pelvic diameters adequate for vaginal breech delivery are shown in Box 19-10.[47]

A prior vaginal delivery of an infant with a weight larger than the estimated weight of the present fetus is a useful criteria for assessing the adequacy of the maternal pelvis. If the past obstetric history contains only deliveries of infants weighing less than that estimated for the present pregnancy, it is better to deliver the baby by cesarean section.

The role of x-ray pelvimetry in the management of breech presentation is highly controversial. Most investigators believe that this method is inadequate for selecting patients who will have difficulties during labor. Therefore x-ray pelvimetry is not used frequently in the management of breech presentations. The mother's height, characteristics of the pubic arch, prominence of ischial spines, shape of the sacrum, station of the presenting part, and characteristics of the Friedman's labor curve are some of the clinical criteria used to assess the size of the maternal pelvis.

Labor in breech presentation should be monitored electronically, and the pregnancy should be delivered by cesarean section if there is evidence of fetal distress or any abnormality of labor. Mild variable decelerations happen frequently in the course of labor when the infant is in breech presentation. Variable decelerations become indicative of fetal distress if they are severe or occur simultaneously with poor beat-to-beat variability. Blood sampling from the buttock to assess fetal pH is feasible in breech infants. In carefully selected patients with breech presentation at term, a trial of labor is a safe procedure that will end in vaginal delivery in approximately 80% of the cases.[48]

A summary of the overall plan of management for breech presentation at the time of labor appears in Figure 19-7.

Persistent occiput posterior position

In about 5% of all term labors, the occiput fails to spontaneously rotate to an anterior position. In the majority of cases the persistent occiput posterior (OP) position resolves spontaneously but in others requires instrumentation with potential fetal and maternal trauma. A persistent OP position usually is manifested by protracted descent or by arrest of descent.

Etiology. There is no clear explanation for the lack of spontaneous internal rotation in cases of persistent OP positions. The problem occurs

---

BOX 19-10

Minimal Pelvic Diameters Adequate for Vaginal Breech Delivery

Inlet

Transverse	11.5 cm
Anteroposterior	10.5 cm

Midpelvis

Transverse	10.0 cm
Anteroposterior	11.5 cm

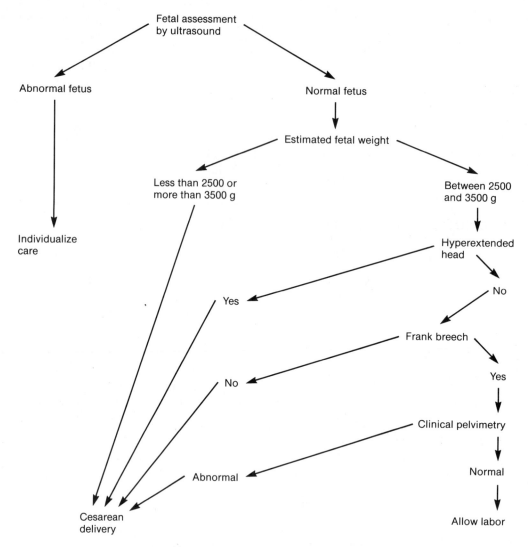

FIGURE 19-7 ◪ Intrapartum management of breech presentation.

more often in small women, in blacks, and when the fetus is large. It seems to be associated with the presence of relatively narrow transverse diameters of the midpelvis.[49] The pelvic shape is not the only factor in the cause of the OP position. OP positions occur up to 3 times more often in patients laboring under conduction anesthesia, a fact that suggests a possible etiologic role for a deficiency of the expulsive forces of labor. There is no association between OP position and CPD.

Associated labor abnormalities. The most common labor abnormalities in patients with

persistent OP position are protracted descent and arrest of descent. Prolonged latent phase, prolonged active phase, and prolonged deceleration phase may also occur, but descent problems are predominant. Malposition of the fetal head should be suspected when the fetal head remains at −1 or 0 station during the last few centimeters of cervical dilation, and the suspicion should be stronger if the presenting part remains at this station after complete cervical dilation. Lack of descent is frequently attributed to incomplete cervical dilation because there is a persistent anterior rim of the cervix that fails to disappear despite adequate uterine contractions. However, the anterior rim of cervix is the result rather than the cause of the labor abnormality. Every time that a patient has a persistent anterior rim of cervix and high presenting part, the presence of an OP malposition should be strongly suspected and the diagnosis confirmed by pelvic and ultrasound examinations.

Management. During the early part of this century several reports described dangers and perils in persistent OP positions. However, most of these complications are unrelated to the fetal position, and the main cause of problems is inadequate intervention.

It is important to rule out the possibility of CPD in patients with persistent OP position and abnormal labor. If the infant is large, the mother is short, and the presenting part is above 0 station, CPD should be strongly suspected. Also, if the Hillis-Müller maneuver fails to show a downward thrust of the fetal head, CPD should be suspected. If CPD is strongly suspected, cesarean delivery is indicated.

In many patients with persistent OP, uterine contractions of poor quality perpetuate the malposition and prolong the labor abnormality. If a deficiency in uterine contractility is suspected, a pressure catheter should be inserted. If the uterine work is deficient, labor augmentation with intravenous oxytocin is the treatment of choice; in many cases this is followed by spontaneous rotation of the head to an occipitoanterior (OA) position and vaginal delivery. In other cases there is no spontaneous rotation, but the improvement in uterine contractility makes the head descend, and it becomes possible to deliver in OP position. In this case episiotomy should be performed to avoid a perineal tear.

The patient with persistent OP malposition should be allowed to labor if there is no evidence of CPD or fetal distress and if the uterine work is adequate. Approximately 59% of these patients will deliver spontaneously in OP position.[50] Other patients rotate spontaneously and deliver in OA position.

An important question in cases of persistent OP presentation is how long a patient may stay in the second stage of labor before there is significant risk of fetal or maternal complications. The upper limit of normal for the duration of the second stage of labor is 2 hours for the nullipara and 50 minutes for the multipara. However, intervention is not necessarily justified when these limits have been reached. Studies[51] have shown that in the absence of fetal distress, the second stage of labor may be prolonged beyond those limits without unfavorable effects on the infant.

If further descent occurs and the fetal head reaches the perineum, a digital rotation to the OA position may be attempted.[52] The following is the technique for digital rotation from OP to OA position:

1. The vertex should be at a low station, visible at the introitus. The exact position of the occiput and the fetal spine should be determined first, clinically and by ultrasound examination.
2. Using the right hand for a left-sided position and the left hand for a right-sided position, the lambdoid suture should be identified and the tip of the middle finger placed exactly at the angle of the lambdoid suture with the tip of the index finger directly alongside the middle finger on the upper lambdoid suture.
3. The hand that is outside the vagina should be applied in the form of a fist against the anterior shoulder of the infant.
4. The two fingers placed on the lambdoid suture should exert a steady rotary motion in a direction at right angles to the sagittal suture (clockwise), and simultaneously the fist should push the fetal shoulder transversely (counterclockwise) in the direction of the occiput. The counterpressure to the rotary motion of the fingers brings about flexion of the head and correction of asynclitism.

If the digital rotation fails, one-blade forceps rotation may be attempted.[53] For this purpose one blade of a Tucker-McLane or similar forceps is introduced upside down in the opposite side of the maternal pelvis. With the second and third fingers, the blade is rotated up and around the pubic symphysis, "wandering" over the fetal ear. When the blade is under the pubic symphysis, the fetal head usually rotates. If the head does not rotate easily, the maneuver is ended. The edge of the blade should not be angled into the fetal head or the maternal pelvis.

If the rotation attempts fail and the maternal expulsive efforts are not enough to achieve spontaneous delivery, low forceps should be applied and the infant delivered in OP.

A summary of the plan of management for persistent OP malposition is shown in Figure 19-8. The emphasis of this plan is on avoiding midforceps rotations. It has been demonstrated that most of the adverse effects of labor abnormalities occur in babies undergoing midforceps operations.[54]

Other abnormal presentations

Shoulder, face, and compound presentations are rare events in obstetrics. Their management is reviewed briefly here.

Shoulder presentation. Shoulder presentation or transverse lie occurs in approximately 0.3% of singleton pregnancies and in approximately 10% of multiple births. Shoulder presentation implies that the long axis of the fetus is perpendicular to the long axis of the mother. In the majority of cases, the shoulder is the presenting part. In other cases the infant has hand and arm prolapsed in the vagina, and occasionally there is no presenting part in the pelvis because the fetal back is above the pelvic outlet. In other cases the fetal back is up against the uterine fundus and the small parts are over the inlet, and the patient presents with the umbilical cord prolapsed in the vagina. An ultrasound examination confirms the diagnosis. Transverse lies are usually associated with multiparity, and more than 80% of the cases occur in patients who are para 3 or more. They also frequently occur in preterm infants and in women with placenta previa.

Cesarean section is the method of choice for the delivery of a fetus in transverse lie with two exceptions, grossly immature fetuses less than 500 g and macerated fetuses up to 1050 g, both of which can be delivered vaginally. In all other circumstances, even in neglected shoulder presentations with fetal death and chorioamnionitis, cesarean section is the recommended procedure.

A low transverse uterine incision is inadequate in most cases of transverse lie. It is difficult to extract an infant in transverse lie through a low transverse incision, especially when the fetal back is over the pelvic inlet. However, if the low

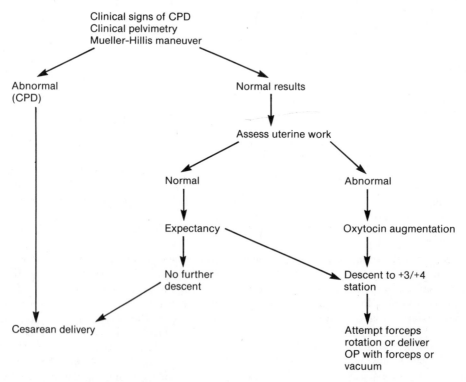

FIGURE 19-8 Management of persistent occiput posterior position.

uterine segment is developed, some transverse lies can be delivered with a low transverse uterine incision.

Face presentation. Face presentation occurs in about 0.2% of all deliveries. It is characterized by extreme extension of the fetal head so that the face rather than the skull becomes the presenting part. Any factor that favors the extension or prevents the flexion of the fetal head, such as congenital goiter or anencephaly, may be an etiologic factor in cases of face presentation. Face presentation is associated with multiparity because the lack of resistance of the anterior abdominal wall allows the fetus to sag forward and extend the cervical spine. Face presentation may occur in association with CPD. A combination of inlet contraction and macrosomic infant is found in up to 39.4% of cases of face presentation.

The diagnosis of a face presentation is made by vaginal examination. The presentation may be confused with a breech, a mistake that is easily avoided by remembering two rules:

1. The anus has sphincter tone; the mouth does not.
2. The anus is in line with the ischial tuberosities; the mouth and the malar prominences form a triangle.

Spontaneous vaginal delivery of face presentations should be expected in 60% to 80% of the cases.[55] Approximately 50% of these patients with the fetal chin in the posterior part of the maternal pelvis rotate spontaneously to mentoanterior position allowing vaginal delivery. This usually happens during the second stage of labor. There is no reason to intervene early in cases of mentoposterior positions if dilation of the cervix and descent of the head are proceeding normally.

Manuevers to convert a face presentation to a vertex or to convert manually or instrumentally a mentoposterior to a mentoanterior position should be avoided. If a patient with a face presentation is making progress during labor, she should be left alone. If arrest of labor occurs, cesarean section is indicated.

Compound presentations. Compound presentations are rather uncommon situations in which one or two of the fetal extremities enter the pelvis simultaneously with the presenting part. The problem occurs in 0.1% of all deliveries. The most common combinations are vertex-hand, breech-hand, and vertex-arm-foot. The

most common associated complication is umbilical cord prolapse, which may occur in up to 20% of the cases. Compound presentations are associated with multiparity, prematurity, twin gestation, and CPD.

In the majority of cases, the prolapsed extremity does not interfere with the normal course of labor and vaginal delivery. In the case of vertex-hand presentation, the hand of the newborn will be swollen and bluish for 24 to 48 hours after birth, but recovery without sequelae is the rule. Breech-hand presentations (the second most common) should be managed with the same criteria used to manage any breech presentation. Vertex-foot and vertex-arm-foot presentations require a gentle attempt at repositioning the lower extremity. If this fails and the foot or arm does not move inside the uterus, cesarean section is necessary unless the fetus weighs less than 800 g.

◼ OPERATIVE VAGINAL DELIVERY

Achievement of a safe vaginal delivery depends, in many cases, on the ability of the obstetrician to effect an operative vaginal delivery with forceps or vacuum. The American College of Obstetricians and Gynecologists[16] recognizes three indications for these procedures: indicated shortening of the second stage of labor, management of prolonged second stage, and presumed fetal jeopardy.

Shortening of the second stage of labor with an outlet forceps is the most common indication for operative vaginal delivery. When the procedure is performed following the conditions required for outlet forceps delivery (Box 19-11), the perinatal outcome is similar to that of spontaneous vaginal delivery.[56,57]

BOX 19-11

Conditions for Shortening the Second Stage Using Outlet Forceps

1. Fetal scalp visible at the introitus without separating labia
2. Fetal skull has reached pelvic floor
3. Sagittal suture in the anteroposterior diameter on right or left occipitoanterior or occipitoposterior positions
4. Rotation does not exceed 45°

The typical example of presumed fetal jeopardy in the second stage of labor is the occurrence of repetitive severe variable decelerations concomitant with contractions and maternal expulsive efforts. In these cases the obstetrician needs to deliver the baby before asphyxia and acidosis become established. For many of these patients, forceps or vacuum delivery can be performed faster and with significantly less maternal and fetal morbidity than cesarean section.

Operative vaginal delivery is an adequate plan of management when the second stage of labor in nulliparous patients lasts more than 3 hours with epidural or 2 hours without epidural anesthesia. For the multipara these limits are 2 hours with epidural and 1 hour without epidural.[58] These time limits are in agreement with the work of Kilpatrick and Laros.[59] These investigators found that the 95th percentiles for the duration of the second stage in nulliparous patients with and without epidural anesthesia were 185 and 132 minutes, respectively. For multiparous patients they were 61 and 85 minutes, respectively. These values reflect the significant impact of regional anesthesia on the duration of the second stage. In patients without epidural anesthesia, the most common cause of prolonged second stage is insufficient expulsive efforts resulting from maternal exhaustion.

In most cases operative vaginal delivery because of suspected fetal jeopardy or because of prolonged second stage of labor can be performed without causing maternal or fetal morbidity. However, in some cases the procedure is a disaster and ends with the delivery of a depressed infant and with maternal complications caused by cervical, vaginal, and perineal trauma. To avoid a poor outcome, it is necessary to comply rigorously with the conditions necessary for low forceps or vacuum application (Box 19-12). The cardinal rule is to perform only simple operative procedures: the biparietal diameter, not the caput, should be at +2 station; the fetal size should be less than 4000 g; clinical pelvimetry should demonstrate a roomy pelvis; and the exact position of the head and the fetal spine should be determined with ultrasound before the procedure. If any difficulty is anticipated or is found during the procedure, the best management is to inhibit uterine activity with terbutaline, administer oxygen to the mother, and deliver promptly by cesarean section.

◪   IMPORTANT POINTS   ◪

1. Labor abnormalities are easily recognized by using the Friedman's curve. Their diagnosis in the absence of graphic analysis is possible but imprecise and frequently in error.

2. Identification of labor abnormalities by means of the Friedman's curve is only the first step in the analysis of this problem. The second step is to decide whether the labor abnormality originates in conditions affecting the power of the expulsive forces, the fetal passenger, or the maternal pelvis.

3. To measure precisely the "work" of the uterus, it is necessary to use an intrauterine pressure catheter. The uterine work may be expressed in Montevideo units.

4. Cephalopelvic disproportion (CPD), also called *dystocia*, is a common cause of labor abnormalities. CPD should not be confused with *lack of progress* or *failure to progress*. The use of the latter terms is strongly discouraged.

5. The diagnosis of CPD requires: (1) documentation of adequate uterine work; (2) presence of clinical signs; (3) abnormal clinical pelvimetry; and (4) negative results of the Hillis-Müller maneuver.

6. Secondary arrest of cervical dilation is the most common abnormality of the active phase of labor. In 20% to 50% of the cases, the cause is CPD. For this reason the first thing to do after this diagnosis is to evaluate the fetal-pelvic relationship.

7. Patients receiving epidural anesthesia during labor have more descent disorders and a higher incidence of operative vaginal deliveries than patients without epidural blocks. These disadvantages are minimized by using a mixture of low-dose bupivacaine, fentanyl, and epinephrine for continuous epidural infusion.

8. There are several methods to promote cervical ripening. The most commonly used are stripping of the membranes, osmotic dilators, mechanical dilators, prostaglandin E_2, and oxytocin.

9. The response to oxytocin is determined by the plasma concentration and the myometrial sensitivity. The plasma concentration depends on the rate of administration and the rate of clearance. The myometrial sensitivity depends on the concentration and affinity of oxytocin receptors. These receptors increase with gestational age.

10. A stable plasma concentration of oxytocin after initiating or changing the rate of administration is achieved in 40 to 60 minutes. Increasing the oxytocin rate at shorter intervals offers no advantages and is associated with hyperstimulation.

11. External cephalic version is a reasonable alternative for patients with persistent breech presentations near term. The procedure reduces the number of cesarean sections resulting from breech presentations. External version is contraindicated in patients with conditions that require cesarean section or that call for vaginal delivery.

12. Every time that a patient in labor has protracted descent and a persistent anterior rim of cervix, the presence of an occiput posterior position should be suspected and the diagnosis confirmed by pelvic and ultrasound examinations.

13. Operative vaginal delivery with forceps or vacuum is indicated when the second stage of labor in nulliparous patients reaches 3 hours with epidural or 2 hours without epidural anesthesia. In multiparas these limits are 2 hours with epidural and 1 hour without epidural.

14. The cardinal rule for avoiding a poor outcome with operative vaginal delivery is to comply rigorously with the norms for outlet and low forceps applications.

REFERENCES

1. Gyselaers W, Vansteelant L, Spitz HJ, et al: Do biphasic uterine contractions imply poor uterine function? *Eur J Obstet Gynecol* 1991;42:111-114.
2. American College of Obstetricians and Gynecologists: *Dystocia,* ACOG technical bulletin 137. Washington, DC, ACOG, 1989.
3. O'Brien WF, Cefalo RC: Evaluation of x-ray pelvimetry and abnormal labor. *Clin Obstet Gynecol* 1982;25:157.
4. Peisner DB, Rosen MG: Transition from latent to active labor. *Obstet Gynecol* 1986;68:448-451.
5. Friedman EA, Sachtleben MR: Dysfunctional labor: I. Prolonged latent phase in the nullipara. *Obstet Gynecol* 1961;17:135.
6. Sokol RS, Stojkov J, Chik L, et al: Normal and abnormal labor progress: I. Quantitative assessment and survey of the literature. *J Reprod Med* 1977;18:47-53.
7. Friedman EA, Sachtleben MR: Dysfunctional labor: II. Protracted active phase dilatation in the nullipara. *Obstet Gynecol* 1961;17:566.
8. Friedman EA, Kroll BH: Computer analysis of labor progression: IV. Diagnosis of secondary arrest of dilatation. *J Reprod Med* 1971;7:176.
9. Friedman EA, Sachtleben MR: Dysfunctional labor: III. Secondary arrest of dilatation in the nullipara. *Obstet Gynecol* 1962;19:576.
10. Bottoms SF, Hirsch VJ, Sokol RJ: Medical management of arrest disorders of labor: A current overview. *Am J Obstet Gynecol* 1987;156:935-939.
11. Friedman EA, Sachtleben MR: Dysfunctional labor: V. Therapeutic trial of oxytocin in secondary arrest. *Obstet Gynecol* 1963;21:13.
12. Friedman EA: *Labor: Clinical Evaluation and Management,* ed 2. New York, Appleton-Century-Crofts, 1978.
13. Friedman EA, Sachtleben MR: Station of the fetal presenting part: V. Protracted descent patterns. *Obstet Gynecol* 1970;36:558.
14. Bates RG, Helm CW, Duncan A, et al: Uterine activity in the second stage of labour and the effect of epidural analgesia. *Br J Obstet Gynaecol* 1985;92:1246.
15. Youngstrom P, Sedensky M, Frankmann D, et al: Continuous epidural infusion of low-dose bupivacaine-fentanyl for labor analgesia. *Anesthesiology* 1988;69:A686.
16. American College of Obstetricians and Gynecologists: *Operative vaginal delivery,* ACOG technical bulletin 152. Washington, DC, ACOG, 1991.
17. Friedman EA, Sachtleben MR: Station of the fetal presenting part: VI. Arrest of descent in nulliparas. *Obstet Gynecol* 1976;47:129.
18. Modanlou H, Yeh SY, Hon EH, et al: Fetal and neonatal biochemistry and Apgar scores. *Am J Obstet Gynecol* 1973;117:942.
19. Kazzi GM, Bottoms SF, Rosen MG: Efficacy and safety of *Laminaria digitata* for preinduction ripening of the cervix. *Obstet Gynecol* 1982;60:440.

20. Schaeyen P, Sherman DJ, Ariely S, et al: Ripening the highly unfavorable cervix with extraamniotic saline instillation or vaginal prostaglandin E_2 application. *Obstet Gynecol* 1989;73:938.
21. Gordon AJ, Calder AA: Oestradiol applied locally to ripen the unfavorable cervix. *Lancet* 1977;7:1319-1321.
22. Deleted.
23. Rayburn WF: Prostaglandin E_2 gel for cervical ripening and induction of labor: A critical analysis. *Am J Obstet Gynecol* 1989;160:529-534.
24. Owen J, Winkler CL, Harris BA, et al: A randomized, double-blind trial of prostaglandin E_2 gel for cervical ripening and meta-analysis. *Am J Obstet Gynecol* 1991;165:991-996.
25. McLanman AH, Green RC, Grant P, et al: Ripening of the human cervix and induction of labor with intracervical purified porcine relaxin. *Obstet Gynecol* 1985;92:693.
26. Seitchik J, Castillo M: Oxytocin augmentation of dysfunctional labor: II. Uterine activity data. *Am J Obstet Gynecol* 1983;145:526-529.
27. Foster TCS, Jacobson JD, Valenzuela GJ: Oxytocin augmentation of labor: A comparison of 15- and 30-minute dose increment intervals. *Obstet Gynecol* 1988;71:147-149.
28. Blakemore KJ, Quin NG, Petrie RH, et al: A prospective comparison of hourly and quarter-hourly oxytocin dose increase intervals for the induction of labor at term. *Obstet Gynecol* 1990;75:757-761.
29. Mercer B, Pilgrim P, Sibai BM: Labor induction with continuous low-dose oxytocin infusion: A randomized trial. *Obstet Gynecol* 1991;77:659-663.
30. Wein P: Efficacy of different starting doses of oxytocin for induction of labor. *Obstet Gynecol* 1989;74:863-868.
31. Brenner WE, Bruce RD, Hendricks CA: The characteristics and perils of breech presentation. *Am J Obstet Gynecol* 1974;118:700.
32. DeCrespigny LJC, Pepperell RJ: Perinatal mortality and morbidity in breech presentation. *Obstet Gynecol* 1979;53:141.
33. Bilodeau R, Marier R: Breech presentation at term. *Am J Obstet Gynecol* 1978;130:555.
34. Lyons ER, Papin FR: Cesarean section in the management of breech presentation. *Am J Obstet Gynecol* 1978;130:558.
35. Sinder A, Wenstler NE: Breech presentation with follow-up. *Obstet Gynecol* 1965;25:322.
36. Jurado L, Miller GL: Breech presentation. *Am J Obstet Gynecol* 1968;101:183.
37. Kauppila O: The perinatal mortality in breech deliveries and observation on affecting factors: A retrospective study of 2227 cases. *Acta Obstet Gynecol Scand (Suppl)* 1975;39:1.
38. Goldenberg RL, Nelson KG: The premature breech. *Am J Obstet Gynecol* 1977;127:240.
39. Galloway WH, Bartholomew RA, Coluin ED, et al: Premature breech delivery. *Am J Obstet Gynecol* 1967;99:975.
40. Potter EL, Adair FL: Clinical pathological study of the infant and fetal mortality for a ten-year period at the Chicago Lying-In Hospital. *Am J Obstet Gynecol* 1943;45:1054.
41. Caterini H, Langer A, Sama JC, et al: Fetal risk in hyperextension of the fetal head in breech presentation. *Am J Obstet Gynecol* 1975;123:632.
42. Wigglesworth JS, Husemeyer RP: Intracranial birth trauma in vaginal breech delivery: The continued importance of injury to the occipital bone. *Br J Obstet Gynaecol* 1977;84:684.
43. Ralis ZA: Birth trauma to muscles in babies born by breech delivery and its possible fatal consequences. *Arch Dis Child* 1975;50:4.
44. Milner RDG: Neonatal mortality of breech deliveries with and without forceps to the aftercoming head. *Br J Obstet Gynecol* 1975;82:783.
45. Van Dorstein JP, Schifrin BS, Wallace RL: Randomized control trial of external cephalic version with tocolysis in late pregnancy. *Am J Obstet Gynecol* 1981;141:417.
46. Cruikshank OP, Pitkin RM: Delivery of the premature breech. *Obstet Gynecol* 1977;50:367.
47. Collea JV, Ratin SC, Weghorst GR, et al: The randomized management of term frank breech presentation: Vaginal delivery vs. cesarean section. *Am J Obstet Gynecol* 1978;131:186.
48. Roumen FJME, Luyben AG: Safety of term vaginal breech delivery. *Eur J Obstet Gynecol* 1991;40:171-177.
49. Holmberg NG, Liliequist B, Magnusson S, et al: The influence of the bony pelvis in persistent occiput posterior position. *Acta Obstet Gynecol Scan (Suppl)* 1977;66:49.
50. Haynes DM: Occiput posterior position. *JAMA* 1954;156:494.
51. Cohen WR: Influence of the duration of second stage labor on perinatal outcome and puerperal morbidity. *Obstet Gynecol* 1977;49:266.
52. Lowenstein A, Zevin R: Digital rotation of the vertex. *Obstet Gynecol* 1971;37:790.
53. Escamilla JO, Carlan SJ: One blade rotation of a persistent posterior vertex. *Am J Obstet Gynecol* 1991; 165:373-374.
54. Friedman EA, Sachtleben MR: Station of the fetal presenting part: VI. Arrest of descent in nulliparas. *Obstet Gynecol* 1976;47:129.
55. Duff P: Diagnosis and management of face presentation. *Obstet Gynecol* 1981;57:105.
56. Dierker LJ, Rosen MG, Thompson K, et al: Midforceps deliveries: Long-term outcome of infants. *Am J Obstet Gynecol* 1986;154:764-768.
57. Hagadorn-Freathy AS, Yeomans ER, Hankins GDV: Validation of the 1988 ACOG forceps classification system. *Obstet Gynecol* 1991;77:356-360.
58. American College of Obstetricians and Gynecologists: *Obstetrics forceps,* ACOG Committee opinion 71. Washington, DC, ACOG, 1989.
59. Kilpatrick SJ, Laros RK: Characteristics of normal labor. *Obstet Gynecol* 1989;74:85-87.

20

BIRTH ASPHYXIA

The potentially dangerous effects of parturition on the fetus have been intuitively recognized for centuries. Labor interferes with the umbilical and uteroplacental blood blow and affects the fetal gas exchange. This results in mild metabolic acidosis during the active phase and early second stage and in respiratory acidosis at the end of the second stage of labor.[1-3] In addition to this normal tendency toward acidosis, the majority of agents that compromise fetal health during labor act by interfering with oxygen-carbon dioxide (O_2-CO_2) exchange and with pH regulation. For these reasons a large part of the current obstetric practice consists of methods to detect fetal asphyxia.

■ DEFINITIONS

Acidosis A pathologic condition characterized by an increased concentration of hydrogen ions in the tissues and in the blood (acidemia).

Hypoxia A pathologic condition characterized by a decreased concentration of oxygen in the tissues and in the blood (hypoxemia).

Asphyxia There is no universally accepted, specific definition of fetal asphyxia. However, most investigators agree that it means a severe abnormality of the fetal gas exchange resulting in hypoxia, hypercarbia, and acidosis.

Fetal asphyxia is frequently confused with meconium staining of the amniotic fluid, low Apgar score, neonatal depression, and neonatal encephalopathy, symptoms that may be indicators of fetal asphyxia but that also have multiple other causes. This confusion in terminology is unfortunate and has had a definite impact in the medico-legal area.

To add to the confusion in definitions, many obstetricians use the term *fetal distress* as an equivalent of fetal asphyxia. The term fetal distress designates an unspecific state of fetal jeopardy that may or may not be caused by asphyxia, and the term should not be used equivalently.

■ INCIDENCE

As many as 20% of all newborns exhibit abnormal arterial oxygen pressure (pO_2), partial pressure of carbon dioxide pCO_2, and pH values at birth.[4,5] However, the majority of these acidotic and hypoxic newborns are vigorous and do not develop abnormalities during the neonatal period. Asphyxia needs to be severe or affect a previously compromised fetus before it translates into end-organ damage.

■ FETAL GAS EXCHANGE AND pH REGULATION

The effects of fetal asphyxia are variable depending on the severity and the duration of the process. Also, the fetal effects of asphyxia are different depending on the mechanism—respiratory or metabolic—that originates the problem. Respiratory acidosis is frequently transient and responds more readily to therapy than metabolic acidosis, which is a more severe condition with a guarded long-term outcome.

CO_2 exchange and respiratory acidosis

The fetal acid-base balance depends on a bicarbonate buffer system that is not as efficient inside the uterus as it is extrauterine because the ability to eliminate carbon dioxide (CO_2) into the atmosphere does not exist. Fetal CO_2 is eliminated by diffusion throughout the placenta as molecular CO_2 and eventually disposed of by the maternal respiration. The diffusion of CO_2 through the placenta is possible because of the existence of a CO_2 gradient between the fetal and maternal circulations. Fetal pCO_2, measured in scalp blood, is 38 to 44 mm Hg, whereas maternal pCO_2 is 18 to 24 mm Hg.

The majority of interferences with the fetal gas exchange affect the ability to eliminate CO_2. This condition is designated as respiratory acidosis. Typical examples are umbilical cord compression and severe maternal asthma. In such cases the initial biochemical change is an increase in fetal pCO_2. The increase in pCO_2 causes an increase in fetal hydrogen (H+) ion concentration and lowering of the pH. This happens because, as shown in Figure 20-1, any interference with CO_2 elimination causes a drive of the bicarbonate buffer equation toward the

left with the formation of H+ ions. Similarly, any excessive H+ ion production by the fetus—metabolic acidosis—drives the equation toward the right and causes an increase in pCO_2. The characteristics of the fetal bicarbonate buffer equation are such that at the beginning of fetal acidosis, it may be possible to find biochemical evidence of the respiratory or metabolic origin of the problem, but in the majority of cases, the clinician encounters a mixed profile.

O_2 exchange and metabolic acidosis

Decreased oxygen (O_2) transfer to the fetus is another important cause of acidosis. A normal fetus requires 5 to 10 ml O_2/kg/min to sustain normal growth, development, and normal pH. Decreased O_2 supply to the fetus may occur suddenly (abruptio placentae, hypertonic labor, spinal shock syndrome), but also it may be a chronic process. In both cases O_2 deficiency causes a switch to anaerobic metabolism with the generation of 2 moles of lactate and 2 moles of H+ ion per each mole of glucose. The H+ ions generated reduce the concentration of buffer base (bicarbonate and protein), producing initially a biochemical picture of metabolic acidosis. Later, however, the excessive H+ ions generate equimolar amounts of CO_2 driving the equation in Figure 20-1 toward the right, resulting in a biochemical profile of mixed metabolic and respiratory acidosis.

When fetal hypoxia is acute and severe such as in abruptio placentae, there is no time for ade-

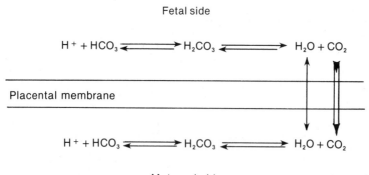

FIGURE 20-1 ◪ Fetal bicarbonate buffer system. The H$^+$ ions produced in the intermediate metabolism of the fetus are transformed into CO_2. This CO_2 is transferred by a pressure gradient into the maternal circulation and eventually eliminated by the maternal lungs. The fetus is easily affected by conditions that impair CO_2 transfer to the placenta, such as cord compression, or interfere with maternal CO_2 elimination, such as severe asthma.

quate adaptation to the sudden decrease in pO_2, and signs and symptoms become readily apparent. If fetal hypoxia is chronic, such as in cases of maternal chronic hypertension, the fetus will temporarily adapt to the situation. However, the inefficient generation of adenosine triphosphate (ATP) caused by the chronic O_2 deprivation will affect fetal growth, and the capacity of the fetus to tolerate stressful situations will be seriously compromised.

Fetal compensating mechanisms can deal more effectively with deficiencies in O_2 supply than with excessive H+ ion production or defects in CO_2 elimination. The high oxygen affinity of fetal hemoglobin allows an adequate saturation of the fetal blood despite significant decreases in maternal pO_2 (Figure 20-2). For ex-

ample, at a maternal pO_2 of 40 mm Hg, the fetus is still capable of keeping about 75% of its hemoglobin saturated with oxygen. In contrast, the compensation for rises in H+ ion or pCO_2 is limited to improving the delivery of CO_2 to the placenta by increasing the heart rate. The rebound tachycardia seen after episodes of cord compression most likely represents such a mechanism of compensation.

In some cases fetal acidosis is caused by an interference with both fetal oxygenation and CO_2 elimination. In that case the effects on the fetus are severe, and the metabolic events occur rapidly. A typical example of this situation is hypertonic labor in which both the availability of oxygen to the fetus and the ability to dispose of the fetal pCO_2 are compromised. The biochemical profile in this situation is that of a mixed respiratory and metabolic acidosis.

◢ CLINICAL INDICATORS OF FETAL ASPHYXIA

The clinical indicators of fetal asphyxia are imprecise and unreliable. They are meconium in the amniotic fluid, low Apgar scores, and poor neurologic outcome of the newborn. Each of them is analyzed separately in the following sections.

Meconium in the amniotic fluid

In the past, the presence of meconium in the amniotic fluid was considered to be a sign of fetal hypoxia. However, most of the recent literature tends to disregard the importance of intrapartum meconium as a sign of fetal hypoxia.[6,7] Meconium is an unspecific finding that may be associated with many other fetal problems different from fetal asphyxia. For example, in one retrospective study[8] the most frequent findings in infants with meconium-stained fluid were cardiovascular malformations (13.9%), Rh isoimmunization (22.4%), chorioamnionitis (37.7%), and preeclampsia (11.1%).

The predictive value of meconium as an indicator of fetal asphyxia is better when it occurs in high-risk patients and when it is dark green or black, thick, and tenacious. Lightly stained, yellow or greenish meconium has a poor correlation with fetal hypoxia.

A study presented a classification of meconium during labor and its correlation with the fetal outcome.[9] Meconium staining was classified as *early* when noted before or during the active

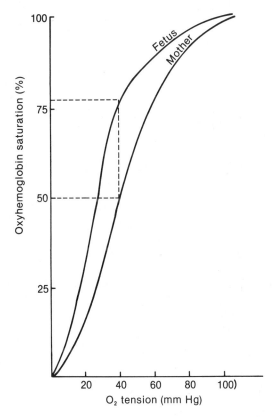

FIGURE 20-2 ◢ Fetal and maternal oxyhemoglobin dissociation curves. The high oxygen affinity of fetal hemoglobin allows the fetus to have an adequate oxygen saturation at O_2 tensions that are inadequate to maintain a normal oxygen concentration in the maternal blood.

phase of labor and *late* when it was passed in the second stage of labor after clear fluid had been noted previously. Early meconium was subdivided into *light* when it was lightly stained yellow or greenish or *heavy* when it was stained dark green or black, usually thick and tenacious. Meconium was observed in 646 pregnancies (22%) in vertex presentation, and it had the following distribution:

Early light	53.6%
Early heavy	25.2%
Late	21.2%

The incidence of 1- and 5-minute Apgar scores below 7 and intrapartum and neonatal deaths was significantly greater in patients with early heavy meconium than in controls matched by age, parity, and birth weight. Early heavy and late meconium were associated with a significantly large incidence of meconium aspiration. From this study it may be concluded that in about 50% of the cases, intrapartum meconium is an insignificant finding. In contrast, early heavy or late meconium is suggestive of fetal hypoxia.

Another study[10] found that the sensitivity and the positive predictive values of moderate or severe meconium staining in the prediction of fetal acidosis were 31% and 5%, respectively. It is obvious that the finding of meconium-stained fluid is an unreliable and inaccurate predictor of fetal acidosis.

Apgar score

Several studies have demonstrated that Apgar scores are a poor predictor of fetal hypoxia and acidosis.[4,5,11-17] This is not surprising since the Apgar score is a system to assess the condition of the neonate at birth, and it may be affected by several factors other than hypoxia and acidosis (Box 20-1).

Sykes et al.[11] found that only 21% of newborns with an Apgar score less than 7 at 1 minute and only 19% of those with Apgar less than 7 at 5 minutes had a pH below 7.10. Luthy et al.[15] studied preterm infants and found that only 10% of those babies with 1-minute Apgar less than 3 had a pH less than 7.2. Silverman et al.[17] concluded that umbilical artery blood gases were not closely related to Apgar scores except in cases of severe acidosis (pH <7.05), hypoxia (pO_2 below 10 mm Hg) and hypercarbia (pCO_2 over 65 mm Hg).

BOX 20-1

Causes of Low Apgar Scores

Prematurity
Medications given during labor
Fetal infection
Fetal congenital abnormalities
Fetal chromosome abnormalities
Fetal neuromuscular disorders
Birth trauma
Inadequate resuscitation
Meconium aspiration
Fetomaternal hemorrhage
Birth asphyxia

An analysis of several published works on this subject gives the following approximate indexes of accuracy for the Apgar score in the prediction of fetal hypoxemia:

Sensitivity	47%
Specificity	89%
Positive predictive value	56%
Negative predictive value	86%

It is clear that the Apgar score is not closely related to and cannot be used to predict the biochemical status of the newborn. The Apgar score provides valuable information about the overall health of the newborn but should not be used as an index of his or her acid-base situation.

Neurologic outcome of the newborn

It was accepted for many years that cerebral palsy (CP) was the result of intrapartum asphyxia. This conviction has been vigorously challenged by research performed during the last 20 years, and today it is clear that intrapartum asphyxia is rarely responsible for neurologic damage in the newborn. The National Institutes of Health has recognized this fact by stating in a recent publication that "birth complications account for a minority of cases of cerebral palsy".[18]

The evidence that perinatal asphyxia causes brain damage is based mainly on animal experiments. In animals, asphyxia must be severe, very close to that causing death, to produce cerebral lesions. In the human, fetal death and survival with an intact brain seem to be the most common outcomes following episodes of severe intrapartum asphyxia. Also, there is compelling evidence indicating that fetuses with conditions af-

---

BOX 20-2

Causes of Cerebral Palsy

Developmental abnormalities
Chromosomal abnormalities
Infection
Prematurity
Trauma
Birth asphyxia

---

fecting the central nervous system may develop hemodynamic alterations during labor as a result of their brain disease. In other words, asphyxia will be the result rather than the cause of their brain damage.

There are multiple causes of cerebral palsy (Box 20-2), and birth asphyxia is responsible only for approximately 8% of the cases.

The consensus today is that neonatal brain damage should be suspected of being caused by perinatal asphyxia only if the following conditions are present:

1. The fetal or neonatal acidemia is severe, with arterial blood pH <7.1 and base excess −20 or less.
2. Neonatal depression with hypotonia and a need for prolonged assisted ventilation are present.
3. There is clinical and laboratory evidence of multiple end-organ dysfunction caused by hypoxic damage.

Since most newborn asphyxia is not followed by cerebral palsy and most infants with cerebral palsy do not show signs of asphyxia at birth, it follows that neurologic damage of the newborn is an extremely poor indicator of fetal asphyxia.

◢ BIOPHYSICAL INDICATORS OF FETAL ASPHYXIA
Fetal heart rate monitoring

Intermittent auscultation of the fetal heart. Intermittent auscultation of the fetal heart rate (FHR) with aural stethoscope was for many years the only available method to evaluate fetal health during labor. This method was abandoned with the advent of continuous electronic monitoring, but it has been resurrected as a result of randomized trials comparing the two techniques.

Auscultation of the fetal heart can be effected with a DeLee fetal stethoscope or with a Dop-

pler device. The auscultation should be performed during and for 30 seconds after a contraction. For high-risk patients, the American College of Obstetricians and Gynecologists (ACOG) recommends evaluating and recording the FHR frequency at least every 15 minutes during the active phase of labor.[19] During the second stage of labor, high-risk patients should be evaluated and recorded every 5 minutes. For low-risk patients, ACOG recommends evaluating and recording FHR at least every 30 minutes during the active phase and at least every 15 minutes during the second stage of labor. ACOG recognizes that there are no data to demonstrate optimal time intervals for intermittent auscultation of low-risk patients.

There are few studies on the use of intermittent auscultation for intrapartum fetal monitoring, and the sensitivity, specificity, and predictive values of the method for the detection of fetal asphyxia are unknown. Most of the information on this technique comes from studies in which intermittent auscultation was compared with electronic monitoring. However, the data from the Collaborative Perinatal Project were obtained before the advent of electronic monitoring and show that intermittent auscultation was unable to anticipate fetal jeopardy.[20] A prior study concluded that intermittent auscultation was equivalent to nonsurveillance.[21]

According to ACOG, an FHR obtained by intermittent auscultation is considered to be nonreassuring if:

1. The average rate between contractions is less than 100 beats/min.
2. The rate is less than 100 beats/min. 30 seconds after a contraction.
3. There is an unexplained average rate of more than 160 beats/min. between contractions, especially in at-risk patients in whom the tachycardia persists through three or more contractions (10-15 minutes) despite corrective measures.

According to ACOG, when a nonreassuring FHR frequency is detected by auscultation, continuous electronic monitoring, fetal scalp sampling, or vibroacoustic stimulation may be helpful in confirming a diagnosis. If the abnormal findings persist despite conservative measurements and other tests are not available or desirable, expedient delivery may be considered.

Despite ACOG endorsement, intermittent auscultation of FHR rate is rarely used in the

United States, and continuous electronic monitoring remains firmly as the current standard of care. There are multiple reasons for the resistance of obstetricians and hospitals to use intermittent auscultation for intrapartum fetal surveillance. Some of these reasons are the need for a 1:1 nurse-to-patient ratio, the lack of studies evaluating the accuracy of this methodology, the lack of adequate definition of the frequency and duration of auscultation in low-risk patients, the intuitive conviction that intermittent auscultation is inaccurate and unreliable, the lack of ability of intermittent auscultation to discriminate benign from ominous FHR changes, and the feeling that a return to intermittent auscultation negates the knowledge acquired during the last 20 years about different types and degrees of FHR alterations during labor.

Continuous electronic FHR monitoring. In the early 1970s continuous electronic heart rate monitoring was introduced and enthusiastically adopted by obstetricians as a significant improvement in intrapartum fetal assessment. Unfortunately, several prospective, randomized studies involving thousands of subjects have failed in demonstrating benefits with respect to perinatal outcome of continuous electronic FHR as compared with intermittent auscultation.[22-28] These studies have involved term and preterm infants, and the perinatal outcome has been determined by the frequency of low Apgar scores, fetal acidosis, admission to intensive care nursery, need for assisted ventilation, incidence of intrapartum stillbirths, and incidence of neonatal seizures. Also, follow-up studies of term and preterm children involved in some of these trials[29,30] have failed to show any long-term benefits with respect to neurologic development. Furthermore, some of these controlled studies have shown an increased rate of cesarean sections and operative vaginal deliveries caused by erroneous diagnoses of fetal distress in electronically monitored patients. In view of these disappointing conclusions, ACOG recommended that either continuous electronic FHR monitoring or intermittent auscultation may be used for intrapartum fetal assessment.[19]

Despite the controversy about its usefulness, it is clear that continuous electronic FHR monitoring provides the obstetrician with information that:

1. Allows reliable determination of the presence of fetal well-being

---

> **BOX 20-3**
>
> ### Characteristics of a Reassuring FHR Pattern
>
> 1. Stable baseline rate between 120 and 160 beats/min.
> 2. Normal short- and long-term variability
> 3. No decelerations
> 4. Accelerations (>15 beats/min. for >15 seconds) with fetal movements and with contractions

2. Allows, with a high degree of reliability, determination of the presence of severe fetal problems
3. Suggests the possibility that fetal problems may be present

The presence of fetal well-being is demonstrated by the presence of a *reassuring* FHR pattern (Box 20-3). This information is highly reliable, and there are no reports of severely asphyxiated fetuses in the presence of a normal FHR pattern. The presence of *ominous* FHR patterns is also highly reliable, and it is uncommon that a healthy neonate is delivered when one of these patterns is present.

The problem with continuous electronic FHR monitoring is the third category of information, the *nonreassuring* patterns, because errors in their interpretation are easily made and result in unnecessary cesarean deliveries.

Reassuring FHR pattern. A reassuring FHR pattern has the characteristics described in Box 20-3. When it is present, the possibility of severe fetal hypoxia or acidosis is very low.

Ominous FHR patterns. Ominous FHR patterns are usually seen when there is a profound alteration of the fetal central nervous system because of developmental anomalies, chromosome abnormalities, or because of a severe derangement of the O_2 and CO_2 exchange between mother and fetus. The alteration in fetal gas exchange causing the ominous pattern is usually the result of a serious obstetric complication such as umbilical cord compression, abruptio placentae, severe fetal growth retardation, severe placental insufficiency, fetal infection, or fetomaternal hemorrhage or is caused by interventions such as oxytocin stimulation or regional anesthesia.

Some fetuses who develop ominous FHR patterns are affected by pathologic conditions during their intrauterine life, particularly placental vascular insufficiency and severe growth retardation. In these cases the stress of labor is the insult that precipitates the appearance of the ominous pattern. How much uterine activity is necessary to produce hypoxemia and how severe will be the effects of the hypoxemia in these fetuses depends to a large extent on the nature and intensity of their antepartum condition.

For the inexperienced physician, it seems paradoxic that continuous electronic FHR monitoring is capable of identifying ominous tracings resulting from fetal asphyxia and at the same time is a poor predictor of fetal brain damage. The answer to that is, first, that ominous tracings reflect an alteration of the fetal central nervous system that may or may not be the result of acute perinatal asphyxia. Second, perinatal asphyxia is an uncommon cause of brain damage, and most severely asphyxiated fetuses either die or survive intact. In fact, despite an incidence of acidosis (pH <7.20) of 12% to 20% at birth,[4,17] the incidence of cerebral palsy is approximately 2 per 1000, and intrapartum fetal death at term in the absence of risk factors occurred in less than 1 per 25,000 patients in the Collaborative Perinatal Study.[31]

The most common ominous FHR patterns are:

1. Absent heart rate variability and shallow late decelerations
2. Absent heart rate variability and mild variable decelerations with overshoot
3. Absent or markedly decreased variability and prolonged bradycardia following severe variable or late decelerations
4. Absent or markedly decreased variability and severe variable decelerations with slow recovery

A fundamental component of ominous FHR patterns is absent or markedly decreased FHR variability.[32,33] Variability may be short term or long term. Short-term variability reflects the duration of the interval between heart beats and varies from 20 to 30 msec, which is equivalent to two to three beats when converted to rate. Long-term variability consists of oscillations with an amplitude of 5 to 20 beats and a frequency of three to five per minute.

FHR variability depends on the interaction between the adrenergic and the cholinergic systems and requires anatomic and functional integrity of the fetal central nervous system. Variability is affected by fetal hypoxemia and acidosis. It is also affected by fetal sleep and by the action of medications that interact with the fetal neurovegetative system.

Nonreassuring FHR patterns. Nonreassuring FHR patterns are a problem for the obstetrician because of their high false-positive rate. Although there are occasional problems with the interpretation of *reassuring* and *ominous* FHR monitoring patterns, overestimation of *nonreassuring* tracings is common, and only one of every five fetuses with nonreassuring patterns has a low pH.

One contributory factor to the over-reading of nonreassuring patterns is the fear of medico-legal problems. The obstetrician prefers intervention despite the high rate of false-positive results rather that the potential consequences of nonintervention in the truly affected fetus. The most common nonreassuring FHR patterns are:

1. Decreased variability without periodic changes
2. Persistent mild and moderate variable decelerations
3. Occasional severe variable decelerations
4. Late decelerations with adequate variability
5. Moderate-to-severe variable decelerations in the second stage of labor
6. Fetal bradycardia

ABSENT OR DECREASED VARIABILITY. FHR variability is one of the most important pieces of information that the obstetrician can obtain from the examination of a monitoring tracing. FHR variability is an index of the fetal reserve or tolerance to hypoxic insults. The presence or absence of FHR variability confers special significance to meconium staining of the amniotic fluid, late decelerations, variable decelerations, and fetal bradycardia. These signs become ominous if they occur concomitantly with decreased or absent beat-to-beat variability.

The best way to evaluate beat-to-beat variability is with a fetal scalp electrode. In all intrapartum high-risk situations, FHR monitoring should be performed with a scalp electrode to observe adequately this important measure of fetal well-being.

In most instances decreased FHR variability is not the result of fetal hypoxemia. The most common cause of decreased variability is fetal sleep. Also, variability decreases under the effect of

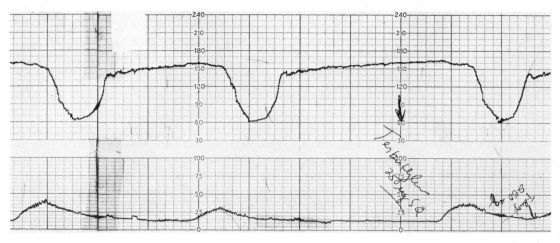

FIGURE 20-3 ◪ Late decelerations. Absent long- and short-term variability and severe late decelerations after each uterine contraction. This is an ominous tracing.

medications such as atropine, propranolol, diazepam, meperidine, butorphanol (Stadol), scopolamine, phenobarbital, and morphine, drugs often used for patients in labor. FHR variability is also dependent on the degree of maturation of the fetal central nervous system and is decreased in preterm infants. Fetal tachycardia decreases the beat-to-beat intervals and FHR variability without necessarily meaning that fetal hypoxia is present. All these variables must be taken into consideration when evaluating an FHR pattern with decreased variability.

LATE DECELERATIONS. Late decelerations (Figure 20-3) have been traditionally considered an indicator of fetal distress. Human and animal studies show significantly greater morbidity and mortality in fetuses with late decelerations during labor than in others not exhibiting the same monitoring pattern.[34-36] However, the association between late decelerations and fetal hypoxemia occurs in only a minority of patients, and in the majority of cases late decelerations are transient and treatable.

Late decelerations may occur in up to 25.8% of all patients receiving epidural anesthesia during labor[35] and may be corrected by repositioning the patient and giving intravenous fluids to compensate for the effect of peripheral blood pooling. Late decelerations are also present in the majority of patients who develop hypertonic labor spontaneously or, more frequently, as a consequence of oxytocin administration. In these cases the decelerations disappear with measures that decrease uterine contractility. Late decelerations often follow maternal administration of hypotensive agents such as diazoxide and hydralazine, but they disappear after elevation of the maternal blood pressure. Also, mild or moderate variable decelerations may occur after the peak of uterine contractions and be confused with late decelerations.

Late decelerations are of concern only when they occur in a context of decreased variability and lack of accelerations. Under other circumstances fetal hypoxia is rare.

SEVERE VARIABLE DECELERATIONS. Variable decelerations are the most common periodic change seen during labor. Their name is derived from the inconsistency of their relationship to the uterine contractions and their variable configuration (Figure 20-4).

There is evidence from animal and human studies that variable decelerations result from compression of the umbilical cord with baroreceptor and chemoreceptor stimulation provoking transient vagal bradycardia. However, in more than 50% of the cases, it is not possible to document entanglement of the cord around the fetal neck or the fetal parts.[37] It is probable that stimuli other than cord compression may also produce the vagal response that causes variable decelerations.

Variable decelerations may be mild, moderate, or severe (Box 20-4). The possibility of fetal hypoxia increases with the severity of decelerations and is larger when variability is decreased and

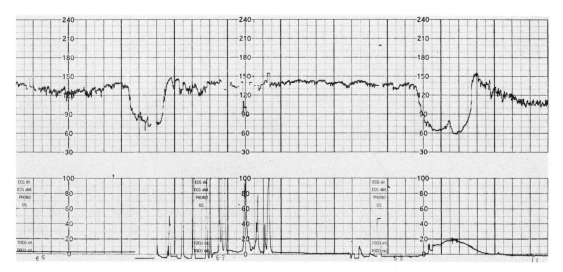

FIGURE 20-4 ▨ Variable decelerations. Two moderate variable decelerations with preserved long- and short-term variability can be seen. Variable decelerations are characterized by the shape of the deceleration and may occur before, during, or after a contraction.

BOX 20-4

Classification of Variable Decelerations

Mild

Less than 30 second's duration and more than 80 beats/min.

Moderate

More than 30 second's duration and less than 80 beats/min.

Severe

Less than 70 beats/min. for more than 60 seconds

---

the return to baseline is slow. In compromised fetuses it is not unusual to see an acceleration, or *overshoot*, following severe variable decelerations.

Severe variable decelerations during the second stage of labor may be a marker of fetal asphyxia or may be benign. To make a differentiation, it is necessary to consider the stability of the baseline frequency, the presence of variability, the characteristics of the return to baseline, and the length of time that they have been present.

FETAL BRADYCARDIA. Fetal bradycardia has a varied significance with respect to fetal well-being, and it is necessary to recognize at least the following different situations:

1. *Baseline bradycardia.* This pattern corresponds to an FHR of less than 120 beats/min without coexistent periodic changes and with adequate beat-to-beat variability. Baseline bradycardia is a benign pattern[38] that does not demand further intervention unless it occurs simultaneously with severe decelerations or with lack of beat-to-beat variability.

2. *Prolonged end-stage deceleration.* This pattern is a sudden, prolonged drop in FHR that happens in some patients who are close to the time of delivery.[39] The FHR during the episode is anywhere from 40 to 90/min. This bradycardia is the product of a vagal reflex caused by head compression and does not have pathologic significance if the patient is low risk, the tracing does not show decelerations, and variability is normal. However, it is alarming and often influences the obstetrician's decision to intervene with cesarean section or operative vaginal delivery.

3. *FHR bradycardia concomitant with lack of beat-to-beat variability.* This ominous pattern occurs mainly in postterm pregnancies

and may or may not be preceded by mild late decelerations.[40]

4. *Prolonged FHR bradycardia following late or severe variable decelerations.* This is another ominous pattern that should be interpreted as a manifestation of exhaustion of the fetal reserve (Figure 20-5).

FHR response to scalp stimulation

It has been known for years that acceleration of the FHR in response to stimuli such as sound, movement, and manual stimulation is an excellent indicator of fetal well-being. For this reason Clark et al.[41] made a retrospective review of their experience with fetal scalp sampling and found that the presence of a FHR acceleration of at least 15 bpm lasting at least 15 seconds at the time of scalp sampling was associated in 95.9% of the cases with a fetal scalp pH of 7.28 or larger. None of the fetuses with pH <7.2 responded to stimulation.

In a subsequent prospective study[42] the same investigators found that an FHR response with acceleration after firm digital pressure and pinching of the fetal scalp with an Allis clamp was uniformly associated with a scalp pH >7.19. The incidence of scalp pH <7.19 was 38% among those fetuses that did not respond to scalp stimulation.

It is clear that scalp stimulation is an important tool to further the fetal assessment in patients with nonreassuring FHR monitoring patterns. Its use has the potential to decrease significantly the need for fetal scalp pH sampling.

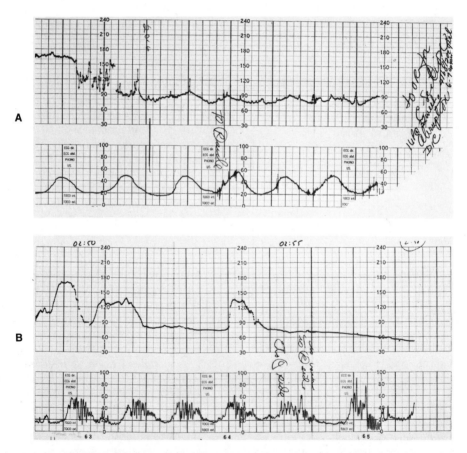

FIGURE 20-5 ◪ Prolonged bradycardia. Prolonged fetal heart rate bradycardia after variable decelerations. In **A,** variability, although decreased, is still present. In **B,** FHR variability is markedly decreased. In both tracings, labor is hypertonic. Both patients were delivered by emergency cesarean section. A partial abruption was found in the patient corresponding to panel **A,** and the baby had Apgar scores of 6 and 7. An occult cord prolapse was the diagnosis in the patient corresponding to panel **B,** and the baby had Apgar scores of 1 and 5.

FHR response to vibroacoustic stimulation

Fetal vibroacoustic stimulation (VAS) has been used for several years as an adjunct to antepartum FHR monitoring. Most recently this technique has been introduced as a test to predict intrapartum asphyxia. Smith et al.[43] found in fetuses with abnormal FHR patterns that a response to VAS with FHR acceleration of at least 15 bpm lasting a minimum of 15 seconds was uniformly associated with a scalp pH >7.25. On the other hand, the incidence of pH <7.25 was 50% among those fetuses that failed to respond to stimulation. Polzin et al.[44] also found that the fetal response to VAS reliably predicted ph <7.2 in fetuses with nonreassuring FHR monitoring patterns.

VAS stimulation also has been found to be useful in the prediction of fetal well-being when it is used at the beginning of labor. Ingemarsson et al.[45] found a 75% incidence of abnormal FHR monitoring tracings during labor when the FHR tracing at the initiation of labor was nonreactive and VAS was negative. Sarno et al.[46] studied 201 patients, 60% of them with complications of pregnancy, and found that those fetuses with a nonreactive response to VAS at the beginning of labor had a significantly high incidence of abnormal FHR patterns, meconium staining, and Apgar scores <7 at both 1 and 5 minutes.

It seems, therefore, that both VAS and scalp stimulation have an important role in reducing the false-positive rate of nonreassuring FHR monitoring and also in reducing the need for fetal scalp sampling. Reactivity to VAS or to scalp pinching with an Allis clamp in fetuses with nonreassuring FHR patterns indicates that the fetal pH is not in the acidotic range and that scalp pH is not necessary.

◪ BIOCHEMICAL INDICATORS OF FETAL HYPOXIA AND ACIDOSIS

In rigorous terms, a fetus is asphyxiated when the arterial blood gases are below the 5th percentile value of a normal population. Table 20-1 shows the mean values and the 5th and 95th percentile limits for umbilical artery and vein blood gases obtained in a population of 147 term, healthy neonates.[47] According to those values, a fetus will be asphyxiated when the pH is 7.12 or below, the pO$_2$ is 6.5 mm Hg or less, the pCO$_2$ is 71.2 mm Hg or more, and the base excess is <−10.

The most commonly used lower limit of nor-

TABLE 20-1 ◪ Normal cord blood gases

		Percentile	
	Mean +/− SD	5th	9th
Umbilical artery			
pH	7.27+/−0.6	7.12	7.33
pCO$_2$	56.0 +/−7.6	44.2	71.2
pO$_2$	15.6 +/−5.7	6.5	26.1
HCO$_3$	24.7 +/−2.3	20.3	28.0
Base excess	−3.3 +/−2.8	−10.1	−0.3
Umbilical vein			
pH	7.35+/−0.05	7.25	7.41
pCO$_2$	42.5 +/−5.9	35.0	50.9
pO$_2$	27.9 +/−7.7	16.3	41.1
HCO$_3$	22.8 +/−2.0	18.7	25.6
Base excess	−2.5 +/−2.2	−7.1	−0.2

From Miller JM, Bernard M, Brown HL, et al: Umbilical cord blood gases for term healthy newborns. *Am J Perinatol* 1990;7:157-159.

mal for fetal pH is 7.20,[48] and there is no universal agreement on the lower limit for fetal pO$_2$. Fetal pH values between 7.20 and 7.24 are in the *preacidotic* range. These numbers are too high. They do not correspond to two standard deviations from normal, which is the scientifically accepted limit for biologic measurements, and do not correlate with the fact that only severe acidosis, pH <7.10, is associated with significant neonatal morbidity.

Fetal scalp blood gases

Measurement of the fetal scalp blood gases is the most accurate method for determining the acid-base balance of the fetus during labor and the respiratory or metabolic type of abnormality responsible for the fetal acidosis. However, the test is not perfect and occasionally does not reflect truly the fetal situation. The following are some of the common causes for false-positive and false-negative fetal scalp measurements:

1. Mother in the dorsal position (falsely low pH)
2. Maternal alkalosis (falsely normal or elevated fetal pH)
3. Slow rate of collection of scalp blood into the collection tube (falsely low pH)

The diagnostic value of fetal scalp pH determinations increases if several sequential measurements are performed to determine the trend of the acid-base status. For example, an isolated pH value of 7.22 does not necessarily mean that the fetus is acidotic. The same pH value has greater significance if in two previous observations the pH was 7.28 and 7.25. In this case the trend is toward progressively lower pH values, and intervention is justified at a pH of 7.22, although this value still is not in the acidotic range.

To obtain a fetal scalp blood sample, the patient is placed in the left lateral knee-chest position with the right leg elevated by the patient with the help of a nurse. This position is preferred to avoid the hemodynamic changes caused by the supine position and the eventual effects on the uteroplacental circulation. An amnioscope (metal or plastic) is introduced into the posterior fornix of the vagina, and its anterior border is guided with the clinician's finger until it is placed inside the cervix. There are amnioscopes with different diameters to be used according to the degree of cervical dilation. Scalp sampling is rarely successful, however, before the cervix has reached 3 to 4 cm of dilation. Once the amnioscope is in contact with the fetal head, a light source is attached to the instrument, and the fetal scalp is cleaned of amniotic fluid and blood using cotton swabs. Next the fetal scalp is sprayed with ethyl chloride to cause hyperemia. This is an important step, since the objective of the procedure is to obtain a sample of *arteriolized* venous blood, which implies the production of vasodilation and hyperemia in the tissue to be sampled. The excess of ethyl chloride is removed with cotton swabs, and an incision of about 3 to 5 mm is made in the scalp using a specially designed guarded blade that is only 2 mm long and is not supposed to penetrate the scalp aponeurosis. The incision must be made in the upper part of the circumferential area of the scalp seen through the amnioscope to facilitate the collection of blood in a preheparinized capillary tube. The instruments for bedside determination of fetal scalp pH require only 15 μl of blood for an accurate pH measurement. Determination of pH, pO_2, pCO_2 and base excess require 30 to 50 μl.

The number of reported complications with fetal scalp sampling is small. The most common are bleeding and infection in the incision site. Bleeding at the time of the procedure usually subsides after a few minutes of pressure with a cotton swab. If the incision is bleeding at the time of delivery, pressure will stop the bleeding in most cases, but if necessary, a small metal clip may be used for suturing. It is probably wise not to use vacuum extraction after scalp sampling to avoid further bleeding and eventual formation of cephalohematoma.

Fetal scalp pH does not have a perfect correlation with Apgar scores: 6% to 20% of patients with fetal scalp pH measurements within normal range have infants with low Apgar scores; also, 8% to 10% of all infants delivered because of low pH values have normal Apgar scores at birth.[49]

A comparison between scalp measurements and electronic monitoring has shown that 32 of 37 fetuses found to be acidotic by scalp pH measurements had abnormalities of the FHR tracing, but only 32 of 138 fetuses with abnormal FHR tracings were found to be acidotic.[38]

The predictive value of acidosis at birth for perinatal brain damage is very poor. Ruth and Rairio[50] investigated this problem by measuring umbilical artery pH in 982 consecutive births. They found an incidence of neonatal acidosis (pH <7.16) of 12%. However, the sensitivity of low pH to detect posterior brain damage was only 21%, and the positive predictive value only 8%. Similar poor predictive value was found for low Apgar scores at 5 minutes and high lactate concentration in umbilical cord.

The use of fetal scalp pH for the assessment of ominous or nonreassuring FHR monitoring patterns is being questioned. It is argued that fetal blood pH measurements provide only an instantaneous reflection of a rapidly changing environment and that only continuous or frequent measurements can yield accurate information. Another criticism is that in the majority of cases the evaluation is limited to the fetal pH, and this makes it impossible to make the important distinction between respiratory and metabolic types of acidosis. Also, it is believed that the development of indirect techniques to evaluate the fetal acid-base balance, such as scalp stimulation and VAS, makes scalp sampling unnecessary. Finally, it is argued that very few well-oxygenated fetuses will be delivered unnecessarily by cesarean section among those that have a combination of nonreassuring or ominous FHR patterns and do not respond to VAS or scalp stimulation.

Umbilical cord blood gases

Umbilical artery and vein blood gases are frequently obtained at the time of delivery to assess the acid-base situation of the newborn at the time of delivery. Initially this modality was limited to depressed newborns because of its potential usefulness for establishing a prognosis and an adequate treatment of acidosis. In the last few years this evaluation has been extended to normal fetuses mainly because of concern about potential litigation if neurologic dysfunction develops later in life. By demonstrating the presence of normal acid-base balance at birth, the obstetrician has evidence that any neurologic dysfunction that may develop is not the result of intrapartum hypoxia. Proponents of this approach list additional advantages such as the potential for a better definition of the degree of asphyxia necessary to cause neurologic damage, the benefit of having an objective end point to judge the efficacy of interventions directed toward prevention of asphyxia, and the therapeutic benefits of a better knowledge about the respiratory or metabolic mechanism of the acidosis.[51]

Opponents of the routine use of umbilical blood gases at delivery observe that the incidence of cerebral palsy is one in 2000 births, whereas the incidence of intrapartum acidosis is 6% to 20% depending on the end point selected. Therefore the probability of finding vigorous babies with acidotic pH is many times greater than the probability of finding babies that are going to develop cerebral palsy and have normal pH. The significant difference in incidence between these conditions makes routine determination of umbilical blood gases more prone to result in incriminating evidence in the patient's chart rather than in useful data for malpractice defense.

As a response to this controversy, ACOG[52] has recommended double clamping and dividing a segment of the umbilical cord following delivery of the baby, placing the segment on the delivery table, and obtaining umbilical artery blood gases if any serious abnormality in the delivery process or problems in the neonatal condition persist beyond the first 5 minutes of life. Venous blood should be obtained if it is not possible to obtain arterial blood. A clamped segment of cord will keep blood stable for blood gas measurements for at least 15 minutes, and a heparinized blood sample in a syringe will be stable for up to 60 minutes. ACOG's recommendation makes sense and will avoid useless, expensive, and potentially incriminatory blood gas measurements in healthy neonates.

◢ MANAGEMENT OF FETAL ASPHYXIA

Prompt delivery by cesarean section is the best management for fetal asphyxia documented by scalp blood examination or suggested by ominous FHR monitoring patterns. However, it is necessary to remember that ominous patterns may occur in the absence of asphyxia in fetuses with developmental abnormalities of the central nervous system.

In the majority of cases, the obstetrician is faced with nonreassuring FHR patterns. In this situation it is important to have in mind that nonreassuring patterns are frequently transient and correctable without the need for emergency cesarean section. The first step in these cases is discontinuation of oxytocin, positional changes, administration of oxygen, and intravascular volume expansion with crystalloid solutions. If these simple measures do not correct the nonreassuring pattern, the next step should be fetal scalp stimulation or VAS. A reactive FHR response to either maneuver indicates that the fetus is not acidotic and labor may be allowed to continue.

If there is no response to scalp or VAS stimulation, the next step should be administration of a tocolytic agent.[53] Inhibition of uterine activity with beta adrenergic drugs is useful for distinguishing between patients with true deficits of the fetal-maternal exchange and patients with transient impairment who have no need for emergency delivery.

Uterine contractions are inhibited by administering an intravenous bolus of 250 μg of terbutaline. The injection may be given subcutaneously if an intravenous line is not available. If the abnormal pattern continues, the possibility of hypoxemia and acidemia is high, and the pregnancy must be delivered by cesarean section. An improvement in the FHR pattern strongly suggests that the fetus has recovered and that continuation of labor is possible. Esteban-Altirriba et al.[54] demonstrated that fetal pH increases after tocolytic therapy in 84.8% of nonreassuring patterns caused by excessive uterine activity, in 72% of cases caused by umbilical cord compression, and in 69.6% of abnormal patterns resulting from other causes. When a nonreassuring FHR pattern is secondary to placental insufficiency, a successful response is observed in only 31.4% of the cases. A favorable response happens in 76.9% of the cases when the fetal pH is between 7.20 and 7.24, but it still occurs in approximately 50% of fetuses with pH less than 7.20.

If a nonreassuring FHR pattern improves following terbutaline administration, it is important to repeat the scalp or VAS stimulation. If the fe-

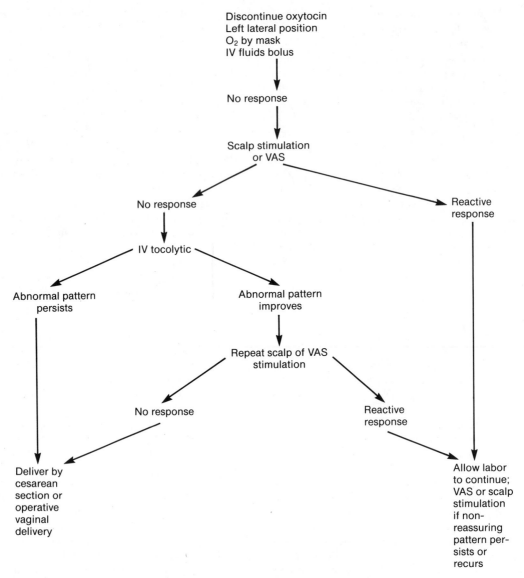

Discontinue oxytocin
Left lateral position
O₂ by mask
IV fluids bolus

↓

No response

↓

Scalp stimulation
or VAS

No response   Reactive
                     response

↓

IV tocolytic

Abnormal pattern   Abnormal pattern
persists   improves

Repeat scalp of VAS
stimulation

No response   Reactive
                     response

Deliver by   Allow labor
cesarean   to continue;
section or   VAS or scalp
operative   stimulation
vaginal   if non-
delivery   reassuring
                          pattern per-
                          sists or
                          recurs

FIGURE 20-6 ◪ Management of nonreassuring FHR patterns during labor.

tus has a reactive response, this indicates that the pH is normal, and labor should be allowed to continue. If there is no response, it means that the fetus is still acidotic, and the best option may be to deliver by cesarean section or by operative vaginal delivery. Figure 20-6 summarizes the steps in the management of nonreassuring FHR patterns during labor.

An alternative management plan makes use of fetal scalp pH in fetuses with abnormal FHR patterns who do not respond to administration of beta adrenergic agents or to scalp or VAS stimulation. If the pH is below 7.20, pregnancy must be terminated by cesarean section. If the pH is between 7.20 and 7.25, a new scalp blood sample must be obtained in 10 to 15 minutes. Either no change in pH or a lower pH value in the second sample is an indication for cesarean section. Improved pH values in the second sample are indicative of fetal recovery, and in that case there is no need for surgical intervention. The management can be more refined if pCO_2 and base excess are measured concomitantly with the pH. A pH within normal range and a decrease in base excess are strongly suggestive of compensated metabolic acidosis and the need for delivery. A low pH and an elevated pCO_2 indicate respiratory acidosis and good prognosis with adequate neonatal resuscitation.

The management of patients with severe variable decelerations is somewhat different. When they occur, the patient must be immediately examined to rule out a cord prolapse or a funic presentation—umbilical cord present in the pelvis before the body of the infant—either of which is an indication for cesarean section. If the pelvic examination is negative, positional changes and tocolytic therapy must be used to correct the deceleration. If the variable deceleration pattern persists or recurs, amnioinfusion should be carried out.

Amnioinfusion

Variable decelerations during labor occur more frequently in patients with ruptured membranes, postterm pregnancies, intrauterine growth-retarded babies, and in any other situations with decreased amniotic fluid volume. In these cases amnioinfusion may eliminate or decrease significantly the severity of the FHR monitoring pattern.[55]

Amnioinfusion is performed with 200 to 500 ml of warm saline solution injected through an intrauterine pressure catheter. The solution is infused in approximately 30 minutes. No significant fetal or maternal complications resulting from the procedure have been reported.

◪ IMPORTANT POINTS ◩

1. There is no universally accepted, specific definition of fetal asphyxia. Most investigators agree that it means severe impairment of the fetal gas exchange resulting in hypoxia (pO_2 less than 6.5 mm Hg), hypercarbia (pCO_2 greater than 65 mm Hg), and acidosis (pH less than 7.10).

2. The majority of interferences with the fetal gas exchange affect the ability to eliminate CO_2, causing respiratory acidosis. This condition responds promptly to neonatal resuscitation.

3. Decreased transfer of oxygen to the fetus resulting in anaerobic metabolism and formation of lactic acid is the mechanism of production of metabolic acidosis.

4. Meconium staining of the amniotic fluid is an unreliable and inaccurate indicator of fetal asphyxia.

5. The Apgar score is an index for assessing the condition of the newborn who may be affected by multiple factors other than hypoxia and acidosis. Only a small percentage of newborns with low 1- and 5-minute Apgar scores have pH below 7.1.

6. Intrapartum asphyxia is rarely responsible for neurologic damage in the newborn. Fetal death or survival with an intact brain are the most common outcomes following severe fetal asphyxia.

7. There are multiple causes of cerebral palsy. Most cases are caused by developmental defects.

8. To suspect perinatal asphyxia as a cause of neonatal brain injury, it is necessary that the following conditions are present: (1) severe neonatal acidemia with pH less than 7.1 and base excess less than −20; (2) neonatal depression with hypotonia and need for prolonged assisted ventilation; and (3) clinical and laboratory evidence of multiple organ dysfunction caused by hypoxic insult.

9. There are few studies on the use of intermittent auscultation for intrapartum fetal monitoring. The sensitivity, specificity, and predictive values of this technique are unknown. It requires a 1:1 nurse-to-patient ratio.

10. Continuous electronic FHR monitoring allows reliable determination of fetal well-being. There are no reports of severely asphyxiated babies born in the presence of a reassuring FHR pattern.

11. Ominous FHR patterns are usually seen when there is a profound alteration of the fetal central nervous system, usually caused by developmental anomalies, chromosome abnormalities, and, rarely, because of severe fetal asphyxia.

12. The problem with electronic FHR monitoring is the high false-positive rate of nonreassuring patterns.

13. The presence of an FHR acceleration of at least 15 bpm lasting at least 15 seconds following pinching of the fetal scalp with an Allis clamp or following vibroacoustic stimulation is uniformily associated with a scalp pH greater than 7.19.

14. Fetal scalp pH should be used in fetuses with abnormal FHR patterns who do not respond to administration of beta adrenergic agents or to scalp or VAS stimulation. However, the use of fetal scalp pH for further assessment of ominous or nonreassuring FHR monitoring patterns is being questioned. Few well-oxygenated fetuses will be delivered unnecessarily among those with a combination of abnormal FHR pattern and lack of response to vibroacoustic or scalp stimulation.

15. The routine determination of umbilical blood gases is unnecessary and should be discouraged. Rather than being useful for malpractice defense, they may become potentially incriminating evidence. Umbilical blood gases should be obtained only if there is any serious abnormality in the delivery process or problems in the neonatal period persist beyond the first 5 minutes of life.

16. Variable decelerations are the most commonly observed FHR abnormality. Amnioinfusion may eliminate or decrease the severity of variable decelerations.

REFERENCES

1. Modanlou HD, Yeh S-Y, Hon EH, et al: Fetal and neonatal biochemistry and Apgar scores. *Am J Obstet Gynecol* 1973;117:942.
2. Bretscher J, Saling E: pH values in the fetus during labor. *Am J Obstet Gynecol* 1967;97:906.
3. Beard RW, Morris ED: Fetal and maternal acid-base balance during normal labor. *J Obstet Gynaecol Br Commonw* 1965;72:496.
4. Josten BE, Johnson TRB, Nelson JP: Umbilical cord blood pH and Apgar scores as an index of neonatal health. *Am J Obstet Gynecol* 1987;157:843-848.
5. Marrin M, Paes BA: Birth asphyxia: Does the Apgar score have diagnostic value? *Obstet Gynecol* 1988;72:120-123.
6. Abramovici H, Brandes JM, Fuchs K, et al: Meconium during delivery: A sign of compensated fetal distress. *Am J Obstet Gynecol* 1974;118:251.
7. Miller FC, Sacks DA, Yeh SY, et al: Significance of meconium during labor. *Am J Obstet Gynecol* 1975;122:573.
8. Fujikura T, Klionsky B: The significance of meconium staining. *Am J Obstet Gynecol* 1975;121:45.
9. Meiss PJ, Hall M, Marshall JR, et al: Meconium passage: A new classification for risk assessment during labor. *Am J Obstet Gynecol* 1978;131:509.
10. Low JA: The role of blood gas and acid-base assessment in the diagnosis of intrapartum fetal asphyxia. *Am J Obstet Gynecol* 1988;159:1235-1240.
11. Sykes GS, Johnson P, Ashworth F, et al: Do Apgar scores indicate asphyxia? *Lancet* 1982;1:494.
12. Lauener PA, Calame A, Janecek P, et al: Systematic pH measurements in the umbilical artery: Causes and predictive value of neonatal acidosis. *J Perinat Med* 1983;11:278.
13. Suidan JS, Young BK: Outcome of fetuses with lactic acidemia. *Am J Obstet Gynecol* 1984;150:33.
14. Fields LM, Entman SS, Boehm FH: Correlation of one-minute Apgar score and the pH of umbilical arterial blood. *South Med J* 1983;76:1477 .
15. Luthy DA, Kirkwood KS, Strickland D, et al: Status of infants at birth and risk for adverse neonatal events and long- term sequelae: A study in low birth weight infants. *Am J Obstet Gynecol* 1987;157:676.
16. Page FO, Martin J, Palmer S, et al: Correlation of neonatal acid-base status with Apgar scores and fetal heart rate tracings. *Am J Obstet Gynecol* 1986;154:1306.
17. Silverman F, Suidan J, Wasserman J, et al: The Apgar score: Is it enough? *Obstet Gynecol* 1985;66:331.
18. Freeman JE: *Prenatal and Perinatal Factors Associated with Brain Disorders,* US Dept of Health and Human Services publication No. (NIH) 85-1149. National Institutes of Health, 1985.
19. American College of Obstetricians and Gynecologists: *Intrapartum Fetal Heart Rate Monitoring,* ACOG technical bulletin 132. Washington, ACOG, September 1989.
20. Benson RC, Shubeck F, Deutschberger J, et al: Fetal heart rate as a predictor of fetal distress: A report from the Collaborative Project. *Obstet Gynecol* 1968;32:259.
21. Walker N: The case for conservatism in the management of fetal distress. *Br Med J* 1959;2:1221.
22. Haverkamp AD, Thompson HE, McFee JG, et al: The evaluation of continuous fetal heart rate monitoring in high-risk pregnancy. *Am J Obstet Gynecol* 1976;125:310-320.
23. Renou P, Chang A, Anderson I, et al: Controlled trial of fetal intensive care. *Am J Obstet Gynecol* 1976;126:470-476.
24. Kelso IM, Parsons RJ, Lawrence GF, et al: An assessment of continuous fetal heart rate monitoring in labor: A randomized trial. *Am J Obstet Gynecol* 1978;131:526-532.
25. Wood C, Renou P, Oats J, et al: A controlled trial of fetal heart rate monitoring in a low-risk obstetric population. *Am J Obstet Gynecol* 1981;141:527-534.
26. McDonald D, Grant A, Sheridan-Pereira M, et al: The Dublin randomized controlled trial of intrapartum fetal heart rate monitoring. *Am J Obstet Gynecol* 1985;152:524-539.
27. Leveno KJ, Cunningham FG, Nelson S, et al: A prospective comparison of selective and universal electronic fetal monitoring in 34,995 pregnancies. *New Engl J Med* 1986;315:615-619.
28. Luthy DA, Shy KK, vanBelle G, et al: A randomized trial of electronic fetal monitoring in preterm labor. *Obstet Gynecol* 1987;69:687-695.

29. Haverkamp AD, Orleans M, Langendoerfer S, et al: A controlled trial of the differential effects of intrapartum fetal monitoring. *Am J Obstet Gynecol* 1979;134: 399-412.

30. Shy KK, Luthy DA, Bennett FC, et al: Effects of electronic fetal-heart-rate monitoring, as compared with periodic auscultation, on the neurologic development of premature infants. *New Engl J Med* 1990;322:588-593.

31. Lilien AA: Term intrapartum fetal death. *Am J Obstet Gynecol* 1970;107:595.

32. Shields JR, Schifrin BS: Perinatal antecedents of cerebral palsy. *Obstet Gynecol* 1988;71:899-905.

33. Langer O, Vega-Rich M, Cohen W: Terminal pattern: Characteristics and management. *Am J Perinatol* 1985;2:300-304.

34. Beard RW, Filshie GM, Knight CA, et al: The significance of the changes in the continuous fetal heart rate in the first stage of labor. *Br J Obstet Gynaecol* 1971;78:865.

35. Cibils LA: Clinical significance of fetal heart rate patterns during labor: II. Late decelerations. *Am J Obstet Gynecol* 1975;123:473.

36. Myers RE, Mueller-Heubach E, Adamsons K: Predictability of the state of fetal oxygenation from a quantitative analysis of the components of late decelerations. *Am J Obstet Gynecol* 1973;115:1083.

37. Tejani JA, Mann LI, Shangavi M, et al: Association of umbilical cord complications and variable decelerations with acid-base findings. *Obstet Gynecol* 1977;49:159.

38. Kubli FW, Hon HE, Khazin HF, et al: Observations on heart rate and pH in the human fetus during labor. *Am J Obstet Gynecol* 1969;104:1190.

39. Bohen FH: Prolonged end-stage fetal heart rate decelerations. *Obstet Gynecol* 1975;45:579.

40. Cibils LA: Clinical significance of fetal heart rate patterns during labor: IV. Agonal patterns. *Am J Obstet Gynecol* 1977;129:833.

41. Clark SL, Gimovsky ML, Miller FC: Fetal heart rate response to scalp blood sampling. *Am J Obstet Gynecol* 1982;144:706-708.

42. Clark SL, Gimovsky ML, Miller FC: The scalp stimulation test: A clinical alternative to fetal scalp blood sampling. *Am J Obstet Gynecol* 1984;148:274-277.

43. Smith CV, Nguyen HN, Phelan JP, et al: Intrapartum assessment of fetal well-being: A comparison of fetal acoustic stimulation with acid-base determinations. *Am J Obstet Gynecol* 1896;155:726-728.

44. Polzin GB, Blakemore KJ, Petrie RH, et al: Fetal vibroacoustic stimulation: Magnitude and duration of fetal heart rate accelerations as a marker of fetal health. *Obstet Gynecol* 1988;72:621-626.

45. Ingemarsson I, Arulkumaran S, Paul RH, et al: Fetal acoustic stimulation in early labor in patients screened with the admission test. *Am J Obstet Gynecol* 1988;158:70-74.

46. Sarno AP, Ahn MO, Phelan JP, et al: Fetal acoustic stimulation in the early intrapartum period as a predictor of subsequent fetal condition. *Am J Obstet Gynecol* 1990;162:762-767.

47. Miller JM, Bernard M, Brown HL, et al: Umbilical cord blood gases for term healthy newborns. *Am J Perinatol* 1990;7:157-159.

48. Saling E, Schneider D: Biochemical supervision of the fetus during labor. *J Obstet Gynaecol Br Commonw* 1967;74:799.

49. Bowe ET, Beard RW, Finster M, et al: Reliability of fetal blood sampling. *Am J Obstet Gynecol* 1970;107:279.

50. Ruth VJ, Rairio KO: Perinatal brain damage: Predictive value of metabolic acidosis and the Apgar score. *Br Med J* 1988;297:24-27.

51. Johnson JWC, Richards DS, and Wagaman RA: The case for routine umbilical blood acid-base studies at delivery. *Am J Obstet Gynecol* 1990;162:621-625.

52. American College of Obstetricians and Gynecologists: *Utility of Umbilical Cord Blood Acid-Base Assessment,* Committee opinion No. 91. Washington, ACOG, 1991.

53. Arias F: Intrauterine resuscitation with terbutaline: A method for the management of acute intrapartum fetal distress. *Am J Obstet Gynecol* 1978;131:39.

54. Esteban-Altirriba J, Cabero L, Calaf F: Correction of fetal homeostatic disturbances, in Aladjem S, Brown AK, Sureau C (eds): *Clinical Perinatology.* St. Louis, Mosby–Year Book, 1980, pp 100-115.

55. Miyazaki FS, Mevarez F: Saline amnioinfusion for relief of repetitive variable decelerations: A prospective randomized study. *Am J Obstet Gynecol* 1985;153:301.

PART SIX

Postpartum Problems

21

POSTPARTUM COMPLICATIONS

This chapter covers some of the complications that occur in the postpartum period. The management of most of these complications does not require a specialist in maternal-fetal medicine, but occasionally, because of their atypical presentation or their unexpected severity, a consultation will be necessary.

The key to the successful management of postpartum problems is the identification of the patient at risk and the adoption of precautions to avoid occurrence of the problem. However, in many cases complications occur unexpectedly, and successful management is based on early recognition and adequate treatment.

◪ POSTPARTUM HEMORRHAGE
Incidence

Postpartum hemorrhage complicates approximately 3.9% of vaginal and 6.4% of cesarean deliveries[1,2] and is responsible for most of the use of blood and blood products in obstetric units. Postpartum bleeding has serious consequences and accounts for approximately 35% of all maternal deaths caused by bleeding during pregnancy.[3]

Definition

There is not a specific, universally accepted definition of postpartum bleeding. Pritchard et al.[4] found that the average blood loss following vaginal delivery and cesarean section was approximately 500 and 1000 ml, respectively. It follows that postpartum hemorrhage should exceed significantly those numbers. The problem is that the estimation of blood loss at delivery is notoriously inaccurate because it is based on the visual observation of the obstetrician rather than on any objective measurement.

In a recent study[1] a hematocrit change of 10% or the need for red cell transfusion was adopted as a definition of postpartum bleeding. This definition has multiple advantages and should be universally accepted.

Patients at risk and preventative measures

A group of investigators at the University of California in San Francisco performed recently an analysis of predisposing factors associated with postpartum bleeding.[1,2] They found that the factors most significantly associated with excessive bleeding following vaginal delivery were:

1. Prolonged third stage of labor
2. Preeclampsia
3. Mediolateral episiotomy
4. Twins
5. Arrest of descent
6. Soft tissue lacerations

7. Augmented labor
8. Forceps or vacuum delivery
9. Asian or Hispanic ethnicity
10. Midline episiotomy
11. Nulliparity

The factors most significantly associated with postpartum bleeding following cesarean section were:

1. General anesthesia
2. Chorioamnionitis
3. Preeclampsia
4. Protracted active phase of labor
5. Arrest of second stage of labor
6. Hispanic ethnicity

Some of these factors—prolonged third stage of labor, episiotomy, forceps, anesthesia—can be prevented or modified by the obstetrician attending the delivery. Others cannot be changed, but their presence should alert the obstetrician to the potential for postpartum bleeding and make him or her take precautionary measures for adequate management of the problem.

General preventative measures. Several measures should be taken in anticipation of problems in patients with risk factors such as preeclampsia, twin gestation, and arrest of descent. The most important is to have a sample of blood sent to the laboratory for determination of the blood type and screening for irregular antibodies in case blood products are needed. Also, it is crucial to obtain adequate intravenous access before the patient starts bleeding. Patients with multiple risk factors for postpartum bleeding should have two intravenous lines before delivery. Similar precautions should be adopted for patients undergoing cesarean section after prolonged labor, chorioamnionitis, or preeclampsia or for patients who are under general anesthesia during the cesarean section.

Management of the third stage of labor. Adequate management of the third stage of labor is important for the prevention of postpartum bleeding in patients undergoing vaginal delivery. Investigators have compared the effect on postpartum bleeding of active versus expectant management of the third stage of labor.[5] In the active management protocol, 5 units of oxytocin and 0.5 mg ergonovine maleate, or 10 units of oxytocin if the mother had elevated blood pressure, were given immediately after delivery of the anterior shoulder. The umbilical cord was clamped 30 seconds after delivery of the baby. When the uterus contracted, the placenta was

delivered by controlled cord traction with a hand on the abdomen to prevent uterine inversion. In the expectant management group, no oxytocin was given, and the umbilical cord was not clamped and remained attached to the baby until delivery of the placenta. The mother was encouraged to push and adopt a posture aiding delivery when she felt contractions or the urge to push. The authors found an incidence of postpartum bleeding of 5.9% in the actively managed group and 17.9% in the physiologically managed group. The conclusion is that active management of the third stage reduces the incidence of postpartum bleeding.

In addition to administration of oxytocin, rapid clamping of the cord, and controlled delivery of the placenta, adequate management of the third stage requires (1) avoiding undue traction on the umbilical cord to prevent uterine inversion, (2) delivering the placenta manually for excessive bleeding or prolonged third stage, (3) performing abdominal compression and massage of the uterus to assure adequacy of contraction, and (4) doing a manual and visual inspection of the birth canal following delivery, especially if an instrumental delivery was performed.

Episiotomy. Another factor associated with postpartum bleeding that is under the control of the obstetrician attending the delivery is the performance of episiotomy. Episiotomies are performed for the following reasons:

1. Perineal laceration seems to be imminent
2. To prevent severe perineal trauma, particularly third- and fourth-degree extensions
3. As prophylaxis against future pelvic relaxation
4. To shorten the duration of the second stage in cases of fetal distress
5. To facilitate vaginal breech delivery

The first reason to perform episiotomy makes sense. When perineal laceration seems imminent, performance of episiotomy will permit a meticulous repair of anatomic structures, avoiding the difficulties and complications inherent to the repair of an irregular break of the tissues. However, this indication is not supported by controlled, randomized studies comparing the short- and long-term effects of episiotomy repair vs. perineal laceration repair.

The second reason to perform episiotomy—prevention of perineal trauma—most likely is not valid. The modern literature indicates that episiotomy rather than protecting against perineal injury, actually predisposes the patient to third- and fourth-degree lacerations.[6,7]

The third reason for the performance of episiotomies—prevention of future pelvic relaxation—is controversial. However, the only comparative study on pelvic relaxation following spontaneous delivery without episiotomy or forceps delivery with episiotomy shows significantly more damage to the anatomic structures of the pelvis following spontaneous delivery.[8] Although it is possible to raise criticisms against some aspects of this work, its conclusions remain unchallenged up to this time.

Routine use of episiotomy is unnecessary. However, episiotomies are justified in a large number of situations, especially in nulliparous patients. However, large episiotomies may result in blood loss approaching that found in cesarean section, about 1000 ml. Blood loss is significantly larger in patients undergoing mediolateral rather than midline episiotomy. Also, mediolateral episiotomies are more painful, and patients experience dyspareunia for a long time after the procedure. However, midline episiotomies are not entirely benign and are associated with significant risk of perineal lacerations that may result in rectovaginal fistulas and anal sphincter incontinency.[9,10] Shiono et al.[7] found that perineal lacerations occurred in 8.3% of primiparous and 1.5% of multiparous patients. Patients with midline episiotomy were approximately 50 times more likely and women with mediolateral episiotomy were over 8 times more likely to suffer a severe laceration than women who did not have episiotomy. Combs et al.[6] found that the factors associated with third- and fourth-degree perineal lacerations were:

1. Midline episiotomy
2. Nulliparity
3. Second-stage arrest
4. Occiput posterior presentation
5. Delivery at low or mid station
6. Use of forceps instead of vacuum
7. Local anesthesia
8. Asian race

To prevent excessive blood loss, midline episiotomy should be the procedure of choice whenever episiotomy is required. However, for patients with one or more risk factors for perineal lacerations—such as nulliparas with occiput posterior positions, Asiatic patients, deliveries with forceps at stations other than outlet—the episiotomy should be mediolateral because

the complications associated with midline episiotomy are more disabling than those resulting from the mediolateral procedure.

Forceps and vacuum. The use of forceps and vacuum is another factor associated with postpartum bleeding. There are multiple indications for the use of these instruments, and the choice between them depends mostly on the skill and training of the obstetrician.

Several investigations[11,12] have concluded that there is less risk of maternal trauma with vacuum than with forceps, but others[13] have found a similar incidence of maternal complications. With respect to the fetus, some investigators[14] have found vacuum as safe as forceps, but others[11,12,15] concluded that infants delivered with vacuum have a higher incidence of cephalic hematomas, intracerebral bleeding, scalp lesions, retinal hemorrhages, and neonatal jaundice requiring phototherapy than babies delivered with forceps.

In summary, it is controversial whether vacuum should be the instrument of choice for operative vaginal delivery. Many obstetricians are ready to accept a relatively small increase in the risk of maternal trauma and blood loss with the use of forceps rather than the increased risk of fetal morbidity caused by vacuum. However, many others prefer to use the vacuum and feel uncomfortable with forceps application.

Causes of postpartum bleeding

There is an unavoidable blood loss during parturition. In a study of more than 9000 patients,[1] it was found that the average admission hematocrit of 36.3% +/- 3.5% decreased to 33.7% +/- 4.3% in the postpartum period. The blood loss is not larger because of two mechanisms that maintain vascular integrity following placental separation. The first involves constriction of uterine blood vessels in the placental bed by myometrial fibers. The second is an intact coagulation system. A disruption of either or both of these mechanisms will result in postpartum bleeding. The causes of this complication are shown in Box 21-1. The most common of them is uterine atony, and the most rare are alterations of the coagulation cascade.

Uterine atony. There are many reasons why the uterus may fail to adequately contract in the immediate postpartum period. They are shown in Box 21-2. Mechanical factors include inability of the uterus to contract because of an intrauter-

---

BOX 21-1

Causes of Postpartum Bleeding

Uterine atony
Retained products of conception
Lacerations of the genital tract
Uterine inversion
Uterine rupture
Abnormalities of the coagulation system

BOX 21-2

Causes of Uterine Atony

Mechanical factors
Retained placental fragments
Retained clots

Extreme uterine dilation
Multiple gestation
Polyhydramnios

Rapid uterine evacuation
Precipitous delivery
Forceps delivery

Metabolic factors
Uterine hypoxia
Sepsis
Hypocalcemia

Pharmacologic factors
Magnesium sulfate
Beta adrenergic agents
Diazoxide
Halothane
Calcium channel blockers

---

ine object, usually placental fragments or blood clots. Also, it has been observed that extreme uterine distention before labor, as in multiple gestation or polyhydramnios, is accompanied by poor uterine tone postpartum. The etiology of this phenomenon is unclear. Overstretching may disrupt the bundles of actin-myosin in individual smooth muscle cells and decrease the efficiency of uterine contractions. Another cause of uterine atony is rapid uterine evacuation as sometimes seen in precipitous forceps delivery. Presumably an orderly evacuation of the uterine contents with adequate opportunity for the myometrium to contract is important.

Metabolic factors may contribute to uterine atony. For effective contraction to be maintained, it is necessary to have an adequate supply of oxygen and fuel to support the aerobic metabolism of myometrial cells. Hypoxia or acidosis from any cause, including acute respiratory insufficiency, diabetic ketoacidosis, and sepsis, may disturb myometrial metabolism. Patients who deliver after difficult or obstructed labor may suffer from uterine atony. The mechanism of uterine atony in these cases is complex, and muscle exhaustion, lactate buildup, and glycogen depletion may be implicated. Because calcium is an important regulator of smooth muscle tone, hypocalcemia can be implicated in some cases of uterine atony.

Drugs may have important effects on postpartum uterine tone. The use of large dosages of oxytocin to stimulate desultory or obstructed labor may result in relative oxytocin insensitivity. It is not clear whether this tachyphylactic effect of exogenously administered oxytocin results from down-regulation of oxytocin receptors or simply from individual variability of oxytocin effects. Magnesium sulfate, administered to prevent or treat seizures in preeclampsia or as a tocolytic agent, may result in uterine atony by impairing the calcium-mediated activation of actin-myosin interaction. Beta-adrenergic tocolytic agents inhibit uterine contractility by increasing intracellular cyclic adenosine monophosphate. These drugs are given to inhibit preterm labor and treat fetal distress, and they may decrease effective uterine contractions for several hours. Diazoxide, a potent antihypertensive agent, is also a powerful tocolytic drug inhibiting uterine contractions for up to 12 hours after an intravenous infusion. Halothane, a volatile anesthetic agent, also causes uterine relaxation and is useful in situations in which rapid, reversible uterine relaxation is desirable. However, obese patients may accumulate this drug, which is fat soluble, and not display the rapid reversibility expected. Calcium channel blockers, such as nifedipine, medication extensively used for the treatment of preterm uterine contractions, also may inhibit effective postpartum uterine contraction.

Retained placenta. There are different clinical presentations of retained placenta. They vary from failure of the placenta to deliver spontaneously, requiring manual removal and causing minor blood loss, to a placenta accreta that cannot be removed and causes severe bleeding requiring massive blood transfusion. Bleeding caused by retained small placental fragments is uncommon in the immediate postpartum period.

Combs and Laros[16] investigated the factors associated with retained placenta and prolonged third stage of labor. They found that the mean duration of the third stage was 6 minutes and that the incidence of complications increased significantly after it was prolonged beyond 30 minutes. They also found that prolonged third stage was strongly associated with preterm delivery, labor induced for medical reasons, augmented labor, amnionitis, and prolonged rupture of the membranes. After controlling for confounding factors, these investigators found that the most important predictor of prolonged third stage was preterm delivery confirming a prior observation by Romero et al.[17] The increase in incidence of retained placenta affects predominantly women with induced preterm labor rather than women who deliver preterm after spontaneous labor. The reason for the failure of the placenta to separate in preterm deliveries is not known.

A placenta abnormally adherent to the uterus, or placenta accreta, is a relatively rare cause of postpartum bleeding. It occurs in one of every 2000 to 4000 deliveries. However, this incidence is increasing because of the increased frequency of cesarean deliveries. In fact, the presence of a scar in the uterus is the most important risk factor associated with placenta accreta.[18]

Lacerations of the low genital tract. Cervical, vaginal, and perineal lacerations are a common cause of postpartum bleeding, which occasionally may be severe. Cervical lacerations are associated mainly with precipitous deliveries, the use of forceps, and with attempts to dilate the cervix manually. Lacerations of the upper vagina are almost always associated with instrumental deliveries. Perineal lacerations usually result from extension of episiotomy incisions.

Uterine rupture. Uterine rupture is a catastrophic obstetric event that usually occurs and is detected in the intrapartum period. On some occasions, however, uterine rupture is manifested by postpartum bleeding. The most common predisposing factors to uterine rupture are prior cesarean section, use of oxytocin, and multiparity.

Uterine inversion. Uterine inversion is a catastrophic complication of the third stage of labor that occurs in approximately 1 of every 2500 deliveries. In most cases it results from efforts to deliver a pathologically adherent placenta implanted in the fundus of the uterus. In a minority of cases, uterine inversion follows excessive fundal compression combined with cord traction for the delivery of a fundal placenta. Blood loss may be severe in patients with uterine rupture, but in many of them, shock seems to be out of proportion to the amount of bleeding.

Abnormalities of the coagulation system. The second major mechanism of postpartum hemostasis involves the blood coagulation system. Coagulation is important in controlling bleeding from all spontaneous or surgical disruptions of the birth canal. Small lacerations of the cervix, vagina, or perineum, which are confined to the mucosa and do not involve large blood vessels, seldom cause significant postpartum blood loss if blood coagulation is normal. However, if coagulopathy is present, even small lacerations may result in exsanguination.

Defects in the coagulation system are rather uncommon. However, it is important to detect them before delivery. The most common are disseminated intravascular coagulation (DIC), von Willebrand's disease, and alterations in platelet number or function.

DIC is the most common bleeding disorder seen in obstetric patients. In molar pregnancy, amniotic fluid embolism, endotoxic shock, and fetal death in utero, DIC is the result of release of material with thromboplastin-like activity into the maternal circulation with subsequent activation of the coagulation and fibrinolytic systems. Consumption of coagulation factors probably initiates DIC in abruptio placentae and hemorrhagic shock. The etiology of DIC in severe preeclampsia is unclear but may involve, as a first step, activation of platelet aggregation at the site of endothelial damage.

The most common clotting-factor deficiency in young women is von Willebrand's disease, an acquired autosomal recessive disorder resulting in a relative, though not absolute, deficiency of factor VIII. Most patients have a family or personal history strongly suggesting coagulopathy, but a few patients who have never experienced serious injury or surgery may be undiagnosed. Fortunately, most patients with von Willebrand's disease have increased factor VIII activity during pregnancy.

Deficiency in platelet number or function may occur in pregnancy. A form of severe preeclampsia, the HELLP (*H*emolytic anemia, *E*levated *L*iver enzymes, *L*ow *P*latelet count) syndrome, has thrombocytopenia among its characteristic features. Fortunately, seldom is the platelet count less than 50,000/mm, a level at which thrombocytopenia results in poor hemostasis. Immune thrombocytopenic purpura, an autoimmune disease often diagnosed in young women, is caused by circulating IgG antibodies to platelet antigens. These patients may have profound thrombocytopenia and are at risk of delivering infants with thrombocytopenia. Defects in platelet function occur with aspirin ingestion. Aspirin inhibits the enzyme cyclooxygenase and prevents the formation of thromboxane and other procoagulants that are potent stimulators of platelet aggregation.

Diagnosis and treatment

The diagnosis of postpartum bleeding is usually obvious, and in the majority of cases the etiology of the problem is also apparent. Excessive bleeding may occur before delivery of the placenta, following delivery of the placenta, or late in the postpartum period. The etiology and the management of the bleeding will be different depending on when the bleeding occurs.

Bleeding before delivery of the placenta. Bleeding during the third stage of labor is usually the result of retained placenta. However, patients also may bleed because of lacerations to the genital tract occurring during delivery of the fetus. The differential diagnosis between these two possibilities is easy because in the majority of cases of retained placenta, bleeding will stop after its removal, whereas patients with lacerations of the genital tract will continue bleeding after the placenta is removed.

When bleeding is brisk and the placenta is still inside of the uterus, the first step should be an attempt to remove the placenta with gentle traction of the cord together with counter pressure on the uterus with a hand placed on the abdomen. If this maneuver is successful and the placenta is delivered, the uterus should be kept compressed between the hand in the vagina and the hand in the patient's abdomen, and a dilute solution of oxytocin should be given intravenously. Bimanual compression of the uterus should be maintained until the uterus is firmly contracted. If gentle pulling of the cord and abdominal pressure fail in provoking separation and delivery of the placenta, the next step is a pelvic examination. The pelvic examination will allow determination of whether the placenta is retained because of a contracted cervix or whether the problem is caused by excessive attachment of the placenta to the uterus.

Retained placenta caused by a contracted cervix. When the placenta is retained because of a contracted cervix, a situation that occurs almost exclusively in preterm deliveries, the pelvic examination will reveal a cervix that does not permit introduction inside the uterus of more than two of the operator's fingers. In this situation it is not advisable or useful to continue attempts to deliver the placenta by traction on the cord, abdominal pressure, or administration of oxytocic agents, and the best approach is the administration of nitroglycerin to relax the cervix and allow manual removal of the placenta.[19]

Nitroglycerin is a powerful vasodilator, hypotensor, and relaxant of the myometrial muscle. Given intravenously in a low dose, it relaxes the uterus without pronounced effects on blood pressure. However, the drug should not be used in patients in shock or with low blood pressure to avoid aggravation of their situation. Before administration of nitroglycerin, it is important to expand rapidly the intravascular volume with 500 to 1000 ml of crystalloid solution. Then 500 µg of nitroglycerin are administered as an intravenous push. Approximately 60 to 120 seconds after administration of the drug, the cervix will relax enough to permit introduction of the operator's hand into the uterus and manual removal of the placenta. In many cases the placenta is expelled spontaneously after cervical relaxation has been achieved. If manual extraction is necessary, supplemental analgesia may be provided by giving 50 to 100 µg of fentanyl intravenously.

Retained placenta caused by abnormal attachment to the uterus. There are degrees in the severity of the placental attachment to the uterine wall. In the majority of cases the placenta can be peeled off of the uterus without major difficulties, and no explanation is found for the delay in its delivery. In a few cases the placenta is firmly attached to the uterine wall, and it is impossible to find an adequate plane of cleavage for its removal. Persistency in attempts to deliver the placenta manually end with the removal of multiple fragments, but a large part of the organ will remain attached to the uterus, and the bleeding frequently becomes profuse. This condition is called placenta accreta, and in the majority of patients the best treatment is to perform a hysterectomy. A review in 1972 of 622 published cases of placenta accreta shows a maternal mortality 4 times larger when conservative treatment consisting of "piecemeal" removal and uterine packing was used instead of hysterectomy.[20] Today, with better antibiotics, chemotherapeutic agents, and means of surveillance, conservative treatment may produce different results and may be indicated in selected patients who desire preservation of their fertility.

Bleeding after delivery of the placenta. Bleeding after delivery of the placenta is usually the result of uterine atony. Other less frequent etiologies are retained placental fragments, genital tract lacerations, uterine inversion, uterine rupture, and abnormalities of the coagulation system.

The first thing to do in response to severe bleeding after delivery of the placenta is vigorous bimanual vaginal and abdominal uterine compression. This maneuver stops the bleeding in many cases, and even if not successful as the sole treatment, it will reduce the rate of blood loss. Next, one or two intravenous lines should be inserted and an oxytocin infusion begun (30 U in 1000 ml of lactated Ringer's solution).

If uterine compression and intravenous oxytocin are not successful in stopping the bleeding, the patient should have an ultrasound examination to rule out the presence of retained products and a rapid but thorough digital examination of the uterine cavity to rule out a uterine rupture. A careful visualization of the cervix and vagina for an undetected laceration is performed next.

Uterine atony. Once the diagnosis of uterine atony is confirmed on the basis of physical and ultrasound examination, blood is crossmatched, and bimanual abdominal and vaginal uterine massage is continued. If blood loss continues, the patient should be moved to an operating room and given methylergonovine maleate, 0.2 mg intramuscularly (IM), if her blood pressure is normal. If the patient is hypotensive, 0.4 mg of methylergonovine maleate should be administered IM. The dose may be repeated in 10 minutes. If the bleeding continues, Hemabate, the 15 methyl derivative of prostaglandin $F_{2\alpha}$ should be given intramuscularly in the deltoid or gluteal area. The dose is 250 mg IM, and it can be repeated every 30 minutes. If Hemabate is not available, bleeding may be controlled with vaginal suppositories[21] or with intrauterine irrigation of prostaglandin E_2.[22] If bleeding persists, intrauterine irrigation with hot saline solution, 40° to 55° C may be tried.[23] Another option at this stage is uterine packing, a method that has enthusiastic supporters and severe censors. For some it has proven to be useful and has avoided several laparotomies.

If bleeding still persists, a second intravenous line should be inserted while bimanual abdominal and vaginal uterine compression is continued. Transfusion of packed red cells is started. A Foley catheter is inserted, and a central venous pressure line may be necessary if the volume replacement is massive. Coagulation studies are sent to the laboratory, and coagulation factors are administered if needed, based on the laboratory and clinical situation. Then a laparotomy should be performed through a vertical midline incision. The uterus should be carefully examined, and if a uterine rupture is present, it should be repaired. If the uterus is intact, there are several options depending on the specific situation.

Bilateral uterine artery ligation is a simple and effective procedure that will control most cases of postpartum bleeding and will preserve the patient's reproductive capacity.[24] The uterine artery is ligated just above the bladder flap using a nonabsorbable suture material (0 Vicryl), including into the ligature some of the underlying myometrium. A second ligature is placed high in the broad ligament just below the insertion of the ovarian ligament in the uterus.

Bilateral hypogastric artery ligation can be used as a treatment of postpartum bleeding or as a first step before hysterectomy.[25] This method is indicated when there are large broad ligament or lateral pelvic hematomas that distort the anatomy and prevent the performance of the more simple uterine artery ligation. The procedure is accomplished by identification of the intersection of the external iliac artery and the ureter, incision of the posterior peritoneum, identification of the hypogastric artery, and passage of a Vicryl or chromic catgut tie around the artery 1 to 2 cm from its origin in the common iliac artery. The pelvic arterial bed is rich in anastomosis, and the uterus still will be perfused after ligating the hypogastric arteries. However, the pressure head will be much lower and without pulsatile properties, and hemostasis can be more reliably achieved with pressure alone.

Hysterectomy is another option for the surgical treatment of uterine atony that should be used when bleeding fails to respond to more conservative measures. If the bleeding is caused by uterine atony and the patient is unstable, it is better to perform a rapid supracervical procedure. If the origin of the bleeding is in the low uterine segment, the cervix should be included in the resection.

Uterine inversion. Most cases of uterine inversion are a complication resulting from a combination of abnormally adherent placenta and uterine atony. The placenta brings down the attached uterus at the time of delivery, and the fundus herniates through the cervix into the vagina and, in extreme cases, prolapses outside of the external genitalia. The placenta may separate or may remain attached to the uterus. These events are usually accompanied by profuse bleeding and shock. Uterine inversion is a serious accident that may cause maternal mortality if it is not treated adequately.

The diagnosis of uterine inversion is obvious when the uterus protrudes outside of the external genitalia. When the placenta has detached and the inverted uterus remains in the vagina, the diagnosis is made by pelvic examination that will reveal a hard muscular mass filling the upper part of the vagina that is easy to confuse with a uterine myoma. The abdominal examination will reveal absence or abnormally small size of the uterus.

The fundamental points in management include rapid recognition of the inversion, uterine replacement, uterotonic agents, and prophylactic antibiotics afterward. It may be possible to replace the inverted uterus as soon as the problem is recognized, but in some cases a strong constriction ring will block the initial efforts, and hydrostatic pressure or general anesthesia with uterine relaxant agents will be necessary. If the placenta is adherent, it is best not to remove it until uterine replacement can be performed, or increased bleeding may ensue.

Before attempting to replace the uterus, a uterine relaxant such as magnesium sulfate, 4 g IV, or terbutaline, 0.25 mg IV, should be given. To replace the uterus, it is necessary to grasp the inverted fundus in the palm of the hand with the fingers pointing posteriorly and the thumb anteriorly and push it upwards toward the umbilicus.[26] It is important that the pressure be exerted below the ring on the portion of the uterus that inverted last because efforts to push the fundus first will create a double thickness of the myometrium and the attempt to replace the uterus will fail.[27] If the initial attempt to replace

the uterus fails, the next step should be to use hydrostatic pressure.

To apply hydrostatic pressure, it is necessary to place the prolapsed uterus, with or without the attached placenta, inside of the vagina. Two enema bags, each filled with 1000 ml of normal saline, are placed several feet above the level of the vagina. The nozzle tips of the enema bags are placed inside the vagina, and the saline solution is infused while the labia are kept tightly together with the hands to avoid spilling the fluid.[28] The vagina begins to distend, and the fundus of the uterus rises.[29] This simple maneuver is usually successful, and it is rare that the patient requires replacement under general anesthesia. When general anesthesia is necessary, the anesthetic of choice is halothane because of its profound relaxing effect on the uterus.

Following uterine replacement and removal of the placenta, it is necessary to administer uterotonic agents to avoid recurrence of the problem. The medication of choice for this purpose is 15-methyl PGE_2, 0.25 mg IM. In some cases it will be necessary to use uterine packing in combination with prostaglandin to avoid recurrences.[30] In some cases the placenta is an accreta, cannot be removed, and the procedure of choice will be hysterectomy.

Uterine rupture. Uterine rupture is an uncommon event that happens in approximately 1 in 1000 to 1 in 6000 deliveries. In the majority of cases this catastrophic event occurs in the antepartum or intrapartum period, and in only a few patients, it manifests initially as postpartum bleeding.

The most common associations of uterine rupture are prior cesarean section, use of oxytocin, multiparity, and abruptio placentae. In the majority of cases the first indication is a nonreassuring fetal heart rate pattern during labor. In a few cases labor and delivery are uneventful, but following placental separation, the patient develops vaginal bleeding, and uterine exploration reveals a complete separation of the wall of the uterus.

The treatment of uterine rupture is a simple repair if the patient wants to preserve her childbearing capacity; otherwise a hysterectomy is performed. The possibilities of recurrence following a simple repair are approximately 10%.

Late postpartum bleeding. Late postpartum bleeding is that occurring 24 hours or more after delivery. The most common causes are retained fragments of placenta and subinvolution of the placental implantation site.

The first thing to do in cases of late postpartum bleeding is to secure an IV line and rapidly expand volume with normal saline or lactated Ringer's solution containing 30 or 40 units of oxytocin per each 1000 ml. Then a pelvic ultrasound examination should be made to rule out retained placental fragments. The sensitivity and specificity of ultrasound for this diagnosis is close to 100%. If placental fragments are present, curettage of the uterine cavity and removal of these fragments is indicated. If no placental fragments are present, treatment should be conservative, using prostaglandins and blood replacement.[31] To perform uterine curettage in the absence of retained placental tissue is ineffective and frequently aggravates the bleeding. Successful control of bleeding following curettage may be achieved by injecting 5 ml of diluted vasopressin (20 U in 30 ml of normal saline) at the 3 o'clock and 9 o'clock positions followed by hysteroscopic coagulation of bleeding points.[32]

◪ PELVIC HEMATOMAS

Pelvic hematomas are caused by injury and rupture of a blood vessel without disruption of the overlying tissues. Because of the increased tissue elasticity and large potential spaces within the pelvis, the likelihood of hematoma development after vessel injury is increased. Sources of injury to pelvic vessels include pressure exerted by the presenting part, forceps, or vacuum extractors and lacerations caused by paracervical or pudendal injection of anesthesia. In addition, hematomas may form at the apex of the episiotomies or lacerations.

Pelvic hematomas are uncommon, with an approximate incidence of 1 in 1000 deliveries. They are potentially lethal and require active management to avoid serious complications.

Classification

Pelvic hematomas may develop in any plane of the pelvis. Usually they are classified as vulvar, vaginal, and retroperitoneal depending on their location in relation to the pelvic diaphragm and the cardinal ligament.[33]

Patients at risk and preventative measures

Patients at risk include those with difficult or obstructed labor, instrumental delivery, or lacerations of the birth canal. Patients with coagulopathy are at increased risk of hematoma forma-

tion. Prevention entails careful use of forceps and vacuum extractors.

Diagnosis and treatment

Any postpartum patient with unusual pelvic or perineal pain should be examined to rule out pelvic hematoma. For most hematomas the predominant symptom is pain, although a few result in such a large blood loss that hypotension is the first sign. Careful abdominal, rectal, and vaginal examination is mandatory for proper diagnosis. Evaluation of the coagulation system is mandatory since many patients that develop postpartum hematomas have coagulation abnormalities.

Opinion varies as to whether all vulvar hematomas should be evacuated. Hematomas in the episiotomy site, those obviously enlarging, those causing disabling symptoms, and those infected should definitely be evacuated. In most cases bleeding vessels cannot be found. Small cavities left after evacuation may be obliterated by mattress sutures, and large cavities should be treated with a pressure dressing.

In the case of vaginal hematomas, it is useless to spend time attempting to find the source of the bleeding. After evacuation no attempts should be made to suture the vaginal mucosa or to pack the hematoma cavity. Instead, a vaginal pack is placed and removed in 24 hours. Catheterization of the urinary bladder is needed when vaginal packing is used.

The presence of a retroperitoneal hematoma should be suspected in patients who develop postpartum hypovolemia without external blood loss. The diagnosis is confirmed by ultrasound and computed tomography (CT) scanning. Such patients, most of whom have had a cesarean section, should have adequate blood replacement and be taken to the x-ray department for angiographic embolization.[34,35]

Embolization should be preceded by catheterization of one or both internal iliac arteries and angiographic demonstration of the sites of bleeding. The most commonly used embolic material is small pieces of surgical gelatin sponge (Gelfoam). This method is successful in more than 90% of the cases and can be used also in patients with abdominal and cervical pregnancies and with hematomas caused by pelvic fractures.

If angiographic embolization cannot be performed or fails in stopping the bleeding, a MAST (Military Anti-Shock Trousers) suit may save the patient's life and avoid surgery. The MAST suit or antigravity suit is extremely effective in stopping pelvic bleeding.[36] It consists of plastic bags that are wrapped around the lower extremities and against the anterior abdominal wall and inflated to a pressure as high as 100 mm Hg. The procedure for using the MAST suit is shown in Box 21-3. In the majority of patients, pelvic bleeding stops shortly after inflation of the devise, concomitantly with improvement of vital signs and urinary output.

Some patients need laparotomy to identify and ligate bleeding vessels. In many cases it is necessary to perform bilateral hypogastric artery ligation. If the bleeding ceases after hypogastric artery ligation, no further surgery or clot evacuation is needed; otherwise, hysterectomy is necessary. Unfortunately, some patients continue bleeding after bilateral hypogastric artery ligation and hysterectomy. In these cases the obstetrician should be prepared to use desperate measures such as filling the pelvis with a pack to tamponade the bleeding areas[37] or postoperative use of angiographic embolization and the MAST suit.

BOX 21-3

Procedure for Use of the MAST Suit

1. Remove clothing below the waist, and place a Foley catheter in the bladder.
2. Move the patient into the deflated trousers.
3. Encase the lower extremities and the abdomen in the suit using the Velcro straps. The upper border of the abdominal portion of the MAST suit should be below the rib cage.
4. Inflate the legs and then the abdominal compartment. Start with a pressure of 10 mm and increase by 10-mm increments. Pressures up to 40 mm are well tolerated. When pressures higher than 40 mm are used, lactic acidosis may occur, and arterial blood gases should be measured periodically.
5. The suit should remain inflated for 12 to 24 hours after bleeding has stopped. Do not use it for more than 48 hours.
6. To deflate, start with the abdominal compartment and deflate gradually infusing IV fluids at each 5-mm level of decompression to maintain blood pressure at the predeflation level. When the abdominal compartment is completely deflated, repeat procedure in leg compartments.

◪ POSTPARTUM ENDOMETRITIS

Postpartum endometritis is the most common obstetric infection. It affects approximately 1% to 3% of women delivering vaginally and 10% to 30% of those delivering by cesarean section. These figures vary widely depending on the patient population, and the problem is much more common in low socioeconomic groups.

Patients at risk and preventative measures

The most common factor associated with postpartum endometritis is cesarean delivery. The complication occurs more frequently in patients undergoing cesarean section after several hours of labor and multiple vaginal examinations than in those who have elective repeated cesarean deliveries.

Other factors traditionally associated with postpartum endometritis are labor, premature rupture of the membranes, number of pelvic examinations, cervical and vaginal lacerations, and anemia. Newton et al.[38] performed a multivariate analysis of several predictive factors using stepwise logistic regression and found that most cases of postpartum endometritis could be explained by only three factors: cesarean section, lack of prophylactic antibiotics, and presence of certain organisms in the amniotic fluid during labor. All the other traditionally recognized predictive factors were eliminated by this analysis, and it is possible that they act by facilitating rather than predicting the development of endometritis.

It is clear that the most important measure for preventing the onset of postpartum endometritis is avoiding the abdominal route of delivery. Unfortunately, this measure seems to be unrealistic in view of the increasing incidence of cesarean deliveries.

Administration of prophylactic antibiotics at the time of cesarean delivery is another important measure for preventing postpartum endometritis. There is universal agreement that antibiotics should be given to those patients undergoing cesarean section that are at high risk for infection, such as after prolonged labor or premature rupture of membranes. A single dose of cefoxitin, cefotetan, or ampicillin/sulbactam given after cord clamping is all that is necessary. More controversial is the administration of prophylactic antibiotics to patients undergoing elective repeat cesarean section. Some authorities do not recommend treatment in those cases because of lack of proof of benefit and fear of gastrointestinal side effects. However, a recent prospective study of 1863 women undergoing cesarean section and considered at low risk for infection revealed a 3.9% incidence of postpartum endometritis among 957 patients who did not receive antibiotics vs. 0.9% in 906 patients that had prophylaxis.[39] There was no diarrhea-gastroenteritis in any of the patients who received prophylactic antibiotics.

A potential preventative measure for postpartum endometritis is the treatment of women with bacterial vaginosis. Antepartum bacterial vaginosis is an important risk factor not only for preterm labor,[40] but also for postpartum endometritis. Pregnant patients with bacterial vaginosis diagnosed by Gram stain are approximately 6 times more likely to develop endometritis than women with normal vaginal Gram stain.[41] Unfortunately there are no studies indicating the best antibiotic treatment, its duration, side effects, and efficacy.

Etiology

Postpartum endometritis is a polymicrobial *ascending* infection of organisms that constitute the normal vaginal flora. Usually a mixture of aerobic and anaerobic organisms is involved (Box 21-4). The most common isolates are *Gardnerella vaginalis*, group B streptococci, *Escherichia coli*, *Bacteroides bivius*, and *Mycoplasma*.

The mechanism responsible for the ascending infection has not been clarified. Most likely there are a series of complex interrelations between the indigenous vaginal bacteria and the host defense mechanisms that can be affected more easily in some patients than in others.

Diagnosis

The most important element in the diagnosis of postpartum endometritis is the development of fever. The temperature should exceed 38° C (100.4° F) on two occasions 4 hours apart. The majority of patients will complain of pain in the lower abdomen. Pelvic examination will reveal an extremely tender uterus. Foul smelling lochia will be present when the infection is predominantly caused by anaerobic bacteria.

The laboratory usually shows leukocytosis with left shift. Blood cultures will be positive in approximately 10% of the patients.

The value of endometrial cultures in the management of patients with postpartum endometritis has been debated for years. Opponents of routine culturing argue that contamination with the vaginal flora is common, that the test is expensive, and that the majority of patients are treated immediately after the onset of symptoms and are feeling better by the time culture results are back. Proponents of routine culturing believe that vaginal contamination can be easily avoided and that the results of the culture are of crucial importance in the management of the 10% to 20% of patients that fail to respond to the initial antibiotic therapy.

Aerobic and anaerobic cultures of the endometrium should be obtained in every patient with postpartum fever. The simplest way to obtain the samples is with the use of a cotton swab grasped with a sponge forceps to facilitate its introduction into the fundus of the uterus. The culture should be obtained after cleaning the cervix with gauze or a cotton ball soaked in povidone-iodine (Betadine) and wiping it off with sterile gauze. The endocervical canal is mantained open with the help of a sponge forceps while the samples are obtained. This technique allows the physician to obtain a fundal sample

---

BOX 21-4

Bacteria Commonly Isolated from Patients with Postpartum Endometritis

Anaerobic bacteria
Bacteroides bivius
Bacteroides fragilis
Peptostreptococcus sp.
Fusobacterium sp.
Clostridium sp.

Mycoplasma
Ureaplasma urealyticum
Mycoplasma hominis

Aerobic bacteria
Gardnerella vaginalis
Group B streptococci
Escherichia coli
Enterococcus
Staphylococcus sp.
Klebsiella pneumoniae

without causing vaginal contamination and is less expensive and yields a larger number of bacterial species than double-lumen catheters or endometrial suction devices.[42]

Treatment

The "gold standard" treatment for postpartum endometritis has been a combination of clindamycin, 900 mg IV every 8 hours, and gentamicin, 2 mg/kg IV initial dose followed by 1.5 mg/kg every 8 hours. The gentamicin maintenance dose should be adjusted to obtain peak levels 30 minutes after a dose, between 5 and 8 μg/ml, and through levels, obtained before the next dose, that should be less than 1 μg/ml.

The problems with clindamycin/gentamicin treatment are several: it cures only 92% of the patients, it does not treat enterococcus, it has significant potential for renal toxicity caused by gentamicin and gastrointestinal toxicity caused by clindamycin, and it has all the inconveniences and increased cost of multiple drug treatment. Because of these problems, multiple studies have been performed with a variety of single antibiotics, mostly cephalosporins and penicillins. Treatment with a single antibiotic offers the advantages of less toxicity, less pharmacy and nursing time, and less cost. Unfortunately, the effectiveness of single antibiotic treatment is on the average only 80%. Treatment with ampicillin/sulbactam, 3 g IV every 6 hours, combined with aztreonam, 2 g IV every 6 to 8 hours, is preferred. This antibiotic combination treats enterococcus and has less potential for severe gastrointestinal or renal side effects.

◪ OVARIAN VEIN THROMBOPHLEBITIS

The ovarian veins increase markedly in size during pregnancy from an average diameter of 9 mm to approximately 25 mm. This increase in diameter is necessary to accommodate the increased blood flow to the pregnant uterus. Thrombosis and infection of this large vascular channel occur during pregnancy, almost exclusively in patients with postpartum endometritis. The condition affects predominantly the right ovarian vein.

Incidence

Ovarian vein thrombophlebitis is a relatively uncommon event. The exact incidence is unknown and varies from institution to institution in direct relationship to the incidence of postpartum endometritis. It may be as high as 1 in 600 deliveries,[43] but a more reasonable figure is 1 in 3000.

Patients at risk and preventative measures

The strongest association of ovarian vein thrombophlebitis is with postpartum endometritis. Therefore the best prevention of this condition is the prevention of postpartum uterine infection. Patients with cesarean section following prolonged premature rupture of membranes, prolonged labor, multiple pelvic examinations, prolonged second stage of labor, and clinical amnionitis are at high risk for postpartum endometritis and ovarian vein thrombosis. They should be aggressively treated with antibiotics and mobilized quickly after delivery. Protracted fever that does not respond to treatment should immediately suggest the possibility of ovarian vein thrombosis, and adequate diagnostic testing should be ordered without delay.

Clinical presentation

Typically, the patient with ovarian thrombophlebitis has a history of delivery by cesarean section after prolonged labor and multiple pelvic examinations. This is followed by postpartum endometritis that does not respond to antibiotic treatment. The patient is febrile and has several episodes of chills and elevated temperature every day. Some patients complain of right lower quadrant pain. Physical examination usually reveals pain on palpation of the right lower quadrant, and on some occasions a mass can be felt.

The onset of symptoms usually occurs between the first and the fourth day postpartum. Usually there is a delay in the diagnosis because of difficulties with the differential diagnosis of acute appendicitis and urinary tract infection. Pulmonary embolization occurs in approximately 13.2% of the cases.[44]

Diagnosis and treatment

A CT[45] or magnetic resonance imaging (MRI)[46] scan of the lower abdomen usually reveals the sausage-shaped, dilated, and thrombosed ovarian vein and in some patients also shows associated thrombosis of the iliac vein and the inferior vena cava. Duplex Doppler may also be used for the diagnosis of this condition.[47] The treatment of ovarian vein thrombosis is full anticoagulation with heparin for a minimum of 7 days and continuation of antibiotic therapy. If ovarian vein thrombophlebitis is found in the course of an exploratory laparotomy, the abdomen should be closed and medical treatment started. Four deaths have been reported as a result of pulmonary embolization in association with surgical manipulation of thrombosed ovarian veins.[46]

◢ MATERNAL CEREBROVASCULAR ACCIDENTS
Incidence

The incidence of cerebrovascular accidents in pregnancy is approximately 1 in 6000 deliveries.[48] However, they account for 5% to 15% of all maternal deaths. Approximately 50% of all cerebrovascular accidents during pregnancy occur in the puerperium.

Pathophysiology

Cerebrovascular accidents may be hemorrhagic or occlusive. Intracranial hemorrhage may be caused by trauma, hypertension, and arterial or venous malformations. Also, cocaine abuse is becoming an important etiologic factor.[49] Berry aneurysms account for approximately one half of the malformations that bleed during pregnancy, and arteriovenous malformations and angiomas account for the other half.[50] Vascular occlusion may be caused by vasculitis, vasospasm, embolism or arteriosclerosis. The majority of pregnant patients have arterial rather than venous thrombosis, usually in the midcerebral artery area.

Patients at risk and possible preventative measures

Box 21-5 lists some of the conditions associated with patients predisposed to cerebrovascular accidents during pregnancy. Antiphospholipid antibodies (anticardiolipin, lupus anticoagulant, false-positive VDRL [Venereal Disease Research Laboratory]) are found with relatively high frequency in pregnant patients with cerebrovascular thrombosis and no other predisposing factors. Antithrombin III, protein C, and protein S deficiencies are rarely found. Insulin-dependent diabetic patients with disease of early onset may have extensive arteriosclerosis at the childbearing age. Patients with connective tissue disorders may develop cerebral vasculitis, especially in the postpartum period. Preeclampsia is a frequent cause of intracranial bleeding, especially when it appears superimposed in chronic hypertension.

BOX 21-5

Conditions Associated with Cerebrovascular Accidents in Obstetric Patients

Cerebral thrombosis

Antiphospholipid antibodies
Insulin-dependent diabetic patients with vascular disease
Connective tissue disorders
Sepsis
Antithrombin III, protein C, and protein S deficiencies

Cerebral hemorrhage

Preeclampsia
Chronic hypertension
Head trauma
Cocaine abuse
Arteriovenous malformations
Berry aneurysms

Recognition and treatment

Most cerebrovascular accidents in pregnancy are of sudden onset and produce major symptoms. The clinical picture is characterized by headaches, convulsions, alterations in consciousness, motor and sensory deficits, papilledema, and disturbances of vision and speech. Lumbar puncture demonstrates elevated cerebrospinal fluid pressure and increased protein and cell concentration. CT of the head and arteriography confirm the diagnosis.

Treatment involves ensuring adequate ventilation with endotracheal intubation as needed, antiseizure medications, and lowering of the intracranial pressure with glucocorticoids and mannitol. The best treatment of a ruptured cerebral aneurysm during pregnancy is surgical clipping.[51]

Patients with chronic hypertension are at increased risk of intracranial bleeding,[52] and management of their blood pressure may be difficult after the cerebrovascular accident occurs. Hypotension can be a sign of imminent brain stem herniation caused by increased intracranial pressure. If the blood pressure is labile and the fetus is viable, it is better to effect delivery.

Puerperal cerebral vein thrombosis usually occurs between the fourth and the twenty-first postpartum days. It usually manifests by headaches and convulsions and is easily confused with postpartum eclampsia. The maternal mortality rate is approximately 25%.

◢ NEONATAL DEPRESSION
Incidence

The incidence of depressed newborns requiring immediate assistance in an unselected population of obstetric patients is approximately 3%. This incidence climbs to 20% to 30% in a population of high-risk gravidas.

Pathophysiology

Neonatal depression results from the inability of the fetus to establish extrauterine homeostasis and may or may not be preceded by hypoxia and acidosis in utero. The failure to establish homeostasis is usually caused by a failure of the fetal circulatory and pulmonary systems to provide the tissues with oxygen and with adequate removal of carbon dioxide (CO_2). The most common causes of neonatal depression are shown in Box 21-6.

Inadequate oxygen delivery and CO_2 removal are usually secondary to structural or functional derangements of the cardiovascular and circulatory systems. Structural problems include airway or pulmonary hypoplasia, diaphragmatic hernia, choanal atresia, tracheoesophageal fistula, and congenital or iatrogenic pneumothorax. Functional pulmonary problems include hyaline membrane disease, pneumonia, or pulmonary edema. Although structural cardiovascular derangements usually become symptomatic some time after birth, some may show up immediately after birth with neonatal depression; this includes anomalies producing shunting around the lung, such as uncompensated transposition of the great vessels or pulmonary atresia. Functional cardiovascular problems appearing in the delivery room include myocardial depression caused by lactic acidosis from in utero asphyxia, sepsis, persistent fetal circulation from significant meconium aspiration, hypocalcemia, and profound anemia. Finally, oxygen may be present in inadequate amounts when demands are especially high, as in sepsis or hypothermia or with incorrect application of ventilatory assist devices, notably face masks and endotracheal tubes.

Deficiency of glucose and calcium may also contribute to neonatal depression. Hypoglycemia is associated with fetal hyperinsulinemia and maternal hyperglycemia, notably maternal diabetes

---

BOX 21-6
Causes of Neonatal Depression

Maternal

Asthma, adult respiratory distress syndrome, severe anemia, vascular disease, drug abuse

Fetal

Structural disease of heart and great vessels
Severe fetal acidosis
Persistent fetal circulation
Sepsis
Anemia
Umbilical cord compression

Placental

Abruptio placentae
Placenta previa
Placental vascular insufficiency

Medications

Magnesium sulfate
Diazepam
Halothane
Morphine and/or meperidine

---

or treatment with beta-adrenergic tocolytic agents. Also, hypoglycemia may be present subsequent to a long and difficult labor. Calcium deficiency may accompany asphyxia, shock from any cause, and extreme prematurity and result in continued neonatal depression until corrected.

Patients at risk and preventative measures

Neonatal depression is exceedingly rare in a healthy fetus who progresses through a normal labor. The fetuses at risk are those with structural defects or acquired disease and those who become hypoxic and acidotic during labor. If any of these conditions are present, the neonatology department should be informed of the potential delivery of a depressed neonate. The neonatologist should be present at the time of delivery, and all the necessary facilitites for neonatal resuscitation must be available in the delivery areas. The objective is to have a rapid, atraumatic resuscitation.

Diagnosis

At the moment of birth, normal newborns have a heart rate over 100. Spontaneous respirations are established in 30 to 60 seconds, and spontaneous movements and crying usually occur during the first minute. Color usually becomes pink with some mild cyanosis of hands and feet within 1 minute. Muscle tone should be present at the time of birth. By 2 minutes of age, the newborn should be breathing quietly with a rate of 50 to 70 per minute, have a heart rate of 130 to 170 bpm, and have good muscle tone. Failure to establish regular respirations, poor muscle tone, bradycardia, the presence of meconium staining, or signs of decreased lung compliance, such as tachypnea, nasal flaring, or retractions, mandates immediate resuscitative efforts.

Treatment

The importance of skilled and immediate intervention for the distressed newborn is well established. The longer the Apgar score remains low and asphyxia persists, the greater the incidence of subsequent neonatal morbidity. Under ideal circumstances, newborn resuscitation requires the presence of one neonatologist and one neonatal nurse practitioner, plus the proper equipment and support personnel. The goal of neonatal resuscitation is to provide ventilatory, circulatory, metabolic, and thermal support. Although these are all administered concurrently, each will be considered separately.

Ventilatory support. In the majority of cases, all that is necessary for the resuscitation of a depressed newborn is adequate ventilation. Most neonates can receive ventilation effectively with a bag and mask. Unfortunately, most clinicians who attend neonates in the delivery room are unfamiliar with the proper technique for doing so and rapidly abandon unsuccessful attempts at mask ventilation for hurried attempts at endotracheal intubation. It is crucial to apply the mask without pressure, elevate the chin with the fingers, and maintain the head in a neutral position because the airway of the newborn is easily occluded by extensive flexion of the head and undue pressure of the mask over the face. It is necessary to perform 30 to 50 ventilations per minute and not to exceed 30 cm H_2O positive airway pressure. The flow of oxygen should not be greater than 30 cm H_2O because it can easily result in iatrogenic pneumothorax, greatly complicating resuscitative efforts. Some infants require a few lung expansions to begin spontaneous respirations and movements and cry soon thereafter, making it possible to discontinue positive pressure ventilation almost immediately. However, if neonatal depression is not immediately reversed, it is necessary to continue ventilatory support until a full neonatal evaluation can be made. Adequacy of ventilation and oxygenation can be assessed clinically by heart rate, breath sounds, and color of lips and tongue, but blood gas determinations should be performed as soon as possible.

If ventilation cannot be established rapidly by bag and mask, it is necessary to proceed to endotracheal intubation. To do that, the fetal head should be in a neutral position with the blade of the laryngoscope pushing the tongue downward toward the patient's feet. Looking straight down, the clinician will view the cords, and a semirigid tube can be passed down easily. Adequate tube placement should be assured by continuous auscultation of lung fields. If the tube is passed too far, it commonly lodges in the right bronchus, blocking ventilation of the left lung. If left lung sounds are diminished, the endotracheal tube should be pulled back 1 to 2 cm. Common errors in endotracheal intubation are hyperextension of the fetal head that obscures the larynx, and persistence in failed attempts for more than 30 to 45 seconds.

If ventilation cannot be performed with a properly placed endotracheal tube, diagnostic possibilities include diaphragmatic hernia, pneumothorax, and pulmonary hypoplasia. If diaphragmatic hernia exists, the bagging attempts may have inflated the bowel present in the thorax, and decompression is necessary to allow adequate ventilation. For this purpose a nasogastric tube should be immediately passed and suction applied. The next step, if ventilation is still unsuccessful, is to rule out the possibility that pneumothorax has occurred and perform bilateral thoracentesis. Each hemithorax should be entered in the midaxillary line at the level of the nipple to avoid liver and spleen, and a 10- or 20-ml syringe should be used to aspirate any air present. A chest x-ray film should be obtained as rapidly as possible.

If particulate or thick meconium staining is noted before delivery, the hypopharynx should be gently suctioned before the thorax is delivered with a bulb syringe or a DeLee catheter. Hageman et al.[53] demonstrated that the bulb syringe was equally as effective as the DeLee catheter in preventing aspiration of meconium into the larynx and trachea. Then the vocal cords should be visualized and endotracheal intubation performed only if there is meconium at the level of or below the cords. In this case the endotracheal tube is used to suck the airway and should be removed while sucking. If meconium is present, the lungs should be reintubated and sucked again. Then the baby's lungs should be gently inflated with 100% oxygen by bag and mask. Infants with significant meconium aspiration may need continued intubation to establish adequate ventilation.

Circulatory support. Indications for immediate circulatory support include heart failure at birth, usually caused by severe asphyxia and manifested by bradycardia in the face of adequate ventilation, shock from any cause, and anemia. Methods to support neonatal circulation include closed chest cardiac massage, intravenous fluid therapy, and drugs.

After ventilation is established, if the heart rate is less than 80 bpm, closed chest massage with thumb and forefingers should be performed at a rate of 120 compressions per minute. Usually, as the oxygen deficit is compensated for by rapid mechanical ventilation, acidosis resolves and heart rate improves. Bradycardia and asystole, which do not respond to compression and ventilation, should be treated with 0.2 to 0.5 ml of 1 per 10,000 epinephrine given via the endotracheal tube.

Shock can be diagnosed with certainty only with measurement of systolic blood pressure by occlusion of the brachial or femoral artery with a pneumatic cuff and auscultation with a Doppler device or by a pressure transducer attached to an umbilical arterial catheter. Clinically, shock should be suspected with pallor, cyanosis, poor apical impulse, distant heart sounds, poor capillary filling, and hypotonia. Newborns in shock should have an immediate determination of central or peripheral hematocrit level. A hematocrit less than 40% suggests partially compensated hypovolemia or normovolemic anemia, both indications for transfusion in the setting of neonatal depression. If shock is diagnosed, the best volume expander is blood, 10 ml/kg, repeated if needed. For this purpose the obstetrician should obtain 10 or 20 ml of cord blood and have it available for transfusion of the newborn in the delivery room when a depressed baby is delivered. Caution should be exercised with volume replacement in preterm infants, especially those less than 34 weeks of gestation, since too vigorous or unnecessary volume expansion can cause rebound hypertension that is associated with intraventricular hemorrhage.

Umbilical vein catheterization can be performed rapidly and safely in the delivery room. For this purpose an umbilical tape is loosely tied around the base of the cord, the skin is prepared with povidone-iodine (Betadine), the cord is cut evenly with a scalpel 3 to 4 cm from the abdominal wall, and a No. 3 to 5 French neonatal feeding tube is inserted into the vein. The catheter is pushed in only far enough to aspirate blood, which signifies success. To prevent blood loss the umbilical tie should be secured with a 3-0 silk suture and tightened.

Thermal support. Hypothermia and hyperthermia may result in increased oxygen and glucose requirements, overwhelming the neonatal reserves. The newborn gains or loses heat in three ways: *conduction* is heat gain or loss by being in contact with an object such as a blanket or the maternal abdomen; *convection* is heat gain or loss by movement of air, usually prevented by the isolette chamber; and *radiation* is heat gain or loss from an object not in direct contact with the neonate, such as the cold glass walls of the isolette. There will be heat loss under a radiant heater if a newborn is wrapped or draped for a procedure. In contrast, in a convection heater, such as an isolette, a naked newborn loses heat through radiation to the cold isolette walls. It is important to provide a neutral thermal environment for the newborn because hypothermic neonates manifest signs indistinguishable from a hypoxic neonate—cyanosis, retractions, hypotension, and hypotonia.

Metabolic support. Indications for metabolic support are limited now to instances of documented substrate deficiency. All depressed newborns should have immediate blood-glucose sampling and administration of 1 g/kg intravenous dextrose in 50% solution if two successive determinations are less than 45 mg/dl. A determination should be repeated every 30 minutes until stable blood glucose is achieved.

With the possible exception of babies born in cardiac arrest, correction of acidosis with bicarbonate should be performed only after adequate oxygenation and circulation have been established and serial blood gas determinations obtained. As a rule, the respiratory component of any acidosis will be corrected rapidly by adequate ventilation. Maintenance of adequate gas exchange will allow elimination of the lactic acid generated by anaerobic metabolism of asphyxiated tissues with eventual correction of meta-

---

BOX 21-7

Treatment of the Depressed Newborn

Ventilatory

Bag and mask

Adequate in almost all situations; do not exceed 30 cm H_2O of pressure; can suffocate neonate if poor technique is used; contraindicated if there is known diaphragmatic hernia

Endotracheal tube

Must be used with meconium, diaphragmatic hernia, chloanal atresia, severe respiratory distress, pneumothorax

Ancillary techniques if ventilation cannot be established:

Gastric decompression

To rule out inflated stomach in the chest

Thoracentesis

To rule out pneumothorax

Circulatory

Cardiac massage

If heart rate is below 80 bpm with adequate ventilation

Endotracheal epinephrine

0.5 to 1.0 ml 1/10,000 solution

Volume expansion

For shock or anemia; 10 ml/kg of blood, crystalloid, or albuminated saline solution

Thermal

Provide neutral thermal environmment

Metabolic

Glucose

For proven hypoglycemia; use 1 g/kg of 50% glucose

Bicarbonate

After correction of respiratory acidosis; give 2-4 mEq/kg if needed

---

bolic acidosis. In some cases severe metabolic acidosis manifested by base deficits greater than −4 to −5 persists despite adequate ventilation, and it may be corrected with $NaHCO_3$, 1 to 2 mEq/kg, diluted to a concentration of 0.5 mEq/ml. Sodium bicarbonate solutions are hypertonic and must be given slowly by the intravenous route. Tris buffer may be used instead of bicarbonate in these situations.

If neonatal depression has been preceded by narcotic administration, it is best to administer naloxone, 0.1 mg/kg IM or by umbilical venous catheter. True asphyxia may also be accompanied by narcotic depression that may complicate resuscitation. Box 21-7 summarizes the treatment for the distressed newborn.

◼ IMPORTANT POINTS: ◼

1. Postpartum bleeding complicates 3.9% of vaginal and 6.4% of cesarean deliveries and accounts for approximately 35% of all maternal deaths caused by bleeding during pregnancy.

2. Some of the factors commonly associated with postpartum bleeding following vaginal delivery are prolonged third stage of labor, multifetal pregnancies, episiotomy, abnormal labor, forceps and vacuum delivery.

3. Some of the factors associated with postpartum bleeding following cesarean delivery are general anesthesia, preeclampsia, chorioamnionitis, and abnormalities of labor.

4. One of the reasons given to justify the routine use of episiotomy is prevention of perineal trauma. Modern studies indicate that episiotomy, rather than protecting against perineal injuries, actually predisposes the patient to third- and fourth-degree lacerations.

5. Most investigations concluded that there is less risk of maternal trauma with vacuum than with forceps delivery. However, most

investigations concluded that there is an increased risk of fetal trauma with vacuum.

6. The most important prediction factor of retained placenta is preterm delivery. The increased incidence of retained placenta affects predominantly women with induced preterm labor rather than women who deliver preterm after spontaneous labor.

7. When the placenta is retained because of a contracted cervix, the best management is manual removal after relaxation of the cervix with intravenous nitroglycerin.

8. Bilateral uterine artery ligation is a simple and effective procedure that preserves the reproductive capacity of patients with postpartum bleeding unresponsive to medical treatment.

9. Hydrostatic pressure replacement is a simple and effective procedure for the treatment of uterine inversion unresponsive to uterine relaxants and manual replacement.

10. Pelvic ultrasound is an excellent technique for ruling out retained placental fragments in patients with postpartum bleeding.

11. In patients with vaginal hematomas, it is useless to attempt finding the source of the bleeding. After evacuation of the hematoma, the vaginal mucosa should not be sutured or the hematoma cavity packed. Instead, a vaginal pack should be placed and removed in 24 hours.

12. The treatment of choice of retroperitoneal hematomas is angiographic embolization. If angiographic embolization cannot be performed, the MAST suit may save the patient's life and avoid dangerous surgery.

13. The most important measures for preventing postpartum endometritis are avoiding cesarean sections and using antibiotic prophylaxis with all cesarean sections.

14. The simplest and cheapest way to obtain adequate postpartum endometrial cultures is with a cotton swab grasped with a ring forceps. The cultures are obtained while the cervical canal is maintained open with a sponge forceps. Vaginal contamination is rare, and the culture yields a larger number of bacterial species than double lumen catheters or endometrial suction devices.

15. Cocaine abuse is an important cause of maternal intracranial hemorrhage during pregnancy.

REFERENCES

1. Combs CA, Murphy EL, Laros RK: Factors associated with postpartum hemorrhage with vaginal birth. *Obstet Gynecol* 1991;77:69-76.
2. Combs CA, Murphy EL, Laros RK: Factors associated with hemorrhage in cesarean deliveries. *Obstet Gynecol* 1991;77:77-82.
3. Kaunitz AM, Hughes JM, Grimes DA, et al: Causes of maternal mortality in the United States. *Obstet Gynecol* 1985;65:605-612.
4. Pritchard JA, Baldwin RM, Dickey JC, et al: Blood volume changes in pregnancy and the puerperium: II. Red blood cell loss and changes in apparent blood volume during and following vaginal delivery, cesarean section, and cesarean section plus total hysterectomy. *Am J Obstet Gynecol* 1962;84:1271-1282.
5. Prendiville WJ, Harding JE, Elbourne DR, et al: The Bristol third stage trial: Active versus physiological management of the third stage of labour. *Br Med J* 1988;297:1295-1297.
6. Combs CA, Robertson PA, Laros RK: Risk factors for third-degree and fourth-degree perineal lacerations in forceps and vacuum deliveries. *Am J Obstet Gynecol* 1990;163:100-104.
7. Shiono P, Klebanoff MA, Carey CJ: Midline episiotomies: More harm than good? *Obstet Gynecol* 1990;75:765-770.
8. Gainey HL: Postpartum observation of pelvic tissue damage: Further studies. *Am J Obstet Gynecol* 1955;70:800-807.
9. Haadem K, Dahlstrom JA, Ling L, et al: Anal sphincter function after delivery rupture. *Obstet Gynecol* 1987;70:53-56.
10. Sorensen SM, Bondesen H, Istre O, et al: Perineal rupture following vaginal delivery: Long-term consequences. *Acta Obstet Gynaecol Scand* 1988;67:315-318.
11. Broekhuizen FF, Washington JM, Johnson F, et al: Vacuum extraction versus forceps delivery: Indications and complications, 1979 to 1984. *Obstet Gynecol* 1987;69,338-342.
12. Meyer L, Mailloux J, Marcoux S, et al: Maternal and neonatal morbidity in instrumental delivery with the Kobayashi vacuum extractor and low forceps. *Acta Obstet Gynaecol Scand* 1987;66:643-647.
13. Punnonen R, Aro P, Kuukankorpi A, et al: Fetal and maternal effects of forceps and vacuum extraction. *Br J Obstet Gynecol* 1986;93:1132-1135.
14. Schenker JG, Serr DM: Comparative study of delivery by vacuum extractor and forceps. *Am J Obstet Gynecol* 1967;98:32-35.
15. Arad I, Fainmesser P, Birkenfeld A, et al: Vacuum extractor and neonatal jaundice. *J Perinat Med* 1982;10:273-277.
16. Combs CA, Laros RK: Prolonged third stage of labor: Morbidity and risk factors. *Obstet Gynecol* 1991;77:863-867.

17. Romero R, Hsu YC, Atanassiadi Ap, et al: Preterm delivery: A risk factor for retained placenta. *Am J Obstet Gynecol* 1990;163:823-826.

18. Clark SL, Koonings PP, Phelan JP: Placenta previa/accreta and prior cesarean section. *Obstet Gynecol* 1985;66:89.

19. Peng AT, Gorman RS, Shulman SM, et al: Intravenous nitroglycerin for uterine relaxation in the postpartum patient with retained placenta. *Anesthesiology* 1989;71:172-173.

20. Fox H: Placenta accreta, 1945-1969. *Obstet Gynecol Surv* 1972;17:475.

21. Hertz RH, Sokol RJ, Dierker LJ: Treatment of postpartum uterine atony with prostaglandin E_2 vaginal suppositories. *Obstet Gynecol* 1980;56:129.

22. Peyser MR, Kupfermine MJ: Management of severe postpartum hemorrhage by intrauterine irrigation with prostaglandin E_2. *Am J Obstet Gynecol* 1990;162:694-696.

23. Fribourg SRC, Rothman LA, Rovinsky JJ: Intrauterine lavage for control of uterine atony. *Obstet Gynecol* 1973;41:876.

24. O'Leary JL: Pregnancy following uterine artery ligation. *Obstet Gynecol* 1980;55:112.

25. Clark LS, Phelan JP, Yeh SY, et al: Hypogastric artery ligation for obstetric hemorrhage. *Obstet Gynecol* 1985;66:353-356.

26. Shah-Hosseini R, Evrard JR: Puerperal uterine inversion. *Obstet Gynecol* 1989;73:567-570.

27. Kitchen J, Thiagarajah S, May H, et al: Puerperal inversion of the uterus. *Am J Obstet Gynecol* 1975;123:51.

28. O'Sullivan JV: Acute inversion of the uterus. *Br Med J* 1945;2:282-283.

29. Momani AW, Hassan A: Treatment of puerperal uterine inversion by the hydrostatic method; Reports of five cases. *Eur J Obstet Gynecol Rep Biol* 1989;32:281-285.

30. Heyl PS, Stubblefield PG, Phillippe M: Recurrent inversion of the puerperal uterus managed with 15(s)-15-methyl-prostaglandin F_2alpha and uterine packing. *Obstet Gynecol* 1984;63:263-264.

31. Andrinopoulos GC, Mendenhall HW: Prostaglandin F_2alpha in the management of delayed postpartum hemorrhage. *Am J Obstet Gynecol* 1983;146:217.

32. Townsend DE, Barbis SD, Mathews RD: Vasopressin and operative hysteroscopy in the management of delayed postabortion and postpartum bleeding. *Am J Obstet Gynecol* 1991;165:616-618.

33. Pieri RJ: Pelvic hematomas associated with pregnancy. *Obstet Gynecol* 1958;12:249-258.

34. Heffner LJ, Mennuti MT, Rudoff JC, et al: Primary management of postpartum vulvovaginal hematomas by angiographic embolization. *Am J Perinatol* 1985;2:204-207.

35. Chin HG, Scott DR, Resnik R, et al: Angiographic embolization of intractable puerperal hematomas. *Am J Obstet Gynecol* 1989;160:434-438.

36. Pearse CS, Magrina JF, Finley BE. Use of MAST suit in obstetrics and gynecology. *Obstet Gynecol Surv* 1984;39:416-422.

37. Robie GF, Morgan MA, Payne GG, et al: Logothetopulos pack for the management of uncontrollable postpartum hemorrhage. *Am J Perinatol* 1990;7:327-328.

38. Newton ER, Prihoda TJ, Gibbs RS: A clinical and microbiologic analysis of risk factors for puerperal endometritis. *Obstet Gynecol* 1990;75:402-406.

39. Ehrenkranz NJ, Blackwelder WC, Pfaff SJ, et al: Infections complicating low-risk cesarean sections in community hospitals: Efficacy of antimicrobial prophylaxis. *Am J Obstet Gynecol* 1990;162:337-343.

40. Gravett MG, Hummel D, Eschenbach DA, et al: Preterm labor associated with subclinical amniotic fluid infection and with bacterial vaginosis. *Obstet Gynecol* 1986;67:229-237.

41. Watts DH, Krohn MA, Hillier SL, et al: Bacterial vaginosis as a risk factor for post-cesarean endometritis. *Obstet Gynecol* 1990;75:52-58.

42. Marteus MG, Faro S, Hammill HA, et al: Transcervical uterine cultures with a new endometrial suction curette: A comparison of three sampling methods in postpartum endometritis. *Obstet Gynecol* 1989;74:273-276.

43. Brown TK, Munsick RA: Puerperal ovarian vein thrombophlebitis: A syndrome. *Am J Obstet Gynecol* 1971;109:253-273.

44. Dunnihoo DR, Gallaspy JN, Wise RB, et al: Postpartum ovarian vein thrombophlebitis: A review. *Obstet Gynecol Surv* 1991;46:415-427.

45. Rezier JC, et al: Diagnosis of puerperal ovarian vein thrombophlebitis by computed tomography. *Am J Obstet Gynecol* 1988;159:737-740.

46. Martin B, Mulopulus GP, Bryan PJ: MRI of puerperal ovarian-vein thrombosis (case report). *AJR* 1986;147:291-292.

47. Baran GW, Frisch KM: Duplex Doppler evaluation of puerperal ovarian vein thrombosis, *AJR* 1987;149:321-322.

48. Simolke GA, Cox SM, Cunningham FG: Cerebrovascular accidents complicating pregnancy and the puerperium. *Obstet Gynecol* 1991;78:37-42.

49. Mercado NA, Johnson G, Calver D, et al: Cocaine, pregnancy, and postpartum intracerebral hemorrhage. *Obstet Gynecol* 1989;73:467-468.

50. Tuttelman RM, Gleicher N: Central nervous system hemorrhage complicating pregnancy. *Obstet Gynecol* 1981;58:651.

51. Dias MS, Sekhar LN: Intracranial hemorrhage from aneurysms and arteriovenous malformations during pregnancy and the puerperium. *Neurosurgery* 1990;27:855.

52. Amias AG: Cerebral vascular disease in pregnancy: I. Hemorrhage. *J Obstet Gynaecol Br Commonw* 1970;77:100.

53. Hageman JR, Conley M, Francis K, et al: Delivery room management of meconium staining of the amniotic fluid and the development of meconium aspiration syndrome. *J Perinatol* 1988;8:127.

INDEX

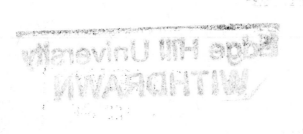